OXFORD MEDICAL PUBLICATIONS

Huntington's Disease

OXFORD MONOGRAPHS ON MEDICAL GENETICS

General Editors

ARNO G. MOTULSKY

MARTIN BOBROW

PETER S. HARPER

CHARLES SCRIVER

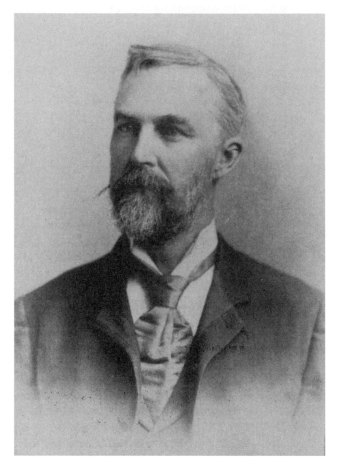

George Huntington (1850–1916). Reproduced by courtesy of the Wellcome Institute for the History of Medicine, from Watson, L.A. (ed.) (1896). Physicians and Surgeons of America (Republican Press Association, Concord)

Huntington's Disease

Third Edition

GILLIAN BATES

*Professor of Neurogenetics, Division of Medical and Molecular Genetics,
GKT School of Medicine King's College, Guy's Hospital, London, UK*

PETER S. HARPER

*Professor of Medical Genetics and Consultant Physician, Institute of Medical Genetics,
University Hospital of Wales College of Medicine, Heath Park, Cardiff, UK*

LESLEY JONES

*Senior Lecturer in Neuropsychiatric Genetics, Institute of Medical Genetics,
and Dept of Psychological Medicine University of Wales College of Medicine
Heath Park, Cardiff, UK*

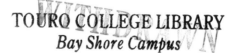
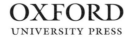

OXFORD

UNIVERSITY PRESS

BS

OXFORD

UNIVERSITY PRESS

Great Clarendon Street, Oxford OX2 6DP

Oxford University Press is a department of the University of Oxford.
It furthers the University's objective of excellence in research, scholarship,
and education by publishing worldwide in

Oxford New York

Auckland Bangkok Buenos Aires Cape Town Chennai
Dar es Salaam Delhi Hong Kong Istanbul Karachi Kolkata
Kuala Lumpur Madrid Melbourne Mexico City Mumbai Nairobi
São Paulo Shanghai Taipei Tokyo Toronto

Oxford is a registered trade mark of Oxford University Press
in the UK and in certain other countries

Published in the United States
by Oxford University Press Inc., New York

A catalogue record for this title is available from the British Library.

Library of Congress Cataloging in Publication Data
(Data available)

ISBN 0 19 851060 8 (Hbk)

10 9 8 7 6 5 4 3 2 1

Typeset by Newgen Imaging Systems (P) Ltd., Chennai, India
Printed in Great Britain
on acid-free paper by
Biddles Ltd, Guildford and King's Lynn

10/29/03

Preface to the third edition

It is now almost a decade since the identification of the Huntington's disease (HD) gene and its mutation; the advances that have occurred in our understanding of the disorder during this time have been truly profound. In 1991, when this book was first published, these advances lay entirely in the future; by the time of the second edition, in 1996, the genetic aspects had become well understood in terms of genetic instability, but we still had almost no insight into the cell biology and pathogenesis of the disorder. Now, we not only have extensive evidence on how the HD mutation actually causes brain pathology, but we also have the experimental tools to take this research further towards new therapeutic approaches.

As a result of these fundamental changes, this is in essence an entirely new book. We have been fortunate in developing an international team of authors, all leaders in their particular fields, to contribute the individual chapters and have tried to ensure, by careful editing, that the unity of the book is not lost. As before, we have aimed to make it of practical value to all clinicians and geneticists working with HD patients and their families, as well as covering the key areas of basic science. The increasing convergence of thought and of both basic and clinical research across the field of neurodegenerative disease should also make the book relevant to workers whose primary focus is on allied disorders.

Readers familiar with previous editions will find that, with few exceptions, the chapters and authors for this new edition are entirely different from before, and that much material in the previous edition has thus been omitted, even though it is not necessarily outdated. Fortunately, the change of publisher has allowed the copyright of that edition to revert to the editors and we have therefore made it available in its entirety electronically (contact PSH – Harper PS@cardiff.ac.uk). In this way, readers who wish to have access to it will still be able to use it. We should especially like to thank those previous contributors who are not included in this new edition, but parts of whose chapters may have been utilized.

We should like to thank all those involved in the production of this book, especially Audrey Budding for organizing and collating the material and Oxford University Press for helping to achieve a rapid production of the book.

Cardiff and London　　　　　　　　　　　　　　　　　　　　　　　　　　　　G. P. B.

2002　　　　　　　　　　　　　　　　　　　　　　　　　　　　　　　　　　　P. S. H.

　　　　　　　　　　　　　　　　　　　　　　　　　　　　　　　　　　　　　L.J.

Preface to the second edition

The isolation of the Huntington's disease (HD) gene, 2 years after the original publication of this book, made it immediately clear that a major revision would be required. The timing for this was not easy to decide, since a flood of new publications has occurred during the past 3 years, which shows no sign of abating. Hopefully, we have chosen a point where genetic research on the HD mutation is now reasonably definitive. Work on the function of the gene remains at a much earlier stage and is only just beginning to affect significantly our detailed understanding of the neurobiology of the disorder, although this is changing rapidly.

As before, the writing of this book has been a team effort involving present and former members of the Cardiff HD unit; many readers have commented that this has resulted in an integrated style and approach that has made the book easy to read, and we hope that we have been able to preserve this in the new edition.

We are grateful to a number of people for their help, including those who pointed out corrections needed in the first edition, and those who kindly supplied new illustrative material; our Cardiff collaborators in Psychiatric Genetics, Professor Peter McGuffin and Professor Mike Owen; colleagues in neurology, neuropathology, psychology, and genetics; Dr Gavin Reynolds, Sheffield, and many others. We also acknowledge the funding support of the Medical Research Council, the Mental Health Foundation, the Hereditary Disease Foundation, the Huntington's Disease Association, and the Welsh Office and Department of Health.

Finally, Michele Thomas undertook most of the arduous task of preparing and coordinating the manuscript, while the staff of W. B. Saunders were of great help in processing and publishing the book rapidly and efficiently.

Preface to the first edition

This book had its origins almost 20 years ago, when one of us (PSH) returned from America to develop medical genetics in Cardiff, Wales, after 2 years working at Johns Hopkins Hospital, Baltimore, where colleagues were involved in a project attempting to map the gene for Huntington's disease (HD). Considerable numbers of referrals of HD families for genetic counselling in Cardiff soon made it clear that the disease was frequent in South Wales, an impression reinforced by a series of family records kept by a neurologist colleague in Cardiff, Dr Charles Wells, who suggested that there might be as many as 20 families in the area and encouraged a systematic survey.

Twenty years later we know of over 200 HD families in Wales and the number is probably still incomplete. If we had known the scale of the project we were undertaking when we were starting, we might well not have had the courage to begin! However, begin we did, and over the years a group of workers has evolved, with a combination of skills that has been able to make a significant contribution to our understanding of HD, as well as providing a service to our families locally.

The decision to write this book came from the realization that our group had a particularly wide range of expertise, including psychiatric and genetic counselling experience, as well as molecular genetic skills and knowledge of the social effects of HD. Four of us had written theses on the disorder, with a considerable amount of information gained and collected that we felt could be valuable to others. Urgency was given to the task by the realization that some of this expertise would soon disperse, with two authors moving to senior posts elsewhere; if a book was to be written, the opportunity had to be seized.

Although we have placed a particular emphasis on the genetic aspects of HD in view of our own work and interests, we have tried to make this a balanced book. The contents list of chapters indicates which authors have been principally responsible for writing the different sections but we should emphasize that they have all been written in close collaboration with the group as a whole, with criticism, additions, and amendments often being made by others. This close consultation, only possible within a single working group, will we hope give a unity of style and content that is often lacking in a multiauthor book.

We had nursed a hope that the HD gene might itself have been isolated in time for inclusion in the book, but while this appears very close at the time of writing (March, 1991), it has not yet happened and its description must await a future edition. In retrospect this is perhaps fortunate as isolation of the gene will lead to a complete reassessment of much of the older work and will radically change both experimental strategies and the practical approach to genetic counselling and prediction. We hope that the present account will give readers an up-to-date assessment of our current knowledge and that it will prove of practical use to clinicians involved with HD families, whether neurologists, psychiatrists, or from other specialities, to geneticists and others in relation to genetic counselling and predictive testing, and to the many scientists in HD research who wish to know about the broader aspects of the disease they are studying.

Many thanks are owed for a book such as this, which encompasses work done over such a prolonged period. Here we can only mention a few of the most conspicuous.

First, to our clinical colleagues in Cardiff, especially those in the Departments of Neurology and Psychiatry, we owe a considerable debt for their close and continuing partnership over a long period. Within the Institute and Department of Medical Genetics there have been numerous major contributors over the years, notably Mrs Pat Jones, Nursing Sister, who has been the mainstay of our service to the HD families in South Wales, along with Mrs Morag Nordin and other fieldworkers. Dr David Walker undertook the original clinical study, while Dr Robert Newcombe was responsible for much of the statistical analysis of various studies up to the present, including the life-table data that have been re-analysed for this book. The HD register has seen the involvement of a number of colleagues, including Valerie McBroom, Mansoor Sarfarazi, Jeff Wolak, Iain Fenton, and Lodewijk Sandkuijl. In the laboratory Russell Snell, Shelley Rundle, Tracey Ford, and Nicole Datson have all been closely involved with our molecular genetics research, while Laz Lazarou and Linda Meredith have been responsible for the diagnostic analyses in predictive testing.

The advice of Dr Benno Müller-Hill has been particularly valuable in handling the difficult and sensitive area of HD in Nazi Germany, while the help of Drs Manuela Koch, Kathy Davies, and Nicole Datson in obtaining and translating material from the German literature is much appreciated.

A number of colleagues have been particularly helpful in reading and criticizing parts of the manuscript, including Drs Niall Quinn, David Turner, David Ball, and Raymund Roos, Professors Mark Wiles, Peter McGuffin, Michael Conneally, and Alan Richens, and Mrs Shirley Dalby. There is no doubt that their comments have improved the end result considerably, though it goes without saying that any remaining defects are our own responsibility.

A number of illustrations have been provided by colleagues where our own material seemed inadequate; they are mentioned individually in the text but we have greatly appreciated their generosity, as we do the permission of those who have allowed us to quote unpublished data. Dr Raymund Roos of Leiden and Dr. J. Neal of Cardiff kindly provided and organized the neuropathological material on HD. Our own department of medical illustration under Professor Ralph Marshall, has been unfailingly helpful in turning our own efforts into high quality drawings and prints.

We thank our hard-pressed secretarial staff, especially Michele Thomas and Karen Evans, for their help in producing the manuscript and in the correspondence involved; as well as the staff of Baillière Tindall and Saunders for their efficiency and their tolerance in allowing late alterations.

Our work has received financial support from many sources over the years, but the Huntington's Disease Association, Mental Health Foundation, Medical Research Council, Wellcome Trust, Department of Health, and Welsh Office, and the Hereditary Disease Foundation deserve special mention.

Finally, this book could not have been written were it not for the HD patients and families in Britain, and especially in Wales, on whom our own studies have been based. Working with them over the years has been a privilege for us all, and it is appropriate that it should be to them that this book is dedicated.

This book is dedicated to
patients with Huntington's disease world-wide
and to their families

Contents

List of Contributors

Thomasin Andrews, MD, MRC Clinical Sciences Centre, Imperial College School of Medicine, Hammersmith Hospital, London, UK

Gillian P. Bates, PhD, F Med Sci, Professor in Neurogenetics, Division of Medical and Molecular Genetics, Guy's, King's, and St Thomas' School of Medicine, Guy's Hospital, London SE1 9RT, UK

Caroline Benn, BSc, Neurogenetics Laboratory, Division of Medical and Molecular Genetics, Guy's, King's, and St Thomas' School of Medicine, Guy's Hospital, London SE1 9RT, UK

David J. Brooks, MD, MRC Clinical Sciences Centre, Imperial College School of Medicine, Hammersmith Hospital, London, UK

Jang-Ho J. Cha, MD, PhD Associate Professor of Neurology, Harvard Medical School Center for Aging, Genetics, and Neurodegeneration Massachusetts General Hospital Charlestown, Massachusetts 02129-4404 USA

David Craufurd, MBBS, MSc, FRCPsych, Academic Unit of Medical Genetics and Regional Genetic Service, St Mary's Hospital, Manchester, UK

Anja Dröge, PhD, Department of Neuroproteomics, Max-Delbrueck-Centre for Molecular Medicine, 13092 Berlin, Germany

Stephen B. Dunnett, Brain Repair Group, School of Biosciences, Cardiff University, Cardiff CF10 3US, Wales, UK

Claire-Anne Gutekunst, Department of Neurology, Emory University School of Medicine, Atlanta, GA 30322 Georgia, USA

Peter S. Harper, MA, DM, FRCP, Professor of Medical Genetics, Consultant Physician and Consultant in Medical Genetics, Institute of Medical Genetics, University of Wales College of Medicine and University Hospital of Wales, Cardiff CF14 4XN, UK

Steve, M. Hersch, MD, PhD, Department of Neurology, Massachusetts General Hospital, Harvard Medical School, Center for Aging, Genetics and Neurodegeneration, Charlestown, MA 02129, USA

Lesley Jones, PhD, Senior Lecturer in Neuropsychiatric Genetics, Institute of Medical Genetics and Department of Psychological Medicine, University of Wales College of Medicine, Heath Park, Cardiff, CF14 4XN, UK

Karl Kieburtz, MD, MPH, Professor of Neurology and Community and Preventive Medicine, University of Rochester, Rochester, New York 14620, USA

Berry Kremer, MD, PhD, Professor of Clinical Neurology, Department of Neurology, University of Nijmegen, PO Box 9101 6500 HB Nijmegen, The Netherlands

Kerry P. S. J. Murphy, PhD, Department of Biological Sciences, The Open University, Walton Hall, Milton Keynes MK7 6AA, UK

Martha A. Nance, MD, Hennepin County Medical Center, Department of Neurology, Minneapolis, Minnesota 55415, USA

Francine Norflus, PhD, Department of Neurology, Massachusetts General Hospital, Harvard Medical School, Center for Aging, Genetics and Neurodegeneration, Charlestown, MA 02129, USA

Anne E. Rosser, Brain Repair Group, School of Biosciences, Cardiff University, Cardiff CF10 3US, Wales, UK.

A.H.V. Schapira, MD, DSc, FRCP, FMedSci, University Department of Clinical Neurosciences, Royal Free and University College Medical School and Institute of Neurology, University College London, London NW3 2PF, UK

Ira Shoulson, MD, Professor of Neurology, Pharmacology, and Medicine, Louis C. Lasagna Professor of Experimental Therapeutics, University of Rochester, Rochester, New York 14620, USA

Julie S. Snowden, PhD, Cerebral Function Unit, Creater Manchester Neuroscience Centre, Salford M6 8HD, UK

Aad Tibben, PhD, Professor of Psychology of Genetic disorders, Departments of Clinical Genetics and Neurology, University of Leiden, 2300 RC Leiden, The Netherlands

C. Turner, BSc, MBChB, MRCP, University Department of Clinical Neurosciences, Royal Free and University College Medical School, University College London, London NW3 2PF, UK

Erich E. Wanker, PhD, Professor of Molecular Medicine, Department of Neuroproteomics, Max-Delbrueck-Centre for Molecular Medicine, 13092 Berlin, Germany

Beryl Westphal, RN, APRN, Hennepin County Medical Center, Department of Neurology, Minneapolis, Minnesota 55415, USA

George J. Yohrling, IV, PhD, Associate Professor of Neurology, Harvard Medical School Center for Aging, Genetics, and Neurodegeneration, Massachusetts General Hospital Charlestown, Massachusetts 02129-4404 USA

Section 1   Clinical aspects of Huntington's disease

1 Huntington's disease: a historical background

Peter S. Harper

Introduction

Huntington's disease (HD) has a particularly rich historical literature, stretching back well over a century and involving some of the most prominent figures in medicine and neurology. Thus, before going into depth on the various clinical and experimental aspects covered by subsequent chapters, it seems appropriate to put them in a historical context so that present-day workers can see how the different areas of work evolved and how their predecessors thought.

When reading the early clinically based descriptions it is often striking how relevant they remain today and how thorough they are, reflecting the fact that detailed and accurate clinical studies were for the most part all that could be done. By contrast, in current publications clinical descriptions are often inadequate in comparison with the more experimental aspects. Early neuropathology studies likewise often show both descriptive and illustrative material of considerable detail and high standards.

As a starting point for outlining the origins and growth of our early knowledge on HD there can be no better source than the original description that gave the disorder its name, and that has served ever since as the foundation for all subsequent work.

The description by George Huntington in 1872 of the disease that has subsequently borne his name is one of the most remarkable in the history of medicine. Subsequent workers, from Osler through to the present, have remarked on its clarity, brevity, and comprehensiveness. It was not the first description of the disorder, as will be seen, but it stands out as the first full delineation of the condition as a specific disease entity, quite separate from other forms of chorea.

George Huntington and hereditary chorea

Huntington's paper was given before the Meigs and Mason Academy of Medicine at Middleport, Ohio, on 15 February 1872 and published only 2 months later in the Philadelphia journal, *The Medical and Surgical Reporter* (Fig. 1.1). While the first part deals with chorea in general and does not contain any particularly original information, the final part, occupying only a single page of printed text, is strikingly different in character; its vividness and authenticity of clinical detail come across as strongly today, more than a century later, as they did to contemporary readers such as Osler. One can do no better than quote it in full here.

And now I wish to draw your attention more particularly to a form of the disease which exists, so far as I know, almost exclusively on the east end of Long Island. It is peculiar in itself and seems to obey

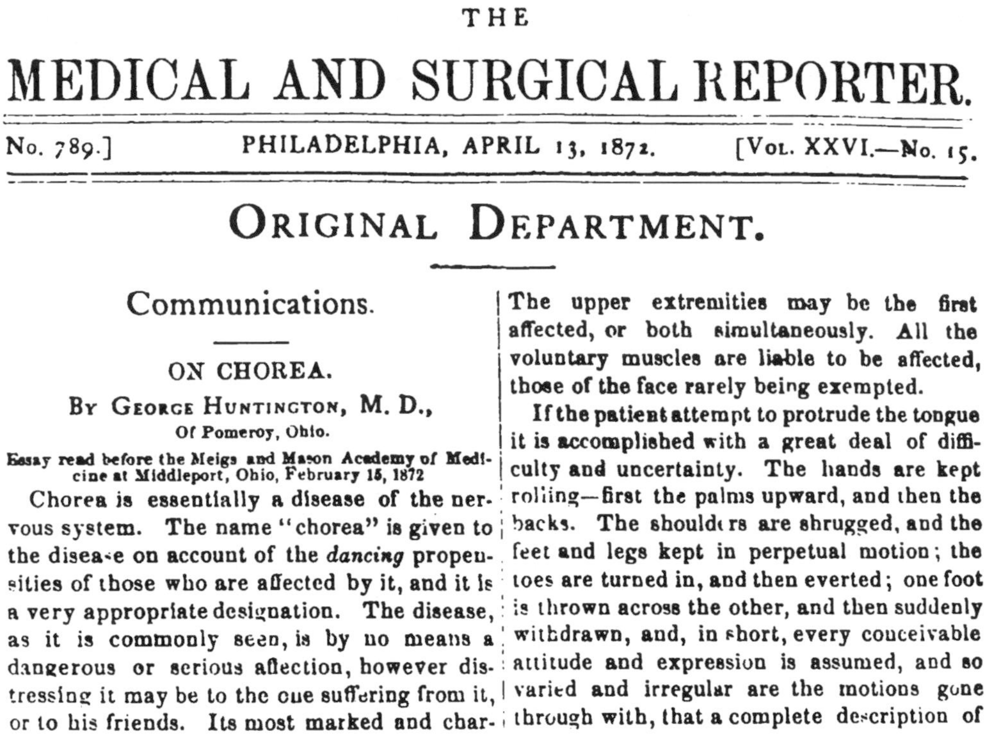

THE

MEDICAL AND SURGICAL REPORTER.

No. 789.]   PHILADELPHIA, APRIL 13, 1872.   [Vol. XXVI.—No. 15.

ORIGINAL DEPARTMENT.

Communications.

ON CHOREA.

By GEORGE HUNTINGTON, M. D.,
Of Pomeroy, Ohio.

Essay read before the Meigs and Mason Academy of Medicine at Middleport, Ohio, February 15, 1872

Chorea is essentially a disease of the nervous system. The name "chorea" is given to the disease on account of the *dancing* propensities of those who are affected by it, and it is a very appropriate designation. The disease, as it is commonly seen, is by no means a dangerous or serious affection, however distressing it may be to the one suffering from it, or to his friends. Its most marked and char-

The upper extremities may be the first affected, or both simultaneously. All the voluntary muscles are liable to be affected, those of the face rarely being exempted.

If the patient attempt to protrude the tongue it is accomplished with a great deal of difficulty and uncertainty. The hands are kept rolling—first the palms upward, and then the backs. The shoulders are shrugged, and the feet and legs kept in perpetual motion; the toes are turned in, and then everted; one foot is thrown across the other, and then suddenly withdrawn, and, in short, every conceivable attitude and expression is assumed, and so varied and irregular are the motions gone through with, that a complete description of

Fig. 1.1 The title page of George Huntington's 1872 paper in the *Medical and Surgical Reporter*.

certain fixed laws. In the first place, let me remark that chorea, as it is commonly known to the profession, and a description of which I have already given, is of exceedingly rare occurrence there. I do not remember a single instance occurring in my father's practice, and I have often heard him say that it was a rare disease and seldom met with by him.

The hereditary chorea, as I shall call it, is confined to certain and fortunately a few families, and has been transmitted to them, an heirloom from generations away back in the dim past. It is spoken of by those in whose veins the seeds of the disease are known to exist, with a kind of horror, and not at all alluded to except through dire necessity, when it is mentioned as 'that disorder'. It is attended generally by all the symptoms of common chorea, only in an aggravated degree hardly ever manifesting itself until adult or middle life, and then coming on gradually but surely, increasing by degrees, and often occupying years in its development, until the hapless sufferer is but a quivering wreck of his former self.

It is as common and is indeed, I believe, more common among men than women, while I am not aware that season or complexion has any influence in the matter. There are three marked peculiarities in this disease: 1. Its hereditary nature. 2. A tendency to insanity and suicide. 3. Its manifesting itself as a grave disease only in adult life.

1. Of its hereditary nature. When either or both the parents have shown manifestations of the disease, and more especially when these manifestations have been of a serious nature, one or more of the offspring almost invariably suffer from the disease, if they live to adult age. But if by any chance these children go through life without it, the thread is broken and the grandchildren and great-grandchildren of the original shakers may rest assured that they are free from the disease. This you

will perceive differs from the general laws of so-called hereditary diseases, as for instance in phthisis, or syphilis, when one generation may enjoy entire immunity from their dread ravages, and yet in another you find them cropping out in all their hideousness. Unstable and whimsical as the disease may be in other respects, in this it is firm, it never skips a generation to again manifest in another; once having yielded its claims, it never regains them. In all the families, or nearly all in which the choreic taint exists, the nervous temperament greatly preponderates, and in my grandfather's and father's experience, which cojointly cover a period of 78 years, nervous excitement in a marked degree almost invariably attends upon every disease these people may suffer from, although they may not when in health be over nervous.

2. The tendency to insanity, and sometimes that form of insanity which leads to suicide, is marked. I know of several instances of suicide of people suffering from this form of chorea; or who belonged to families in which the disease existed. As the disease progresses the mind becomes more or less impaired, in many amounting to insanity, while in others mind and body both gradually fail until death relieves them of their sufferings. At present I know of two married men, whose wives are living, and who are constantly making love to some young lady, not seeming to be aware that there is any impropriety in it. They are suffering from chorea to such an extent that they can hardly walk, and would be thought, by a stranger, to be intoxicated. They are men of about 50 years of age, but never let an opportunity to flirt with a girl go past unimproved. The effect is ridiculous in the extreme.

3. Its third peculiarity is its coming on, at least as a grave disease, only in adult life. I do not know of a single case that has shown any marked signs of chorea before the age of thirty or forty years, while those who pass the fortieth year without symptoms of the disease are seldom attacked. It begins as an ordinary chorea might begin, by the irregular and spasmodic action of certain muscles, as of the face, arms, etc. These movements gradually increase, when muscles hitherto unaffected take on the spasmodic action, until every muscle in the body becomes affected (excepting the involuntary ones), and the poor patient presents a spectacle which is anything but pleasing to witness. I have never known a recovery or even an amelioration of symptoms in this form of chorea; when once it begins it clings to the bitter end. No treatment seems to be of any avail, and indeed nowadays its end is so well-known to the sufferer and his friends that medical advice is seldom sought. It seems at least to be one of the incurables.

Dr Wood, in his work on the practice of medicine, mentions the case of a man, in the Pennsylvania Hospital, suffering from aggravated chorea, which resisted all treatment. He finally left the hospital uncured. I strongly suspect that this man belonged to one of the families in which hereditary chorea existed. I know nothing of its pathology. I have drawn your attention to this form of chorea gentlemen, not that I considered it of any great practical importance to you, but merely as a medical curiosity, and as such it may have some interest.

It can be seen that all the cardinal features of HD are recognized in this description: the adult onset, progressive course, and eventually fatal outcome; the choreic movements combined with mental impairment, and risk of suicide; even the pattern of inheritance, with 'the thread broken' once a person had gone through life without developing it. A description of this nature could have been written only by one whose observations were based on direct and continued contact with affected patients. George Huntington's role as a family doctor, following his father and grandfather to give a 78-year total period of observation, gave him this perspective to a unique degree.

The active involvement of the two older generations of the family was acknowledged by George Huntington himself (1910) and is attested by the presence of pencil notes and corrections by his father on the original manuscript (Winfield 1908; De Jong 1937). The paper was prepared while George Huntington was working in his father's practice before leaving for

Ohio, so that it can indeed be regarded as a distillation of the observations of three generations of family doctors.

Huntington was more fortunate than many authors who have given classical description to a disease; his paper was widely appreciated from the outset and soon became internationally recognized. Browning (1908a) discussed the reasons why this was so.

There were good reasons why his paper succeeded in drawing general attention to this disorder and in securing for it permanent recognition.

Huntington was the first to give definitely the location of his cases and thus positively establish a verifiable record.

The abstracting of his original article by Kussmaul and Nothnagel in Virchow Hirsch's 'Jahrbuch' for 1872.

Thanks to the work of Friedreich on hereditary ataxia, as well as the growing interest in heredity, the time was ripe for its appreciation. Only work of unusual, incisive and wide reaching interest could attract such a share of attention.

A further factor was the interest and appreciation of William Osler, Professor of Medicine at Philadelphia and then Johns Hopkins Hospital, Baltimore. Osler remarked that 'there are few instances in the history of medicine in which a disease has been more accurately, more graphically or more briefly described' (Osler 1894, 1908).

George Huntington—life and background

The intimate connection between George Huntington's description of HD and his background in family practice gives a particular interest to knowing more about his life. Fortunately, this had already become a subject of interest during his lifetime; the 'Huntington's number' of *Neurographs*, edited by William Browning (1908a–d), provides much detail (Fig. 1.2), with a valuable biographical sketch by Winfield (1908). Further information and accounts from family members have recently been collected by Durbach and Hayden (1993). It should also be noted that there has been confusion in some accounts with George Sumner Huntington, an apparently unrelated nineteenth century American anatomist (Van der Weiden 1989, 1993).

Huntington's ancestors came, as did those of the families he studied, from the East Anglian region of England. Simon Huntington, of Norwich, is recorded as sailing to America in 1633 with his wife and children; he died on the voyage, but a son settled in Connecticut, from where Abel Huntington, grandfather of George, moved in 1797 to practise medicine in East Hampton, Long Island. Dr Abel Huntington was a distinguished physician and was the first on Long Island to perform the operation of lithotomy. He was also interested in infectious diseases and personally prepared and preserved the variola virus. His interests were not confined to medicine. He held several important public offices: in 1820, he was Presidential Elector; in 1821, he was elected New York City Senator; he was elected congressman for two terms; in 1845, he was appointed Collector of Customs for Sag Harbour; and in 1846 he was a member of the committee to revise the constitution of the State of New York. Dr Abel Huntington's son, George Lee Huntington, succeeded him in his practice, and George Huntington the younger was born at East Hampton in 1850.

George Huntington's upbringing would seem to have been a quiet and stable one, in a respectable small town in rural surroundings. He accompanied his father on his rounds and

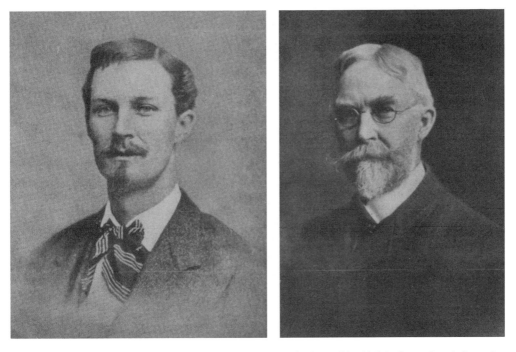

Fig. 1.2 George Huntington as a young man (left) and in later life (right). Reproduced from the 'Huntington number' of *Neurographs* (Browning 1908a).

began his medical studies with him before graduating at Columbia University, New York, in 1871. In present-day medical education, where originality is often stifled by an excessive number of facts, it is salutary to note that he qualified aged 21 and wrote his paper at the age of 22.

Although George Huntington initially returned to East Hampton to practise, he soon moved to Pomeroy, Ohio, where he married, but apparently found Pomeroy 'abundantly supplied with Physicians', causing him to move again, first to Dutchess County, New York, then to Asheville, North Carolina. He had serious health problems during this time, principally asthma, but by 1903 was able again to return to Dutchess County, where he remained in practice until 1915. In this year he retired to live with his son not far away, dying in 1916 at the age of 65 years.

George Huntington never published further papers after his 1872 description, either on chorea or on other topics. This would seem to have been due not just to his health, nor to his practice commitments, but to his removal from the environment that had resulted in his single, but remarkable, contribution to medicine—the presence of the patients studied by three generations of his family, suffering from the disorder that has so appropriately preserved the name of Huntington. Durbach and Hayden (1993) have also shown how his devotion to country medical practice and his interests in rural pursuits, along with his poor health, would have been factors against him working in an urban academic setting. An additional factor, illustrated by Huntington himself (Fig. 1.3), must have been his family commitments. Workers today

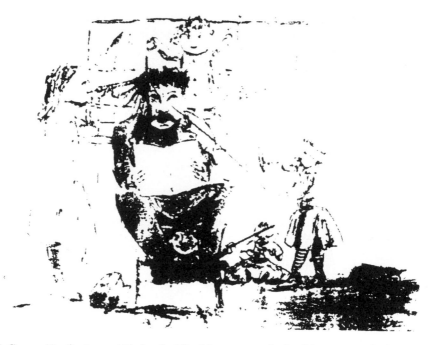

Fig. 1.3 George Huntington and his family. Was this a reason why he did not pursue further research on the disorder? A drawing by George Huntington himself (from Durbach and Hayden 1993, with kind permission).

will sympathize with him—though it has to be said that the other side of this picture, the long-suffering family of the dedicated HD researcher, equally needs to be recognized!

Perhaps the clearest insight into how George Huntington's background affected his description of the disorder is seen in an address that he gave in 1909 to the New York Medical Society.

Over fifty years ago, in riding with my father on his professional rounds, I saw my first cases of 'that disorder', which was the way in which the natives always referred to the dreaded disease. I recall it as vividly as though it had occurred but yesterday. It made a most enduring impression upon my boyish mind; an impression every detail of which I recall today, an impression which was the very first impulse to my choosing chorea as my virgin contribution to medical lore. Driving with my father through a wooded road leading from East Hampton to Amagansett, we suddenly came upon two women, mother and daughter, both tall, thin, almost cadaverous, both bowing, twisting, grimacing. I stared in wonderment, almost in fear. What could it mean? My father paused to speak with them and we passed on. Then my Gamaliel-like instruction began; my medical education had its inception. From this point on my interest in the disease has never wholly ceased.

Descriptions of HD before 1872

There can be few diseases in medicine where the description that has given the author's name to the condition is truly the first. HD is no exception, and there is no doubt that others had recognized and to some extent described the condition before George Huntington published his 1872 paper. Not surprisingly, there have been a number of claims of such descriptions (De Jong 1937; Bruyn 1968; Stevens 1972), but few stand up to critical examination. Thus Elliotson's (1832) mention of chronic adult chorea, noting that 'I have often seen it hereditary', might or might not have referred to HD, while Husquinet's interesting finding (1975) that the case described in 1873 by Landouzy could be traced to Belgium and linked to records from the previous century can hardly be regarded as a prior description.

The first definite record of HD was in a letter by Charles Oscar Waters (1816–92) in 1841 and published by Dunglison in the first edition of his *Practice of medicine* in 1842. It is worth reproducing this in detail, as it gives such a clear picture of the clinical features and natural history.

It consists essentially in a spasmodic action of all the voluntary muscles of the system, of involuntary and more or less irregular motions of the extremities, face and trunk. In these involuntary movements the upper part of the air passages occasionally participate as is witnessed by the 'clucking' sound in the glottis and in a manifest impediment to the powers of speech. The expression of the countenance and general appearance of the patients are very much such as are described as characteristic of chorea.

The disease is markedly hereditary, and is most common among the lower classes, though cases of it are not infrequent among those who by industry and temperance have raised themselves to a respectable rank in society. These involuntary movements of the face, neck, extremities and body cease entirely during sleep.

The singular disease rarely, very rarely indeed makes its appearance before adult life, and attacks after forty-five years of age are also very rare. When once it has appeared, however, it clings to its suffering victim with unrelenting tenacity until death comes to his relief. It very rarely or never ceases while life lasts.

The first indications of its appearance are spasmodic twitching of the extremities generally of the fingers which gradually extend and involve all the voluntary muscles. This derangement of muscular action is by no means uniform; in some it exists to a greater, in others to a less extent, but in all cases it gradually induces a state of more or less perfect dementia.

When speaking of the manifestly hereditary nature of the disease, I should perhaps have remarked that I have never known a case of it to occur in a patient, one or both of whose ancestors were not, within the third generation at farthest, the subject of this distressing malady.

In 1846, a further description occurred in the form of a thesis submitted to Jefferson Medical College, Philadelphia, by Dr Charles Gorman (1817–96) entitled 'On a form of chorea, vulgarly called magrums'. Although the thesis is lost, it is mentioned in the third edition (1848) of Dunglison's book: 'an inaugural dissertation, presented before the Faculty of Jefferson Medical College of Philadelphia by Charles R, Gorman of Luzerne County, Pa., the writer states that this affection prevails also in other portions of the country. According to him, it seems to be circumscribed by neighbourhood boundaries, and to be confined to sections of the country, the inhabitants of which are intimately connected in their Social or Business relations.'

A valuable account of these early American descriptions of hereditary chorea is given by Browning (1908a–d) in the 'Huntington number' of *Neurographs*, along with the location of the families and biographical details of Waters, Gorman, and other early workers.

The other independent early description that undoubtedly represented HD is that of Johan Christian Lund, written in Norwegian and generally appreciated only since relevant parts were translated by Ørbeck (1959), although recognized in Scandinavia before that. Lund was public health physician in the region of Saetersdal, Norway, and wrote in his medical report for 1860:

As recorded in the previous medical report, chorea St Vitus [which is Lund's term for St Vitus's dance] seems to recur as an hereditary disease in Saetersdal. It is commonly known as the 'twitches', occasionally as the 'inherited disease'. It usually occurs between the ages of 50 and 60, generally starting with less obvious symptoms, which at times only progress slowly, without becoming violent, so that the patient's normal activities are not particularly hindered: but more often after a few years they increase to a considerable degree, so that any form of work becomes impossible and even eating becomes difficult and circuitous. The entire body, though chiefly the head, arms, and trunk, is in constant jerking and flinging motion, except during sleep, when the patient is usually motionless. A couple of the severely affected patients have during the last days of their lives become Fatui [i.e. demented]. The disease occurs in two families which are registered below. Information is not as complete as could be desired though enough to start with, as long as doctors in Saetersdalen are mindful of the disease in future. [Lund 1860; quoted by Ørbeck 1959].

Lund gave further details on family members in later reports and, according to Ørbeck, descendants with HD still exist today. It seems that Lund was doubly unlucky in not gaining recognition, since not only was the original source restricted in readership by being written in Norwegian, but subsequent commentators on it confused the disorder with Parkinson's disease.

One further description of HD before 1872 is widely quoted, namely that of Lyon (1863), who reported three families from New York State with hereditary chorea under the title 'Chronic hereditary chorea' in the *American Medical Times*. Lyon's families do not seem to have been connected with those of Waters, but were also called 'megrim families' locally. Browning (1908d) traced the localization of the families to Bedford, on the New York–Connecticut border, but no subsequent clinical evaluation of the patients or their descendants has been carried out. However, a critical look at the description of these cases suggests that Lyon's families 1 and 2 (family 3 was not described in detail) were far from typical for HD and much more suggestive of benign familial chorea (see Chapter 2). So that readers can decide for themselves, these cases are quoted here.

CASE I. Mr A., residing in the town of ——, county of ——, NY, has well marked chorea, which is quite general; so that he is constantly, when awake, making irregular movements with the upper and lower extremities, facial muscles, and more or less with those of the body. This condition has existed for many years, but seems not to interfere materially with his general health, the vegetative functions being well performed. Mr A has two brothers and three sisters; the two brothers have themselves never had choreal symptoms, but one of them has two children in whom well defined chorea has existed for many years; of the three sisters, two have had chorea for the most of their lives, being now past the middle age.

The progenitors of Mr A., on the male side, were perfectly free from chorea, but not so on the maternal side; his mother had well developed choreal manifestations from early life, which continued till her decease; she had also a brother who died during adult life from the severity of the disease; but to go still further, both the grandfather and great-grandfather of Mr A., on the maternal side, had the same disorder which we find in their children: whether collateral instances of the affection occurred in the families we are not advised.

CASE II. Mrs K., of the town of ——, Ct and a descendant from a family which has long been known and designated as migrim, had chorea for the most of her life, being about seventy-five years old at the date of death. She had a family of two sons and three daughters: of these one son and two daughters had chorea, with which disease they attained an advanced age; no satisfactory information can be readily obtained in relation to the offspring of the son and one of these daughters so affected; but the other daughter married, and had a son, who is now forty years of age, in whom chorea has exhibited itself from puberty.

In particular, the fact that the proband of family 1 is stated to have had chorea for many years, but that the condition had not interfered with his general health, while his two affected sisters 'had chorea for most of their lives' and their mother from early life, is most unlike HD. So is the fact that the grandson in family 2, then 40 years old, had had chorea since puberty. There is no mention of progression or of general deterioration apart from the one individual of family 1, who is stated to have 'died during adult life from the severity of the disease'.

Thus it would seem that Lyon's families should not be accepted as having HD, but are rather characteristic of benign familial chorea. Such a situation has an interesting precedent in the myotonic disorders, where the non-progressive and much rarer myotonia congenita was described by Thomsen in 1876 considerably before the recognition of the more common myotonic dystrophy by Steinert and by Batten and Gibb in 1909.

William Osler and HD

The rapid spread and wide distribution of knowledge concerning HD was in no small measure due to the interest that William Osler (1849–1919) took in it. Osler had a lifelong interest in chorea and his monograph *On chorea and choreiform affections* (1904) contains a wealth of personally collected data on rheumatic (Sydenham's) chorea. However, he included a separate chapter on hereditary chorea in this, as well as a brief section in his *The principles and practice of medicine* (1892), and dealt specifically with Huntington's chorea in several case reports and papers (1890, 1893, 1894). (Surprisingly and most atypically, he misspells the eponym as 'Huntingdon' in some of these.)

Osler made attempts to reassess Huntington's original family during the summer of 1887 but Huntington wrote back indicating that they would not welcome this, although Osler was sent notes on these patients the following year. He was able to gain personal experience from patients seen at Johns Hopkins Hospital of both English and German origin; his case reports are a model of clarity and detailed observation, and ring as true today as a century ago.

When sitting in a chair, at ease, the arms and hands are in more or less constant irregular motion. The fingers are extended and flexed alternately; sometimes the entire set. At other times the whole hand will be lifted, or there are constant movements of pronation and supination. For half a minute or so they may be perfectly motionless. The head and trunk present occasional slow movements; in the latter more of a swaying character. The legs jerk irregularly and the feet are flexed or extended; but the movements are not so frequent as in the arms. The face in repose is usually motionless, but the lips are occasionally brought together more tightly and the chin elevated or depressed. There is an occasional movement of the zygomatic and of the frontal muscles. He puts out the tongue, with tolerably active associated movements of the face, and it is usually quickly withdrawn or rolled from side to side. It is impossible for him to hold it out for any length of time. There are no irregular movements of the palate muscles.

He walks with a curious irregular gait, displaying distinct incoordination, swaying as he goes, hesitating a moment in a step, keeping the arms out from the body and in constant motion. The legs are spread wide apart; the steps are unequal in length and he seems rather to drag the feet. He stands well with the heels close together and the eyes shut. [From Osler 1894]

The spread of knowledge on HD

The rapid spread of awareness of George Huntington's 1872 paper has already been mentioned, but from the work on hereditary chorea discussed so far it could be imagined that most of the interest and activity was in America, not in Europe. Such an impression would be entirely wrong, for not only was the topic of chorea in general one of great interest among European physicians and neurologists, but many of the early reports and studies of HD in the last quarter of the nineteenth century were European in origin. The monograph of Petit (1970) and the review of Bruyn (1968) are especially valuable in giving appropriate recognition to these early European workers.

Table 1.1, based on the bibliography of Bruyn *et al.* (1974), gives a picture of how widely diffused information on HD soon became. Some of these reports (for example, that of Landouzy in 1873) were described before being aware of Huntington's description, but international communication seems to have been remarkably rapid at that time (perhaps because the number of investigators and volume of literature were limited). Medicine, neurology, and pathology had not yet become fully demarcated specialties, and in reading the early descriptions one gains the impression of an actively communicating body of workers whose interests ranged over a wide variety of disorders. The names of some of these workers who published on HD, including Landouzy (1873), Bourneville (1874), Golgi (1874), Déjerine (1886), and Hoffmann (1888), are now better remembered in relation to other neurological disorders than in connection with HD.

It is also relevant to note that HD was described early in a number of countries, such as Cuba and Brazil, in which the disorder is not today recognized as a frequent occurrence,

Table 1.1 The spread of information on HD. First reports from different countries, based on Bruyn *et al.* (1974)

Country	Date of report*	Author*
USA	(1842), 1872	(Waters), Huntington
Norway	(1860)	(Lund)
France	1873	Landouzy
Italy	1874	Golgi
Germany	1877	Meynert
United Kingdom	1880	Harbinson
Russia	1889	Kornilowa
Cuba	1890	Arostegui
Netherlands	1890	Beukers
Poland	1890	Biernacki
Brazil	1891	Couto
Denmark	1892	Friis
Argentina	1894	Costa
Czechoslovakia	1895	Ganghofner
Yugoslavia	1900	Gutschy
Australia	1902	Hogg
Canada	1904	Mackay

*Entries in parentheses indicate a description before George Huntington's 1872 report.

reinforcing the impression, discussed further in Chapter 6, that HD has been a widespread condition for a considerable time.

HD in New England—history and origins

While the recognition of HD was spreading rapidly throughout the world during the last decades of the nineteenth century, laying the foundations of our detailed knowledge of the natural history of the disease, there was considerable activity also in tracing and attempting to connect the various families in the New England region that had been responsible for most of the original descriptions. Jelliffe (1908) and Davenport and Muncey (1916) were able to compile extensive pedigrees and to link them into groups that could be traced back to possible founding members. Most of these appeared to originate in the early seventeenth century from the East Anglian areas of England (from which George Huntington's ancestors had also come), and which had seen extensive migration to the USA.

Unfortunately, the attempts to identify specific individuals as the source of the gene for HD all seem to have stretched the evidence far beyond what actually exists. Vessie (1932) claimed to have traced one large HD grouping back over a 300-year period to three individuals from the village of Bures in Suffolk. He gave these individuals pseudonyms but the actual names were used by Critchley (1934, 1964, 1973) who extended the tracing in East Anglia, as did van Zwanenberg (1974); Vessie (1932, 1939) and later Maltsberger (1961) developed a further aspect of these families during the early colonial period in New England—their possible involvement in the notorious witchcraft trials of that time. Their papers, especially that of Maltsberger, are more notable for their lurid and exaggerated descriptions than for their scientific approach and do not actually show any direct involvement of likely HD patients in these episodes.

Subsequent investigation has shown that the whole of this work is based on inadequate and probably erroneous foundations. Caro and Haines (1975) and Caro (1977), themselves based in East Anglia, traced the genealogical evidence in both England and America, and found that the principal person named by Critchley as most likely to have introduced the HD gene did not actually exist; additionally they noted numerous errors and discrepancies in the previous accounts. The previous conclusions associating carriers of the HD gene with witchcraft and criminality were also invalidated. Despite this, Critchley (1984) was still giving essentially the original account 10 years later. In view of the frequent tendency to stigmatization of patients and families with HD, which has existed from the beginning and still remains a problem, it seems especially important to correct this much cited chapter of history and to exhort workers on HD to be as cautious in their historical conclusions as in their scientific work.

Regardless of the precise details, New England has clearly played a pivotal role in receiving HD genes from Europe and distributing them throughout the USA. It is possible also that it may have been responsible for a wider spread of the disorder, as described in Chapter 6. It seems likely that the HD gene in some Pacific Island communities may have been brought by visiting New England whaling ships in the early nineteenth century (Scrimgeour 1983). If this can be confirmed (a possibility now with molecular haplotypes), it will provide a particularly interesting example of how a genetic disorder may not only contribute to a chapter of history but also leave long-term effects that persist after the original events of the Pacific whaling industry are all but forgotten, except as literature.

Evolution of the clinical picture

Compared with most original descriptions of a disease, that given by George Huntington in 1872 was remarkably complete, despite its brevity. This was largely due to the all-round view that he was able to obtain as a general practitioner and the length of time over which his own family had observed the patients for whom they cared. Subsequent work over the next three decades thus served mainly to give more detail to the neurological and psychiatric symptoms, to extend awareness of the range and variation seen in the disorder, and to attempt to analyse the pathological and genetic aspects.

The numerous case and family reports following the original description have already been mentioned and, in the case of Osler, quoted. The existence of HD as a specific entity of chronic, progressive, hereditary chorea of adult onset soon became widely accepted. The detailed clinical picture that emerged will be described in Chapters 2 and 3 but it is worth examining here some of the more important aspects that had not been fully appreciated in the initial descriptions already given.

Psychiatric syndromes

Huntington in his original paper recognized that mental deterioration was one of the characteristic features of the disorder that was to bear his name; he noted 'the tendency to insanity, and sometimes that form of insanity that leads to suicide'. Most of the subsequent case reports, however, concentrated on the chorea rather than the psychiatric manifestations of HD.

One of the more systematic of the early studies on mental disorder in HD was conducted by Phelps (1892) at Rochester, Minnesota. He found five patients with HD, or one in 600 (out of the 3000 admissions) who had been admitted to the Second Minnesota Hospital for the Insane. In addition, he wrote to the superintendents of 50 psychiatric institutions all over the United States asking for details on patients with HD. Thirteen cases were reported to him in replies from 24 hospitals, so that he had the largest series up to that time. He described many of the major forms of psychiatric disorder, including psychotic symptoms, 'melancholia', suicide, irritability, and 'steady mental degeneration'.

In the early literature on HD, there are clear descriptions of psychosis. Delusions of grandeur figure prominently in a number of clinical descriptions. One inpatient said that 'God is my lawyer' (Phelps 1892), while another called her mental hospital a 'castle' (Eager and Perdrau 1910). Delusions of royalty in HD have also been reported (Phelps 1892; Eager and Perdrau 1910). An interesting American case of delusions of special ability was described in a man who said he was getting 'a million dollars for standing back and allowing Harrison to be President instead of himself' (Phelps 1892). Some of these patients may have had concurrent general paresis, which is a well-known cause of grandiose delusions.

Cognitive decline was described in the early reports (for example, Osler 1893) and indeed in the opinion of Sinkler (quoted by Mitchell 1895) 'nearly all cases of Huntington's chorea terminate in dementia'. Perhaps the most perceptive of the early accounts of impaired intellectual functioning was provided by Edward Mapother (1911) from Dublin.

As the disease progresses the most marked noteworthy and constant feature comes to be a failure of the power of sustained attention. Often there is no marked deficit of memory. There is no disorientation either in regard to place or time. Comprehension of speech is good and the capacity for simple judgements and deduction is unimpaired. But if one gives the patient a somewhat complex order involving the performance of several successive actions or the observation of a series of phenomena, his capacity for sustained attention is immediately manifested.

Bower and Mills (1890) also commented on higher mental functions in HD, especially abnormalities of speech and handwriting. Although dementia was thus well recognized in HD, early authors also observed that there were exceptions and that some patients remained 'mentally clear' (Fisher 1906).

Juvenile Huntington's disease and the rigid form

The paper of Lyon (1863) is commonly quoted as the first description of childhood HD but, as mentioned earlier, the lack of clear progression and the early onset in his families make it likely that he was dealing with a separate disorder such as benign familial chorea. A number of other early childhood cases are discussed by Bruyn (1968) in his review, but the most detailed of these is the report of Hoffmann (1888). In this three-generation family with HD, there were two daughters who had onset at 4 and 10 years, showed rigidity, hypokinesia, and seizures, as well as choreic movements, both showing prolonged survival. This report showed clearly that not only could childhood onset occur within a typical HD family, but that the clinical features might be strikingly different to those normally seen in the adult disorder.

The recognition of juvenile HD was closely linked with the realization that chorea was not the only motor disorder in HD, and that some patients showed a predominance of rigidity and hypokinesia. The term 'Westphal variant' has often been used for this clinical presentation, but in describing his 18-year-old patient with these features, Westphal (1883) attributed them to a separate cause rather than to HD. The family of Hoffmann (1888) already mentioned, together with those reported by Curschmann (1908), Freund (1911), and many others, reinforced the existence of the rigid form of HD as an important clinical picture, usually in young adults or children, but occurring in the same families as cases with more typical chorea as the presenting feature.

Thus by the end of the nineteenth century, as a result of a very large number of careful and detailed descriptions, the clinical picture of HD was, if not complete, at least well established in terms of its main neurological features, its psychiatric involvement, and its natural history. It was already quite clear that it was a specific disorder with well defined, though variable, clinical features; the universal adoption of the title 'Huntington's chorea' or 'Huntington's disease' reinforced the degree to which the disorder was accepted as an entity, as well as the contribution that George Huntington had made to its original description.

Neuropathology

The search for neuropathological abnormalities in HD began early. Lewis (1876) was forced to conclude that 'no definite portion of the cerebrospinal system can at present be chosen as the site of lesions peculiar to chorea'. However, Meynert (1877) was more successful in detecting the post-mortem changes in HD. He proposed that chorea could be explained by lesions in the corpus striatum, but this remained contentious for many years. Osler (1893) found no specific changes, as already mentioned, and could give no clear explanation for the clinical features. Some workers thought that brain inflammation was a neuropathological characteristic of HD (Oppenheim 1887; Phelps 1892; Sinkler 1892), whereas others believed that the disorder was caused by a congenital malformation of the motor cortex (Stier 1902; Müller 1903). These reports were disputed by other investigators who thought that vascular sclerosis and the overgrowth of neuroglia were the pathological changes in HD (see Mapother 1911).

Perhaps the most influential of the early neuropathological studies was that conducted by Jelgersma (1908). He described generalized shrinkage of the HD brain and atrophy of the caudate nucleus (reduced to one-third of its original volume). These findings were confirmed by later workers (Alzheimer 1911; Pfeiffer 1913), but it was not until the 1920s that there was general agreement that the brain changes in HD were primarily degenerative and atrophic, and that the caudate nucleus was preferentially involved in the process.

Neuropathological studies have recently again become of central importance in HD research, first with the advent of detailed quantitative analyses, and now with the recognition of neuronal inclusions as a key element in the pathology of both human HD and in the transgenic mouse models, as discussed in later sections of the book.

Early forms of treatment

At the time of Huntington's report, there was little in the therapeutic armamentarium for most diseases. Nonetheless, several authors tried drug treatment for HD and some animal trials were also conducted. In the 1890s, strychnia was injected into dogs until they were 'violently choreic' (Wood 1893). Quinine 3 was found to 'arrest these movements' and, in a clinical trial on a patient with pronounced chorea, the drug was reported to be effective (Wood 1893). After administration of bromide of potassium, it was noted that 'twitchings decreased remarkably' in another case report (McFaren 1874). Other drugs were less successful, such as hyoscamine (Lewis 1876) and arsenic (Eager and Perdrau 1910). MacFaren (1874) was probably the first investigator to recommend a nutritional diet for weight loss in HD. None the less, admission to an asylum was the only significant intervention that could be offered. Now we are at last on the threshold of more definitive therapy, as indicated in Chapters 15, 16, and 17.

Inheritance

The later part of this book is largely devoted to a detailed description of the genetic and molecular basis of HD (Chapters 5, 12, and 13) and the practical applications of this knowledge in genetic counselling and prediction (Chapter 7). The main features of the inheritance pattern were already well recognized by George Huntington in his original description.

When either or both parents have shown manifestations of the disease, and more especially when these manifestations have been of a serious nature, one or more of the offspring almost invariably suffers from the disease, if they live to adult age. But if by any chance these children go through life without it, the thread is broken, and the grandchildren and great-grandchildren of the original shakers may rest assured that they are free from the disease. Unstable and whimsical as the disease may be in other respects, in this it is firm; it never skips a generation to manifest itself in another; once having yielded its claims, it never regains them. [From Huntington 1872]

Reading this passage today, it is as clear a description of Mendelian dominant inheritance as one could wish. However, although Mendel had published his work in 1865, it was rediscovered only in 1900, so no theoretical basis could be provided for the pattern that had been observed until after this time. It did not take long, however, for workers looking for possible human examples of Mendelian inheritance to recognize that HD provided a likely instance. In February 1908, Punnett, a close colleague of Bateson whose work was primarily on poultry, cited HD as likely to follow dominant inheritance, while later in the same year Jelliffe (who had read Punnett's paper) also mentioned this. Neither was very definite, both preferring to cite brachydactyly as a more conclusive example.

By 1911, Davenport was able to be much more confident in listing HD as an autosomal dominant disorder, along with other conditions illustrating autosomal recessive and sex-linked inheritance. Interestingly, he also cited other forms of chorea as being dominantly inherited. By the time of this later collection of material specifically on HD (Davenport and Muncey 1916), the mode of inheritance was beyond doubt, and detailed analysis could begin.

In any discussion of the early development of our concepts of the genetics of HD, the work of Charles Davenport (Davenport 1911; Davenport and Muncey 1916) requires special discussion. Davenport's prejudiced attitude to the disorder, his advocacy of radical eugenic views (Davenport 1911), and later political association with the German race-hygienists make it difficult to assess his work objectively, as does his tendency to overinterpret Mendelian principles, especially in relation to other disorders involving intelligence and mental characteristics. Despite this, though, and bearing in mind the early time at which he was working, he must not only be acknowledged as the person who made it clear beyond doubt that HD followed Mendelian dominant inheritance, but also for his documentation of such important aspects as age at onset, variation between families, possible anticipation and its biases, and the reasons for apparent skipped generations. Clinically, too, he recognized the variability in degree and type of mental involvement and the variety of motor disturbance that might occur. His compilation of data on almost 1000 affected individuals, mainly in the New England area and descended from a small number of original progenitors, provided the foundation for much of the work that was to come and should be recognized for this, even though many of the conclusions drawn may have been flawed.

The development of research into HD

Until recently, the history of research on HD has been one of gradual progress, rather than of sudden leaps. The main discoveries in the different fields of work are recorded in the specific chapters and have been shared by many different disciplines in addition to the neurosciences, genetics having been a major contributor from the beginning to the present.

A broad picture of the early activity relating to the study of HD can be obtained from the bibliography of Bruyn *et al.* (1974). By 1890 up to 20 papers each year were being published on HD, with a peak just before World War I only reached again in the mid-1930s, falling again during World War II, but rising sharply and continuously thereafter. Understandably, the main topics have changed over the years, with studies of neuropathology prominent in the earlier phases, while pharmacological and biochemical topics have been more abundant in recent years, clinical and genetic reports remaining relatively constant, at least until 1972.

Table 1.2 lists some of the landmarks in the development of our understanding of HD. Easily the most notable recent landmark has been the identification of the HD gene, together with the recognition of the specific mutation as an expanded trinucleotide (CAG) repeat,

Table 1.2 Landmarks in the study of HD

1841	First definite description of HD (Waters)
1872	George Huntington's definitive description
1888	Juvenile HD clearly described (Hoffman)
1908	Mendelian dominant inheritance recognized
1934	Systematic study of inheritance (Bell)
1958–59	First detailed genetic-epidemiological survey in specific region (Michigan)
1967	Committee to Combat Huntington's Disease formed
1967	World Federation of Neurology research group formed
1972	Centennial Symposium, Columbus, Ohio
1983	Localization of HD gene on chromosome 4
1987	First applications of DNA markers in prediction
1993	Isolation of HD gene; identification of mutation as expanded CAG repeat
1994	Polyglutamine repeat recognized as important in neuronal pathology (Perutz)
1996	Neurological phenotype produced in transgenic mouse with expanded HD repeat
1997	Neuronal inclusions recognized in transgenic mouse and human HD brain

encoding polyglutamine. Without this finding, much of the later work detailed in Chapters 11–14 would not have been possible. These arguably represent the most important advances in the history of the disease.

HD in the scientific literature

Modern information technology has greatly simplified the analysis and retrieval of published literature relating to HD, but a valuable resource for earlier publications is the HD centennial bibliography (Bruyn *et al.* 1974), which lists all known publications on HD up to 1972, the 100th anniversary of George Huntington's original publication, with a supplement extending the work to 1978.

The critical approach taken, the extensive cross-indexing, and informative comment accompanying the bibliography not only make this the definitive collection of material on HD, but give a clear picture of the pattern of research, its progress and evolution into different subjects, as well as the geographical distribution of work on the disorder. It was used extensively during the writing of earlier editions of this book as a source of reference for older papers (particularly those written in languages other than English) that would otherwise have been difficult to obtain.

The importance of monographs in bringing together and synthesizing information on HD deserves recognition. In addition to the present work and its earlier editions (Harper 1991, 1996), the monograph of Hayden (1981) contains many original data, while that of Folstein (1989) is especially important in being written from the perspective of the psychiatrist.

An important focus and forum for discussion of new work on HD over the past 20 years has been the World Federation of Neurology Research Group on Huntington's Disease. Founded by Dr André Barbeau, this group first met in Montreal in 1967 and has since held a succession of valuable workshops at about 2-yearly intervals. It has helped to create a community of research workers involved with HD who have developed close and continuing links, and collaborations spanning a number of different disciplines.

Lay groups and HD research

A striking feature of the medical scene during the past 30 years has been the development of self-help groups run by sufferers and their families. Fund-raising for research, improvement of services, and greater public awareness have all been major aims. In the case of HD, progress would undoubtedly have been slower had such societies not been developed, and it is unlikely that the disorder would have the high public profile internationally that it does today.

The initial development in this area arose from the illness of Woody Guthrie, the American folk singer (Fig. 1.4), who developed HD symptoms around 1952 and died in 1967 at the age of 55. The remarkable biography by Klein (1981) gives considerable insight into the interplay between personality, creativity, and disease in Guthrie's life. His widow Marjorie devoted the later part of her life to promoting all aspects of HD, and in 1967 the

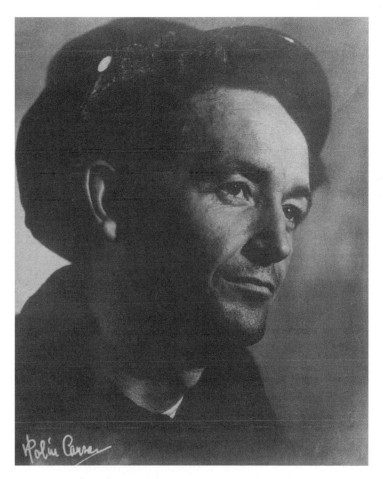

Fig. 1.4 Woody Guthrie, the American folk singer affected with HD, whose illness was the catalyst for the founding of the first lay society involved with HD, the Committee to Combat Huntington's Disease. (Courtesy of Woody Guthrie Publications.)

HD COMMITTEE TO COMBAT HUNTINGTON'S DISEASE, INC.
Suite 1304 · 200 West 57 Street · New York, N.Y. 10019

NEWSLETTER

NUMBER 1   ©1968, Committee to Combat Huntington's Disease, Inc.   SPRING 1968

Purposes of the Committee to Combat Huntington's Disease, Inc.

The Committee's Charter contains a statement of the purposes for which the Committee was organized. Briefly, these purposes are:

Educational. To collect information about all aspects of Huntington's disease and distribute it to interested individuals, "for the purpose of increasing public awareness;"

Assistance. "To assist those afflicted with Huntington's disease and their families in meeting the social, economic, and emotional problems resulting from such affliction;"

Financial. The Committee will raise funds to help support "the advancement

The day-to-day work of the Committee to Combat Huntington's Disease, Inc. is carried out by six operating committees working within the framework of the larger organization. Any member is welcome to join the operating committee whose work interests him most. These committees are:

Financial Committee. Responsible for fund-raising activities and for dispensing the funds that are raised.

Membership Committee. Handles all questions of membership: eventually, this committee will be instrumental in contacting other groups interested in Huntington's disease to form national or international organizations.

Administrative Committee. Works with the Executive Secretary to perform various daily activities of the Committee.

Family Counseling Committee. Helps to determine the needs of families involved in Huntington's disease, and plans action to aid these families and individuals.

Publications and Publicity Committee. Prepares the Newsletter and other publications; makes sure that the work of the Committee receives attention in newspapers, magazines, etc.

Program Committee. Plans general meetings in advance; makes arrangements such as getting speakers, etc.

Fig. 1.5 The initial newsletter of the Committee to Combat Huntington's Disease.

Committee to Combat Huntington's Disease (later the Huntington's Disease Association) was formed with objectives to provide services for families and to promote education and research (Fig. 1.5).

Marjorie Guthrie was also largely responsible for the initiation of comparable organizations in other countries, resulting in 1978 in the International Huntington's Association, a body that now involves 27 member countries. Close links with medical groups, such as the World Federation of Neurology (WFN) Research Group, have ensured that the lay societies have played a constructive role in developing policies in such critical areas as predictive testing.

An organization with entirely different aims but of equal importance has been the Hereditary Disease Foundation, initiated by Dr Milton Wexler after his wife developed the disorder, and continued by his daughter Nancy Wexler. The Hereditary Disease Foundation was instrumental in the collection and analysis of the large Venezuelan kindreds that were so important in the cloning of the HD gene. A fascinating account of these activities seen from the perspective of a family member has been written by Alice Wexler (1995).

The Venezuela project

The remarkable concentration of patients with HD living in the Zulia region of Venezuela, by the shores of Lake Maracaibo (Fig. 1.6), represents the largest cluster of cases derived from a single ancestor that has remained geographically localized. This pedigree contains

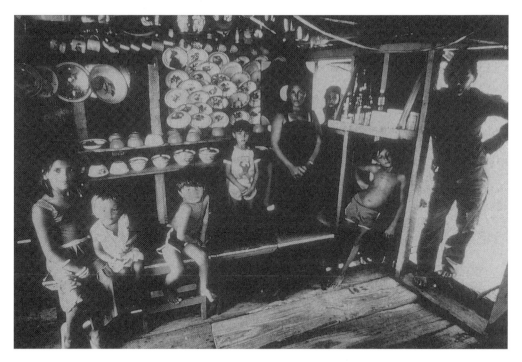

Fig. 1.6 HD in Venezuela. The concentration of the disorder in the villages around Lake Maracaibo and the occurrence there of probable homozygotes for the disorder has led to a major longitudinal study of the disease and to studies of the HD gene. (Courtesy of Dr Nancy Wexler.)

over 10 000 members with over 100 living affected subjects. Some of the epidemiological aspects of this concentration are described in Chapter 6, but the wider significance of HD in Venezuela for the development and understanding of the disease deserves a special mention here.

The high frequency of the disorder in some of the small and isolated lakeside communities was first documented by Negrette (1963), and was brought to general attention by his colleague Avila-Giron (1973), who presented details at the Centennial Symposium on HD. It was then recognized that this isolate could be of special significance, particularly in studying possible homozygotes, because several families had both parents affected; visits by Dr André Barbeau and others confirmed this, but the key development was the decision of the Hereditary Disease Foundation to mount a systematic study of the population. After an initial visit in 1979, comprehensive studies were carried out by an annual visiting team beginning in 1981; detailed pedigrees were drawn up, allowing a full genealogy of the different branches to be pieced together, while accurate clinical assessment of both affected members and relatives at risk was carried out, concentrating on families with two affected parents containing possible homozygotes. Blood samples were taken for DNA analysis and cell lines set up, allowing their long-term study. At the same time the workers tried to provide as much practical help as possible to these poor and deprived communities. The background to the work is well described in a number of general readership articles (Drake 1984; Kolata 1984; Pines 1984;

Steinmann 1987); a full account of this remarkable project has yet to be written, although it is touched on in the book of Alice Wexler (1995).

The most spectacular result of the Venezuela project has been its crucial role in locating and isolating the HD gene, outlined below and described further in Chapter 5. Almost as important, however, have been the clinical studies, which provide a unique longitudinal documentation of HD in a population without access to medication for the disease, as well as clearly showing that the likely homozygotes for HD are no more severely affected than are those with a single copy of the gene. The Venezuela project is a striking example of the value of a long-term clinically based project and there is no doubt that this value will increase further when, as seems imminent, understanding the function of the gene leads to therapy that can significantly alter the natural history of the disorder.

Isolation of the HD gene

It may seem premature for an event as recent as 1993 to be classed as 'history', but there can be no doubt that isolation of the HD gene is already perceived as a historic point in HD research. The scientific aspects and the consequences for our understanding of the disorder are described in Chapter 5, but the background deserves to be noted here. The book by Alice Wexler (1995) gives a fuller account, from a different perspective.

The Huntington's Disease Collaborative Research Group was formed as a direct outcome of the Venezuela project described above, following the realization that this extended kindred held great potential for mapping and isolating the gene. Supported again by the Hereditary Disease Foundation, it developed into a close collaboration of six teams in the United States and Britain. Central to the function—and ultimate success—of the group was an agreement to share fully all resources and to share in any credit by publishing the paper reporting isolation of the gene under the name of the group, as indeed was done (Huntington's Disease Collaborative Research Group 1993). Equally important was the complementary nature of the teams involved, with all members able to offer some particular skill or resource, and to bring in the new techniques or ideas from basic molecular research or from work on other disorders.

It can be imagined that maintaining such close collaboration over a prolonged period (it took 10 years from the initial localization to isolation of the gene itself) was a challenging task, and the Hereditary Disease Foundation deserves great credit for its role in this, as do the scientists involved, who in some cases invested many years of their career in this joint effort—with no guarantee that it would be the Collaborative Research Group itself that was ultimately successful.

The historic nature of the isolation of the HD gene was reflected in the explosion of research that has followed the publication of the full gene sequence and nature of the mutation in the paper by the Collaborative Research Group. This publication allowed the world research community, including many not previously involved in HD research, to join in the field on equal terms, and thus inevitably brought to an end the Collaborative Research Group in its original closed form. Perhaps its best justification has been that its very success should result in its conclusion; happily, the close links formed during its existence, and the continuing support of the Hereditary Disease Foundation, have resulted in most of the teams involved continuing in HD research and maintaining and developing their productive collaborations. In this, as in many other ways, HD has provided an example for those working on other disorders.

HD research after isolation of the gene

The isolation of the HD gene, while marking the end of an era, has provided the starting point for numerous new research approaches to the pathogenesis of the disorder, which are the subject of the later chapters of this book. One of these, however, deserves particular mention at this point; this is the hypothesis, now strongly supported by experimental data, of the late Dr Max Perutz, that the polyglutamine sequence in the HD protein, huntingtin, translated from the CAG repeat in the gene, might itself be the key to disease pathology. Perutz *et al.* (1994) suggested on the basis of molecular modelling that the protein molecules containing this expanded polyglutamine repeat could form a 'polar zipper' structure (Fig 1.7) resulting in aggregates that might themselves produce neuronal damage.

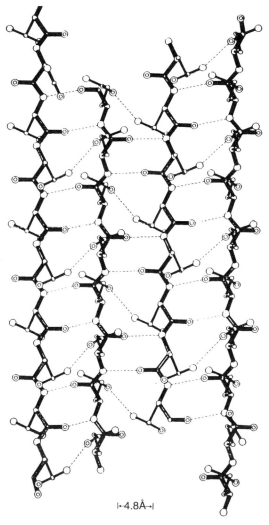

|←4.8Å→|

o – Cα, o – C, O – N, ◎ – O

Fig. 1.7 The 'polar zipper' model for polyglutamine repeats (from Harper and Perutz 2001 and Perutz 1994, with permission).

The detection of neuronal inclusions in HD brain and that of transgenic mice, as well as direct biochemical studies, both indicate that expanded glutamine repeats in the huntingtin protein do indeed lead to aggregation. This work was brought together recently at a Royal Society symposium in London (Perutz *et al.* 2000; Harper and Perutz 2001). The concept also has a particular historical resonance, linking directly with Perutz' comparable studies on haemoglobin and other key molecules originating more than 50 years earlier.

This also provides a striking example of how HD research has repeatedly attracted the interest and involvement of outstanding scientists whose main field of work has been in apparently unrelated areas, but whose insights into basic processes has thrown light on HD also. Now that we are starting to understand the key elements of the molecular pathology of HD and related trinucleotide repeat disorders, there is increasing need and opportunity for such lateral involvement, which has proved rewarding for all concerned.

References

Alzheimer A (1911) Uber die anatomische Grundlage der Huntington'schen Chorea und der choreatis- chen Bewegungen überhaupt. *Zeitschrift für die gesamte Neurologie und Psychiatrie* **3**:566–567.

Avila-Giron R (1973) Medical and social aspects of Huntington's chorea in the State of Zulia, Venezuela. In: *Advances in Neurology* (eds A Barbeau, TN Chase, and GW Paulson), pp. 261–266. New York: Raven Press.

Barbeau A, Chase TN and Paulson GW (1973) *Huntington's Chorea, 1872–1972.* New York, Raven Press.

Batten FE and Gibb HP (1909) Myotonia atrophica. *Brain* **32**:187–205.

Bell J (1934) Huntington's chorea. In: *Treasury of Human Inheritance* (ed. RA Fisher) Vol. IV, part 1, pp. 1–67. Cambridge: Cambridge University Press.

Bourneville DM (1874) De l'emploi thérapeutique du monobromure de camphre. *Progrès Médical (Paris)* **2**:456–459.

Bower JL and Mills CK (1890) Notes on some cases of chorea and tremor. *Journal of Nervous and Mental Disease* **15**:131–142.

Browning W (1908a) Huntington number. *Neurographs* **1**:1–164.

—— (1908b) Rev Charles Oscar Waters MD. I. Biographic sketch. II. Location of his cases. *Neurographs* **1**:137–144.

—— (1908c) Dr Charles Rollin Gorman. I. Personal sketch. II. His relation to the chorea question. *Neurographs* **1**:144–147.

—— (1908d) Irving Whitehall Lyon MD. I. Personal sketch. II. Location of his cases. *Neurographs* **1**:147–149.

Bruyn GW (1968) Huntington's chorea. Historical, clinical and laboratory synopsis. In: *Handbook of Neurology* (eds PJ Vinken and GW Bruyn) Vol. 16, pp. 298–378. Amsterdam: Elsevier.

—— Baro F and Myrianthopoulos NC (1974) *A centennial bibliography of Huntington's chorea 1872–1972.* The Hague: Martinus Nijhoff.

Caro A (1977) A genetic problem in East Anglia. Huntington's chorea. PhD thesis, University of East Anglia.

—— Haines S (1975) The history of Huntington's chorea. *Update* **11**:91–95.

Critchley M (1934) Huntington's chorea and East Anglia. *Journal of State Medicine* **42**:575–587.

—— (1964) Huntington's chorea: historical and geographical considerations. In: *The Black Hole and other essays*, pp. 210–219. London: Pitman Medical.

—— (1973) Great Britain and the early history of Huntington's chorea. In: *Huntington's chorea, 1872–1972* (eds A Barbeau, TN chase, and GW Paulson), pp. 115–122. New York: Raven Press.

—— (1984) The history of Huntington's chorea. *Psychology and Medicine* **14**:725–727.

Curschmann H (1908) Eine neue Chorea-Huntingtonfamilie. *Deutsche Zeitschrift für Nervenheilkunde* **35**:293–305.

Davenport CB (1911) *Heredity in relation to eugenics*. New York: (republished by Arno Press, 1972).

—— and Muncey EB (1916) Huntington's chorea in relation to heredity and eugenics. *Eugenics Record Office Bulletin* **17**:195–222.

Déjerine J (1886) *L'Hérédité dans les maladies du système nerveaux*. Paris: Thèse Aggreg.

De Jong RN (1937) George Huntington and his relationship to the earlier descriptions of chronic hereditary chorea. *Annals in Medical History* **9**:201–210.

Drake DC (1984) The curse of San Luis. *Philadelphia Inquirer* August 26.

Dunglison R (1842) *Practice of medicine*, 1st edn. Philadelphia: Lee and Blanchard.

—— (1848) *Practice of medicine*, 3rd edn. Philadelphia: Lee and Blanchard.

Durbach N and Hayden M (1993) George Huntington: the man behind the eponym. *Journal of Medical Genetics* **30**:406–409.

Eager R and Perdrau JR (1910) Notes on four cases of Huntington's chorea. *Journal of Mental Science* **56**:506–509.

Elliotson J (1832) St Vitus's dance. *Lancet* **i**:162–165.

Fisher ED (1906) A case of Huntington's chorea. *Journal of Nervous and Mental Disease* **33**:781.

Folstein S (1989) *Huntington's disease: A disorder of families*. Baltimore, Johns Hopkins University Press.

Freund CS (1911) Zwei Brüder mit Huntingtonscher Chorea. *Berliner klinische Wochenschrift* **48**:735.

Golgi C (1874) Sulla alterazioni deglia organi centrali nervosi in uno caso di corea gesticulatoria assoziata ad alienazione mentale. *Rivista Clinicale Bologna* **4**:361.

Gorman CR (1848) In: *Practice of medicine*, 3rd edn, Vol. 2 (ed. R Dunglison), p. 218. Philadelphia: Lee and Blanchard.

Harper PS (ed) (1991) *Huntington's disease*, 1st edn. London: W B Saunders.

—— (ed) (1996) *Huntington's disease*, 2nd edn. London: W B Saunders.

—— Perutz MF (ed) (2001) *Glutamine repeats and neurodegenerative diseases: molecular aspects.* Oxford: Oxford University Press.

Hayden MR (1981) *Huntington's chorea*. Berlin: Springer.

Hoffmann J (1888) Uber Chorea chronica progressiva (Huntingtonsche Chorea, Chorea hereditaria). *Virchows Archiv für pathologische Anatomie* **111**:513–548.

Huet E (1889) *De la chorée chronique*. Paris.

Huntington G (1872) On chorea. *Medical and Surgical Reporter* **26**:320–321.

—— (1910) Recollections of Huntington's chorea as I saw it at East Hampton, Long Island, during my boyhood. *Journal of Nervous and Mental Disorders* **37**:255–257.

Huntington's Disease Collaborative Research Group (1993) A novel gene containing a trinucleotide repeat that is expanded and unstable in Huntington's disease chromosomes. *Cell* **72**:971–983.

Husquinet H (1975) Premières descriptions de la chorée de Huntington en France et en Belgique. *Clin Medica* **10**:197–204.

Jelgersma G (1908) Die anatomische Veranderungen bei Paralysis agitans und chronischer Chorea. *Verhandlungen der Gesellschaft deutscher Naturforscher und Arzte* **2**(2):383–388.

Jelliffe SE (1908) A contribution to the history of Huntington's chorea: a preliminary report. *Neurographs* **1**:116–124.

Klein J (1981) *Woodie Guthrie. A life*. London: Faber and Faber.

Kolata G (1984) Closing in on a killer gene. *Discover* March:83–87.

Landouzy LTJ (1873) Mouvements choréiques des membres inférieurs. *Gazette Médical de Paris* **48**:329–330.

Lewis B (1876) A case of chorea associated with mania, terminating fatally by cerebellar apoplexy. *Medical Times and Gazette* **2**:280–282.

Lund JC (1860) *Chorea St Vitus dance in Saetersdalen. Report of health and medicine and medical conditions in Norway in 1860*, p. 137. (Quoted by Ørbeck, 1959.)

Lyon IW (1863) Chronic hereditary chorea. *American Medical Times* **7**:289–290.

MacFaren J (1874) A case of chorea. *Journal of Mental Science* **20**:97–99.

Maltsberger JT (1961) Even unto the twelfth generation—Huntington's chorea. *Journal of the History of Medicine and Allied Sciences* **16**:1–17.

Mapother E (1911) Mental symptoms in association with choreiform disorders. *Journal of Mental Sciences* **57**:646–661.

Mendel G (1865) Versuche über Pflanzenhybriden. *Proceedings of the Natural History Society of Brunn* **4**:3–47. (English translation reprinted 1965. Edinburgh: Oliver and Boyd.)

Meynert T (1877) Discussion to Fritsch. *Psychiatry* Clb **4**:47.

Mitchell JK (1895) Huntington's chorea. *Journal of Nervous and Mental Disorders* **22**:395–397.

Müller LTR (1903) Uber drei Falle von Chorea chronica progressiva (Chorea hereditaria, Chorea Huntington). *Deutsche Zeitschrift für Nervenheilkunde* **23**:315–335.

Negrette A (1963) *Corea de Huntington (Estudio de una sola familia investigade, través de varias generaciones)*. Talleros Graticos. University of Zulia, Maracaibo, Venezuela.

Oppenheim H (1887) Eine seltene Motilitatsneurose (chorea hereditaria?). *Berliner klinische Wochenschrift* **24**:309–310.

Ørbeck AL (1959) An early description of Huntington's chorea. *Medical History* **3**:165–168.

Osler W (1890) Hereditary chorea. *Johns Hopkins Hospital Bulletin* **I**:110.

—— (1892) *The principles and practice of medicine*, pp. 944–945. Edinburgh: Young J. Pentland.

—— (1893) Remarks on the varieties of chronic chorea and a report upon two families of the hereditary form with one autopsy. *Journal of Nervous and Mental Disorders* **18**:97–111.

—— (1894) Case of hereditary chorea. *Johns Hopkins Hospital Bulletin* **5**:119–129.

—— (1904) *On chorea and choreiform affections*, pp. 96–112. Philadelphia: Blakiston and Son.

—— (1908) Historical note on hereditary chorea. *Neurographs* **1**:113–116.

Perutz MF, Johnson T, Suzuki M, and Finch JT (1994) Glutamine repeats as polar zippers: their possible role in inherited neurodegenerative diseases. *Proceedings of the National Academy of Sciences, USA* **9**:3555–3787.

Petit H (1970) La maladie de Huntington. In: C.R. 67e. *Congress de Psychiatre et Neurologie. Langue Franc* (ed. P Warot), pp. 901–1058. Paris: Masson.

Pfeiffer JAF (1913) A contribution to the pathology of chronic progressive chorea. *Brain* **35**:276–292.

Phelps RM (1892) A new consideration of hereditary chorea. *Journal of Nervous and Mental Disorders* **19**:765–776.

Pines M (1984) In the shadow of Huntington's disease. *Science* (May):32–39.

Punnett RC (1908) Mendelian inheritance in man. *Proceedings of the Royal Society of Medicine* **1**:135–168.

Scrimgeour EM (1983) Possible introduction of Huntington's chorea into Pacific Islands by New England whalemen. *American Journal of Medical Genetics* **15**:607–613.

Sinkler W (1892) On hereditary chorea with a report of three additional cases and details of an autopsy. *Medical Record (NY)* **41**:281–285.

Steinert H (1909) Myopathologische Beitrage. 1. Uber das klinische und anatomische Bild des Muskelschwunds der Myotoniker. *Deutsche Zeitschrift für Nervenheilkunde* **37**:58–104.

Steinmann M (1987) In the shadow of Huntington's disease. *Columbia*:14–19.

Stevens DL (1972) The history of Huntington's chorea. *Journal of the Royal College of Physicians* **6**:271–282.

Stier E (1902) Zur pathologischen Anatomie der Huntington'schen Chorea. *Münchener medizinische Wochenschrift* **49**:770.

Thomsen J (1876) Tonische krämpfe in Willkurlich bewUglichen muskeln. *Archiv Psychiatric Nervenheilkunde* **6**:702–718.

Van der Weiden RMF (1989) George Huntington and George Sumner Huntington. A tale of two doctors. *Hist Phil Life Sci* **11**:297–304.

—— (1993) George Huntington: the man behind the eponym. *Journal of Medical Genetics* **30**:1042.

Van Zwanenberg F (1974) The geography of disease in East Anglia. *Journal of the Royal College of Physicians, London* **8**:145–153.

Vessie PR (1932) On the transmission of Huntington's chorea for 300 years. The Bures family group. *Journal of Nervous and Mental Disorders* **76**:553–573.

—— (1939) Hereditary chorea: St Anthony's dance and witchcraft in colonial Connecticut. *Journal of the Connecticut State Medical Society* **3**:596–600.

Waters CO (1842) In: *Practice of medicine*, Vol. 2 (ed. R Dunglison), p. 312. Philadelphia: Lee and Blanchard.

Westphal C (1883) Uber eine dem Bilde der cerebrospinalen grauen Degeneration-ähnliche Erkrankung des zentralen Nervensystems ohne anatomischen Befund, nebst einigen Bemerkungen über paradoxe Kontraktion. *Archiv für Psychiatric und Nervenkrankheiten* **14**:87–96, 767–773.

Wexler A (1995) *Mapping fate*. New York: Times Books.

Winfield JM (1908) A biographical sketch of George Huntington, M.D. *Neurographs* **1**:89–91.

Wood HC (1893) The choreic movements. *Journal of Nervous and Mental Disorders* **4**:241.

2   Clinical neurology of Huntington's disease

Diversity in unity, unity in diversity

Berry Kremer

Introduction

As highlighted in the previous chapter, the core clinical features of Huntington's disease (HD) were outlined by George Huntington in his 1872 paper. For those not familiar with the disease, his description still summarizes most of the clinical characteristics that we recognize today as relevant and important: the hereditary nature of the disease; the prominent movement disorder; the psychiatric and cognitive aspects; the onset usually in adulthood; and its relentlessly progressive natural course. As in George Huntington's time, no cure is yet available.

The hereditary chorea as I shall call it is confined to certain and fortunately few families and has been transmitted to them as an heirloom from generations way back in the dim past. It is spoken of by those in whose veins the seeds of the disease are known to exist with a kind of horror and not at all alluded to except through dire necessity with it being mentioned as 'that disorder'. It is attended generally by all the symptoms of common chorea, only in an aggravated degree, hardly ever manifesting itself until adult or middle life and then coming on gradually but surely, increasing by degrees and often occupying years in its development until the hapless sufferer is but a quivering wreck of his former self. There are three marked peculiarities in this disease: (1) its hereditary nature; (2) a tendency to insanity and suicide; and (3) its manifesting itself as a grave disease only in adult life.
 . . . Its third peculiarity is its coming on, at least as a grave disease, only in adult life. I do not know of a single case that has shown any marked signs of chorea before the age of thirty or forty years, while those who pass the fortieth year without symptoms of the disease are seldom attacked. I have never known a recovery or even an amelioration of symptoms in this form of chorea; when once it begins it clings to the bitter end. No treatment seems to be of any avail, and indeed nowadays its end is so well known to the sufferer and his friends that medical advice is seldom sought. It seems at least to be one of the incurables. [Huntington 1872]

However, although this suggests a fairly straightforward and well recognizable clinical presentation, over the past century we have come to appreciate the wide spectrum of signs and symptoms that the disorder may present. The identification of the HD gene and its pathogenic mutation (Huntington's Disease Collaborative Research Group 1993), in particular, has allowed clinicians to recognize more accurately the multiple manifestations of the disease. Due to molecular diagnostics, a diagnosis of HD is no longer based on characteristic clinical features with ultimate neuropathological confirmation, but a laboratory-based definite diagnosis can be made during life. From a clinical point of view, one of the most interesting aspects of the genotype–phenotype relationship in HD is to understand how what is apparently one single type of mutation can lead to such a remarkable variety in clinical phenotypic appearances. Underlying this phenotypic variation must be a specific progressive brain deterioration affecting the structure and architecture of the brain that can be to some extent variable and is ultimately different in each individual.

The best known determinant of clinical variability is the length of the pathological CAG repeat that causes the disease. Numerous groups have confirmed the initial observation that the length of the CAG repeat explains 50–70 per cent of statistical variance in onset age (Andrew *et al.* 1993; Snell *et al.* 1993; Duyao *et al.* 1993). Details will be given in Chapter 5. Repeat length, however, is not indicative of any other clinical phenotype, as there is no independent association between any particular clinical feature of the illness and the number of repeats. These topics are discussed in detail in Chapter 5.

It has been suggested that additional genetic factors play a role in age of onset determination and in how the disease presents. None have yet been identified unambiguously. One early publication suggested the length of the CAG repeat on the non-HD chromosome as a co-determinant, particularly in individuals who inherited this chromosome from their fathers (Snell *et al.* 1993). This finding has not been replicated. Genotype variation in the kainate GluR6 receptor has been reported as an additional determinant of onset age variation explaining part of the residual variance (Rubinsztein *et al.* 1997; MacDonald *et al.* 1999).

A clinical observation that supports the notion of additional disease phenotype modifier genes is the impression that disease manifestations tend to look similar and run a similar course in affected family members. Within-family variability seems smaller than between-family variability. This observation has been confirmed for psychosis as a manifestation of the disease in some families but it has never been formally tested with respect to other clinical features (Tsuang *et al.* 2000).

As the disease progresses, signs and symptoms change—thus, the duration of the disease is an additional important factor in the clinical presentation. This variation over time will be one of the themes of this chapter.

Onset and early disease

A broad consensus exists among clinicians that a clinical diagnosis of HD can only be made with certainty in the presence of the specific motor disorder. Thus, fixing the onset of the motor disorder in this way yields a more or less reproducible way to conduct, for example, onset age surveys or genotype–phenotype correlation studies. But it should be realized that the onset of the motor abnormalities is not a sensitive measure of disease onset. Prior to these manifestations mood disorder and mild cognitive problems have often already appeared, accompanied or followed by mild motor abnormalities that only gradually evolve into a full blown recognizable extrapyramidal syndrome.

HD may start at any age. The youngest patient ever described had an age of onset of 2 years, while some patients have been noted to develop first signs of the disease in their mid-80s (Huntington's Disease Collaborative Research Group 1993; Hayden 1981; Osborne *et al.* 1982). Even within families, remarkable differences in disease onset between individuals have been observed. Although in a majority of families the onset of affected individuals tended to be similar, many individual families were observed in whom the disease occurred earlier in successive generations, a phenomenon called anticipation (Höweler *et al.* 1989). We now know that the single most important determinant of both onset age and of anticipation is the length of the pathological CAG repeat (see Chapter 5).

It used to be stated that the age at which the first symptoms of HD occur has a normal distribution with a mean of around 40 and a standard deviation of approximately 10 years (Hayden 1981). However, three factors have been raised more recently that modify this statement.

The first is that the onset age distribution does not follow a normal distribution (in a statistical sense) and so it is more useful to assess different measures of dispersion, such as median age and percentiles. The second factor is the problem of truncated intervals of observation. By straightforward observation of onset age in a population, those who are still alive but will develop the disease later in life do not count towards the observed onset age distribution. This will bias the results of such a study towards younger onset ages. When, for example, in the study of Newcombe (1981) sampling was limited to persons born before 1909, the mean age of onset was 48.4 years. A successive decrease in the mean age of onset occurred as the observation interval moved closer to the current time of analysis. Similarly, in the study of Adams *et al.* (1988) the mean age of onset in the total sample of 611 patients was 38.6 years. However, restricting the analysis to persons born in 1920 resulted in a mean age at onset of 43.7 years. Such corrected studies consistently show that the mean age of onset is between 43 and 48 years of age. However, in a series of 800 deceased Dutch patients, a much higher mean onset age, of 55.8 years (standard deviation (S.D.), 13.5 years) was observed (Roos *et al.* 1993).

Since the advent of DNA diagnostics a third factor has become apparent: the number of individuals being diagnosed with late-onset HD (past age 60) has risen, as a family history is no longer required for diagnosis (McCusker *et al.* 2000a). Modelling the distribution of the expanded HD gene and its mutational flow indeed suggests underascertainment of small expanded repeats and the consequent underdiagnosis of late-onset cases (Falush *et al.* 2000). No epidemiological study that addresses all these considerations has been published, so the true distribution of age at onset is not yet known. But we probably should think of HD as a disorder with a median onset age in the late forties or early fifties and a large variation in age of onset.

The most comprehensive way of assessing the early signs and symptoms of HD is to follow a cohort for an extended period of time. The longitudinal study of the Venezuelan kindred is the only published large-scale follow-up study to date (Penney *et al.* 1990). It was conducted prior to the identification of the gene, but its conclusions are still valid. It demonstrated that patients pass through a zone of onset, which represents a transitional state from the normal presymptomatic phase to the time at which the diagnosis can be clearly made on neurological examination. This zone of onset is frequently accompanied by changes in metabolic rates of glucose in the caudate as seen on positron emission tomography (PET) (Hayden *et al.* 1987; Grafton *et al.* 1990). Currently ongoing longitudinal follow-up studies of identified presymptomatic gene-carriers will provide the best and most unbiased assessment of the earliest phases of the disease, that is, the transition from truly asymptomatic to very mildly affected.

There is no single presenting sign or symptom in HD. In the earliest phases, there is an insidious and slow deterioration of intellectual functions as well as mild personality change. The clear appearance of extrapyramidal signs such as chorea, hypokinesia, rigidity, or dystonia marks a phase in the disease progression, not the beginning of disease. Prior to these signs, most individuals will display minor motor abnormalities (Penney *et al.* 1990). These include general restlessness, abnormal eye movements or impaired optokinetic nystagmus, hyperreflexia, impaired finger tapping or rapid alternating hand movements, and excessive and inappropriate movements of the fingers, hands, or toes during emotional stress, as well as mild dysarthria. Minor motor abnormalities usually precede the obvious signs of extrapyramidal dysfunction by at least 3 years. Persons with a completely normal neurological examination have a 3 per cent chance of being diagnosed within the next 3 years (Penney *et al.* 1990).

While data from longitudinal studies are still lacking, our knowledge about early disease comes from two other sources. Retrospective assessment of disease progression can be gained through questionnaires filled out by affected individuals already several years into the disease and by their family members. This has revealed that involuntary movements are among the earliest symptoms experienced and that, somewhat later, mental and emotional symptoms, including sadness, depression, irritability, and episodes of verbal and physical abuse, can develop (Kirkwood *et al.* 2001). These mental and emotional symptoms are discussed at length in the next chapter. Such results, however, are subject to recall bias of the enrolled persons, which may be an important caveat in light of the recent discovery of impairment of disease awareness in HD patients (Snowden *et al.* 1998). In samples of patients who entered predictive testing programmes, and thus still considered themselves free of disease, many abnormalities have been found upon neurological testing (see also Chapter 7). In one series of 171 tested so-called presymptomatic carriers (too little affected to warrant a diagnosis), individuals performed significantly worse than non-carriers on neuropsychological tests such as the digit symbol, picture arrangement, and arithmetic. Mild impairment was noticed on button tapping, auditory reaction time, visual reaction time with decision, and various movement time paradigms (Kirkwood *et al.* 2000). Although in none of the carriers could a formal diagnosis of HD be made on clinical examination, some of them had possible or definite abnormality of oculomotor function, chorea, muscle stretch reflexes, gait and stance, and rapid alternating movements. Such persons probably should be considered to have reached the transitional phase, rather than being truly asymptomatic. Discussing the clinical concerns regarding their true status with such persons should be an essential element of the pre- and post-predictive test-counselling process. This may be all the more urgent as the number of so-called presymptomatic individuals with mild motor abnormalities may be as high as 61 per cent (McCusker *et al.* 2000b). A point of concern, however, is that even trained neurological examiners may overinterpret and overdiagnose mild motor abnormalities. One study found poor interobserver agreement in assessing the presence of these signs (De Boo *et al.* 1998).

Various groups have addressed the issue as to whether so-called asymptomatic gene carriers do in fact display subtle cognitive defects. It has been found that cognitive defects may precede the recognizable motor abnormalities by years. Individuals with an expanded CAG repeat have been identified who perform poorly on tests of executive functions and memory tasks, and their performance is related to the size of their CAG expansion (Campodonico *et al.* 1996). These individuals had a complete absence of motor or psychiatric signs. Other groups who performed neuropsychological assessment of presymptomatic gene carriers found abnormalities on specific tests, such as attentional set shifting and semantic verbal fluency (Lawrence *et al.* 1998), or other executive functions and verbal learning (Hahn-Barma *et al.* 1998). It should be realized, however, that the subjects in such studies do not represent an unbiased, randomly drawn, representative sample of gene carriers. It is important to realize, therefore, that many individuals with expanded repeats may perform just as well or better than matched controls. It is only when an individual is close to the estimated age of onset, as predicted by CAG repeat length (Brinkman *et al.* 1997), that minor deficits in selected cognitive domains can become apparent (Campodonico *et al.* 1996). These findings illustrate two issues: individual gene carriers probably pass through a truly asymptomatic phase, and HD may start with nonspecific cognitive abnormalities, rather than the motor abnormalities that allow a definite diagnosis. Thirdly, it is important to realize that only adequate longitudinal studies of an unbiased sample of gene carriers will reveal the true evolution of the early disease.

Mid-course disease: the classic phenotype

This is the best known manifestation of HD and the form to which George Huntington referred. This phase is visibly dominated by motor abnormalities—both extrapyramidal signs and a more general but nonspecific impairment of skilled movements, such as gait, speech, swallowing, and other essential motor skills.

Extrapyramidal motor abnormalities

Chorea is the major motor sign of the disease, hence the old name 'Huntington's chorea'. Care should be taken to avoid the word 'chorea' as a *pars pro toto* for the disease. The term will be used purely as a phenomenological description of a distinct type of involuntary motor action. One definition of chorea is: 'A state of excessive, spontaneous movements, irregularly timed, randomly distributed and abrupt. Severity may vary from restlessness with mild, intermittent exaggeration of gesture and expression, fidgeting movements of the hands, unstable, dance-like gait to a continuous flow of disabling, violent movements' (Barbeau *et al.* 1981). Choreic movements are continuously present during waking hours, cannot be voluntarily suppressed by the patient, and worsen during stress. Although the pattern of the movements may differ between affected patients, they occur in individual patients in a stereotyped manner. Chorea of the face is common and presents as pouting of the lips, irregular grimacing, twitching of the cheeks, and alternate lifting of the eyebrows and frowning (Fig. 2.1). The neck is often involved, causing forward or backward bending of the head, or rotation. Chorea of the trunk moves the body in different directions. Breathing is often irregular, although patients never complain of breathlessness. In the limbs, there is frequent flexion and extension of the fingers. The legs may be alternately crossed and uncrossed and the toes flexed and extended. Patients who are overtly choreic, particularly early in the disease, tend to have decreased muscle tone, in contrast to those who develop pronounced chorea farther into the disease. Figure 2.2 shows a woman with a dance-like quality of her gait.

Chorea is a feature of HD in over 90 per cent of patients, increasing during the first phase (~10 years) of the patients' illness. A characteristic of true chorea is a decrease in muscle tone. However, hypertonic rigidity and dystonia are often found in conjunction with chorea, particularly in patients with a somewhat longer disease duration. As the disease advances, chorea will tend to disappear, to be replaced by the more disabling movement disorders mentioned below (Bruyn 1968; Hayden 1981; Young *et al.* 1986). Chorea is seen less frequently in patients with juvenile onset (Hayden 1981; Young *et al.* 1986) and may rarely be absent in adult-onset cases (Folstein 1989). The severity and extent of chorea may vary from barely perceptible to the observer and only localized in the distal extremities, to gross, exhausting, and severely disabling for the patient. Ballismus, the most severe form of chorea, is the ultimate level of severity of this disorder (see Fig. 2.3). Interestingly, mild and intermittent choreic movements seem not be noticed by many patients, while lay people tend to describe them as 'nervousness'.

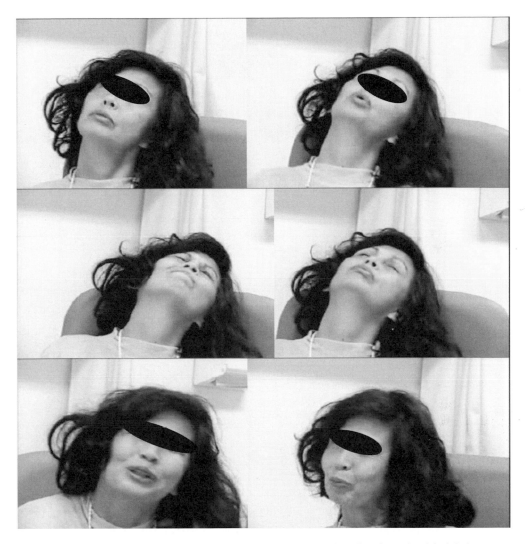

Fig. 2.1 Patient with classical HD, age 52. Dystonia of the neck and orobuccal and facial chorea.

Bradykinesia (or slow movements) and *rigidity*, best known as the core features of parkinsonism, are infrequent in the early phases of adult-onset Huntington disease. However, they appear gradually and often dominate the final stages of the illness in which the patient will become severely rigid and grossly akinetic (Bruyn 1968; Young *et al.* 1986; Penney *et al.* 1990). Early in the illness, bradykinesia alone may contribute to impairment in voluntary motor performance (Thompson *et al.* 1988). Some patients display a significant decrease in overall daytime motor activity, suggestive of hypokinesia, or paucity of movements (Van Vugt *et al.* 1996). A minority of adult patients—about 10 per cent—will start with rigidity and severe hypokinesia, which has been described as the Westphal variant of the disease

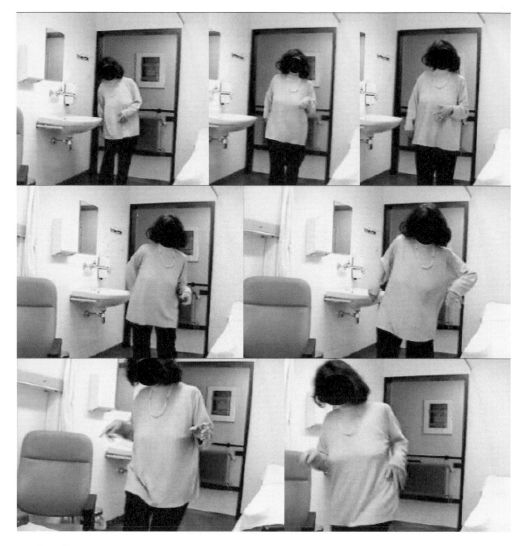

Fig. 2.2 Same patient as in Fig. 2.1. Dance-like choreatic gait while walking towards the camera.

(Westphal 1883; Bittenbender and Quadfasel 1962; Louis *et al*. 2000). In both juvenile and adult rigid cases a coarse resting tremor, distinct from a parkinsonian tremor, may complement the clinical picture (Bittenbender and Quadfasel 1962; Folstein 1989). The use of neuroleptic drugs, intended to suppress choreic movements, may aggravate the existing bradykinesia and rigidity.

Dystonia, characterized by slow abnormal movements and abnormal posturing with increased muscle tone, is again infrequent in the early symptomatic period but worsens and becomes a prominent feature towards the later stages of the illness (Bittenbender and Quadfasel 1962; Young *et al*. 1986). Dystonia may be encountered in chorea-predominant patients where it is

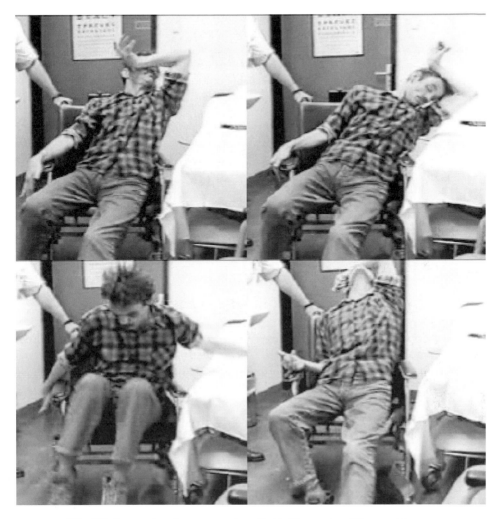

Fig. 2.3 Severe choreic movements, called ballismus, in a 27-year-old man.

primarily seen as abnormal posturing of extremities and the head within the context of the choreic movements. In a recent study of patients who attended an HD specialty clinic, the prevalence of dystonia of any severity was found to be 95 per cent, while in seven of 42 patients (17 per cent) the dystonia was severe and constant. Types of dystonia included internal shoulder rotation, sustained fist clenching, excessive knee flexion, and foot inversion. Disease duration and the taking of antidopaminergic drugs were associated with the severity of the dystonia. It was noted that the abnormal movements and postures were not typical of idiopathic torsion dystonia, and not bothersome to most patients (Louis *et al.* 1999). From a clinical point of view, it is important to realize that it may be hard to differentiate whether an individual movement or a fragment of a movement should be considered dystonic or choreic. These movement disorders easily merge into one another. Therefore it is probably best to assess whether a more prolonged period of involuntary movements represents 'chorea' or 'dystonia'.

Dystonia is particularly closely related to the so-called rigid forms of the disease, as seen in juvenile-onset patients, in patients with the adult-onset rigid Westphal variant, and in patients with late-stage disease. The dystonia-predominant adult-onset form of the disease, which was recently reported to constitute 11.8 per cent of an adult population seen at an HD specialty clinic, may, in fact, be indistinguishable from what is traditionally called the Westphal variant (Louis *et al.* 2000). Perhaps it is time to start talking about the rigid-dystonic form of the disease with hypertonia versus the choreic form of the disease with hypotonia. The first form then would represent a more severe motor abnormality and a more severe form of disease than the second manifestation.

These are by far the most common extrapyramidal motor abnormalities in HD and the most specific signs of the disease, which in most clinical situations will prove reliable disease indicators. Other extrapyramidal movement disorders such as tourettism (Angelini *et al.* 1998), tremor, and myoclonus (Vogel *et al.* 1981; Carella *et al.* 1993) have been reported far less frequently. It may be that their presence and recognition present diagnostic problems.

Other motor abnormalities

Oculomotor disturbances are among the earliest signs and are present in the vast majority of affected patients (Oepen *et al.* 1981; Beenen *et al.* 1986; Lasker and Zee 1997). Saccades display the earliest abnormalities, with inability to suppress reflexive glances to suddenly appearing novel stimuli, and delayed initiation of voluntary saccades (Lasker and Zee 1997). Later in the disease, slowing of saccades may be seen in up to 75 per cent of symptomatic individuals, especially in early-onset cases, more particularly affecting vertical rather than horizontal movements (Oepen *et al.* 1981; Beenen *et al.* 1986; Lasker *et al.* 1988; Lasker and Zee 1997). Impaired pursuit with saccadic intrusions, impairment of gaze fixation due to distractability, slowing of optokinetic nystagmus, and inability to suppress blinking during saccades may also occur (Oepen *et al.* 1981; Beenen *et al.* 1986; Penney *et al.* 1990; Tian *et al.* 1991; Lasker and Zee 1997). Conjugate gaze disturbances may be prominent in rigid cases, which are manifested by the 'bird head phenomenon'. On rapid lateral gaze affected people tend to rotate the head in an exaggerated manner, in order to compensate for the slowness of their saccades (Beenen *et al.* 1986). It is known that antichoreic medication (neuroleptics) influences motor performance in HD patients, but these drugs do not seem to slow or alter saccades (Dursun *et al.* 2000).

A nonspecific but early sign is impairment of *voluntary motor function* (Folstein *et al.* 1983; Hefter *et al.* 1987; Thompson *et al.* 1988). Patients and their families describe clumsiness in common daily activities. Clear abnormalities of rapid alternating movements may already be observed in the transitional phase. Disturbances in motor speed, fine motor control, and gait correlate with disease progression and appear to be better measures of duration of illness than chorea (Folstein *et al.* 1983). Clumsiness may increase with deterioration of functional capacity (Young *et al.* 1986). The true nature of this nonspecific motor impairment is as yet unknown, as chorea alone is not sufficient to impair dexterity. For example, patients with benign hereditary chorea do not suffer from clumsiness. Mechanisms proposed include bradykinesia and impaired internal motor cueing (Thompson *et al.* 1988; Phillips *et al.* 1996;

Curra *et al.* 2000), impairment in constructing and refining internal representations of movement (Georgiou *et al.* 1997), or a reduced ability to process relevant tactile afferent input (Schwarz *et al.* 2001).

Hyperactive reflexes occur early in up to 90 per cent of patients, while clonus and extensor plantar responses occur late and are less frequent (Hayden 1981; Young *et al.* 1986). Again, these latter phenomena are predominant in juvenile and advanced adult cases (Young *et al.* 1986). Frontal release reflexes like snouting, sucking, or grasping typically accompany significant cognitive decline.

Gait disturbances ultimately result in severe disability. Subtle changes in gait may be observed early in the illness, including difficulty with tandem walking, sudden stopping on command, and turning (Koller and Trimble 1985). With more advanced disease walking difficulties are more pronounced. As a consequence, patients experience frequent falls with significant associated morbidity, and often ultimate confinement to a wheelchair. Gait disturbances exist, at least in part, independently from chorea, as neuroleptic treatment, which suppresses choreic movements, does not improve the gait disturbance (Koller and Trimble 1985).

Most patients display *speech abnormalities*, which are present early in the illness (Hayden 1981; Young *et al.* 1986; Podoll *et al.* 1988; Coleman *et al.* 1990). Initially mild disturbance of clarity appears, which becomes aggravated by changes in rate and rhythm of speech as the disease progresses. *Dysphagia*, or swallowing impairment, generally occurs at a later stage in the illness. Initially, this may primarily affect fluid intake but later will also affect intake of solids. Choking with aspiration secondary to dysphagia is a common cause of morbidity.

Cognitive disturbances and psychiatric problems

These are so prominent in the clinical symptomatology of the disease and so complex that they are dealt with separately in the next chapter.

Advanced-stage disease and causes of death

Patients do not die of HD: they die of causes associated with the disease. As a result of the inexorable progression of the disease, disability increases up to the point at which patients are no longer able to support themselves. The same neurological abnormalities that ultimately make independent living and self-support impossible—severe motor impairment and severe cognitive slowing—also render patients susceptible to systemic problems that may ultimately prove fatal. The characteristics of patients in this final stage of the diseases have only rarely been described systematically (Nance and Sanders 1996), but the scant literature may be complemented by clinical experience, and further discussion of the clinical management of this stage of the disease is given in Chapter 15.

Clinical neurology of advanced-stage disease

The final years of most HD patients are dominated by loss of independence, severe restrictions in functioning, and dependence upon others for activities of daily living. During this phase most patients live in nursing homes.

From a clinical neurologist's perspective, advanced-stage disease is dominated by hypokinesia, bradykinesia, rigidity, and dystonia, although choreic movements are often still visible, particularly in the orobuccal region or in the distal extremities. Speech is often severely dysarthric and anarthria or mutism may impair communication to a great extent. Swallowing is equally impaired, which requires very careful assistance by the nursing staff during meals, or, alternatively, feeding through a nasogastric tube or a percutaneous endoscopic gastrostomy (PEG) tube. Examination of eye movements reveals severe slowing of initiation and execution of saccades, and patients tend to display a characteristic 'bird's head' phenomenon. Attempts at lateral gaze result in an exaggerated head turn towards the side of interest, in order to assist and speed up the slowed saccades. The hypokinesia and bradykinesia result in loss of manual dexterity. Patients lose independent gait and spend their days in a chair, a wheelchair, or bed. The increase in muscle tone may result in secondary joint contractures, while immobility increases the risk of pressure sores. Reflexes tend to be brisk, but hyporeflexia is also often seen. Sometimes a combination of muscle hypertonia and increased tendon reflexes suggests upper motor neurone dysfunction. In patients in whom weight loss is prominent, it may be hard to judge whether lower motor neurone pathology with muscle atrophy is present, or just plain malnourishment. One observation, which has never been formally confirmed, is that people with end-stage HD tend to smoke excessively—many patients have a characteristic yellow-brown tarring of the first three fingers.

Upon cognitive examination severe slowing of all cognitive processes ('bradyphrenia') is apparent. Timed tasks are often not executable but, if given enough time, the patient may be able to perform quite well on memory tasks such as a three-word test or retrieval of recent events. Perseverative thinking and utterances also interfere with cognitive tasks. It may be hard to judge whether a patient is depressed. Agitation, on the other hand, may cause nursing problems.

Although the reasons for referral to a nursing home or a long-term care facility may be different in different cultures and health care systems, referral probably occurs when psychiatric problems become too much of a burden, or when the physical strain of nursing becomes unbearable for the care-givers. The majority of patients are still ambulatory on admission but nearly all have lost this basic form of independence by the end of their lives (Nance and Sanders 1996). The combination of often still relatively young patients, with severe psychiatric problems, who require major nursing care, presents quite a burden to many general nursing home facilities or long-term care psychiatric hospitals. As a solution to this problem, specialized long-term care units, exclusively devoted to HD patients, have been established in a number of countries.

The vast majority of patients in nursing homes use psychotropic medication: either benzodiazepine sedatives, antidepressants, or neuroleptics prescribed as sedatives or antichoreic drugs. This latter group of drugs, in particular, is associated with adverse effects such as increased rigidity, balance, and gait problems, as well as swallowing difficulties. We have also observed several cases of medication-induced hyperthermic syndromes (neuroleptic malignant syndrome, serotoninergic syndrome), a complication that has been reported only sparsely in the literature but that may be more common in advanced-stage HD patients than most clinicians realize (Burke *et al.* 1981; Mateo *et al.* 1992; Ossemann *et al.* 1996).

Systemic abnormalities in advanced-stage disease

Weight loss and striking emaciation are features of late-stage HD (Bruyn 1968). Clinical follow-up and anthropometric studies, with dietary assessment, all show that the vast majority of HD patients lose weight in the course of the disease (Sanberg *et al.* 1981; Farrer and Yu 1985; Morales *et al.* 1989). This weight loss may occur in conjunction with adequate dietary intake or even increased carbohydrate intake (Sanberg *et al.* 1981; Farrer and Yu 1985; Morales *et al.* 1989). Weight loss is most prominent during the later stages of the disease, but weight gain may be seen even in late-stage disease patients, probably as a result of improved attention to intake (Nance and Sanders 1996; Kirkwood *et al.* 2001). Swallowing difficulties must be a major cause of weight loss, and a recent study showed that, in mild to moderately affected HD patients, sedentary energy expenditure is higher than in controls in proportion to the severity of the movement disorder. Total free-living energy expenditure is not higher, however, because patients with HD appear to engage in less voluntary physical activity (Pratley *et al.* 2000). Intriguingly, a relationship has been found between weight at initial examination and rate of progress of the disease (Myers *et al.* 1991).

Sleep is often disturbed in advanced disease. Polysomnographic studies have revealed reversal of the normal day–night sleep pattern, increased sleep onset latency, reduced sleep efficiency, frequent nocturnal awakenings with more time spent awake, and reduced rapid eye movement (REM) and slow-wave sleep (Hansotia *et al.* 1985; Wiegand *et al.* 1991; Silvestri *et al.* 1995). In early disease, sleep is essentially normal (Hansotia *et al.* 1985; Bollen *et al.* 1988; Emser *et al.* 1988). Chorea was said to disappear during sleep, but many partners of patients will attest to the fact that nocturnal involuntary movements do occur. Polysomnographic studies have definitely supported this observation, but it should be noted that the movements seem to occur most often during lighter sleep stages, or during awakening (Fish *et al.* 1991; Silvestri *et al.* 1995).

Approximately 20 per cent of all patients are *incontinent* of urine and faeces in the terminal phases of the illness, while in early symptomatic persons incontinence rarely occurs (Hayden 1981). In incontinent patients with frequency, urgency, and nocturia, detrusor hyperreflexia without sphincter dyssynergia is apparent. Choreatic contractions have been electromyographically recorded from perineal musculature in affected patients (Wheeler *et al.* 1985).

Probably no special precautions have to be taken when HD patients have to undergo *anaesthesia* for surgical procedures. It has been suggested that patients are abnormally sensitive to barbiturate anaesthesia and may exhibit prolonged apnoea, but these reports have been disputed (Davies 1966; Gualandi and Bonfanti 1968; Farina and Rauscher 1977; Browne and Cross 1981; Blanloeil *et al.* 1982; Browne 1982). Weight loss and poor general condition may render patients susceptible to adverse effects of anaesthesia, while regurgitation and an increased likelihood of pulmonary aspiration require increased postoperative surveillance, particularly in those with severe motor impairment, such as juvenile patients (Gupta and Leng 2000).

Age at death and causes of death

Studies of death certificates have confirmed the experience of every clinician who cares for HD patients. Pneumonia, choking, nutritional deficiencies, and chronic skin ulcers as causes of death occur significantly more often in patients than in controls (Lanska *et al.* 1988a). The leading causes of death in persons with HD were pneumonia (33 per cent) and heart disease (24 per cent), this latter cause being somewhat surprising and perhaps the result of inadequate reporting (Haines and Conneally 1986; Lanska *et al.* 1988a). Pneumonia occurs five times more commonly in HD than in controls and is likely to be secondary to the significant dysphagia, which results in choking and aspiration pneumonia.

HD is one of the conditions associated with an increased risk of suicide (Harris and Barraclough 1994). Estimated suicide rates vary from 1 to 7.3 per cent but suicide is likely to be underreported (Farrer 1986; Lanska *et al.* 1988b; Di Maio *et al.* 1993). The number of suicide attempts in symptomatic patients may greatly exceed this rate; up to 27.6 per cent of patients have been reported to attempt suicide at least once (Farrer 1986). If one assumes death due to suicide in all cases in which accidental poisonings and violence were reported, this would account for approximately 8 per cent of deaths (Lanska *et al.* 1988b). Suicide may cluster in some families (Di Maio *et al.* 1993).

Mortality is higher in HD patients than in age-matched controls. A study of 10 HD families that collected mortality data from 1800 onwards and encompassed 257 gene carriers and 474 at-risk individuals (or 25 013 person-years) found a standardized yearly mortality ratio of 1.5, with excess mortality particularly in the age range of 40 to 70 years (Hille *et al.* 1999). These numbers are in good agreement with death certificate surveys (Lanska *et al.* 1988b).

It is hard to pinpoint a distribution of age of death in HD patients. In an individual the age of death depends on the age at onset of the disease. In fact, like age at onset, age at death correlates significantly with CAG size (Andrew *et al.* 1993; Sieradzan *et al.* 1997). Surveys of the mean ages of death in a population have been subject to the same biases of ascertainment as age of onset assessment, that is, the assessment of a recent cohort would not include those with late onset or who are longer survivors. Thus, older studies tended to underestimate the mean age of death, for example, 51.4 years in a 1964 study from Australia (Brothers 1964). Data from the US National Center for Health Statistics for the period 1971–78, based on 3058 death certificates, yielded a mean age of death of 56.5 years (Lanska *et al.* 1988b). A mean age of death in Tasmania of 62.9 years was consistent with the finding of mean age at onset of 48.3 years in that region (Pridmore 1990a,b). In all instances those studies with lower ages of death have had lower ages of onset suggesting that this does not reflect variation in duration of the disease.

Duration of HD and rate of progression

The median duration of HD, that is, the difference between age at onset and age of death, is similar in various modern studies and is about 15 to 20 years with no differences between the sexes (Roos *et al.* 1993; Foroud *et al.* 1999). For example, in a retrospective study of a cohort of 1106 patients a median disease duration of 16.2 years (range 2–45 years) was found. Almost 20 per cent of the patients survived the onset of choreatic movements for more than 23 years (Roos *et al.* 1993). In another cohort of 2494 affected persons the median duration was 21.4 years (range 1.2 to 40.8 years; Foroud *et al.* 1999). From a clinical point of view the main lesson from these studies would be that there are marked individual variations, with disease course extending up to as much as 45 years from time of onset. It would appear that, in some families, HD follows a milder course with longer survival.

The factors that are associated with longer survival and disease progression in families are not yet clear, but again CAG size may play a role. Age at death was found to be significantly correlated to CAG size (Andrew *et al.* 1993), but this reflected earlier death in those with earlier onset. It is not clear whether earlier onset is also associated with more rapid disease progression as measured in terms of survival time or disease duration. Although it has been claimed that there is no relation between disease duration and onset age (Roos *et al.* 1993), the relation graph may in fact be bell-shaped, with those with early- and those with late-onset disease having shorter disease duration (Foroud *et al.* 1999). This is discussed further in Chapter 5.

Whether disease progression as measured by functional deterioration is determined by CAG size is similarly under debate (see Chapter 5). In a 2-year longitudinal study, patients with repeat sizes of 37 to 46 were found to deteriorate less rapidly on a quantified neurological examination score, daily living assessment, and a cognitive measurement than those with CAG repeat sizes of 47 and over (Brandt *et al.* 1996). Whether this more rapid deterioration also leads to earlier death is unclear. But other authors using different measurements of decline were unable to observe such a correlation (Ashizawa *et al.* 1994; Claes *et al.* 1995). For example, in a cohort of 50 patients who were prospectively followed for at least a few years, the major index of disease progression, a total functional capacity scale, did not reveal a relationship between functional deterioration and CAG repeat size (Kieburtz *et al.* 1994). In a 30-month duration drug study, again no correlation between CAG size and functional deterioration was found (Kremer *et al.* 1999). Apparently, disease progression over relatively brief follow-up periods of a few years cannot be easily related to CAG size.

Assessment of neurological and functional decline

Although clinical deterioration may be well documented in a qualitative way in the patient's file, long-term follow-up studies and the advent of experimental therapeutics have necessitated a more quantitative description of disease progression. Early attempts at measuring progression focused upon the severity of the motor disorder, but investigators soon turned to the assessment of functional status as a relevant, reliable, and reproducible indicator of disease progression (Shoulson and Fahn 1979; Myers *et al.* 1985; Bylsma *et al.* 1993). The Total Functional Capacity (TFC) scale introduced by Shoulson and Fahn in 1979 (Shoulson and Fahn 1979; Shoulson 1981) has been extensively used. This rating scale with a range from 0 (minimal) to 13 (maximal) is simple to score, more or less linear in its downward slope over the early and mid stages of the disease, and correlates strongly with various other clinical parameters of disease progression (Young *et al.* 1986; Penney *et al.* 1990; Shoulson *et al.* 1989; Kremer *et al.* 1999). The scale is summarized in Table 2.1. During early and mid-disease stages the average annual deterioration is about 0.6 to 0.7 points per year, irrespective of age at onset of HD, body weight, gender of affected parent, or history of neuroleptic use (Feigin *et al.* 1995; Marder *et al.* 2000). However, decline is fastest in the early stages, while it slows down, in terms of TFC score, in later disease stages (Marder *et al.* 2000). This phenomenon represents a floor effect of the scale, rather than a true biological correlate.

Which factors determine deterioration of functional capacity as measured by such scales? The most important one is cognitive deterioration, while depression may also play an important role (Mayeux *et al.* 1986). In contrast, chorea, unless very severe, does not appear to constitute a major impairment to normal function. Neuroleptic drugs that suppress choreic movements do not improve the functional ratings and may in fact even worsen them (Shoulson 1981). Furthermore, during advanced stages, a diminished severity of choreatic

Table 2.1 Total functional capacity (TFC) scale* (Shoulson and Fahn 1979)

Domain	Level of functioning	Score
Occupation	Normal	3
	Reduced capacity for usual job	2
	Marginal work only	1
	Unable	0
Finances	Normal	3
	Slight assistance	2
	Major assistance	1
	Unable	0
Domestic chores	Normal	2
	Impaired	1
	Unable	0
Activities of daily living	Normal	3
	Minimal impairment	2
	Gross tasks only	1
	Total care	0
Care level	Home	2
	Home with chronic care	1
	Full-time skilled nursing	0

*The appropriate level of functioning on each of the five individual domains is scored and, by adding the numbers obtained, a functional capacity score that may range from 0 to 13 can be generated.

movements without improvement of function, is apparent. These findings caution against the liberal use of neuroleptic medication in the later stages of illness.

Apart from quantitative functional capacity assessments, pure motor assessment scales specifically developed for HD are available, for example, the Quantified Neurological Examination, first described in 1983 (Folstein *et al.* 1983). This rating instrument has provided the model for the motor section of the Unified Huntington's Disease Rating Scale (UHDRS; see below) and has been supplanted by its successor in studies of the effects of particular drugs on the motor manifestations of the disease.

For the assessment of the cognitive and psychiatric effects of the disease no HD-specific instruments have ever been developed. Existing psychometric and psychiatric questionnaires have always been used in explorative and interventional studies, depending on the interests and inclinations of the neurologist, (neuro)psychologist, or psychiatrist who planned the study.

In order to provide a comprehensive assessment of motor performance, cognitive functioning, behavioural and psychiatric problems, and functional status of an individual, the UHDRS was developed by the US-based Huntington Study Group in 1994 (Huntington Study Group 1996). This UHDRS has quickly become the standard assessment instrument for drug studies aimed at ameliorating disease progression. Scores on the motor, cognitive, and functional subscales show high correlations, while, interestingly, the behavioural/psychiatric domain is not predictable from the other scores (Huntington Study Group 1996). In assessing the UHDRS, it should be borne in mind that it was never intended to provide an all-encompassing description of every possible manifestation of HD but rather a comprehensive, rapid, and efficient survey that is highly sensitive to disease progression over relatively brief periods of time, for example, 1 year. Its main intended use was as an instrument suitable for quantifying progression in intervention studies.

Clinical variants

In genetic and neurological diseases the existence of clinical variants often points towards multiple types of mutation or to differences in underlying disease pathophysiology. In contrast, HD is a truly genetically homogeneous disease in which the only variation between the disease alleles in the population is a quantitative one, that is, the length of the CAG repeat. Thus, although clinical subtypes different from the classical choreic variant have been extensively described and discussed in the literature, these subtypes should be regarded as representing extremes of the different dimensions of the disease rather than as qualitatively separate entities. Studying the genotypes of these patients has partially explained why and how the clinical subtypes occur. For example, juvenile cases can now be characterized as representing patients with the longest CAG repeats (Telenius *et al.* 1993), while late-onset cases typically represent relatively short expanded repeats. However, as patients with such nonclassical clinical features may present diagnostic problems for nonspecialists, a separate description of these phenotypes seems warranted. Moreover, in discussing the problems and prognosis of their illness with patients and their care-givers, variant types of the disease may require management decisions that differ from those that are generally appropriate for HD patients.

From a scientific perspective, the recognition and study of variant clinical phenotypes sheds light on how the length of the pathognomonic CAG repeat is related to the severity of the disease. A general concept seems to be the following. Long CAG repeats cause an early-onset, severe rigid-dystonic form of the disease with early and severe cognitive impairment. Shorter repeat lengths start with a less severe choreatic hypotonic disease that gradually progresses over the years to the severe rigid-dystonic form. This progression is paralleled by a gradual cognitive deterioration over the years. Finally, the shortest repeat lengths cause a mild choreatic hypotonic movement disorder late in life with only mild cognitive impairment and with death often resulting from totally unrelated causes.

If this general concept turns out to be correct, then at least two major issues need to be resolved. First, how should the deviations from this general rule be explained, for example, patients with adult-onset rigid-dystonic disease, or patients with choreatic hypotonic disease and early severe cognitive problems, and, second, how does the psychiatric disease fit into this model?

Juvenile disease

Juvenile cases with onset before age 20 constitute approximately 10 per cent of all patients with HD. About 2 per cent show the first signs of the disease before age 10 (Rasmussen *et al.* 2000). The youngest patient described in the literature had onset at age 2 (Huntington's Disease Collaborative Research Group 1993; Hayden 1981; Osborne *et al.* 1982). In line with the inverse correlation between onset age and length of the CAG repeat, juvenile cases have the longest repeats, with sizes typically exceeding 50 CAGs (Telenius *et al.* 1993; Sanchez *et al.* 1996; Alonso *et al.* 1997). The longest repeat size ever described in such a juvenile patient was around 250 CAGs (Nance *et al.* 1999).

The earliest manifestations of the disease in children are often a decline in school performance and nonspecific behavioural problems. In those with onset prior to or around age 20, psychiatric problems often interpreted as schizophrenia (because of the similar onset age) may dominate the clinical picture (Woldag *et al.* 1997). The motor disorder often appears a few years later. In contrast to adult cases, bradykinesia and rigidity are conspicuous from early in the illness, dominating the neurological findings in about 50 per cent of the cases (Markham and Knox 1965; Bruyn 1968; Oliver and Dewhurst 1969; Hayden 1981; Osborne *et al.* 1982). Chorea is present in almost all cases but is often mild, of short duration and quickly superseded by rigidity. Frequent falls, dysarthria, clumsiness, hyperreflexia, and oculomotor disturbances are frequent in children with HD and occur early. Although it has been suggested that cerebellar dysfunction as elicited from the neurological examination might be observed in juvenile patients (Hayden 1981; Young *et al.* 1986), we ourselves have never seen true cerebellar ataxia in HD. Mental deterioration is first manifested by declining school performance. Over the years a severe progressive dementia develops.

Epileptic seizures, occurring with a frequency in adult HD patients similar to that in the general adult population (1 per cent; Hayden 1981), are more common in early-onset cases with an estimated 30–50 per cent of the juvenile patients affected (Jervis 1963; Brackenridge 1980; Hayden 1981; Osborne *et al.* 1982). Partial or generalized, tonic–clonic or absence seizures may all appear. Seizures should be differentiated from myoclonic jerks, which also occur rarely in adult cases (Vogel *et al.* 1991). The epilepsy of juvenile HD patients is often difficult to control with the common anti-epileptic drugs. No data on modern anti-epileptic drugs are available.

Thus, the overall clinical picture of juvenile HD suggests more severe disease than in adult cases, and this clinical impression is supported by the presence of longer triplet repeat sizes in the HD gene.

The adult-onset rigid subtype or Westphal variant

The original description by Westphal of the rigid, not overtly choreic, phenotype of the disease that bears his name was of an 18-year-old patient from an HD family (Westphal 1883). However, as the concept evolved that juvenile disease (often) starts with such a rigid variant, attention was drawn to those adult cases that manifest with early rigid rather than choreic disease. For those adult cases the eponym of the Westphal variant of HD became commonly accepted (Bittenbender and Quadfasel 1962; Bruyn 1968). The proportion of such cases is unknown: they probably represent about 10 per cent of all adult-onset cases, if late-onset cases are excluded. Patients with the Westphal variant are almost all quite young: mostly in their twenties, rarely in their thirties. A patient with a Westphal variant and a disease onset after age 50 should be considered exceptional, warranting publication. This relatively early onset age again seems to fit in the concept that such rigid dystonic forms represent a more severe form of the disease that is associated with relatively longer CAG repeats.

Late-onset disease

In contrast to juvenile disease, the manifestations in late-onset disease are often surprisingly mild. Approximately 25 per cent of all known patients will display first signs and symptoms after age 50, and in these patients the disease will follow a slower progression than usual, although the number of years they survive after disease onset may not be much different from that of earlier-onset cases (Myers *et al.* 1985; James *et al.* 1994). Chorea is the presenting motor disorder and gait disturbances and dysphagia are common, though not severe. Cognitive impairment, although invariably present, may be less debilitating and less prominent than in younger patients, while psychiatric manifestations may occur less often (Myers *et al.* 1985; James *et al.* 1994). Families have been described in whom cognitive deterioration and mental changes seemed to be totally absent, chorea in old age being the exclusive manifestation of the disease (Britton *et al.* 1995). An older onset is associated with a slower disease progression, as measured by functional disability (Myers *et al.* 1985).

Patients with sporadic late-onset chorea and an expanded CAG repeat in the HD gene may be clinically indistinguishable from those without such a mutation, the latter being classified as 'senile chorea' (Garcia Ruiz *et al.* 1997). Late-onset HD presenting as levodopa (L-dopa)-responsive parkinsonism with cardiovascular dysautonomia was recently described in four patients and initially misdiagnosed as multiple system atrophy (MSA) in three. L-dopa treatment did not unmask significant chorea (Reuter *et al.* 2000).

This generally milder late-onset form of the disease is associated with shorter repeat lengths, typically shorter than 40 repeats, but repeat lengths up to 48 have been described (Kremer *et al.* 1993; James *et al.* 1994). In quite a few cases, a family history of affected parents is lacking, either because of parental death prior to disease onset, because of misdiagnosis of mild late-onset signs in affected persons from such earlier generations, or because the CAG repeat length in earlier generations was in the intermediate range (30 to 35 CAGs—see Chapter 5). Theoretical considerations about the mutational flow of CAG repeats in the HD population, in fact, suggest a substantial underascertainment of CAG repeats smaller than 40 and therefore underdiagnosis of late-onset cases (Falush *et al.* 2000).

Interestingly, the perception of HD as a severe disorder that heavily interferes with normal life expectancy may be ameliorated in at-risk individuals from families in whom such late-onset disease is common. This perception, in turn, may have consequences for the willingness of family members to seek medical attention or to undergo predictive testing, and thus contributes to underdiagnosis of late-onset cases.

Mental and psychiatric manifestations as sole manifestations of HD

Given the observation that HD may vary tremendously in its clinical manifestations of motor, cognitive, and psychiatric abnormalities, is it conceivable that the disease manifests without motor abnormalities, that is, as an exclusively mental and psychiatric disorder? Depression, mood alterations, behavioural abnormalities, and alterations in personality have been detected preceding the onset of the motor disorder in many individuals. However, as the view has been held that the motor abnormalities are the most specific signs of the disease, and disease onset tends to be equated with onset of motor signs, these exclusively mental and psychiatric stages of the disease are poorly represented in the literature.

Although psychiatric problems are very common in HD patients (see Chapter 3), it seems somewhat surprising that no psychiatric manifestations of the disease, either in terms of onset time, severity, or in terms of their nature, have ever been demonstrated to correlate with CAG length (Weigell-Weber *et al.* 1996). Thus, it is clear that psychiatric signs are not simply or linearly correlated to the progressive neurodegeneration that occurs in the brains of HD patients. Rather, any type of HD-related neurodegeneration may predispose affected individuals to psychiatric problems. In addition, non-neurological factors, such as previous life events, relationships, the environment in which the affected persons live, as well as putative additional genetic factors, may play a much more prominent role in the pathophysiology of particular psychiatric symptoms, than in the pathophysiology of the motor and the cognitive disorder (see Chapter 5).

Can a diagnosis of HD be made in a person with exclusively mental or psychiatric symptoms, for example, depression, who is a proven gene carrier? Many clinicians would feel reluctant under such circumstances to tell a person who consults them that the disease has begun. At that point a too narrow emphasis on the technical question of disease onset may distract from more pressing needs, such as adequate treatment of the mood disorder. If an at-risk person with exclusively psychiatric manifestations requested DNA testing, we in our group would consider this as a request for predictive testing rather than diagnostic testing. Such people would not be enrolled in drug trials to test compounds aimed at retarding disease progression.

Making a diagnosis of HD: differential diagnostic considerations

Prior to the discovery of the HD gene, a definite diagnosis of HD would be made in the presence of: (1) a positive family history consistent with autosomal dominant inheritance; (2) progressive motor disability involving both involuntary and voluntary movement; and (3) mental disturbances including cognitive decline, affective disturbances, and/or changes in personality. Despite these criteria, misdiagnoses occurred fairly frequently. In a community-based survey in the state of Maryland, 11 per cent of 212 patients had previously received another (incorrect) diagnosis, while 15 per cent could not be confirmed to have HD on closer examination (Folstein *et al.* 1986). In an older unselected autopsy series, 7 per cent of the cases diagnosed as having HD had some other neurological condition (Bird 1978). In addition, making a diagnosis of HD in the absence of family history, was difficult (Bateman *et al.* 1992).

The discovery of the HD gene and its pathogenic mutation has changed this situation. Molecular DNA diagnosis, based on polymerase chain reaction (PCR) amplification of the expanded repeat, has allowed a diagnostic test with a sensitivity and specificity of almost 100 per cent (Kremer *et al.* 1994). At present, a diagnosis can be made with virtually 100 per cent certainty when the clinical demonstration of signs that are consistent with HD can be matched by the demonstration of an expanded CAG repeat in the HD gene. Even in the absence of positive family history, this approach will lead to the correct diagnosis. HD cannot currently be diagnosed if DNA diagnostics fails to demonstrate an expanded repeat. On the other hand, demonstration of the presence of an expanded CAG repeat in an as yet completely asymptomatic person should never be confounded with making a diagnosis of HD—this is predictive testing. Such people do not suffer from disease.

When patients demonstrate minor motor abnormalities, subtle cognitive changes, or psychiatric episodes, while lacking the specific extrapyramidal motor abnormalities, there may be a question about whether the disease has begun. In such cases the assessment of CAG repeat expansion can demonstrate that the patient will develop the clinical features of HD at some future time, but such a test should not be equated with making a diagnosis of clinical disease. A clinician may express his or her concern regarding the possibility of disease and more certainty may perhaps be obtained by performing imaging studies such as 2-(^{18}F)-fluoro-2-deoxyglucose (FDG) or D2 receptor ligand PET, magnetic resonance imaging (MRI) morphometry, or functional MRI, which are able to demonstrate the neurobiological correlates of the disease (Grafton *et al.* 1990; Antonini *et al.* 1996; Harris *et al.* 1999). Single-photon emission computerized tomography (SPECT) is probably less sensitive to early changes (Martin *et al.* 1995). These methods will be discussed in Chapter 4. Imaging studies are primarily of scientific interest at present. From a clinical perspective it should be pointed out that the diagnostic value of these methods in detecting incipient disease has never been formally assessed for routine clinical use. We know nothing about positive or negative predictive value. In a study of chorea-free at-risk individuals with psychiatric disorders that was conducted prior to the discovery of the gene, imaging studies were not able to discriminate lower-risk from higher-risk persons (Baxter *et al.* 1992).

Differential diagnosis

The advent of CAG assessment has greatly facilitated the diagnosis of HD, to the point at which a diagnosis of HD in an individual with an extrapyramidal movement disorder can be made unambiguously, even if a family history is lacking. Problems that confront the clinician nowadays are either patients with a nontypical motor disorder who turn out to have HD (see above), or patients with chorea and perhaps cognitive or psychiatric problems who turn out not to have an expanded CAG repeat.

Non-inherited chorea

Many different conditions are associated with chorea (Padberg and Bruyn 1986), but most are rare and can easily be excluded in a patient with suspected HD. The most common cause of isolated chorea to be considered is *tardive dyskinesia* associated with the use of neuroleptics. Many different medications may induce chorea, including *medication-induced dyskinesias in parkinsonism* (L-dopa), *anticonvulsant drugs* (particularly carbamazepine in children), *noradrenergic stimulant drugs* (cocaine, amphetamine, aminophyline), *digoxin intoxication*, and *oral contraceptives*. Other causes of chorea, including *thyrotoxicosis*, cerebrovascular disease of arteriolosclerotic or vasculitic origin such as *bilateral lacunar infarcts* of the striatum, *cerebral lupus erythematosus* (associated with the lupus anticoagulant), and *polycythaemia* can easily be excluded based on family history, associated findings, and the course of the illness.

Senile chorea, or chorea of late onset in the elderly person without a family history of other affected individuals may clinically resemble HD or any of the aforementioned disorders (Shinotoh *et al.* 1994; Garcia Ruiz *et al.* 1997). In fact, senile chorea of unknown origin and late-onset HD may be clinically indistinguishable, requiring CAG repeat length assessment to produce a diagnosis (Garcia Ruiz *et al.* 1997). The cause of non-HD senile chorea is a clinical diagnostic challenge. All of the non-inherited causes that are discussed in the previous paragraph should be considered.

In contrast, *Sydenham's chorea* occurs in young patients—children or young adults, in association with streptococcal rheumatic fever. Up to 25 per cent of patients with this severe and potentially life-threatening disease may develop the movement disorder (Cardoso *et al.* 1997). The acute onset of the disease and a much finer aspect to the choreic movements allows clinical differentiation from HD especially as chorea as a presenting sign in a young HD patient is rare. However, like HD, Sydenham's chorea may be associated with prominent psychiatric and mental alterations. In this era of acronyms the term PANDAS (paediatric autoimmune neuropsychiatric disorder associated with streptococcus) has been introduced to emphasize this association (Murphy *et al.* 2000). Sydenham's chorea may manifest as a monophasic episodic disease, as recurrent episodes, or as a prolonged movement disorder after a streptococcal infection (Cardoso *et al.* 1999).

Inherited chorea
Choreo-acanthocytosis, or neuroacanthocytosis, is one of a heterogeneous group of neurological disorders associated with irregular spiny erythrocytes, or acanthocytes, which can be detected in a peripheral blood smear. Among the neurological disorders with acanthocytes, two groups may be distinguished. The first may additionally be characterized by low serum betalipoproteins and includes: Bassen Kornzweig disease (abetalipoproteinaemia, a recessive disease with vitamin E dependent polyneuropathy and ataxia); a form of hypobetalipoproteinaemia (Mars *et al.* 1969); and the HARP syndrome—hypoprebetalipoproteinaemia, acanthocytosis, retinitis pigmentosa, and pallidal degeneration (Higgins *et al.* 1992). A second group comprises those with normal serum betalipoproteins and, apart from a few patients with Hallervorden–Spatz-like disease, includes patients with neuromuscular and basal ganglia disease with or without the McLeod bloodgroup phenotype. This latter group is known as choreo-acanthocytosis, neuroacanthocytosis, familial amyotrophic chorea with acanthocytosis, or the Levine–Critchley syndrome (Critchley *et al.* 1967). Choreo-acanthocytosis is a slowly progressive neurodegenerative disorder that affects the basal ganglia, peripheral nerves, and muscle. In a review of 19 sporadic and familial British cases, as well as 26 cases from the literature, Hardie and co-authors found onset varying between 8 and 62 years, with a mean of about 32.5 years. Of these 45, 8 were reported to have died between 7 and 24 years after onset of the disease (mean 13.9 years) (Hardie *et al.* 1991). The clinical manifestations may resemble those of HD, and often patients with this disorder have first been diagnosed as having HD. Mild cognitive impairment and psychiatric symptoms may manifest early in the disease. Dementia will develop in most patients, but early in the disease frontal lobe dysfunction dominates. Personality changes, impulsive and distractable behaviour, mood disorder, paranoid delusions, and obsessive–compulsive features may necessitate psychiatric help. In contrast to adult patients with HD, epilepsy occurs much more frequently than in the general population, with about half of the reported cases affected. Choreic movements of the limbs and face are present in almost all cases: they usually start in the legs. Orofacial dyskinesia may lead to tongue and lip biting and offer a strong clue to diagnosis. Orofacial dyskinesia may cause severe problems with speaking and swallowing. Apart from chorea, dystonia, parkinsonism and tics may occur in the course of the disease. Vocalizations and, rarely, coprolalia may resemble those seen in Tourette's disease. Computerized tomography (CT) or MRI studies of the brain may reveal atrophy of the caudate nucleus. In addition, in a number of cases, focal symmetrical abnormalities can be demonstrated in various parts of the basal ganglia that consist of hyperintense lesions in T_2-weighted sequences. These lesions can be found in the caudate, putamen, or globus pallidus, where they may resemble the 'eye of the tiger' sign in Hallervorden–Spatz disease. The clinical feature that distinguishes neuroacanthocytosis from HD is the presence of neuromuscular abnormalities, consisting of hypo- or areflexia of tendon reflexes and distal amyotrophy. Serum creatine kinase (CK)

activity is elevated in the majority of cases, while nerve conduction studies reveal reduced sensory action potentials in about 50 per cent of cases. In contrast, motor nerve conduction studies are generally uninformative, and electromyography reveals denervation only in a minority of cases (Hardie *et al.* 1991). The neuropathology of neuroacanthocytosis is distinct. In the central nervous system, the caudate nucleus, the putamen, and the globus pallidus consistently show atrophy with marked neuronal loss and gliosis. The substantia nigra, the thalamus, and the motor neurones in the spinal cord may atrophy (Rinne *et al.* 1994). In peripheral nerves axonal loss primarily affects the large-diameter myelinated fibres distally, with signs of regeneration after axonal degeneration. But unmyelinated axons may not escape destruction (Hardie *et al.* 1991). Choreo-acanthocytosis is probably inherited as a recessive trait, although autosomal dominant transmission has been suggested (Vance *et al.* 1987; Hardie *et al.* 1991). Genetic analysis of 11 families of different origin found evidence for a recessive locus at 9q21 (Rubio *et al.* 1997). A few candidate genes from this region have already been excluded (Rubio *et al.* 1999).

Benign hereditary chorea (BHC, also known as chronic juvenile hereditary chorea) is much rarer than HD. The earliest descriptions date from 1966 and 1967 (Haerer *et al.* 1967; Pincus and Chutorian 1967), but few series of patients and families have been described (Harper 1978). A complete review of the literature up to 1985, presented by Bruyn and Myrianthopoulis (1986), summarizes the clinical features of the disease. BHC starts before the age of 5 in the vast majority of cases, although onset shortly after birth or around age 10 may occur. Males and females seem equally affected. The severity of the choreic movements may reach its maximum between ages 10 and 20, but then tends to decrease. Apart from choreic movements that may affect the limbs (both proximally and distally), the neck, and the face, not many additional features occur. Dysarthria is rare, while tremor has been described in a few families. Motor development may be somewhat slow and some patients manifest clumsiness. Although some were reported to be mentally retarded, the majority seem to be of normal intelligence and cognitive development. Similarly, psychiatric manifestations are not part of the usual clinical course. Other findings, such as hypospadias and minor digital abnormalities, have been found in single families and may be chance occurrences. BHC is inherited as an autosomal dominant trait with reduced penetrance in females. The HD locus on 4p16–3 has been excluded as the locus of the BHC gene (Quarrell *et al.* 1988). Recently, a locus has been found at 14q, in a region that spans approximately 20.6 cM and contains several interesting candidate genes involved in the development and/or maintenance of the central nervous system (CNS): glia maturation factor-beta, guanosine 5′-triphosphate (GTP) cyclohydrolase 1, and the survival of motor neurones (SMN)-interacting protein 1 (De Vries *et al.* 2000).

Dentatorubro-pallidoluysian atrophy (DRPLA) is a disorder that received its name from its neuropathological characteristics. The initial reports from 1946 described sporadic cases, but in 1982 Naito and Oyanagi identified five Japanese families with multiple affected members and an autosomal dominant pattern of inheritance (Naito and Oyanagi 1982). The disease is more common (although still very rare) in Japan than in other countries. Three clinical phenotypes are evident. The first is dominated by initial ataxia and subsequent choreo-athetosis. The second was called the pseudo-Huntington type, with choreatic movements and dementia, and only mild cerebellar ataxia. The third consists of progressive myoclonus-epilepsy: initial myoclonus, and generalized seizures with progressive mental deterioration. Different phenotypes may occur in one family (Iizuka *et al.* 1984; Warner *et al.* 1994), but cerebellar ataxia could be elicited to some extent in almost all cases (Iizuka *et al.* 1984). Age of onset ranges from 6 to 69 years and death occurs between age 20 and 75. Disease duration is approximately 10 years. Anticipation was noted in some families, with early onset associated with myoclonus epilepsy and ataxia, and later onset with dementia and choreo-athetosis (Iizuka *et al.* 1984). The disease seems to be extremely rare in patients of non-Japanese descent and only a few non-Japanese families have been described. In the course of the disease multiple CNS neuronal systems degenerate, consistently including the globus pallidus (especially its lateral part), the subthalamic nucleus, or nucleus of Luys, the cerebellar dentate nucleus, and the red nucleus. In addition, several other structures in the brainstem and spinal chord may be affected. As in HD, neuronal loss and gliosis constitute the main microscopic findings, with secondary demyelination of affected tracts. DRPLA is caused by a CAG expansion in a novel gene on chromosome 12 (Koide *et al.* 1994; Nagafuchi *et al.* 1994). The expansion is strongly correlated with age of onset (Koide *et al.* 1994). Haw River syndrome, which has a clinical similarity to typical DRPLA but lacks myoclonic epilepsy and basal ganglia degeneration, has been shown to be caused by expansion of the same CAG tract (Burke *et al.* 1994). A comparison of the other polyglutamine-related trinucleotide repeat disorders is given in Chapter 14.

Paroxysmal hyperkinesias or *dyskinesias* present short-lasting (minutes to hours) episodes of dystonia or chorea, often with an identifiable precipitating event, without any signs of movement disorder in between. Although the dystonia and chorea of HD, choreo-acanthocytosis, or DRPLA may wax and wane with emotion, fatigue, and other exogenous factors, these involuntary movements are still considered to present a more or less static movement disorder. In contrast, in the so-called paroxysmal dyskinesias intermittent movement abnormalities, interspersed by prolonged periods of completely normal movements, constitute the core clinical feature. These paroxysmal dyskinesias encompass various disorders, such as 'familial paroxysmal choreoathetosis', 'familial paroxysmal dystonic choreoathetosis', 'paroxysmal kinesigenic choreoathetosis', and others (Fahn 1994; Demirkiran and Jankovic 1995). A clinically useful classification has been proposed by Demirkiran and Jankovic (1995) who used as the classifying factors the duration of the attacks, the inducing factor, and whether they are primary—familial or sporadic—or secondary. The most important classifying criterion, in their opinion, is whether or not attacks are induced by voluntary movements. The resulting categories are kinesiogenic, non-kinesiogenic, and exertion–induced paroxysmal involuntary movements. A secondary subdivision can be made to take into account the duration of the attacks—lasting longer or shorter than 5 minutes. Various loci that segregate with familial paroxysmal disease have been identified (Fouad *et al.* 1996; Auburger *et al.* 1996; Raskind *et al.* 1998; Tomita *et al.* 1999), but a diagnosis of these conditions is still primarily a clinical one. None of the paroxysmal movement disorders is associated with mental alterations.

In the *autosomal dominant cerebellar ataxias*, particularly SCA3 or Machado–Joseph disease, dystonia and, rarely, chorea may occur. A neurological examination will however always elicit ataxia, long tract signs, and typical eye movement abnormalities that are completely distinct from those seen in HD. *Mitochondrial myoencephalopathies* may occasionally present with an extrapyramidal syndrome (Truong *et al.* 1990). Wilson's disease should also be considered as this has significant therapeutic implications.

Finally, chorea may be a manifestation of a large group of metabolic (often recessive) disorders that start at young age and lead to progressive neurological impairment.

Rare or unnamed diseases with inherited chorea that resemble HD
A consanguineous family affected by an autosomal recessive, progressive neurodegenerative HD-like disorder was recently described in Saudi Arabia (Kambouris *et al.* 2000). The disease manifests at approximately 3–4 years and is characterized by both pyramidal and extrapyramidal abnormalities, including chorea, dystonia, ataxia, gait instability, spasticity, seizures, mutism, and intellectual impairment. Juvenile-onset HD was ruled out by genotyping. Linkage with a LOD score of 3.03 was initially achieved with a marker at 4p15.3 (Kambouris *et al.* 2000).

In one large family of Swedish descent, disease onset was between ages 28 and 41, while those who died did so between ages 42 and 52 (Xiang *et al.* 1998). Clinically, patients displayed a motor disorder (chorea, rigidity, myoclonic jerks, gait disturbances, dysarthria, sometimes cerebellar coordination problems) as well as psychiatric (depression, aggressiveness, personality changes) and global cognitive alterations. Several individuals suffered from epilepsy. Imaging studies and post-mortem examination revealed both basal ganglia disease and more global atrophy, particularly of the frontal and temporal lobes. Thus, this disorder could be one of the large group of frontotemporal dementias. In this family a significant LOD-score of 3.01 was obtained with markers on chromosome 20p.

Creutzfeldt–Jakob disease, which can be familial and is inherited as an autosomal dominant trait in some families, progresses much more rapidly than HD. The major involuntary movements are myoclonus. In older patients in whom dementia is insidious, *Alzheimer's disease* (AD) deserves consideration, as it sometimes presents with myoclonus. Abnormalities typical for AD may be found in the brains of older HD patients. The simultaneous occurrence of AD and HD in the same individual is not unexpected from their relative frequencies.

Frontotemporal dementias, including Pick's disease, may present as an insidious deterioration of social conduct, with apathy and cognitive impairment. Several forms exist, including those with parkinsonian features that are caused by mutations in the microtubule-associated protein tau (Foster *et al.* 1997; Wilhelmsen 1997; Hutton *et al.* 1998).

If affective disturbances or psychosis dominate the initial syndrome, an incorrect diagnosis of schizophrenia may be applied. Chorea in these patients may be wrongly considered to represent *tardive dyskinesia*. A carefully taken family history and a neurological examination can lead to a correct diagnosis. On the other hand, a patient with tardive dyskinesia and defect schizophrenic features may be wrongly considered to suffer from HD—raising the question of the true diagnosis if DNA diagnostics fails to show an expanded CAG repeat.

The diagnosis of HD in children should present no problems if the details of the clinical phenotype are recognized and the family is known, but it may be extremely difficult in isolated cases, for example in the case of adopted children. The complex tics of *Gilles de la Tourette syndrome* should be quite distinguishable from the motor disorder in HD. *Hallervorden–Spatz syndrome* is a very rare condition that can be diagnosed by its clinical features and rather characteristic MRI abnormalities (Swaiman 1991), many other rare metabolic diseases should be considered. *Lesch–Nyhan syndrome* is associated with hyperuricacmia.

Although the combination of progressive chorea and cognitive dysfunction in a patient with a positive family history establishes the diagnosis of HD, those in whom a family history is lacking pose a special diagnostic challenge. The most obvious causes may be nonpaternity, adoption, nonrecognition of the existence of the disorder in family members, or early death or late-onset in the affected parent. The availability of a DNA diagnostic test means that an absent family history no longer confounds the process of making a correct diagnosis.

Neuropathology

The most characteristic neuropathological abnormalities are neuronal loss and concomitant gliosis in the caudate nucleus and, to a somewhat lesser extent, the putamen (together called the neostriatum). But the pathology is not restricted to the neostriatum. The globus pallidus, various cortical areas, and several subcortical structures are also affected. The evolution of the neuropathological striatal abnormalities follows a characteristic course, while the sequence of extrastriatal neurodegeneration has yet to be established. The relationship that has been established between CAG length and clinical course is reflected (and, in all likelihood, has its origin) in the relationship between CAG length and the neuropathological alterations. Recently, the emphasis of HD neuropathological descriptions has shifted from the distribution of disease-related neuronal loss to the detection and the distribution of abnormal depositions of *huntingtin* fragments: abnormal fibrillar aggregations of cleaved protein fragments that become deposited in the nuclei and the cytoplasm of central nervous system neurones. This topic forms the subject of Chapter 8 where there is a detailed discussion of the classical and molecular neuropathology of HD.

Diagnostic accuracy of the neuropathological examination

The combination of clinical signs and neuropathological examination traditionally provided a sensitive and specific approach to the diagnosis of HD. Indeed, before the advent of DNA testing, post-mortem neuropathological examination was considered the gold standard of HD diagnostic testing. The accuracy of previous neuropathological diagnoses has been confirmed by recent studies of CAG repeat lengths in clinically and neuropathologically diagnosed cases. Sensitivity was illustrated in a series of 157 cases in which a clinical diagnosis was confirmed by a post-mortem detection of CAG expansion. A correct neuropathological diagnosis was obtained in 153 of these 157 (Xuereb *et al.* 1996). However, it should be noted that, even in patients with a choreic movement disorder from HD families, the routine neuropathological examination may be completely normal—so-called grade 0 neuropathology in the terminology introduced by Vonsattel *et al.* (Vonsattel *et al.* 1985; Xuereb *et al.* 1996). In *in situ* hybridization studies of such grade 0 cases, decreased dopamine D1 and D2 receptor mRNA expression was demonstrated (Augood *et al.* 1997). Thus, neuronal functional alterations precede the actual cell loss.

In terms of specificity, neuropathological diagnosis may reach a level of accuracy that is similar to its level of sensitivity. In a series of 310 cases diagnosed neuropathologically as HD, 307 cases turned out to harbour an expanded repeat (Persichetti *et al.* 1994). Rare cases with clinical features, a family history, and neuropathology consistent with HD, but without a CAG repeat, have been reported in other series as well (Xuereb *et al.* 1996). Such cases should be considered true phenocopies of the disease. Either a different gene or a different mutation in the *huntingtin* gene could be held responsible for the HD-like disorder in such families (see Chapter 5).

Since the advent of DNA diagnostics, however, neuropathological confirmation of a diagnosis of HD is no longer required unless the clinical features have been atypical, suggesting that an alternative or additional condition might be present. CAG repeat length assessment in affected individuals is considered to be the gold standard upon which a clinical diagnosis can be based, and a characteristic combination of clinical signs with an expanded repeat is sufficient for a diagnosis of HD (Kremer *et al.* 1994).

Neuropathological changes in presymptomatic individuals

Neuropathological examination is now primarily used to resolve atypical cases, as noted above, as well as for scientific purposes. A major issue of scientific interest has always been the question of how long before the onset of clinical signs the first structural brain alterations actually occur. In presymptomatic individuals, that is, individuals with an expanded CAG repeat but without clinical signs of the disease, the routine neuropathological examination may be completely normal, and is probably so in the vast majority of cases (Persichetti *et al.* 1994). However, with advanced morphological techniques, such as receptor-binding studies of *N*-methyl-D-aspartate (NMDA) and DL-alpha-amino-3-hydroxy-5-methyl-isoxazole proprionate (AMPA) receptors, and *in situ* hybridization studies of such receptors, abnormalities of striatal projection neurones have been detected in presymptomatic individuals (Albin *et al.* 1990, 1991).

   Neuropathological examination of six presymptomatic confirmed gene carriers did show some minor but interesting changes (Gomez-Tortosa *et al.* 2001). In the tail of the caudate nucleus, one of the earliest affected structures, neither neuronal nor astrocytic nor microglial cell counts differed from those in non-carriers. In contrast, the density of oligodendroglial cells was double the density in controls. In addition, although the number of neurones was still normal, using ubiquitin staining, neuronal inclusions were found in these presymptomatic brains, including the brain of a person who died 3 decades before the expected age for onset of the clinical syndrome (Gomez-Tortosa *et al.* 2001).

Relationship between CAG repeat length and neuropathological changes

The relation between CAG and the clinical characteristics of the disease was established immediately after the discovery of the gene (see Chapter 5 for details). As the clinical features of HD are ultimately determined by the changes in brain function, a relation between CAG size and neuropathological changes can be postulated. Simple correlations are not obvious (Sieradzan *et al.* 1997). But when CAG repeat size was related to striatal neuronal counts or to neuropathological grade corrected for age at death or for duration of disease, strong correlations were indeed detected (Furtado *et al.* 1996; Penney *et al.* 1997). CAG length typically explained about 80 per cent of the variance in neuropathological alterations, which is a remarkably strong biological effect. Cortical atrophy has also been found to correlate with repeat size (Halliday *et al.* 1998).

Conclusions

The recognition of HD, based on the classic triad of symptoms recognized by Huntington (1872) plus a family history of the disease, remains at the core of clinical diagnosis of the disease. The recent discovery of the HD gene and its mutation have led to refinements in diagnosis, in particular a recognition of the previous underascertainment of late-onset disease. Knowledge of the mutation has also led to a consideration of the length of the CAG repeat tract in relation to disease symptoms, with strong correlations seen for age at onset and neuropathological changes and very little correlation for symptom type or disease duration. The symptoms of the disease remain, to a large extent, as distressing and incurable as they were in Huntington's time, although the advances gained through knowledge of the gene and its mutation offer hope of therapies in the future. These recent advances in our knowledge of the pathogenesis of HD are outlined in the further chapters of this volume.

References

Adams P, Falek A, Arnold J. Huntington disease in Georgia: age at onset. *Am J Hum Genet* 1988; **43**: 695–704.

Albin RL, Young AB, Penney JB, Handelin B, Balfour R, Anderson KD, Markel DS, Tourtellotte WW, Reine A. Abnormalities of striatal projection neurons and N-methyl-D-aspartate receptors in presymptomatic Huntington's disease. *New Engl J Med* 1990; **322**: 1293–1298.

—— Qin Y, Young AB, Penney JB, Chesselet MF. Preproenkephalin messenger RNA-containing neurons in striatum of patients with symptomatic and presymptomatic Huntington's disease: an *in situ* hybridization study. *Ann Neurol* 1991; **30**: 542–549.

Alonso ME, Yescas P, Cisneros B, Martinez C, Silva G, Ochoa A, Montanez C. Analysis of the (CAG)n repeat causing Huntington's disease in a Mexican population. *Clin Genet* 1997; **51**: 225–230.

Andrew SE, Goldberg YP, Kremer B, Telenius H, Theilmann J, Adam S, Starr E, Squitieri F, Lin B, Kalchman MA, *et al*. The relationship between trinucleotide (CAG) repeat length and clinical features of Huntington disease. *Nat Genet* 1993; **4**: 398–403.

Angelini L, Sgro V, Erba A, Merello S, Lanzi G, Nardocci N. Tourettism as clinical presentation of Huntington's disease with onset in childhood. *Ital J Neurol Sci* 1998; **19**: 383–385.

Antonini A, Leenders KL, Spiegel R, Meier D, Vontobel P, Weigell-Weber M, Sanchez-Pernaute R, de Yebenez JG, Boesiger P, Weindl A, Maguire RP. Striatal glucose metabolism and dopamine D2 receptor binding in asymptomatic gene carriers and patients with Huntington's disease. *Brain* 1996; **119**: 2085–2095.

Ashizawa T, Wong LJ, Richards CS, Caskey CT, Jankovic J. CAG repeat size and clinical presentation in Huntington's disease. *Neurology* 1994; **44**: 1137–1143.

Auburger G, Ratzlaff T, Lunkes A, Nelles HW, Leube B, Binkofski F, Kugel H, Heindel W, Seitz R, Benecke R, Witte OW, Voit T. A gene for autosomal dominant paroxysmal choreoathetosis/ spasticity (CSE) maps to the vicinity of a potassium channel gene cluster on chromosome 1p, probably within 2 cM between D1S443 and D1S197. *Genomics* 1996; **31**: 90–94.

Augood SJ, Faull RL, Emson PC. Dopamine D1 and D2 receptor gene expression in the striatum in Huntington's disease. *Ann Neurol* 1997; **42**: 215–221.

Barbeau A, Duvoisin RC, Gerstenbrand F, Lakke JP, Marsden CD, Stern G. Classification of extrapyramidal disorders. Proposal for an international classification and glossary of terms. *J Neurol Sci* 1981; **51**: 311–327.

Bateman D, Boughey AM, Scaravilli F, Marsden CD, Harding AE. A follow-up study of isolated cases of suspected Huntington's disease. *Ann Neurol* 1992; **31**: 293–298.

Baxter LR Jr, Mazziotta JC, Pahl JJ, Grafton ST, St George-Hyslop P, Haines JL, Gusella JF, Szuba MP, Selin CE, Guze BH, *et al*. Psychiatric, genetic, and positron emission tomographic evaluation of persons at risk for Huntington's disease. *Arch Gen Psychiatry* 1992; **49**: 148–154.

Beenen N, Buttner U, Lange HW. The diagnostic value of eye movement recordings in patients with Huntington's disease and their offspring. *Electroencephalogr Clin Neurophysiol* 1986; **63**: 119–127.

Bird ED. The brain in Huntington's chorea. *Psychol Med* 1978: **8**: 357–360.

Bittenbender JB, Quadfasel FA. Rigid and akinetic forms of Huntington's chorea. *Arch Neurol* 1962; **7**: 275–288.

Blanloeil Y, Bigot A, Dixneuf B. Anaesthesia in Huntington's chorea. *Anaesthesia* 1982; **37**: 695–6.

Bollen EL, Den Heijer JC, Ponsioen C, Kramer C, Van der Velde EA, Van Dijk JG, Roos RA, Kamphuisen HA, Buruma OJ. Respiration during sleep in Huntington's chorea. *J Neurol Sci* 1988; **84**: 63–68.

Brackenridge CJ. Factors influencing dementia and epilepsy in Huntington's disease of early onset. *Acta Neurol Scand* 1980; **62**: 305–311.

Brandt J, Bylsma FW, Gross R, Stine OC, Ranen NG, Ross CA. Trinucleotide repeat length and clinical progression in Huntington's disease. *Neurology* 1996; **46**: 527–531.

Brinkman RR, Mezei MM, Thielmann J, Almqvist E, Hayden MR. The likelihood of being affected with Huntington disease by a particular age for a specific CAG size. *Am J Hum Genet* 1997; **60**: 1202–1210.

Britton JW, Uitti RJ, Ahlskog JE, Robinson RG, Kremer B, Hayden MR. Hereditary late-onset chorea without significant dementia: genetic evidence for substantial phenotypic variation in Huntington's disease. *Neurology* 1995; **45**: 443–447.

Brothers CRD. Huntington's chorea in Victoria and Tasmania. *J Neurol Sci* 1964; **1**: 405–420.

Browne MG, Cross R. Huntington's chorea. *Br J Anaesthesia* 1981; **53**: 1367.

—— Anaesthesia in Huntington's chorea. *Anaesthesia* 1982; **38**: 65–66.

Bruyn GW. Huntington's chorea. Historical, clinical and laboratory synopsis In: *Diseases of the basal ganglia. Handbook of clinical neurology* (ed. PJ Vincken and GW Bruyn), Vol. 6, pp. 298–378. Amsterdam: North Holland: 1968.

—— Myrianthopoulos NC. Chronic juvenile hereditary chorea (benign hereditary chorea of early onset). In: *Handbook of clinical neurology*, revised series, Vol 5 (49). *Extrapyramidal disorders* (ed. PJ Vincken, GW Bruyn, and HL Klawans), pp. 335–348. Amsterdam: Elsevier: 1986.

Burke JR, Wingfield MS, Lewis KE, Roses AD, Lee JE, Hulette C, Pericak-Vance MA, Vance JM. The Haw River syndrome: detatorubropallidoluysian atrophy (DRPLA) in an African-American family. *Nat Genet* 1994; **7**: 521–524.

Burke RE, Fahn S, Mayeux R, Weinberg H, Louis K, Willner JH. Neuroleptic malignant syndrome caused by dopamine-depleting drugs in a patient with Huntington disease. *Neurology* 1981; **31**: 1022–1026.

Bylsma FW, Rothlind J, Hall MR, Folstein SE, Brandt J. Assessment of adaptive functioning in Huntington's disease. *Movement Dis* 1993; **8**: 183–190.

Campodonico JR, Codori AM, Brandt J. Neuropsychological stability over two years in asymptomatic carriers of the Huntington's disease mutation. *J Neurol Neurosurg Psychiatry* 1996; **61**: 621–624.

Cardoso F, Eduardo C, Silva AP, Mota CC. Chorea in fifty consecutive patients with rheumatic fever. *Movement Dis* 1997; **12**: 701–703.

—— Vargas AP, Oliveira LD, Guerra AA, Amaral SV. Persistent Sydenham's chorea. *Movement Dis* 1999; **14**: 805–807.

Carella F, Scaioli V, Ciano C, Binelli S, Oliva D, Girotti F. Adult onset myoclonic Huntington's disease. *Movement Dis* 1993; **8**: 201–205.

Claes S, Van Zand K, Legius E, Dom R, Malfroid M, Baro F, Godderis J, Cassiman JJ. Correlations between triplet repeat expansion and clinical features in Huntington's disease. *Arch Neurol* 1995; **52**: 749–753.

Coleman R, Anderson D, Lovrien E. Oral motor dysfunction in individuals at risk of Huntington disease. *Am J Med Genet* 1990; **37**: 36–39.

Critchley EMR, Clark DB, Wikler A. An adult form of acanthocytosis. *Trans Am Neurol Assoc* 1967; **92**: 132–137.

Curra A, Agostino R, Galizia P, Fittipaldi F, Manfredi M, Berardelli A. Sub-movement cueing and motor sequence execution in patients with Huntington's disease. *Clin Neurophysiol* 2000; **111**: 1184–1190.

Davies DD. Abnormal response to anaesthesia in a case of Huntington's chorea. *Br J Anaesthesia* 1966; **38**: 490.

De Boo G, Tibben A, Hermans J, Maat A, Roos RA. Subtle involuntary movements are not reliable indicators of incipient Huntington's disease. *Movement Dis* 1998; **13**: 96–99.

Demirkiran M, Jankovic J. Paroxysmal dyskinesias: clinical features and classification. *Ann Neurol* 1995; **38**: 571–579.

De Vries BB, Arts WF, Breedveld GJ, Hoogeboom JJ, Niermeijer MF, Heutink P. Benign hereditary chorea of early onset maps to chromosome 14q. *Am J Hum Genet* 2000; **66**: 136–142.

Di Maio L, Squitieri F, Napolitano G, Campanella G, Trofatter JA, Conneally PM. Suicide risk in Huntington's disease. *J Med Genet* 1993; **30**: 293–295.

Dursun SM, Burke JG, Andrews H, Mlynik-Szmid A, Reveley MA. The effects of antipsychotic medication on saccadic eye movement abnormalities in Huntington's disease. *Prog Neuropsychopharmacol Biol Psychiatry* 2000; **24**: 889–896.

Duyao M, Ambrose C, Myers R, *et al.* Trinucleotide repeat length instability and age of onset in Huntington disease. *Nat Genet* 1993; **4**: 387–392.

Emser W, Brenner M, Stober T, Schimrigk K. Changes in nocturnal sleep in Huntington's and Parkinson's disease. *J Neurol* 1988; **235**: 177–179.

Fahn S. The paroxysmal dyskinesias. In: *Movement disorders*, Vol 3 (ed. CD Marsden and S Fahn), pp. 310–345. Oxford: Butterworth–Heinemann: 1994.

Falush D, Almqvist EW, Brinkmann RR, Iwasa Y, Hayden MR. Measurement of mutational flow implies both a high new-mutation rate for Huntington disease and substantial underascertainment of late-onset cases. *Am J Hum Genet* 2000; **68**: 373–385.

Farina J, Rauscher LA. Anaesthesia and Huntington's chorea. A report of two cases. *Br J Anaesthesia* 1977; **49**: 1167–1168.

Farrer LA, Yu PL. Anthropometric discrimination among affected, at-risk, and not-at-risk individuals in families with Huntington disease. *Am J Med Genet* 1985; **21**: 307–316.

—— Suicide and attempted suicide in Huntington disease: implications for preclinical testing of persons at risk. *Am J Med Genet* 1986; **24**: 305–311.

Feigin A, Kieburtz K, Bordwell K, Como P, Steinberg K, Sotack J, Zimmerman C, Hickey C, Orme C, Shoulson I. Functional decline in Huntington's disease. *Movement Dis* 1995; **10**: 211–214.

Fish DR, Sawyers D, Allen PJ, Blackie JD, Lees AJ, Marsden CD. The effect of sleep on the dyskinetic movements of Parkinson's disease, Gilles de la Tourette syndrome, Huntington's disease, and torsion dystonia. *Arch Neurol* 1991; **48**: 210–214.

Folstein SE, Jensen B, Leigh RJ, Folstein M. The measurement of abnormal movement: methods developed for Huntington's disease. *Neurobehav Toxicol Teratol* 1983; **5**: 605–609.

—— Leigh RJ, Parhad IM, Folstein MF. The diagnosis of Huntington's disease. *Neurology* 1986; **36**: 1279–1283.

—— *Huntington's disease. A disorder of families*. Baltimore: Johns Hopkins University Press: 1989.

Foroud T, Gray J, Ivashina J, Conneally PM. Differences in duration of Huntington's disease based on age at onset. *J Neurol Neurosurg Psychiatry* 1999; **66**: 52–56.

Foster NL, Wilhelmsen K, Sima AA, Jones MZ, D'Amato CJ, Gilman S. Frontotemporal dementia and parkinsonism linked to chromosome 17: a consensus conference. *Ann Neurol* 1997; **41**: 706–715.

Fouad, GT, Servidei S, Durcan S, Bertini E, Ptacek LJ. A gene for familial paroxysmal dyskinesia (FPD1) maps to chromosome 2q. *Am J Hum Genet* 1996; **59**: 135–139.

Furtado S, Suchowersky O, Rewcastle B, Graham L, Klimek ML, Garber A. Relationship between trinucleotide repeats and neuropathological changes in Huntington's disease. *Ann Neurol* 1996; **39**: 132–136.

Garcia Ruiz PJ, Gomez-Tortosa E, del Barrio A, Benitez J, Morales B, Vela L, Castro A, Requena I. Senile chorea: a multicenter prospective study. *Acta Neurol Scand* 1997; **95**: 180–183.

Georgiou N, Phillips JG, Bradshaw JL, Cunnington R, Chiu E. Impairments of movement kinematics in patients with Huntington's disease: a comparison with and without a concurrent task. *Movement Dis* 1997; **12**: 386–396.

Gomez-Tortosa E, MacDonald ME, Friend JC, Taylor SA, Weiler LJ, Cupples LA, Srinidhi J, Gusella JF, Bird ED, Vonsattel JP, Myers RH. Quantitative neuropathological changes in presymptomatic Huntington's disease. *Ann Neurol* 2001; **49**: 29–34.

Grafton ST, Mazziotta JC, Pahl JJ, St George-Hyslop P, Haines JL, Gusella J, Hoffman JM, Baxter LR, Phelps ME. A comparison of neurological, metabolic, structural, and genetic evaluations in persons at risk for Huntington's disease. *Ann Neurol* 1990; **28**: 614–621.

Gualandi W, Bonfanti G. A case of prolonged apnea in Huntington's chorea. *Acta Anaesthesiol* 1968; **19** (suppl. 6): 235–238.

Gupta K, Leng CP. Anaesthesia and juvenile Huntington's disease. *Paediatr Anaesth* 2000; **10**: 107–109.

Haerer AF, Currier RS, Jackson JF. Hereditary non-progressive chorea of early onset. *New Engl J Med* 1967; **276**: 1220–1224.

Hahn-Barma V, Deweer B, Durr A, Dode C, Feingold J, Pillon B, Agid Y, Brice A, Dubois B. Are cognitive changes the first symptoms of Huntington's disease? A study of gene carriers. *J Neurol Neurosurg Psychiatry* 1998; **64**: 172–177.

Haines JL, Conneally PM. Causes of death in Huntington disease as reported on death certificates. *Genet Epidemiol* 1986; **3**: 417–423.

Halliday GM, McRitchie DA, Macdonald V, Double KL, Trent RJ, McCusker E. Regional specificity of brain atrophy in Huntington's disease. *Exp Neurol* 1998; **154**: 663–672.

Hansotia P, Wall R, Berendes J. Sleep disturbances and severity of Huntington's disease. *Neurology* 1985; **35**: 1672–1674.

Hardie RJ, Pullon HWH, Harding A, Owen JS, Pires M, Daniels GL, Imai Y, Misra VP, King RH, Jacobs JM, *et al*. Neuroacanthocytosis. A clinical, haematologic and pathological study of 19 cases. *Brain* 1991; **114**: 13–49.

Harper PS. Benign hereditary chorea—clinical and genetic aspects. *Clin Genet* 1978; **13**: 85–95.

Harris EC, Barraclough BM. Suicide as an outcome for medical disorders. *Medicine (Baltimore)* 1994; **73**: 281–296.

Harris GJ, Codori AM, Lewis RF, Schmidt E, Bedi A, Brandt J. Reduced basal ganglia blood flow and volume in pre-symptomatic, gene-tested persons at-risk for Huntington's disease. *Brain* 1999; **122**: 1667–1678.

Hayden MR. *Huntington's chorea*. London, Berlin, Heidelberg, Springer Verlag, 1981.

—— Hewitt J, Stoessel AJ, Clark C, Moennich D, Martin WR. The combined use of positron emission tomography and DNA polymorphisms for preclinical detection of Huntington's disease. *Neurology* 1987; **37**: 1441–1447.

Hefter H, Hömberg V, Lange HW, Freund HJ. Impairment of rapid movement in Huntington's disease. *Brain* 1987; **110**: 585–612.

Higgins JJ, Patterson MC, Papadopoulos NM, Brady RO, Pentchev PG, Barton NW. Hypoprebetalipoproteinemia, acanthocytosis, retinitis pigmentosa, and pallidal degeneration (HARP syndrome). *Neurology* 1992; **42**: 194–198.

Hille ET, Siesling S, Vegter-van der Vlis M, Vandenbroucke JP, Roos RA, Rosendaal FR. Two centuries of mortality in ten large families with Huntington disease: a rising impact of gene carriership. *Epidemiology* 1999; **10**: 706–710.

Höweler CJ, Busch HF, Geraedts JP, Niermeijer MF, Staal A. Anticipation in mytonic dystrophy: fact or fiction? *Brain* 1989; **112**: 779–797.

Huntington G. On chorea. *Med Surg Rep* 1872; **26**: 317–321.

Huntington's Disease Collaborative Research Group. A novel gene containing a trinucleotide repeat that is expanded and unstable on Huntington's disease chromosomes. *Cell* 1993; **72**: 971–983.

Huntington Study Group. Unified Huntington's Disease Rating Scale: reliability and consistency. *Movement Dis* 1996; **11**: 136–142.

Hutton M, Lendon CL, Rizzu P, Baker M, Froelich S, Houlden H, Pickering-Brown S, Chakraverty S, Isaacs A, Grover A, Hackett J, Adamson J, Lincoln S, Dickson D, Davies P, Petersen RC, Stevens M, de Graaff E, Wauters E, van Baren J, Hillebrand M, Joosse M, Kwon JM, Nowotny P, Heutink P, *et al*. Association of missense and 5'-splice-site mutations in tau with the inherited dementia FTDP-17. *Nature* 1998; **393**: 702–705.

Iizuka R, Hirayama K, Maehara K. Dentato-rubro-pallido-luysian atrophy: a clinico-pathological study. *J Neurol Neurosurg Psychiatry* 1984; **47**: 1288–1298.

James CM, Houlihan GD, Snell RG, Cheadle JP, Harper PS. Late-onset Huntington's disease: a clinical and molecular study. *Age Ageing* 1994; **23**: 445–448.

Jervis GA. Huntington's chorea in childhood. *Arch Neurol* 1963; **9**: 244–257.

Kambouris M, Bohlega S, Al-Tahan A, Meyer BF. Localization of the gene for a novel autosomal recessive neurodegenerative Huntington-like disorder to 4p15.3. *Am J Hum Genet* 2000; **66**: 445–452.

Kieburtz K, MacDonald M, Shih C, Feigin A, Steinberg K, Bordwell K, Zimmerman C, Srinidhi J, Sotack J, Gusella J, *et al*. Trinucleotide repeat length and progression of illness in Huntington's disease. *J Med Genet* 1994; **31**: 872–874.

Kirkwood SC, Siemers E, Hodes ME, Conneally PM, Christian JC, Foroud T. Subtle changes among presymptomatic carriers of the Huntington's disease gene. *J Neurol Neurosurg Psychiatry* 2000; **69**: 773–779.

Kirkwood SC, Su JL, Conneally P, Foroud T. Progression of symptoms in the early and middle stages of Huntington disease. *Arch Neurol* 2001; **58**: 273–278.

Koide R, Ikeuchi T, Onodera O. Unstable expansion of CAG repeat in hereditary dentatorubral-pallidoluysian atrophy (DRPLA). *Nat Genet* 1994; **6**: 9–13.

Koller WC, Trimble J. The gait abnormality of Huntington's disease. *Neurology* 1985; **35**: 1450–1454.

Kremer B, Squitieri F, Telenius H, Andrew SE, Theilmann J, Spence N, Goldberg YP, Hayden MR. Molecular analysis of late onset Huntington disease. *J Med Genet* 1993; **30**: 991–995.

—— Goldberg P, Andrew SE, Theilmann J, Telenius H, Zeisler J, Squitieri F, Lin B, Bassett A, Almqvist E, *et al*. A worldwide study of the Huntington's disease mutation. The sensitivity and specificity of measuring CAG repeats. *New Engl J Med* 1994; **330**: 1401–1406.

—— Clark CM, Almqvist EW, Raymond LA, Graf P, Jacova C, Mezei M, Hardy MA, Snow B, Martin W, Hayden MR. Influence of lamotrigine on progression of early Huntington disease: a randomized clinical trial. *Neurology* 1999; **53**: 1000–1011.

Lanska DJ, Lanska MJ, Lavine L, Schoenberg BS. Conditions associated with Huntington's disease at death. A case-control study. *Arch Neurol* 1988a; **45**: 878–80.

—— Lavine L, Lanska MJ, Schoenberg BS. Huntington's disease mortality in the United States. *Neurology* 1988b; **38**: 769–772.

Lasker AG, Zee DS, Hain TC, Folstein SE, Singer HS. Saccades in Huntington's disease: slowing and dysmetria. *Neurology* 1988; **38**: 427–431.

Lasker AG, Zee DS. Ocular motor abnormalities in Huntington's disease. *Vision Res* 1997; **37**: 3639–3645.

Lawrence AD, Hodges JR, Rosser AE, Kershaw A, ffrench-Constant C, Rubinsztein DC, Robbins TW, Sahakian BJ. Evidence for specific cognitive deficits in preclinical Huntington's disease. *Brain* 1998; **121**: 1329–1341.

Louis ED, Lee P, Quinn L, Marder K. Dystonia in Huntington's disease: prevalence and clinical characteristics. *Movement Dis* 1999; **14**: 95–101.

—— Anderson KE, Moskowitz C, Thorne DZ, Marder K. Dystonia-predominant adult-onset Huntington disease: association between motor phenotype and age of onset in adults. *Arch Neurol* 2000; **57**: 1326–1330.

MacDonald ME, Vonsattel JP, Shrinidhi J, Couropmitree NN, Cupples LA, Bird ED, Gusella JF, Myers RH. Evidence for the GluR6 gene associated with younger onset age of Huntington's disease. *Neurology* 1999; **53**: 1330–1332.

Marder K, Zhao H, Myers RH, Cudkowicz M, Kayson E, Kieburtz K, Orme C, Paulsen J, Penney JB Jr, Siemers E, Shoulson I. Rate of functional decline in Huntington's disease. Huntington Study Group. *Neurology* 2000; **54**: 452–458.

Markham CH, Knox JW. Observations on Huntington's chorea in childhood. *J Pediatr* 1965; **67**: 46–57.

Mars H, Lewis LA, Robertson AL, Butkus A, Williams GH Jr. Familial hypobetalipoproteinemia—a genetic disorder of lipid metabolism with nervous system involvement. *Am J Med Genet* 1969; **46**: 886–900.

Martin WR, Hoskinson M, Kremer B, Maguire C, McEwan A. Functional caudate imaging in symptomatic Huntington's disease: positron emission tomography versus single-photon emission computed tomography. *J Neuroimaging* 1995; **5**: 227–232.

Mateo D, Munoz BJ, Gimenez RS. Neuroleptic malignant syndrome related to tetrabenazine introduction and haloperidol discontinuation in Huntington's disease. *Clin Neuropharmacol* 1992; **15**: 63–68.

Mayeux R, Stern Y, Herman A, Greenbaum L, Fahn S. Correlates of early disability in Huntington's disease. *Ann Neurol* 1986; **20**: 727–731.

McCusker EA, Casse RF, Graham SJ, Williams DB, Lazarus R. Prevalence of Huntington disease in New South Wales in 1996. *Med J Australia* 2000a; **173**: 187–190.

McCusker E, Richards F, Sillence D, Wilson M, Trent RJ. Huntington's disease: neurological assessment of potential gene carriers presenting for predictive DNA testing. *J Clin Neurosci* 2000b; **7**: 38–41.

Morales LM, Estëvez J, Suarez H, Villalobos R, Chacin de Bonilla L, Bonilla E. Nutritional evaluation of Huntington disease patients. *Am J Clin Nutrition* 1989; **50**: 145–150.

Murphy TK, Goodman WK, Ayoub EM, Voeller KK.On defining Sydenham's chorea: where do we draw the line? *Biol Psychiatry* 2000; **47**: 851–857.

Myers RH, Schoenfeld M, Bird ED, Wolf PA, Vonsattel JP, White RF, Martin JB. Late onset of Huntington's disease. *J Neurol Neurosurg Psychiatry* 1985; **48**: 530–534.

—— Sax DS, Koroshetz WJ, Mastromauro C, Cupples LA, Kiely DK, Pettengill FK, Bird ED. Factors associated with slow progression in Huntington's disease. *Arch Neurol* 1991; **48**: 800–804.

Nagafuchi S, Yanagisawa H, Sato K, Shirayama T, Ohsaki E, Bundo M, Takeda T, Tadokoro K, Kondo I, Murayama N, *et al*. Dentatorubral and pallidoluysian atrophy: expansion of an unstable CAG trinucleotide on chromosome 12p. *Nat Genet* 1994; **6**: 14–18.

Naito H, Oyanagi S. Familial myoclonus epilepsy and choreoathetosis: hereditary dentatorubral-pallidoluysian atrophy. *Neurology* 1982; **32**: 798–807.

Nance MA, Sanders G. Characteristics of individuals with Huntington disease in long-term care. *Movement Dis* 1996; **11**: 542–548.

—— Mathias-Hagen V, Breningstall G, Wick MJ, McGlennen RC. Analysis of a very large trinucleotide repeat in a patient with juvenile Huntington's disease. *Neurology* 1999; **52**: 392–394.

Newcombe RG. A life table for onset of Huntington's chorea. *Ann Hum Genet* 1981; **45**: 375–385.

Oepen G, Clarenbach P, Thoden U. Disturbance of eye movements in Huntington's chorea. *Arch Psychiatrie Nervenkr* 1981; **229**: 205–213.

Oliver J, Dewhurst K. Childhood and adolescent forms of Huntington's disease. *J Neurol Neurosurg Psychiatry* 1969; **32**: 455–459.

Osborne JP, Munson P, Burman D. Huntington's chorea. Report of 3 cases and review of the literature. *Arch Dis Child* 1982; **57**: 99–103.

Ossemann M, Sindic CJ, Laterre C. Tetrabenazine as a cause of neuroleptic malignant syndrome. *Movement Dis* 1996; **11**: 95.

Padberg G, Bruyn GW. Chorea—differential diagnosis. In: *Handbook of clinical neurology*, revised series, Vol 5 (49). *Extrapyramidal disorders* (ed. PJ Vincken, GW Bruyn, and HL Klawans), pp. 549–564. Amsterdam: Elsevier: 1986.

Penney JB, Jr, Young AB, Shoulson I, Starosta-Rubenstein S, Snodgrass SR, Sanchez-Ramos J, Ramos-Arroyo M, Gomez F, Penchaszadeh G, Alvir J, *et al*. Huntington's disease in Venezuela: 7 years of follow-up on symptomatic and asymptomatic individuals. *Movement Dis* 1990; **5**: 93–99.

—— Vonsattel JP, MacDonald ME, Gusella JF, Myers RH. CAG repeat number governs the development rate of pathology in Huntington's disease. *Ann Neurol* 1997; **41**: 689–692.

Persichetti F, Srinidhi J, Kanaley L, Ge P, Myers RH, D'Arrigo K, Barnes GT, MacDonald ME, Vonsattel JP, Gusella JF, *et al*. Huntington's disease CAG trinucleotide repeats in pathologically confirmed post-mortem brains. *Neurobiol Dis* 1994; **1**: 159–166.

Phillips JG, Bradshaw JL, Chiu E, Teasdale N, Iansek R, Bradshaw JA. Bradykinesia and movement precision in Huntington's disease. *Neuropsychologia* 1996; **34**: 1241–1245.

Pincus JH, Chutorian A. Familial benign chorea with intention tremor: a clinical entity. *J Pediatr* 1967; **70**: 724–729.

Podoll K, Caspary P, Lange HW, Noth J. Language functions in Huntington's disease. *Brain* 1988; **111**: 1475–1503.

Pratley RE, Salbe AD, Ravussin E, Caviness JN. Higher sedentary energy expenditure in patients with Huntington's disease. *Ann Neurol* 2000; **47**: 64–70.

Pridmore SA. Age of onset of Huntington's disease in Tasmania. *Med J Australia* 1990a; **153**: 135–137.

Pridmore SA. Age of death and duration in Huntington's disease in Tasmania. *Med J Australia* 1990b; **153**: 137–139.

Quarrell OWJ, Youngman S, Sarfarazi M, Harper PS. Absence of close linkage between benign hereditary chorea and the locus D4510. *J Med Genet* 1988; **25**: 191–194.

Raskind WH, Bolin T, Wolff J, Fink J, Matsushita M, Litt M, Lipe H, Bird TD. Further localization of a gene for paroxysmal dystonic choreoathetosis to a 5-cM region on chromosome 2q34. *Hum Genet* 1998; **102**: 93–97.

Rasmussen A, Macias R, Yescas P, Ochoa A, Davila G, Alonso E. Huntington disease in children: genotype–phenotype correlation. *Neuropediatrics* 2000; **31**: 190–194.

Reuter I, Hu MT, Andrews TC, Brooks DJ, Clough C, Chaudhuri KR. Late onset levodopa responsive Huntington's disease with minimal chorea masquerading as Parkinson plus syndrome. *J Neurol Neurosurg Psychiatry* 2000; **68**: 238–241.

Rinne JO, Daniel SE, Scaravilli F, Pires M, Harding AE, Marsden CD. The neuropathological features of neuroacanthocytosis. *Movement Dis* 1994; **9**: 297–304.

Roos RA, Hermans J, Vegter-van der Vlis M, van Ommen GJ, Bruyn GW. Duration of illness in Huntington's disease is not related to age at onset. *J Neurol Neurosurg Psychiatry* 1993; **56**: 98–100.

Rubinsztein DC, Leggo J, Chiano M, *et al*. Genotypes at the GluR6 kainate receptor locus are associated with variation in the age of onset of Huntington disease. *Proc Nat Acad Sci USA* 1997; **94**: 3872–3876.

Rubio JP, Danek A, Stone C, Chalmers R, Wood N, Verellen C, Ferrer X, Malandrini A, Fabrizi GM, Manfredi M, Vance J, Pericak-Vance M, Brown R, Rudolf G, Picard F, Alonso E, Brin M, Nemeth AH, Farrall M, Monaco AP. Chorea-acanthocytosis: genetic linkage to chromosome 9q21. *Am J Hum Genet* 1997; **61**: 899–908.

—— Levy ER, Dobson-Stone C, Monaco AP. Genomic organization of the human galpha14 and Galphaq genes and mutation analysis in chorea-acanthocytosis (CHAC). *Genomics* 1999; **57**: 84–93.

Sanberg PR, Fibiger HC, Mark RF. Body weight and dietary factors in Huntington's disease patients compared with matched controls. *Med J Australia* 1981; **1**: 407–409.

Sanchez A, Castellvi-Bel S, Mila M, Genis D, Calopa M, Jimenez D, Estivill X. Huntington's disease: confirmation of diagnosis and presymptomatic testing in Spanish families by genetic analysis. *J Neurol Neurosurg Psychiatry* 1996; **61**: 625–627.

Schwarz M, Fellows SJ, Schaffrath C, Noth J. Deficits in sensorimotor control during precise hand movements in Huntington's disease. *Clin Neurophysiol* 2001; **112**: 95–106.

Shinotoh H, Calne DB, Snow B, Hayward M, Kremer B, Theilmann J, Hayden MR. Normal CAG repeat length in the Huntington's disease gene in senile chorea. *Neurology* 1994; **44**: 2183–2184.

Shoulson I. Huntington disease: functional capacities in patients treated with neuroleptic and antidepressant drugs. *Neurology* 1981; **31**: 1333–1335.

—— Fahn S. Huntington disease: clinical care and evaluation. *Neurology* 1979; **29**: 1–3.

—— Odoroff C, Oakes D, Behr J, Goldblatt D, Caine E, Kennedy J, Miller C, Bamford K, Rubin A, *et al*. A controlled clinical trial of baclofen as protective therapy in early Huntington's disease. *Ann Neurol* 1989; **25**: 252–259.

Sieradzan K, Mann DM, Dodge A. Clinical presentation and patterns of regional cerebral atrophy related to the length of trinucleotide repeat expansion in patients with adult onset Huntington's disease. *Neurosci Lett* 1997; **225**: 45–48.

Silvestri R, Raffaele M, De Domenico P, Tisano A, Mento G, Casella C, Tripoli MC, Serra S, Di Perri R. Sleep features in Tourette's syndrome, neuroacanthocytosis and Huntington's chorea. *Neurophysiol Clin* 1995; **25**: 66–77.

Snell RG, MacMillan JC, Cheadle JP *et al*. Relationship between trinucleotide repeat expansion and phenotypic variation in Huntington's disease. *Nat Genet* 1993; **4**: 393–397.

Snowden JS, Craufurd D, Griffiths HL, Neary D. Awareness of involuntary movements in Huntington disease. *Arch Neurol* 1998; **55**: 801–805.

Swaiman KF. Hallervorden–Spatz syndrome and brain iron metabolism. *Arch Neurol* 1991; **48**: 1285–1293.

Telenius H, Kremer HP, Theilmann J, Andrew SE, Almqvist E, Anvret M, Greenberg C, Greenberg J, Lucotte G, Squitieri F, *et al*. Molecular analysis of juvenile Huntington disease: the major influence on (CAG)n repeat length is the sex of the affected parent. *Hum Mol Genet* 1993; **2**: 1535–1540.

Thompson PD, Berardelli A, Rothwell JC, Day BL, Dick JP, Benecke R, Marsden CD. The coexistence of bradykinesia and chorea in Huntington's disease and its implications for theories of basal ganglia control of movement. *Brain* 1988; **111**: 223–244.

Tian JR, Zee DS, Lasker AG, Folstein SE. Saccades in Huntington's disease: predictive tracking and interaction between release of fixation and initiation of saccades. *Neurology* 1991; **41**: 875–881.

Tomita H, Nagamitsu S, Wakui K, Fukushima Y, Yamada K, Sadamatsu M, Masui A, Konishi T, Matsuishi T, Aihara M, Shimizu K, Hashimoto K, Mineta M, Matsushima M, Tsujita T, Saito M, Tanaka H, Tsuji S, Takagi T, Nakamura Y, Nanko S, Kato N, Nakane Y, Niikawa N. Paroxysmal kinesigenic choreoathetosis locus maps to chromosome 16p11.2–q12.1. *Am J Hum Genet* 1999; **65**: 1688–1697.

Truong DD, Harding AE, Scaravilli F, Smith SJ, Morgan-Hughes JA, Marsden CD. Movement disorders in mitochondrial myopathies. A study of nine cases with two autopsy studies. *Movement Dis* 1990; **5**: 109–117.

Tsuang D, Almqvist EW, Lipe H, Strgar F, DiGiacomo L, Hoff D, Eugenio C, Hayden MR, Bird TD. Familial aggregation of psychotic symptoms in Huntington's disease. *Am J Psychiatry* 2000; **157**: 1955–1959.

Vance JM, Pericak-Vance MA, Bowman MH, Payne CS, Fredane L, Siddique T, Roses AD, Massey EW. Chorea-acanthocytosis: a report of three new families and implications for genetic counselling. *Am J Med Genet* 1987; **28**: 403–410.

Van Vugt JP, van Hilten BJ, Roos RA. Hypokinesia in Huntington's disease. *Movement Dis* 1996; **11**: 384–388.

Vogel CM, Drury I, Terry LC, Young AB. Myoclonus in adult Huntington's disease. *Ann Neurol* 1991; **29**: 213–215.

Vonsattel JP, Myers RH, Stevens TJ, Ferrante RJ, Bird ED, Richardson EP Jr. Neuropathological classification of Huntington's disease. *J Neuropathol Exp Neurol* 1985; **44**: 559–577.

Warner TT, Lennox GG, Janota I, Harding AE. Autosomal-dominant dentatorubropallidoluysian atrophy in the United Kingdom. *Movement Dis* 1994; **9**: 289–296.

Weigell-Weber M, Schmid W, Spiegel R. Psychiatric symptoms and CAG expansion in Huntington's disease. *Am J Med Genet* 1996; **67**: 53–57.

Westphal CFO. Über eine dem Bilde der cerebrospinalen grauen Degeneration ähnliche Erkrankung des centralen Nervensystems ohne anatomischen Befund, nebst einigen Bemerkungen über paradoxe Contraction. *Arch Psychiatrie Nervenkr* 1883; **14**: 87–95 and 767–773.

Wheeler JS, Sax DS, Krane RJ, Siroky MB. Vesico-urethral function in Huntington's chorea. *Br J Urol* 1985; **57**: 63–66.

Wiegand M, Moller AA, Lauer CJ, Stolz S, Schreiber W, Dose M, Krieg JC. Nocturnal sleep in Huntington's disease. *J Neurol* 1991; **238**: 203–208.

Wilhelmsen KC. Disinhibition–dementia–parkinsonism–amyotrophy complex (DDPAC) is a non-Alzheimer's frontotemporal dementia. *J Neural Transm Suppl* 1997; **49**: 269–75.

Woldag H, Strenge S, Weise K. Diagnostic problems in juvenile Huntington chorea. *Nervenarzt* 1997; **68**: 667–670.

Xiang F, Almqvist EW, Huq M, Lundin A, Hayden MR, Edstrom L, Anvret M, Zhang Z. A Huntington disease-like neurodegenerative disorder maps to chromosome 20p. *Am J Hum Genet* 1998; **63**: 1431–1438.

Xuereb JH, MacMillan JC, Snell R, Davies P, Harper PS. Neuropathological diagnosis and CAG repeat expansion in Huntington's disease. *J Neurol Neurosurg Psychiatry* 1996; **60**: 78–81.

Young AB, Shoulson I, Penney JB, Starosta-Rubinstein S, Gomez F, Travers H, Ramos-Arroyo MA, Snodgrass SR, Bonilla E, Moreno H, *et al.* Huntington's disease in Venezuela: neurologic features and functional decline. *Neurology* 1986; **36**: 244–249.

3 Neuropsychological and neuropsychiatric aspects of Huntington's disease

David Craufurd and Julie Snowden

General introduction

Huntington's disease (HD) is characterized by a triad of motor, cognitive, and psychiatric symptoms. Although the motor symptoms are most immediately evident, there is little doubt that it is the non-motor symptoms that have greatest impact on patients' daily lives and contribute most to patients' loss of independence.

The cognitive changes in HD have traditionally been referred to as a dementia. This is an appropriate descriptor when used purely to denote that changes (1) are progressive and (2) encompass more than one area of cognitive function. Nevertheless, the dementia label has led to considerable misunderstanding of HD. Historically, the term has carried the notion of a generalized intellectual impairment affecting all aspects of cognition in a diffuse, undifferentiated way. This is not an accurate portrayal of degenerative brain disorders in general; it is particularly inaccurate in the case of HD. People with HD have specific and characteristic cognitive difficulties, with other aspects of cognitive function remaining well preserved, a point often argued vociferously by patients' relatives. This chapter aims to characterize the nature of those impairments.

The importance of psychiatric aspects of HD has been recognized since the time of Huntington. In his original description of the disease Huntington (1872) wrote that '. . . In all the families, or nearly all in which the choreic taint exists, the nervous temperament greatly predominates, and . . . nervous excitement in a marked degree almost invariably attends upon every disease these people may suffer from . . . The tendency to insanity, and sometimes that form of insanity which leads to suicide, is marked.' However, the psychiatric symptoms associated with HD are more variable than the motor and cognitive changes, and do not follow the same progressive course. We describe the principal neuropsychiatric features. Problem behaviours in HD are influenced by cognitive and psychiatric as well psychosocial changes. We conclude the chapter with a consideration of the biological and non-biological factors that underpin the behavioural problems of HD.

Cognitive changes in HD

Overview

Cognitive changes are an invariable feature of HD; they are present early in the course of the disease (Butters *et al.* 1978; Brandt and Butters 1986) and become more severe as the disease progresses. Although an intrinsic part of HD, cognitive changes vary in severity. In some affected individuals impairments are readily apparent to family members and are evident at clinical interview. In other people changes are subtle and detected only on formal neuropsychological examination.

In the past it was assumed that, whereas the motor changes in HD reflected striatal dysfunction, the cognitive changes resulted from independent (and generally later) pathological changes in the neocortex. It is now recognized that many of the cognitive changes in HD stem from disruption to striatal–frontal circuits, and that cognitive and as well as motor changes can be ascribed to striatal pathology. Cognitive deficits lie particularly in the realm of executive functions, which include the abilities to plan, organize, and monitor behaviour, to show mental flexibility, and to switch from one way of responding to another (mental set shifting) (Brandt and Butters 1986; Brandt 1991). In addition, procedural memory and psychomotor skills are impaired. Primary tools of cognition, such as language, that are dependent on neocortical function are relatively preserved.

It should be said that, although deficits in HD are circumscribed, those deficits may have a secondary impact on performance across a wide range of cognitive tasks. A problem in monitoring performance might lead to errors, for example, on a dot-counting task, even though the spatial requirements for carrying out that task are not primarily affected. Similarly, psychomotor slowing may result in poorer than normal scores on, for example, a timed naming test, even though language skills themselves are not primarily disordered. This is an important conceptual point; neuropsychological tests do not always measure what the task intends them to measure and identical test scores may reflect different underlying deficits. It is the literal interpretation of scores that has in the past reinforced the misconception of cognitive change in HD as a global impairment. Typically, qualitative characteristics and performance profiles across tasks provide clues to the underlying difficulty, and enable HD to be distinguished from cortical dementias such as Alzheimer's disease (Brandt *et al.* 1988). Profile differences between HD and Alzheimer's disease have been demonstrated at all stages of disease (Paulsen *et al.* 1995a), indicating that, even in the advanced stages, cognitive impairment is not global.

Executive function

Executive function is a generic term that encompasses diverse functions relating to the regulation or control of cognitive performance (Fig. 3.1). In non-neurologically impaired individuals, most behaviour is planned and goal-directed. Actions are organized and carried out in an efficient sequence. People attend to what is relevant, ignore what is not relevant, and shift attention when necessary. They can abstract pertinent information from a conversation or situation and integrate it with their own prior experience. They can monitor performance in relation to the intended goal and self-correct errors. They also have the flexibility to change goal if external circumstances change. It is in these domains of function, which are highly dependent upon the frontal lobes and frontostriatal circuits, that impairments in HD are most prominent.

In their daily lives, people with HD often exhibit poor planning and judgement. They may appear impulsive and show an absence of forethought, their actions being governed by immediate rather than long-term considerations. Actions are disorganized, a feature that contributes to early occupational and domestic inefficiency. People with HD have difficulty coping with multiple tasks simultaneously, suggesting difficulty in the allocation and switching of attention. Difficulty with simultaneous tasks may extend to ostensibly nondemanding activities

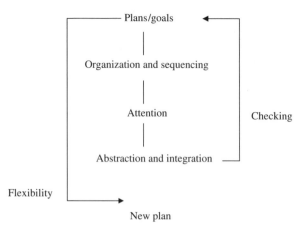

Fig. 3.1 Schematic representation of executive functions. Deficits are present in HD, demonstrable by clinical history and neuropsychological evaluation.

such as talking and walking. HD patients are often noted to stop walking in order to answer a question. Such activities appear to require more conscious attention in HD patients than they do in neurologically intact individuals, suggesting that overload of attentional resources may contribute to the multiple-task difficulty. People with HD show impaired ability to self-monitor and often fail to notice errors that are apparent to others, sometimes creating a false impression of a lackadaisical attitude or indolence. People with HD are often reported by relatives to be inflexible, rigid in their thinking, with difficulty seeing another's point of view. They are poorly adaptable to altered circumstances and may prefer routine.

A substantial body of empirical neuropsychological evidence has accumulated to support these clinical observations of executive deficits in HD. Several investigators (Lange *et al.* 1995; Lawrence *et al.* 1996; Watkins *et al.* 2000) have demonstrated impaired planning, on the basis of patients' poor performance on a problem-solving task (Tower of London) that requires the ability to plan a sequence of actions. Impaired sequencing has been demonstrated on a picture-ordering task (Snowden *et al.* 2000). Sprengelmeyer *et al.* (1995) demonstrated impairments in several aspects of attention, including self-generated maintenance of attention, simultaneous monitoring of different input channels, response suppression, and shifting of attention. Impairments have been demonstrated on tasks (Georgiou *et al.* 1995; Cope *et al.* 1996) in which the subject is required to shift and direct attention away from naturally expected stimulus–response linkages and inhibit a prepotent response. A number of studies have demonstrated impaired cognitive flexibility and difficulty in shifting attentional set. Studies have used the Wisconsin Card Sorting test (Josiassen *et al.* 1983; Weinberger *et al.* 1988; Pillon *et al.* 1991; Paulsen *et al.* 1995b), a computer analogue of the Card Sort test (Lange *et al.* 1995; Lawrence *et al.* 1996), or other related tasks (Hanes *et al.* 1995). HD patients have been found to show impairment on a spatial working memory task (Lawrence *et al.* 1996) that requires the subject to plan, to hold information 'on line', and to use feedback from earlier trials to guide subsequent responses. HD patients show poor use of strategy and, as in the Card Sorting test people, do not make effective use of feedback. People with HD typically perform poorly on verbal fluency tasks, involving generation of words belonging to a specified category or beginning with a specified letter (Butters *et al.* 1978; Monsch *et al.* 1994; Rosser and Hodges 1994; Rich *et al.* 1999; Rohrer *et al.* 1999). Impairments have been attributed to defective strategies for retrieval (Rosser and Hodges 1994) and impaired ability to switch search strategies (Rich *et al.* 1999) secondary to patients' reduced cognitive flexibility.

Executive deficits and striatal change
A number of studies have shown a relationship between patients' performance on executive tasks and changes in the striatum, measured by structural or functional brain imaging. Folstein *et al.* (1992) showed a correlation between attention, sequencing, and sustaining thoughts and atrophy of the caudate. Backman *et al.* (1997) used positron emission tomography (PET) and magnetic resonance imaging (MRI) data as predictors of performance on executive, as well as spatial, memory, fluency, perceptual speed, and reasoning tasks. Dopamine neurotransmission parameters (D1 and D2 receptor density and dopamine transporter density) and volumetric measurements for caudate and putamen accounted for substantial portions of the variance across the majority of tasks. Lawrence *et al.* (1998a) found that performance on executive tasks, including verbal fluency, spatial span, planning, and sequence generation, correlated with PET measures of striatal D1 and D2 receptor binding levels. These findings are consistent with the view that executive deficits in HD result from pathological changes in frontostriatal circuitry.

Psychomotor function

The executive deficits seen in HD bear similarities to those seen in frontal neocortical disorders, such as frontotemporal dementia (Neary *et al.* 1988). A feature that distinguishes the primarily subcortical disorder of HD from cortical degenerative disease is rate of performance. Psychomotor slowing is a distinguishing feature of subcortical forms of dementia (Albert *et al.* 1974; Dubois *et al.* 1988) and it is prominent in HD. Slowing is most frequently demonstrated by clinical tests, such as the Stroop, Digit symbol substitution, and Trail making tests (Bamford *et al.* 1989; Starkstein *et al.* 1992; Snowden *et al.* 2000). It has also been demonstrated by experimental studies of simple and choice reaction time (Jahanshahi *et al.* 1993). Although in many time-based tasks cognitive and motor speed are compounded, cognitive slowing is present even when motor speed is controlled (Snowden *et al.* 2000). Cognitive slowing is likely to contribute to HD patients' impaired performance in a variety of timed tasks including verbal fluency (Rohrer *et al.* 1999). Psychomotor speed has been shown to correlate with measures of caudate atrophy (Bamford *et al.* 1989; Starkstein *et al.* 1992).

Language

HD patients are not aphasic. They understand words and speak in grammatically correct sentences. In general conversation they do not typically show word-finding difficulties, nor do they make paraphasic errors. These features distinguish HD from cortical degenerative disorders, such as Alzheimer's disease, in which linguistic deficits are prominent. Even in advanced disease HD patients produce sentences that are syntactically correct, albeit simplified in grammatical structure (Podoll *et al.* 1988).

Performance on language tasks is not, however, invariably normal. In the later stages of disease patients may show increasing difficulty following complex instructions (Folstein and McHugh 1983). On picture-naming tests HD patients have been found to be slower than normal to produce the correct name (Bayles and Tomoeda 1983; Caine *et al.* 1986; Hodges *et al.* 1991), and they make more errors. On word generation tests, involving production of exemplars of a specified category or words beginning with a specified letter, they produce fewer words (Rich *et al.* 1999; Rohrer *et al.* 1999). Nevertheless, deficits are generally attributable to factors that are not primarily linguistic and that reflect patients' executive impairments or other cognitive deficits. Picture-naming errors are commonly visually based (Bayles and Tomoeda 1983; Podoll *et al.* 1988; Hodges *et al.* 1991), suggesting misperception of stimulus material. Rohrer *et al.* (1999) ascribed poor category fluency to slowed retrieval. Rich *et al.* (1999) attributed poor fluency performance to impaired ability to switch search strategies, reflecting patients' reduced cognitive flexibility. It is likely that attentional demands and the requirement for active mental effort play a role in accounting for the difficulty of patients in the advanced stages of illness to assimilate complex utterances.

Language, which is relatively preserved in HD, needs to be distinguished from speech, which is impaired. Communication is increasingly compromised in HD patients as a result of problems in motor production of speech (Gordon and Illes 1987; Podoll *et al.* 1988). Patients exhibit articulatory and prosodic impairments, leading to increasing unintelligibility over the course of the disease. Dysarthria may be present even in early-stage disease. People with HD often become taciturn, a feature that may be a consequence of the mental effort required for discourse and the apathy associated with advancing disease (Folstein and McHugh 1983).

Perceptual and spatial skills

In their daily lives HD patients recognize objects, do not have difficulty locating objects in their visual field, and are spatially oriented in their external surroundings. They do not exhibit the frank misperceptions, impaired localization skills, and gross spatial disorientation that are common features of Alzheimer's disease in which there is severe involvement of temporoparietal neocortex. People with HD do, however, perform poorly on some perceptual, spatial, and visuoconstructional tasks, indicating that at least some aspects of perception and spatial functioning are compromised.

Within the perceptual domain, impairments have been demonstrated most commonly on perceptual matching and discrimination tasks (Brouwers *et al.* 1984; Lawrence *et al.* 1996), on the Hooper test of perceptual integration (Bamford *et al.* 1989; Gomez Tortosa *et al.* 1996), and on tests of face perception and facial affect (Jacobs *et al.* 1995; Sprengelmeyer *et al.* 1996). What these tasks have in common is that they are relatively high-level tasks that require attention to multiple parts of the stimulus or involve complex visual integration and manipulation of information. That is, they make significant executive demands. Performance has also been found to be impaired on visuoconstructional tasks, such as drawing (Rouleau *et al.* 1992) and block design (Bamford *et al.* 1989), tasks that also require planning and organization.

In the spatial domain there is converging evidence that people with HD have deficits in personal or 'egocentric' space but not extrapersonal space. Potegal (1971) showed that HD patients demonstrated normal localization in external space, except when their own position in relation to the target had been altered, suggesting defective manipulation of personal space. Impaired performance in HD has commonly been demonstrated on a road map test (Brouwers *et al.* 1984; Bylsma *et al.* 1992; Mohr *et al.* 1991, 1997). Subjects track a dotted line through a diagrammatic road map and, at each turn on the map, state whether they would be turning left or right. It is on turns that require the subject to make 90° or 180° mental manipulations that performance is notably impaired (Brouwers *et al.* 1984). Deficits have also been reported on a mental rotation test that requires the subject to mentally rotate complex geometric patterns represented three-dimensionally and to compare them with a target design (Mohr *et al.* 1997). Thus, it is on tasks that require manipulation of egocentric space that performance is impaired. By contrast, performance on tasks involving extrapersonal orientation has been shown to be preserved (Bylsma *et al.* 1992; Brouwers *et al.* 1984). This pattern of findings is in direct contrast to that found in Alzheimer's disease (Brouwers *et al.* 1984), in which tasks involving extrapersonal perception and construction are particularly impaired. The findings indicate that there are different components of spatial processing. It is in the domain of person-centred space, in which mental manipulation of information is required, that performance in HD is particularly compromised. Deficits have typically been ascribed to striatal pathology or damage to frontostriatal pathways (Potega 1971; Bylsma *et al.* 1992). Potegal (1971) argued that the caudate may play a role in updating the perceived position in space to compensate for self-induced movements.

Memory

Memory problems are a ubiquitous feature of HD, present early in the course of the disease, and are often noted by patients themselves. Indeed, if HD patients are probed about cognitive symptoms, it is in the realm of memory and concentration that they most commonly report a subjective change. Symptoms typically have the quality of absent-mindedness, such as forgetting to turn off the gas after cooking or forgetting to pick the children up from school at the appointed time. Those same patients may demonstrate impressive recall of a news item that caught their interest or of a remark made by the clinician more than a year ago. That is, people with HD have inefficient memories, but they are not amnesic in the classical sense of having a fundamental inability to lay down new memories and retain information over time.

A variety of empirical studies have confirmed that memory failures in HD arise largely because of strategic or organizational failures at the time that information is acquired and retrieved, and not because of a primary disorder of retention. Several investigators have shown that recognition memory performance is less impaired than free recall (Butters *et al.* 1985, 1994; Lundervold *et al.* 1994; Pillon *et al.* 1993). HD patients have been shown to demonstrate poor acquisition of information and more use of passive learning strategy than controls, but normal retention over time (Lundervold *et al.* 1994). A comparative study by Pillon *et al.* (1993) showed that HD patients performed as poorly as patients with Alzheimer's disease on free recall of items in a list-learning task, but significantly better with cued recall.

A parallel study of our own used a paired associated learning task, involving unrelated word pairs (for example, gold–sugar; friend–train). Whereas recall improved over successive trials in controls (Fig. 3.2), neither the HD nor the Alzheimer group demonstrated improvement. However, when patients were actively encouraged to form an associative link between words (for example, imagine a gold bar in a bowl of sugar; imagine a friend getting off a train), recall improved dramatically in HD but showed no change in Alzheimer's disease. The data suggest that HD patients do not spontaneously adopt active strategies for learning, such as mentally linking words, but, when such strategies are provided, then performance can improve.

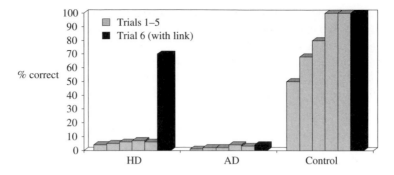

Fig. 3.2 Paired-associate learning in HD, Alzheimer's disease (AD), and controls. HD patients improve after provision of a strategy for learning (trial 6); AD patients do not.

The quality of memory change in HD, characterized by poor use of active strategies for learning and information retrieval, is similar to that found in patients with frontal lobe disease, and suggests disruption in striatal–frontal connections. Complementing these findings, Brandt *et al.* (1995) identified impairments in source memory in HD. Patients recalled facts as well as controls, but they had more difficulty in attributing the source of those facts, a pattern similar to that found in patients with frontal lobe disease. Correlation with MRI volumetric measures of caudate suggested that caudate or its neocortical projections played a role in the encoding of context.

Semantic memory

Semantic memory refers to a person's store of facts and knowledge about the world. It includes knowledge of the meanings of words and objects, as well as encyclopaedic knowledge, such as knowing that Paris is the capital of France. Loss of such conceptual knowledge is predominantly associated with damage to temporal neocortices, and is a feature of cortical dementias. By contrast, semantic memory loss is not a notable clinical feature of HD. Indeed, normally taciturn HD patients may surprise their family by their impressive demonstration of factual knowledge when watching television quiz programmes. Performance on putative tests of semantic knowledge such as picture-naming and word generation may be impaired (Hodges *et al.* 1991; Rich *et al.* 1999; Rohrer *et al.* 1999). However, performance failures typically arise for reasons that are not primarily semantic. HD patients may show poor mental effort and poor use of strategy for accessing information. Factual information may potentially be available, but executive problems lead to inefficient information retrieval.

Skill learning and priming

Conventional memory tests, such as list-learning or paired-associative tasks, require explicit recall or recognition of information (declarative memory). However, some aspects of learning, such as acquisition of a new motor skill or procedure, are not dependent upon explicit recall (procedural or nondeclarative memory). Patients with classical amnesia may demonstrate as much improvement as control subjects over successive trials on a mirror-writing task, even though they have no explicit memory for earlier attempts at the task. This dissociation between learning a skill and explicit recall of learning episodes suggests that nondeclarative and declarative aspects of memory depend upon different brain regions. The basal ganglia appear to play an important role in some but not all aspects of nondeclarative memory, and HD patients show impairment on some but not all nondeclarative tasks.

Impairments have most commonly been demonstrated on tasks involving motor skill learning. HD patients have, for example, shown impairment on a rotary pursuit task (Heindel *et al.* 1988; Gabrieli *et al.* 1997) that involves tracking a rotating target with a stylus and on a serial reaction-time task (Knopman and Nissen 1991). By contrast, normal performance has been demonstrated on a non-motor skill learning task, involving the learning of an artificial grammar (Knowlton *et al.* 1996). Moreover, perceptual priming tasks are typically performed normally. In these tasks, the subject's response to a stimulus (for example, a degraded letter, word, or picture) is 'primed' by earlier exposure to the same or a related stimulus (for example, the complete letter, word, or picture). Under normal circumstances, performance is facilitated, in terms of speed and accuracy of identification, in a primed compared to a nonprimed condition. This is the case too in patients with classical amnesia, who are able to derive benefit from prior exposure to a stimulus (and therefore must have some implicit memory of it), even though they have no explicit recollection of the earlier exposure. Patients with HD also show normal facilitation (Heindel *et al.* 1990; Bylsma *et al.* 1991). They can recognize a fragmented picture more easily when the complete picture has been presented in an earlier unrelated naming test (Heindel *et al.* 1990). HD patients have, however, shown abnormal priming on a weight judgement task. In normal subjects weight judgements are biased by earlier handling of heavy or light weights. HD patients do not show the normal bias (Heindel *et al.* 1991).

The foregoing conveys the impression that it is the motor nature of the task that determines whether HD patients show abnormal performance on skill learning and priming tasks. However, that is an oversimplification. HD patients have demonstrated normal mirror-tracing performance (Gabrieli *et al.* 1997), suggesting that some motor skills can be learned normally. Moreover, Knowlton *et al.* 1996 demonstrated impaired performance in HD on a probabilistic classification learning task, suggesting that some non-motor skill learning is impaired. Willingham and Koroshetz (1993) and Willingham *et al.* (1996) have helped to clarify the core factors that determine success or failure. They noted differential impairment in motor skill acquisition across different tasks. Some motor skills depend on learning to map a perceptual cue with an appropriate motor response (perceptual–motor integration). For example, in learning to use a computer mouse it is necessary to map a movement of the cursor in the coronal plane to an appropriate hand movement in the horizontal plane. It is not dependent upon a particular sequence of stimuli or movements. By contrast, other tasks, such as the rotary pursuit task, involve the learning of a repeated sequence of movements. Willingham and colleagues noted that people with HD have difficulty on the latter but not the former tasks. Patients showed no difficulty, for example, learning to track a moving target on computer with a joystick (Willingham *et al.* 1996), provided that the target moved randomly. However, they were impaired relative to normal when the target moved in a repeated sequence. Willingham *et al.* emphasized that performance was not governed by subjects' awareness of the sequence, since it was immediately evident. The findings suggest that the striatum plays a role when participants learn a repeating sequence of movements, but does not contribute when they learn a new mapping between perceptual cues and the appropriate motor response (perceptual–motor integration task). Knowlton *et al.* interpreted their patients' poor performance on a non-motor skill learning task in parallel terms, suggesting that their task was akin to a habit-learning task and thus dependent upon the striatum.

The data suggest that it is in the domain of cognitive and motor routines, involving a repetitive sequence of actions, that learning in HD is particularly impaired. Snowden *et al.* (2000) have highlighted the breakdown of cognitive and motor routines as a prominent feature in the evolution of HD. These authors have also identified subtle deficits in the implementation of routines in preclinical carriers, interpreted as reflecting early changes in the striatum.

Relationship between cognition and motor function

Most studies indicate significant correlations between cognitive performance and motor functioning. Correlations are greatest for voluntary aspects of motor functioning (Brandt *et al.* 1984; Girotti *et al.* 1988; Heindel *et al.* 1988, 1989; Brandt 1994; Zappacosta *et al.* 1996; Snowden *et al.* 2000). Cognitive performance is more weakly related to chorea (Brandt *et al.* 1984; Snowden *et al.* 2000). The strong correlation with motor function provides indirect support for the view that cognitive changes in HD are attributable more to alterations in the striatum and frontostriatal pathways than to independent pathological changes in the neocortex. Motor impairment has been found to be a better correlate of cognitive decline than illness duration (Brandt *et al.* 1984).

Cognitive impairment and functional disability

Patients' cognitive impairment is a major factor underlying functional disability in HD (Mayeux *et al.* 1986; Bamford *et al.* 1989; Rothlind *et al.* 1993a). Indeed, it has been argued that functional disability is more due to cognitive impairment (Mayeux *et al.* 1986; Bamford *et al.* 1989) and depression (Mayeux *et al.* 1986) than to patients' movement difficulties, particularly chorea. Standard measures of disability such as Total Functional Capacity (Shoulson and Fahn 1979; Shoulson 1981) and scales of activities of daily living have been shown to correlate more closely with both cognitive impairment and loss of voluntary movement than with chorea (Brandt and Butters 1996).

Cognitive change over time

Cognitive functioning declines over the course of the disease. Nevertheless, the rate of decline is variable so that duration of illness *per se* is a relatively poor indicator of cognitive performance (Brandt *et al.* 1984). Moreover, different domains of cognitive function do not decline in a uniform fashion (Bamford *et al.* 1995; Snowden *et al.* 2000). Bamford *et al.* showed most significant and consistent decline over time in psychomotor skills. Snowden *et al.* showed that, over a 1-year period, significant decline could be detected on low-level psychomotor tasks, object recall, and verbal fluency. By contrast, there was no change in performance even over 3 years on a test of executive function (Wisconsin Card Sorting Test) and egocentric spatial function (Road map test). It is worth emphasizing that HD is slowly progressive and cognitive changes over 1 year are typically relatively small. Therapeutic trials that seek to slow the natural course of disease will need to evaluate performance over years rather than months in order to demonstrate efficacy.

Cognitive decline and CAG repeat length

Brandt *et al.* (1996) demonstrated greater decline in cognitive functioning over 2 years in HD patients with long ($\geq$47) compared to short (37–46) repeat length, indicating that CAG repeat length was a strong predictor of decline in cognitive function. However, correlations have not invariably been demonstrated (see Chapter 5). Snowden *et al.* (2000) showed no association between repeat length and cognitive decline in a group of 87 HD patients. It may be that, where correlations exist, they arise largely from inclusion of atypical juvenile cases with very large repeat lengths.

Cognition in preclinical HD

Symptoms of HD develop insidiously and it is well recognized that subtle changes may be present before individuals would conventionally be regarded as clinically affected. The introduction of predictive testing for HD, following isolation of the HD gene (Huntington's Disease Collaborative Research Group 1993), has made it possible to investigate the evolution of cognitive changes in HD by studying presymptomatic individuals who have the HD mutation. A number of studies have addressed the question whether cognitive deficits are present in people with the mutation before they show overt neurological signs of HD. Some studies have identified deficits, whereas others have not (Table 3.1). A number of factors are likely to contribute to the disparate findings. Studies vary greatly in terms of group size, thus affecting the statistical power to detect subtle differences. Some studies have focused on a single domain of cognitive functioning such as visual perceptual and spatial skills (Bylsma *et al.* 1992; Gomez *et al.* 1996) or memory (De Boo *et al.* 1999). Cognitive functions may differ in their vulnerability to early

Table 3.1. Studies of cognition in preclinical gene carriers

Reference	Number of gene-positive subjects	Deficits identified
Strauss and Brandt 1990	12	None
Bylsma *et al.* 1992	14	None
Rothlind *et al.* 1993b	20	None
Blackmore *et al.* 1995	13	None
Giordani *et al.* 1995	8	None
Campodonico *et al.* 1996	22	None
Gomez Tortosa *et al.* 1996	15	None
de Boo *et al.* 1997	9	None
de Boo *et al.* 1999	9	None
Jason *et al.* 1988	7	Visual memory, category generation, spatial function
Diamond *et al.* 1992	7	Verbal memory
Foroud *et al.* 1995	120	Psychomotor speed, picture sequencing
Hahn-Barma *et al.* 1998	42	Verbal memory
Rosenberg *et al.* 1995	14	Attention, learning, and planning
Siemers *et al.* 1996	103	Psychomotor speed
Gray *et al.* 1997	15	Emotion recognition (disgust)
Lawrence *et al.* 1998b	22	Attentional set shifting, category generation
Kirkwood *et al.* 1999	12	Psychomotor speed
Snowden *et al.* 2002	51	Psychomotor speed

change. Perhaps the single most important factor underlying differences in findings is varia-tion in the closeness of people with the HD mutation to clinical onset of HD. Most studies, whether or not group differences reach statistical significance, show that people with the mutation, as a group, achieve numerically poorer scores than people without the mutation. Within the mutation group, however, performance is typically variable. Whereas some individuals perform similarly to controls, others perform poorly, thus reducing the overall group mean score. The variability in performance has been highlighted (Lundervold and Reinvang 1995), and several authors have suggested that deficits are present only in persons approaching the clinical onset of disease (Campodonico *et al.* 1996; De Boo *et al.* 1997; Hahn-Barma *et al.* 1998). Our own studies suggest that functional deficits may not evolve uniformly: very subtle changes in psychomotor function may be present several years before clinical onset, whereas memory deficits emerge only close to the time of clinical onset (Snowden *et al.* 2002). Future longitudinal studies are likely to clarify the time course of cognitive change.

Anatomical basis of cognitive changes in preclinical HD

There is evidence from structural (Aylward *et al.* 1994; 1996) and functional (Antonini *et al.* 1996; Andrews *et al.* 1999) neuroimaging of striatal changes in preclinical HD. Moreover, studies have shown correlations between striatal change and cognitive performance (Campodonico *et al.* 1998; Lawrence *et al.* 1998a).

Psychiatric aspects of HD

Affective disorders

Depression is a common complication of HD, and can occasionally become a severe and intractable problem. It can be difficult to diagnose, because patients with HD may not spon-taneously complain of sadness or low mood, and many of the characteristic symptoms of depression can be masked by other clinical features of HD. For example, the loss of appetite expected in someone with depression may be offset by the increase in appetite that is common in HD. Conversely, HD patients frequently display inactivity and insomnia, whether or not they are depressed. It is important to recognize and treat depression when it occurs in the course of HD, because even a mild degree of depression can significantly exacerbate prob-lems such as apathy, social withdrawal, and weight loss, resulting in a further diminution in quality of life for the patient.

   The high frequency of depression in HD has been recognized from the earliest descriptions of this condition, beginning with Huntington's own reference to 'that form of insanity which leads to suicide' (Huntington 1872). Much of the early psychiatric literature on HD originated from Germany (reviewed by Morris 1991) and emphasized the importance of affective symp-toms. Minski and Guttmann (1938) found that 11 of their 43 cases showed affective emotional reactions, depressive in type, in some instances with suicidal tendencies. Heathfield (1967) reported that the most common psychiatric disorder in his study of HD patients, ascertained from mental hospitals in northeast London and Essex, was an endogenous or reactive depres-sion, occurring in 10 of the 80 cases. Dewhurst *et al.* (1970) studied 102 affected individuals in Oxfordshire, of whom 15 were admitted to hospital with a diagnosis of depression. In seven of these cases an episode of depression antedated the onset of HD, while Oliver (1970) reported that depression was the presenting symptom in 9 of his series of 100 patients from Northamptonshire. Bolt (1970) found evidence of depression affecting 20 per cent of the men and 29 per cent of the women in a study of 334 HD patients from the west of Scotland.

These early studies can all be criticized for methodological reasons. Most were carried out using populations ascertained from mental hospitals, and lacked systematic methods for eliciting clinical information or defined diagnostic criteria. In many cases the patients were not even examined in person, the data being gleaned from clinical records. However, there have been several more recent studies that allow a better estimate of the prevalence of affective symptoms in HD. Caine and Shoulson (1983) found five individuals with major depressive disorder and six with dysthymic disorder defined by DSM-III diagnostic criteria (from the *Diagnostic and statistical manual of mental disorders*, 3rd edn: American Psychiatric Association 1980) in a study of 24 patients with HD, although the patients were not randomly ascertained and the study cannot give a true estimate of the prevalence. Folstein *et al.* (1983, 1987) attempted to ascertain all cases in the state of Maryland, USA, who were alive on 1 April 1980, and to examine all of them using a structured psychiatric interview, the Diagnostic Interview Schedule (Robbins *et al.* 1981). Diagnosis was based on DSM-III criteria (American Psychiatric Association 1980). Affective disorder was diagnosed in 61 (33 per cent) of the 186 cases, with a further 9 (5 per cent) meeting the criteria for dysthymic disorder). One interesting aspect of this study was the discovery that the 50 patients of Black African ancestry had lower rates of depression than the 136 White patients; affective disorder was present in 41 per cent of the White cases but only 10 per cent of the patients of Black ethnic origin. Pflanz *et al.* (1991) attempted to identify all cases of HD that had come into contact with psychiatric, general hospital, or genetic counselling services in the Grampian region of Scotland between 1970 and 1987, and identified 86 cases, of whom 53 per cent had the syndrome of simple depression according to the Present State Examination.

The study of Folstein *et al.* (1987) was carried out at the same time as a community survey in the same area using similar diagnostic criteria, which established that the lifetime prevalence of major affective disorder was 4.3 per cent. The figure of 33 per cent in patients with HD was therefore well in excess of the rate that might be expected by chance. Many authors have suggested that depression in people with HD might well be reactive in nature; as Heathfield (1967) put it, '. . . the depression was due to realisation by a patient that he was suffering from an incurable disease from which a parent had died in a mental hospital.' However, the available evidence suggests that this intuitive explanation may be incorrect. Mindham *et al.* (1985) compared the frequency of depression in 27 patients with HD and 27 with Alzheimer's disease, using the Diagnostic Interview Schedule. The prevalence of major affective disorder in the HD patients was twice that of the controls with Alzheimer's disease, even though the implications for the patient of the two diagnoses are quite similar. Furthermore, some early studies reported that depression can be the initial presenting feature of the illness (Oliver 1970) and may precede the onset of motor symptoms by many years (Dewhurst *et al.* 1970). In the Maryland study, affective symptoms preceded chorea and dementia in 23 of the 34 patients for whom accurate onset data were available, by an average of 5.1 years (Folstein *et al.* 1983). In order to further investigate the causes of depression in HD patients, these authors interviewed first- and second-degree relatives of five consecutively ascertained probands with both HD and affective disorder from the Maryland case series, and five with HD but no associated psychiatric disorder. The average interval between onset of affective disorder and onset of HD was 9.9 years in the 26 relatives with both diagnoses with accurate data about age at onset. Among the affected relatives of probands with HD and affective disorder 20 of 23 were found to have affective disorder themselves, while only 5 of 23 relatives of probands with HD alone had affective disorder, a highly significant difference. Among the spouses, non-HD parents, and 'in-laws' of the 10 probands, the lifetime prevalence of major affective disorder was 2 per cent.

The authors concluded that the high rate of affective disorder in their case series was unlikely to represent a psychological reaction to the illness, given that affective disorder may precede HD by many years and can occur in persons who are not even aware of their risk for HD. They postulated that the observed association between HD and affective disorder in some families but not in others might be due to genetic heterogeneity at the HD locus or, alternatively, to a gene predisposing for affective disorder and closely linked to that for HD. The subsequent discoveries that HD is invariably caused by a triplet repeat expansion in the HD gene (HD Collaborative Research Group 1993) and that psychiatric symptoms do not correlate with CAG repeat length have ruled out the first explanation, and the second now appears less likely in view of the mounting evidence that the genetic basis of affective disorder is multi-factorial. However, the findings of Folstein et al. strongly suggest a genetic contribution to depression in HD, perhaps caused by an interaction between genes predisposing to affective disorder and the underlying neurodegenerative process of the disease. Cummings (1995) pointed out that depression is common in disorders associated with caudate nucleus dysfunction, and that the ventral striatum is involved in reward and reinforcement of behaviours. He therefore hypothesized that neuronal loss in this region would diminish the effectiveness of reward-mediated behaviours and contribute to anhedonia and depression, as well as loss of motivation and apathy. However, in the absence of a direct relationship between affective symptoms and the severity of motor and cognitive changes (Craufurd et al. 2001), it is clear that the relationship is a complex one.

There have been very few satisfactory clinical trials of antidepressant treatment for HD (Leroi and Michalon 1998). However, clinical experience suggests that depressed HD patients respond to the same treatments as do the general population, although care should be taken with doses because HD patients can be very sensitive to side-effects such as sedation. Tricyclic antidepressants, selective serotonin re-uptake inhibitors (SSRI), and monoamine oxidase inhibitors such as moclobemide have all been used successfully; however, it has been suggested that bipolar disorder in HD may be unresponsive to lithium therapy (Ranen et al. 1993).

Suicide

Huntington was correct when he drew attention to the increased frequency of suicide among those affected with HD. His reference to the '. . . form of insanity which leads to suicide' suggests that he thought of it as a manifestation of mental illness secondary to the disease, rather than a reaction to adversity. However, it is often assumed that the high rate of suicide is an understandable response to an almost intolerable situation, and it is certainly true that many people with HD talk about the option of suicide if their situation were to become unbearable; in one survey of 35 at-risk individuals, approximately half indicated that they would commit suicide if they became ill (Wexler 1979). It may be that the possibility of suicide helps the individual to retain a sense of control in the face of an illness that progressively robs them of it. In the authors' experience, suicidal thoughts of this kind are generally perceived by patients as comforting, and differ from the distressing thoughts that usually lead to suicidal acts. Experience suggests that patients who have previously expressed an intention to kill themselves when the condition becomes more advanced seldom actually do so, possibly because the will to live remains strong in spite of appalling circumstances, but perhaps also because cognitive and personality changes such as apathy and affective blunting become more severe as the disease progresses and make suicide less likely. As Minski and Guttmann (1938) put it, '. . . It might be expected that the incidence of suicide among the families of such hereditary diseases, which might be likened to the sword of Damocles, would be extremely high. But if one considers only those cases which must really be attributed to the fear of the disease one finds a comparatively low incidence. Perhaps this may be explained by the progressive deterioration with lack of initiative, loss of insight and emotional facility, that is met with in . . . the condition.'

Most of the published studies concerning psychiatric symptoms in HD have commented on the number of suicides in their sample, but the majority cannot be used to estimate the prevalence of suicide among HD patients because the subjects were ascertained mainly from psychiatric hospitals and may be biased towards those with mental health problems. However, Schoenfeld *et al.* (1984) attempted to ascertain all known families with HD in New England, and found 20 documented cases of suicide out of 506 deceased individuals with definite or probable HD, a prevalence of 4 per cent. This was significantly greater than the 1 per cent occurrence of suicide reported for the general population of Massachusetts at that time, and the third most common cause of death in the HD patients. Comparison with the Massachusetts population using age-specific rates of suicide revealed that the proportion of deaths due to suicide in HD patients and the general population did not differ in those dying before 50 years of age, but was significantly greater (odds ratio (OR) = 8.19) in the 50–69 year age group. The excess of suicides among the HD patients was even more striking if comparison was limited to those for whom a precise cause of death could be established; this was known in only 157 of the 506 cases, and, if the remaining 349 individuals are excluded, the proportion who committed suicide rises to 12.7 per cent, significantly more than the general population in both the 10–49 year age group (OR = 2.7) and the 50–69 year age group (OR = 23). However, it is not clear whether the rate of suicide in HD patients is disproportionately greater than for patients with other medical disorders, since there is a well-established association between suicide and serious illness generally.

Broadly similar findings emerged from a study of HD patients known to the US National HD Research Roster at Indiana University (Farrer 1986). There were 25 cases of suicide out of 440 affected individuals for whom the cause of death was stated, a frequency of 5.7 per cent. In keeping with the New England study, this was the third most common cause of death in HD patients after pneumonia and cardiovascular disease. The figure of 5.7 per cent may well be an underestimate, because the cause of death was simply listed as 'Huntington disease' in 92 cases, without any further details. However, the author noted that a rate of 5.7 suicides per 100 deaths was almost four times greater than the reported rate of 1.5 per cent for the US population as a whole, and was consistent with the rate of 3.35 per cent calculated for the HD population in South Africa (Hayden *et al.* 1980). A further 27.6 per cent of affected individuals known to the roster had attempted suicide on at least one occasion.

Both studies attempted to address the timing of suicide in relation to the disease onset. Farrer (1986) noted that the suicides in the Indiana study occurred mainly in the middle stages of the disease; on average, those who took their own lives died 7 years earlier and had been affected for 5.8 years fewer than those who died by natural causes. On the other hand, Schoenfeld *et al.* (1984) pointed out that in their New England sample the rate of suicide was four times greater in those with suspected HD than among the diagnosed cases, which they interpreted as evidence that patients early in the disease are at greater risk. An alternative explanation might be that persons having the greatest difficulty adjusting psychologically to the onset of the illness, and actively avoiding confirmation of the diagnosis in spite of evident symptoms, are more likely to kill themselves than those who seek medical help.

While the evidence suggests that HD sufferers are more likely to commit suicide than the general population, the causes are complex and poorly understood. It is possible that some instances of suicide in this group of patients may represent 'a rational response to an intolerable situation' (Farrer 1986), and it is very likely that demoralization, social isolation, and poor self-esteem secondary to the loss of economic and social roles as the disease progresses all contribute to the increased risk. The high incidence of affective disorder is also an obvious risk factor, but it would be an oversimplification to blame the increased suicide rate only on the increased prevalence of depression associated with HD. Many other neuropsychiatric manifestations of HD such as irritability, emotional lability, and impulsiveness significantly increase the risk of suicidal behaviour. Prevention of suicide in this high-risk group therefore requires vigorous treatment of psychiatric symptoms such as depression and irritability, combined with careful attention to maintaining and strengthening social support networks and appropriate efforts to foster an optimistic outlook towards the future. While it may be unfair to encourage unrealistic expectations of an imminent cure for the disease, it is possible to offer the prospect of good symptomatic treatment and care and a much better quality of life than was available to previous generations of sufferers.

Mania

Although symptoms of depression are common in HD, the prevalence of mania or hypomania is less certain. Mania, occurring alone or as part of a bipolar manic depressive psychosis, is relatively uncommon in the general population, and some of the early studies of psychiatric disorders in HD appear to suggest an increased frequency. Heathfield (1967) described 4 patients out of 80 with hypomania and delusions of grandeur, while Bolt (1970) reported grandiose ideas in 11 of her 334 cases, religiosity in 4, and elation in 3. Two of the 100 patients described by Oliver had 'emotional instability, expressed as excitement'. However, none of the cases reported by Dewhurst *et al.* (1970) were described as manic or hypomanic, and there was only one out of 199 with a diagnosis of 'affective disorder, manic phase' in the study of Saugstad and Ødegård (1986) from Norway. Since most of the patients were ascertained from mental hospital populations, and none of the studies used operational diagnostic criteria or systematic methods of data collection, it is not possible to use these reports to estimate the prevalence of mania or hypomania in HD patients.

Some of the more recent studies using reliable methods of diagnosis have also reported increased rates of hypomania. Folstein *et al.* (1987) using DSM-III diagnostic criteria (American Psychiatric Association 1980) found that major affective disorder was the most common psychiatric syndrome among their patients in Maryland, with a lifetime prevalence of 33 per cent. Although frank mania with delusions of grandeur and flight of ideas was uncommon, brief episodes of hypomania were observed in about 10 per cent of the patients (Folstein *et al.* 1987); symptoms included increased levels of activity, pressured speech, uncharacteristic cheerfulness, large and inappropriate purchases, and a return of sexual interest after a long period of anhedonia or impotence. Caine and Shoulson (1983) did not find any cases among the 24 patients in their study, but Pflanz *et al.* (1991) using the Present State Examination (PSE) reported the PSE syndrome of hypomania in 33 per cent of their 86 patients and found that manic or mixed affective psychosis was the most common diagnosis according to the CATEGO classification system.

Interpretation of these findings is difficult. Strictly speaking, the rules employed by diagnostic systems such as DSM-III prohibit the diagnosis of bipolar affective disorder (or any other functional psychiatric disorder) in the presence of an organic condition such as HD. Studies using these operational diagnostic criteria to shed light on the psychiatric manifestations of HD therefore have to set aside this rule and apply the criteria as if the patient did not have organic brain disease. Unfortunately, mood states such as emotional lability, irritability, and what is sometimes termed 'vacuous euphoria', which in the absence of organic impairment would certainly indicate the possibility of hypomania, are also seen in many patients with brain injury or disease who do not otherwise have features to suggest bipolar affective disorder. Similarly, behaviours such as inappropriate sexual activity, or making impulsive, ill-judged, and unnecessary purchases, would contribute to the suggestion of hypomania in someone who does not have acquired cognitive impairment, but not necessarily in a person with HD. This is especially problematic with systems that use computer algorithms to avoid subjective bias when assigning diagnostic categories. If the diagnosis of bipolar affective disorder is restricted to patients who have episodes of uncharacteristically increased activity (severe enough to cause some practical problems for the patient or carers) alternating with periods of depression, we have seen only one case out of more than 130 affected individuals, and one more out of 82 asymptomatic individuals with the HD mutation, attending our HD clinic in Manchester. This clinical observation is supported by data from a colleague who provides a neuropsychiatric service in a neighbouring region of England, and has yet to see an HD patient with bipolar disorder (K Barrett, personal communication). Clinical impressions such as these can never be a substitute for systematic scientific investigations, but the difficulties outlined above illustrate the potential problems of reliance on rigid diagnostic algorithms that may not adequately take account of the complexities involved. Further research is required to elucidate the relationship between HD and mania, but on the presently available evidence the authors are not convinced that a syndrome that genuinely resembles bipolar affective disorder is much more common in HD patients than in the general population. This is in marked contrast to schizophrenia-like symptoms (see below), which do seem to occur with considerably increased frequency in patients with HD.

Irritability

Irritability and bad-tempered outbursts are among the most common and troublesome behavioural manifestations of HD. Often, the spouse or another household member will complain that the patient becomes irritable for no very obvious reason, and that during these periods the slightest provocation—such as a minor disagreement or trivial inconvenience—will provoke an outburst of angry or violent behaviour. Such spells can go on for hours or even days at a time, during which the family will describe life as being 'like walking on eggshells', never quite knowing when an innocuous remark will trigger another eruption. Families frequently remark that the irritable behaviour is directed mainly towards one particular member of the household, often the spouse or child who is closely involved in the care of the patient. This can sometimes develop into a persistent and apparently irrational hostility from which the patient cannot be dissuaded. In other cases, the patients themselves will complain that they have become subject to sudden and uncharacteristic upsurges of anger that often surprise them by their ferocity and lack of warning, but subside equally quickly leaving the individual feeling shaken and filled with remorse. Patients often report periods of suicidal ideation after such episodes.

The prevalence of irritable behaviour in HD is difficult to determine in view of the lack of agreed definitions and reliable methods of assessment. Heathfield (1967) noted the high frequency of aggressive traits and irritability, including 'attacking people and throwing things', among patients with HD, in contrast to the other presenile dementias. Bolt (1970) noted that approximately 50 per cent of the patients in her study showed some degree of ill humour, ranging from irritability to actual violence, and that the prevalence of this symptom was very similar in both sexes. She also reported that approximately 10 per cent of both sexes were said to have been difficult, moody, irritable, or 'strange' throughout their lives, while Oliver (1970) described 'emotional instability', expressed as irritability, quarrelsomeness, childish tantrums, violent outbursts, or abusiveness, as the most common psychiatric presenting symptom of the disorder, occurring in 13 of 94 patients. Using a structured psychiatric interview and DSM-III diagnostic criteria, Folstein *et al.* (1987) found a prevalence of 31 per cent for 'intermittent explosive disorder' during an epidemiological study of HD in Maryland. A further study from this group, using a specially constructed scale to measure aggression and irritability, found that HD patients were more aggressive and had more severe aggressive outbursts than a comparison group of patients with Alzheimer's disease (Burns *et al.* 1990). Pflanz *et al.* (1991) using the PSE found that 'irritability' was the second most common PSE syndrome after 'organic impairment', affecting 69 per cent of male and 60 per cent of female HD patients. This is consistent with the findings from our own HD clinic population (Craufurd *et al.* 2001), where clinically significant irritability was found in 57 per cent of males and 49 per cent of females, while 40 per cent of patients had displayed verbal outbursts of temper, and 22 per cent threatening behaviour or actual violence, in the 4 weeks prior to interview.

Irritable behaviour and episodes of verbal or physical aggression directed towards close family or friends will inevitably have a damaging effect on personal relationships, and often contribute to marital breakdown or to rejection of the patient by the relatives and carers he or she most relies on to look after him. Aggressive behaviour directed towards strangers is less common, but can place the patient at risk of violence or in trouble with the law. Management of this particular symptom is therefore crucial to the overall welfare of the patient, and can make the difference between successful care in the community and institutional care. Carers are sometimes reluctant to mention irritable or aggressive behaviour in front of the patient for fear of recriminations afterwards, so it is therefore essential in the clinic to provide the carer with an opportunity to talk confidentially to a member of the clinical team. Fortunately, irritability can usually be treated very successfully. Before resorting to pharmacological methods of treatment, efforts should be made to identify predisposing and precipitating factors (see below). Educating family members and carers about the nature and causes of this behaviour (Ranen *et al.* 1993) can go a long way to solving the problem. However, pharmacological treatment of irritability is often required at some stage in the course of the illness and, although there have been no published clinical trials (Leroi and Michalon 1998), case reports and clinical experience suggest a number of approaches that sometimes prove helpful.

Propranolol can be useful even in low dosage (up to 80 mg daily) to reduce irritability, while serotonin re-uptake inhibitors such as paroxetine or citalopram are also frequently effective but may require larger doses than those used for the treatment of depression. Carbamazepine and sodium valproate can reduce the frequency of explosive outbursts, but their usefulness is often limited by side-effects such as sedation. If these measures fail, low doses of neuroleptics such as sulpiride or olanzapine are usually effective, but again the benefits tend to be offset by the occurrence of side-effects such as sedation and bradykinesia.

Alcoholism

It is not uncommon for the symptoms of HD to be mistaken for drunkenness. The slurred speech, clumsiness, and staggering gait all contribute to this impression, especially if the patient is also irritable or aggressive. However, opinion is divided as to whether alcohol abuse and dependence are actually more common in those with HD than in the general population. Hans and Gilmore (1968) commented on the high incidence of alcoholism in a study of hospitalized HD patients in Albany, New York, but did not provide figures to support this assertion, while Oliver (1970) implied that alcoholism was frequent among the patients and their unaffected relatives. Dewhurst *et al.* (1970) found 19 cases of alcoholism among 80 patients with HD, and suggested that this may be an underestimate because of misleading information from relatives. On the other hand, Bolt (1970) commented that excessive drinking was recorded in the notes of only 11 men and 2 women out of 334 case records examined in the west of Scotland, an area where alcoholism and heavy drinking are common.

King (1985) identified a random selection of 42 patients (25 male, 17 female) from the Maryland HD project, and interviewed a close relative about each proband using the relevant part of the Diagnostic Interview Schedule. Seven (6 male, 1 female) met the DSM-III criteria for alcoholism; 5 of these could also be classified as alcohol-dependent. The overall lifetime prevalence of alcohol abuse in the HD patients was therefore 16.7 per cent, while a community survey of an inner city population in East Baltimore carried out at roughly the same time and using very similar methods identified a lifetime prevalence rate for alcohol abuse of 13.7 per cent (Robbins *et al.* 1984). King therefore concluded that the rate of alcohol abuse in sufferers from HD was little different from prevailing rates in the community, and noted that 5 of the 7 were already abusing alcohol when the first symptoms of HD appeared. The only other published study using a systematic approach to determine rates of substance abuse in HD patients was that of Pflanz *et al.* (1991) who identified alcohol or drug abuse in 16 per cent of males and 9 per cent of females using the PSE. The available evidence therefore suggests that rates of alcohol abuse and dependence in HD patients are probably no worse than the (admittedly high) levels in the general population. However, there is no doubt that excessive drinking can give rise to considerable problems when it does occur because the effects of alcohol exacerbate the motor, cognitive, and psychiatric symptoms of this disorder.

Disorders of sexual function

It is widely believed that promiscuous behaviour and sexual deviations are common in people with HD. In his original description of the disorder, Huntington (1872) wrote of '. . . two married men, whose wives are living, and who are constantly making love to some young lady, not seeming to be aware that there is any impropriety in it . . . They are men of about 50 years of age, but never let an opportunity to flirt with a girl go past unimproved.' Dewhurst *et al.* (1970) in their study of the sociopsychiatric consequences of HD reported that 30 of 102 patients displayed abnormal sexual behaviour, of whom 19 showed hypersexuality while 11 were described as hyposexual. They listed morbid sexual jealousy, indecent exposure, homosexual assault, incestuous sodomy, voyeurism, assault on females, and promiscuity among the sexual aberrations observed in their study, and noted that patients' wives often complained 'that their husbands were demanding an inordinate amount of sexual fulfilment at odd times or in inappropriate places, and whenever these desires were rebuffed they became vindictive, abusive and frequently violent.' Although Dewhurst's paper has been frequently cited in subsequent publications, it should be noted that other contemporary authors reported lower rates of psychosexual disorders. Bolt (1970) found that 20 (6 per cent) of 334 patients had increased libido or sexual deviations, while Oliver (1970) also reported 6 per cent and Heathfield (1967) only 2 (2.5 per cent) of 80 patients displaying similar behaviours.

There is only one published report of a study using modern interviewing methods and defined diagnostic criteria to investigate this issue. Fedoroff *et al.* (1994) examined 39 HD patients in Baltimore and their 32 partners using a semistructured interview schedule designed to elicit symptoms of sexual dysfunctions and paraphilias according to DSM-III-R diagnostic criteria. Eighty-two per cent of the HD patients and 66 per cent of the partners had one or more sexual disorders by DSM-III-R criteria, a statistically significant difference. Hypoactive sexual desire was the most common diagnosis in both male and female patients (63 and 75 per cent, respectively). Inhibited orgasm was the second most common diagnosis in both sexes, and was significantly more common in both male and female HD patients than the non-HD partners (56 per cent of HD males versus 0 per cent of non-HD males; 42 per cent of HD females versus 9 per cent of non-HD females). Excluding patients taking tricyclic antidepressants, neuroleptics, lithium, or antihypertensive medications did not alter this finding. Thirty per cent of the HD males and 25 per cent of the HD females had experienced increased sexual interest, defined as a marked increase of sexual interest over a period of at least a week that could not be attributed to a loss of interest by the person's partner. There was a numerically greater frequency of paraphilias in the HD cases than in the partners (19 per cent of HD males versus 10 per cent of non-HD males; 8 per cent of HD females versus 0 per cent of non-HD females) but this was not a statistically significant difference. Although some participants in the study had been sexually abused as children, the HD patients did not differ from their non-HD partners in this respect (9 per cent versus 8 per cent) and there were no cases of patients who had molested or abused children.

Although the Fedoroff study confirms previous reports that sexual disorders are common in patients with HD, it is apparent that hyposexuality is far more common than hypersexuality in this group of patients. The finding is supported by our own study (Craufurd *et al.* 2001) of patients attending an HD clinic in which 62 per cent experienced a loss of libido, corroborated by their partners, while only 6 per cent reported sexually disinhibited or demanding behaviour. The most remarkable finding of Fedoroff *et al.* was the very high frequency of inhibited male orgasm, the least common male sexual disorder in the general population. The authors suggest that both motor and cognitive aspects of HD may interfere with patients' ability to achieve orgasm; damage to the striatum disrupts the automatic execution of learned patterns of movement, while difficulty in maintaining attention and concentration may also cause problems during intercourse. They also noted that, although the excess of paraphilias among the HD participants was not statistically significant, significantly more men who had both increased sexual interest and inhibited orgasm also had paraphilias, suggesting that the paraphilias may have emerged in the face of increased sexual urges combined with difficulty achieving orgasm by conventional means.

Although loss of libido and cessation of sexual activity appears to be the most common pattern in HD patients, there is no doubt that hypersexual behaviours can become a very difficult problem in the small proportion of cases where they do occur. The combination of mild disinhibition, increased libido, and reduced awareness of emotional responses in other people sometimes leads to the kind of sexually demanding behaviour referred to by Dewhurst in his 1970 paper, made all the more difficult to cope with if the patient is also irritable and prone to aggressive outbursts when his advances are refused. The situation is frequently compounded by the partners' reaction to the personality changes and physical deterioration caused by the disease. It is common for spouses to remark that the patient is 'no longer the person I married' and to admit privately to feelings of relief when the patient ceases to initiate sexual activity. This situation requires great care in order to avoid further damage to the patient's already vulnerable self-esteem, but can usually be greatly improved by effective treatment of the irritability and aggressive behaviour. It is also important to remember that many patients (and their partners) will be too embarrassed to mention psychosexual problems of this sort in the clinic, unless in response to a tactful enquiry by the doctor.

Psychotic symptoms

There have been many reports of schizophrenia-like symptoms in people with HD. Minski and Guttmann (1938) described one patient with a frank schizophrenic illness and three with paraphrenic reactions in their cohort of 43 HD patients admitted to mental hospitals in London. Heathfield (1967) reported 6 cases of paranoid schizophrenia and 3 of schizophrenia simplex in his sample of 80 patients with HD. Folstein *et al.* (1979) found two patients with auditory hallucinations, neither of whom met all the research diagnostic criteria for schizophrenia, out of 11 affected individuals referred to out-patient clinics for diagnosis or genetic counselling.

The diagnosis of schizophrenia, as with most other psychiatric disorders, presents difficulty in HD patients because there are many symptoms such as social withdrawal, emotional blunting, and loss of volition that are common to both conditions. Furthermore, it has been recognized for many years that psychotic symptoms such as delusions and auditory hallucinations can occur in organic brain disorders, and that sometimes schizophrenic illnesses that are typical in every respect can turn out to have an underlying organic basis (Lishman 1998). For this reason, diagnostic systems such as DSM-III or the Research Diagnostic Criteria (RDC) of Spitzer *et al.* (1977) do not allow the diagnosis of schizophrenia to be made in a patient known to suffer from HD or another similar organic brain disease. From a practical point of view, the importance of schizophrenia-like symptoms in HD arises partly from the additional burden for both patient and carer imposed by their presence, and partly because the medications usually prescribed to treat such symptoms tend to exacerbate both the cognitive and motor features of the illness.

In some cases, the onset of delusions and hallucinations may precede the onset of motor symptoms of HD, with the result that the patient is misdiagnosed as suffering from schizophrenia. If dopamine-blocking drugs are used to treat the psychotic symptoms, these will tend to suppress any involuntary movements, while clumsiness or bradykinesia will be attributed to side-effects of the medication, with the result that the underlying diagnosis of HD gets overlooked until the degree of motor disability can no longer be explained away as drug-induced parkinsonism. Saugstad and Ødegård (1986) carried out a retrospective case record study of 199 HD patients admitted to psychiatric hospitals in Norway between 1916 and 1975, and found that only 60 per cent were correctly diagnosed on first admission, the most common alternative diagnoses (in 39 cases) being schizophrenia and paranoid psychosis. In Oxfordshire, Dewhurst et al. (1970) found that 7 of the 102 HD patients in his study had initially been given a diagnosis of schizophrenia on admission to hospital, while Bolt (1970) reported that 8 per cent of her patients in Scotland were at first thought to have schizophrenia or paranoid psychosis. Saugstad and Ødegård noted that the misdiagnosis of schizophrenia was sometimes preserved during 3–4 admissions, and that the records showed a recent reduction in the amount of information recorded about family history of mental disorders, underlining the importance of paying attention to hereditary factors during history-taking.

Estimates of the prevalence of schizophrenia or schizophrenia-like symptoms in HD patients vary widely between studies and are difficult to compare because of the differing methodologies employed and the absence of clearly defined diagnostic criteria in the earlier studies. The evidence from more recent studies using unbiased methods of ascertainment and standardized diagnostic criteria suggests that episodes closely resembling schizophrenia in patients with HD are much less common than was previously thought. Caine and Shoulson (1983) evaluated 30 HD patients using the Schedule for Affective Disorders and Schizophrenia (Spitzer and Endicott 1978), and found that three fulfilled DSM-III criteria for schizophrenic syndrome while two more met the criteria for atypical psychotic syndrome. However, many of the subjects had been referred because of 'substantial behavioural disturbances' and were not necessarily representative of HD patients in general. In their case series of 88 patients from Maryland, assessed using the Diagnostic Interview Schedule, Folstein et al. (1983) found only 3 cases meeting the DSM-III criteria for schizophrenia, a prevalence of just 3 per cent. Baxter et al. (1992) administered the lifetime version of the Schedule for Affective Disorders and Schizophrenia (SADS-L) to 52 at-risk individuals with an affected first-degree relative and did not find any meeting RDC criteria (Spitzer et al. 1977) for schizophrenia or schizoaffective disorder. However, isolated psychotic symptoms may be much more common. For example, a case-record study of 86 patients from the Grampian region of Scotland using the PSE (Wing et al. 1984) found that 25 per cent of the females and 19 per cent of the males had delusions of persecution (Pflanz et al. 1991).

The cause of the psychotic symptoms seen in some people with HD is not known. The lifetime prevalence of schizophrenia in the general population is approximately 1 per cent, so the research findings cited above suggest that schizophrenia-like symptoms occur more often in HD than would be expected by chance. However, psychotic symptoms are certainly not an invariable feature of the disorder, and are seen in only a minority of cases; furthermore, there is no evidence to suggest a relationship between the occurrence of psychotic phenomena and the severity of the underlying neurodegenerative disease. The question arises as to why some patients are affected in this way, while others are not. Heathfield (1967) described a family in which identical paranoid schizophrenic psychoses were seen in a brother and sister with HD, while a further brother suffered from this mental disorder without developing choreiform movements. More recently, Lovestone *et al.* (1996) described a very similar HD family where all four affected individuals presented with a severe psychiatric disorder, in three cases schizophreniform in nature, and in which one other so far unaffected family member had been treated for schizophrenia. In the three affected family members, schizophrenia had preceded the onset of motor symptoms by up to 9 years. Tsuang *et al.* (1998) also reported a patient with juvenile-onset HD whose father and paternal grandmother both exhibited schizophrenia-like symptoms in addition to HD, contrasting this case with an otherwise very similar affected individual with no schizophrenia-like symptoms and no family history of psychotic illnesses. The authors could not find any difference in age at onset of HD, number of CAG repeats, or sex of transmitting parent between those with psychotic symptoms and those with HD alone. In both these case reports the affected individuals had a CAG repeat number in the abnormal range, and in the absence of any other evidence for genetic heterogeneity in HD it seems relatively unlikely that the psychotic symptoms were caused by other, as yet undetected changes in the HD gene. Lovestone *et al.* (1996) speculate that there may be additional familial factors in the kindred they described that influence the clinical presentation of HD. It may be that genes predisposing to schizophrenia are more likely to be expressed in the phenotype of someone who also carries the genetic mutation responsible for HD. This interpretation is supported by a case from our own clinic, in which two siblings with HD and a history of schizophrenia-like episodes have a half-sibling (the child of their unaffected parent) who suffers from chronic schizophrenia. The prevalence of psychotic symptoms with respect to genetic factors is discussed further in Chapter 5.

Apathy

Alterations in behaviour such as irritability, social withdrawal, and loss of motivation are often referred to collectively as 'personality changes' in the literature on HD. Some of these changes are sufficiently common and typical of the disorder that early German writers used the term 'choreopathy' to describe them (see Morris 1991 for a review). Such changes can occur many years before the onset of definite motor and cognitive symptoms. Dewhurst *et al.* (1970) reported that 14 of 102 patients had 'personality disorders' antedating the onset of HD, and in 10 of these cases personality disorder was the initial diagnosis. Oliver (1970) described personality changes as the earliest sign of HD in 19 of 100 cases, with a further 4 who displayed 'apathy, expressed as loss of interest', which he listed as a symptom of depression. The most frequent and characteristic personality change associated with HD is a loss of motivation, initiative, and spontaneous expression, which has been termed 'situational apathy' (Caine *et al.* 1978; Caine and Shoulson 1983). This is particularly common in the middle and later stages of the disease. In the study of Caine and Shoulson (1983), only 4 of the 10 mildly affected individuals, but 13 of 15 moderately impaired and all 5 severely disabled patients manifested a lack of self-initiated activities. In all but the most severe cases this was setting-dependent, in that apathy would disappear when stimulating input and structure were present. Apathy was present in 48 per cent of the HD patients studied by Burns *et al.* (1990).

As Oliver suggested in 1970, apathy may sometimes be secondary to depression. However, Mayberg *et al.* (1992) found no correlation between apathy and depression, while the setting-dependent nature of the phenomenon and the almost universal occurrence of apathy in the later stages of the illness, regardless of whether the patient exhibits other signs of affective disorder, suggest a more complex aetiology. This is discussed further below.

Relationship of psychiatric changes to CAG repeat length

Two studies looking at the presenting symptoms of HD (chorea, cognitive impairment, or psychiatric disturbances) found no relationship between this and the number of CAG repeats (Andrew *et al.* 1993; MacMillan *et al.* 1993). Similarly, Weigell-Weber *et al.* (1996) using a classification based on DSM-III criteria found no relationship between CAG repeat length and psychiatric symptoms; however, personality changes were more often associated with maternal transmission of HD, an observation attributed by the authors to psychosocial factors related to the mother's illness. Zappacosta *et al.* (1996) found no correlation between psychiatric symptoms as measured by the Hamilton Anxiety and Depression Scales and the Brief Psychiatric Rating Scale and either cognitive impairment, motor deterioration, or CAG repeat length. They concluded that psychiatric disorders in HD patients progress nonlinearly, perhaps because of differential degeneration of striatocortical circuits. The topic is discussed further in Chapter 5.

The basis of behavioural problems in HD

Behavioural problems in HD are common and varied. Figure 3.3 shows the prevalence of a range of behavioural problems in a cross-sectional sample of 134 people with mild to moderate HD attending our own regional HD outpatient clinic (Craufurd *et al.* 2001). Many of these behaviours are mood-based. However, it might be anticipated that others relate to altered cognition, as noted above. People with HD frequently show a loss of drive and a lack of initiative. If left to their own devices they may spend all day in bed or watching television. They react to events but are no longer proactive. Under normal circumstances a great

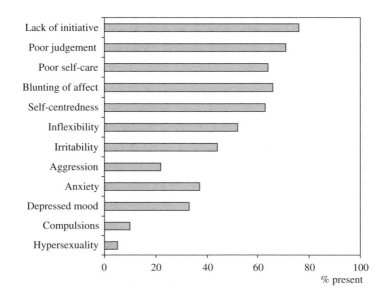

Fig. 3.3 Frequency of behavioural changes in HD. The figures are based on our own study of 134 people in the early and middle stages of HD.

behavioural motivator is the capacity for forward thinking: we see what needs to be done and this provides the stimulus for action. Since HD patients have an impaired capacity for planning and forethought, this might contribute to their passivity and loss of initiative. Similarly, an inability to think plans through and see the consequences of one's own actions might be expected to be largely responsible for HD patients' poor judgement and the increased prevalence of minor offences (Jensen *et al.* 1998).

Impaired self-generated maintenance of attention (Sprengelmeyer *et al.* 1995) would compromise the ability to persist in tasks. Impaired self-monitoring would lead to reduced quality of performance and an increase in errors. Decreased mental flexibility would make it difficult for someone with HD to see alternative points of view—hence the increased self-centredness, mental rigidity, and loss of sympathy and empathy reported in many HD patients.

The assumption that some problem behaviours in HD relate to patients' cognitive deficits whereas others are mood-based and independent of cognitive change is borne out by our own investigations (Craufurd *et al.* 2001; Thompson *et al.* 2002). A factor analysis of behavioural symptoms identified three principal factors. The first, termed the apathy factor, included symptoms of loss of initiative, poor judgement, lack of perseverance, and reduced self-care, and was strongly correlated with measures of cognitive function. The second factor included symptoms related to irritability and temper control, and the third factor was related to depression. Neither the irritability nor the depression factor correlated with degree of cognitive change. These findings complement those of others. Correlative studies of 'behavioural' symptoms of HD that have focused on mood changes such as depression and irritability (Folstein *et al.* 1979; Caine and Shoulson 1983; Mayberg *et al.* 1992; Huntington Study Group 1996; Zappacosta *et al.* 1996) have found no correlation with cognition.

The basis for individual behavioural symptoms is only beginning to be understood and it is likely that many behaviours are multifactorial. It would be reasonable to suppose, for example, that the commonly reported neglect of self-care is linked to patients' loss of initiative and general apathy, and this is supported by the factor analysis. However, a number of studies have shown impaired detection and identification of odours in HD patients (Nordin *et al.* 1995; Bacon-Moore *et al.* 1999; Hamilton *et al.* 1999), raising the possibility that impaired sense of smell contributes to reduced concern for personal hygiene. Affective changes might also play a part. There is evidence that people with HD have difficulty discriminating emotions, particularly the emotion of disgust (Sprengelmeyer *et al.* 1996). If people with HD also have reduced subjective experience of the emotion of disgust, then this too might contribute to patients' apparent lack of concern.

Similarly, the aetiology of irritable behaviour in HD may be complex. In some cases, irritability may be secondary to another psychiatric disorder such as depression. Frustration due to clumsiness or difficulties with communication, and physical factors such as hunger and fatigue may also contribute to the problem. Irritability might, in some instances occur as a secondary consequence of cognitive difficulties. A difficulty in switching attention between two ongoing tasks might lead to irritable outbursts, as a result of the patient feeling cognitively overwhelmed, in much the same way as normal individuals become irritable when subjected to excessive stress. Sometimes, irritability occurs in the context of self-centred, demanding behaviour and patients become upset and angry if their requests are not immediately satisfied (Ranen *et al.* 1993).

A question that is often asked is whether altered behaviour is an integral part of HD, arising as a result of structural brain changes, or occurs as a secondary reaction to a distressing and debilitating illness. The brain basis for much altered behaviour has been emphasized throughout this chapter and should not be underestimated, not least because it fosters awareness that difficult behaviour is not the 'fault' of patients or under their voluntary control. Nevertheless, it would be reasonable to suppose that reactive factors might also play a part. HD imposes profound life changes on a person, with adverse effects on mobility, employment prospects, social life, and functional independence. Moreover, involuntary movements and slurring of speech are commonly misinterpreted by the general public as signs of drunkenness, leading to social ostracism. Feelings of frustration under such circumstances are understandable. In reality, it is likely that behaviour reflects a combination of intrinsic and reactive changes. A patient with HD who, for example, assaults a policeman who falsely accuses him of being drunk, is showing an appropriate sense of outrage (reaction to consequence of illness), combined with a failure both to foresee the consequences of his actions and to suppress the surge of anger (action of HD).

Insight

The distinction between the direct effects of disease and the reaction to it is particularly pertinent in relation to insight. Insight is not an all or nothing phenomenon, perhaps accounting for the absence of a consensus view with respect to insight in HD. Some authors (Caine *et al.* 1978) have reported preservation of insight, on the grounds that most patients in their study admitted to reduced mental ability. Most investigators would concur that many HD patients complain of mental change, particularly difficulties in concentration and memory. However, a feature that is also common in HD is lack of acceptance of illness. People with overt clinical symptoms of HD may refuse to accept that they have HD and may deny that anything is wrong. As a result patients are commonly labelled as 'in denial'. Psychological (reactive) factors might contribute to individuals' unwillingness to confront a devastating illness, particularly if they have had a painful experience of HD through other affected family members. However, other factors are likely to play a major role. Executive deficits compromise the ability to self-monitor and to check performance in relation to an intended goal, so that people with HD may genuinely be oblivious of errors in their own performance. Executive deficits thus inevitably lead to reduced capacity for self-reflection and insightfulness. In the motor domain, people with HD may deny experiencing involuntary movements. The fact that they nevertheless accurately report consequences of their movement disorder such as dropping things, bumping into furniture, and falls (Snowden *et al.* 1998) suggests that a psychodynamic explanation in terms of illness denial is inadequate. They may genuinely have no subjective experience of the choreiform movements that are so apparent to others. Indeed, people with HD who watch themselves on video film frequently express surprise that their involuntary movements are so pronounced. The distinction between impaired egocentric and preserved extrapersonal space in HD may be relevant in accounting for the findings. Patients may have impaired awareness of changes in spatial position with respect to their own body, preventing subjective experience of involuntary movements, yet have no difficulty detecting such changes in external space, permitting normal appreciation of involuntary movements depicted on film.

Just as insight is not all or none, so too there is variation across individuals. Although the capacity for self-reflection is commonly reduced relatively early in the disease, some individuals retain a surprising ability to comment on their disability and the way that this affects them physically and mentally. Whether such differences reflect the magnitude of disruption to frontal lobe function, secondary to damage to frontal striatal pathways remains to be determined.

Conclusion

Cognitive and psychiatric changes are a prominent and integral part of HD and greatly affect patients' functional capacity. Recognition of those changes is essential for successful management. People with HD sustain cognitive changes that place limitations on their capabilities, but they also have areas of strength that need to be harnessed. Psychiatric changes are distressing for patients and carers alike, but many changes are amenable to symptomatic treatment, so that early detection is vital. Behavioural problems in HD are, however, complex. The multiple factors underlying patients' altered behaviour are beginning to be unravelled, providing scope for improved patient care and better understanding of HD.

References

Albert ML, Feldman RG, and Willis AL (1974). The 'subcortical dementia' of progressive supranuclear palsy. *Journal of Neurology, Neurosurgery and Psychiatry* **37**: 121–130.

American Psychiatric Association (1980). *Diagnostic and statistical manual of mental disorders*, 3rd edn. Washington DC: American Psychiatric Association.

Andrew SE, Goldberg YP, Kremer B, Telenius H, Theilmann J, Adam S, Starr E, Squitieri F, Lin B, Kalchman MA, Graham RK, and Hayden MR (1993). The relationship between trinucleotide (CAG) repeat length and clinical features of Huntington's disease. *Nature Genetics* **4**: 398–403.

Andrews TC, Weeks RA, Turjanski N, Gunn RN, Watkins LHA, Sahakian B, Hodges JR, Rosser AE, Wood NW, and Brooks DJ (1999). Huntington's disease progression: PET and clinical observations. *Brain* **122**: 2353–2363.

Antonini A, Leenders KL, Spiegel R, Meier D, Vontobel P, Weigell-Weber M, Sanchez-Pernaute R, deYebenez JG, Boesiger P, Weindl A, and Maguire RP (1996). Striatal glucose metabolism and dopamine D2 receptor binding in asymptomatic gene carriers and patients with Huntington's disease. *Brain* **119**: 2085–2095.

Aylward EH, Brandt J, Codori AM, Mangus RS, Barta PE, and Harris GJ (1994). Reduced basal ganglia volume associated with the gene for Huntington's disease in asymptomatic at-risk persons. *Neurology* **44**: 823–828.

—— Codori AM, Barta PE, Pearlson GD, Harris GJ, and Brandt J (1996). Basal ganglia volume and proximity to onset in presymptomatic Huntington disease. *Archives of Neurology* **53**: 1293–1296.

Backman L, Robins-Wahlin TB, Lundin A, Ginovart N, and Farde L (1997). Cognitive deficits in Huntington's disease are predicted by dopaminergic PET markers and brain volumes. *Brain* **120**: 2207–2217.

Bacon-Moore AS, Paulsen JS, and Murphy C (1999). A test of odor fluency in patients with Alzheimer's disease and Huntington's disease. *Journal of Clinical and Experimental Neuropsychology* **21**: 341–351.

Bamford KA, Caine ED, Kido DK, Plassche WM, and Shoulson I (1989). Clinical–pathologic correlation in Huntington's disease: a neuropsychological and computed tomography study. *Neurology* **39**: 796–801.

—— Caine ED, Kido DK, Cox C, and Shoulson I (1995). A prospective evaluation of cognitive decline in early Huntington's disease: functional and radiographic correlates. *Neurology* **45**: 1867–1873.

Baxter LR, Mazziotta JC, Pahl JJ, Grafton ST, St. George-Hyslop P, Haines JL, Gusella JF, Szuba MP, Selin CE, Guze BH, and Phelps ME (1992). Psychiatric, genetic and positron emission tomographic evaluation of persons at risk for Huntington's disease. *Archives of General Psychiatry* **49**: 148–154.

Bayles KA and Tomoeda CK (1983). Confrontation naming impairment in dementia. *Brain and Language* **19**: 98–114.

Blackmore L, Simpson SA, and Crawford JR (1995). Cognitive performance in UK sample of presymptomatic people carrying the gene for Huntington's disease. *Journal of Medical Genetics* **32**: 358–362.

Bolt JMW (1970). Huntington's chorea in the West of Scotland. *British Journal of Psychiatry* 116: 259–270.

Brandt J (1991). Cognitive impairments in Huntington's disease: insights into the neuropsychology of the striatum. In *Handbook of neuropsychology* (ed. F. Boller and J. Grafman), Vol. 5, pp. 241–264. Amsterdam: Elsevier Scientific Publications.

—— (1994). Cognitive investigations in Huntington's disease. In *Neuropsychological explorations of memory and cognition*: *essays in honor of Nelson Butters* (ed. L. Cermak), pp. 135–146. New York: Plenum Press.

Brandt J and Butters N (1986). The neuropsychology of Huntington's disease. *Trends in Neurosciences* **9: 118–120.**

—— Butters N (1996). Neuropsychological characteristics of Huntington's disease. In *Neuropsychological assessment of neuropsychiatric disorders* (ed. I. Grant and K.M. Adams), pp. 312–341. New York: Oxford University Press.

—— Strauss ME, Larus J, Jensen B, Folstein SE, and Folstein MF (1984). Clinical correlates of dementia and disability in Huntington's disease. *Journal of Clinical Neuropsychology* **6**: 401–412.

—— Folstein SE, and Folstein MF (1988). Differential cognitive impairment in Alzheimer's disease and Huntington's disease. *Annals of Neurology* **23**: 555–561.

—— Bylsma FW, Aylward EH, Rothlind J, and Gow CA (1995). Impaired source memory in Huntington's disease and its relation to basal ganglia atrophy. *Journal of Clinical and Experimental Neuropsychology* **17**: 868–877.

—— Bylsma FW, Gross R, Stine OC, Ranen N, and Ross CA (1996). Trinucleotide repeat length and clinical progression in Huntington's disease. *Neurology* **46**: 527–531.

Brouwers P, Cox C, Martin A, Chase T, and Fedio P (1984). Differential perceptuo-spatial impairment in Huntington's disease and Alzheimer's dementias. *Archives of Neurology* **41**: 1073–1076.

Burns A, Folstein S, Brandt J, and Folstein M. (1990). Clinical assessment of irritability, aggression and apathy in Huntington and Alzheimer disease. *Journal of Nervous and Mental Disease* **178**: 20–26.

Butters N, Sax D, Montgomery K, and Tarlow S (1978). Comparison of the neuropsychological deficits associated with early and advanced Huntington's disease. *Archives of Neurology* **35**: 585–589.

—— Wolfe J, Martone M, Granholm E, and Cermak LS (1985). Memory disorders associated with Huntington's disease: verbal recall, verbal recognition and procedural memory. *Neuropsychologia* **23**: 729–743.

—— Salmon D, and Heindel WC (1994). Specificity of the memory deficits associated with basal ganglia function. *Revue Neurologique Paris* **150**: 580–587.

Bylsma FW, Rebok GW, and Brandt J (1991). Long-term retention of implicit learning in Huntington's disease. *Neuropsychologia* **29**: 1213–1221.

—— Brandt J, and Strauss ME (1992). Personal and extrapersonal orientation in Huntington's disease patients and those at risk. *Cortex* **28**: 113–122.

Caine ED and Shoulson I (1983). Psychiatric syndromes in Huntington's disease. *American Journal of Psychiatry* **140**: 728–733.

—— Hunt RD, Weingartner H, and Ebert MH (1978). Huntington's dementia. Clinical and neuropsychological features. *Archives of General Psychiatry* **35**: 377–384.

—— Bamford KA, Schiffer RB, Shoulson I, and Levy S (1986). A controlled neuropsychological comparison of Huntington's disease and multiple sclerosis. *Archives of Neurology* **43**: 249–254.

Campodonico JR, Codori AM, and Brandt J (1996). Neuropsychological stability over two years in asymptomatic carriers of the Huntington's disease mutation. *Journal of Neurology, Neurosurgery and Psychiatry* **61**: 621–624.

—— Ayward E, Codori A-M, Young C, Krafft L, Magdalinski M, Ranen N, Slavney PR, and Brandt J (1998). When does Huntington's disease begin? *Journal of the International Neuropsychological Society* **4**: 467–473.

Cope MT, Georgiou N, Bradshaw JL, Iansek R, and Phillips JG (1996). Simon effect and attention in Parkinson's disease: a comparison with Huntington's disease and Tourette's syndrome. *Journal of Clinical and Experimental Neuropsychology* **18**: 276–290.

Craufurd D, Thompson J, Snowden JS (2001). Behavioural changes in Huntington's disease. *Journal of Neuropsychiatry, Neuropsychology and Behavioral Neurology* **14**: 219–226.

Cummings JL (1995). Behavioural and psychiatric symptoms associated with Huntington's disease. In *Behavioural neurology of movement disorders* (ed. W.J. Weiner and A.E. Lang), pp. 179–186. New York: Raven Press.

de Boo GM, Tibben A, Lanser JBK, Jennekens-Schinkel A, Hermans J, Maat-Kievit A, and Roos RAC (1997). Early cognitive and motor symptoms in identified carriers of the gene for Huntington's disease. *Archives of Neurology* **54**: 1353–1357.

—— Tibben AA, Hermans JA, Jennekens-Schinkel A, Maat-Kievit A, and Roos RAC (1999). Memory and learning are not impaired in presymptomatic individuals with an increased risk of Huntington's disease. *Journal of Clinical and Experimental Neuropsychology* **21**: 831–836.

Dewhurst K, Oliver JE, and McKnight AL (1970). Socio-psychiatric consequences of Huntington's disease. *British Journal of Psychiatry* **116**: 255–258

Diamond R, White RF, Myers RH, Mastromauro C, Koroshetz WJ, Butters N, Rothstein DM, Moss MB, and Vasterling J (1992). Evidence of presymptomatic cognitive decline in Huntington's disease. *Journal of Clinical and Experimental Neuropsychology* **14**: 961–975.

Dubois B, Pillon B, Legault F, Agid Y, and Lhermitte F (1988). Slowing of cognitive processing in progressive supranuclear palsy. A comparison with Parkinson's disease. *Archives of Neurology* **45**: 1194–1199.

Farrer LA (1986). Suicide and attempted suicide in Huntington's disease: implications for preclinical testing of persons at risk. *American Journal of Medical Genetics* **24**: 305–311.

Fedoroff JP, Peyser C, Franz ML, and Folstein SE (1994). Sexual disorders in Huntington's disease. *Journal of Neuropsychiatry and Clinical Neuroscience* **6**: 147–153.

Folstein MF and McHugh PR (1983). The neuropsychiatry of some specific brain disorders. In *Mental disorders and somatic illness. Handbook of Psychiatry*, Vol. 2 (ed. M.H. Lader), pp. 107–118. Cambridge: Cambridge University Press.

—— Brandt J, and Starkstein S (1992). Cognition in Huntington's disease: characteristics and correlates. In *Function and dysfunction in the basal ganglia* (ed. A.J. Franks, J.W. Ironside, R.H.S. Mindham, R.J. Smith, E.G.S. Spokes, and W. Winlow), pp. 218–223. Oxford: Pergamon.

Folstein SE (1989). The emotional disorder. In *Huntington's disease. A disorder of families* (ed. T. Foroud, J. Gray, J. Ivashing, and P.M. Conneally) pp. 49–64. Baltimore: Johns Hopkins University Press.

—— Folstein MF, and McHugh PR (1979). Psychiatric syndromes in Huntington's disease. In *Huntington's disease. Advances in neurology* (ed. T.N. Chase, N.S. Wexler, and A. Barbeau), Vol. 26, pp. 281–289. New York: Raven Press.

—— Abbott MH, Chase GA, Jensen BA, and Folstein MF (1983). The association of affective disorder with Huntington's disease in a case series and in families. *Psychological Medicine* **13**: 537–542.

—— Chase GA, Wahl WE, McDonnell AM, and Folstein MF (1987). Huntington disease in Maryland: clinical aspects of racial variation. *American Journal of Human Genetics* **41**: 168–179.

Foroud T, Siemers E, Kleindorfer D, Bill DJ, Hodes ME, Norton JA, Conneally PM, and Christian JC (1995). Cognitive scores in carriers of Huntington's disease gene compared to noncarriers. *Annals of Neurology* **37**: 657–664.

Gabrieli JDE, Stebbins GT, Singh J, Willingham DB, and Goetz CG (1997). Intact mirror-tracing and impaired rotary-pursuit skill learning in patients with Huntington's disease. *Neuropsychology* **11**: 272–281.

Georgiou N, Bradshaw JL, Phillips JG, Bradshaw JA, and Chiu E (1995). The Simon effect and attention deficits in Gilles de la Tourette's syndrome and Huntington's disease. *Brain* **118**: 1305–1318.

Giordani B, Berent S, Boivin MJ, Penney JB, Lehtinen S, Markel DS, Hollingsworth Z, Butterbaugh G, Hichwa RD, Gusella JF, and Young AB (1995). Longitudinal neuropsychological and genetic linkage analysis of persons at risk for Huntington's disease. *Archives of Neurology* **52**: 59–64.

Girotti F, Marano R, Soliveri P, Geminiani G, and Scigliano G (1988). Relationship between motor and cognitive disorders in Huntington's disease. *Journal of Neurology* **235**: 454–457.

Gomez Tortosa E, del Barrio A, Barroso T, and Garcia Ruiz PJ (1996). Visual processing disorders in patients with Huntington's disease and asymptomatic carriers. *Journal of Neurology* **243**: 286–292.

Gordon WP and Illes J (1987). Neurolinguistic characteristics of language production in Huntington's disease: a preliminary report. *Brain and Language* **31**: 1–10.

Gray JM, Young AW, Barker WA, Curtis A, and Gibson D (1997). Impaired recognition of disgust in Huntington's disease gene carriers. *Brain* **120**: 2029–2038.

Hahn-Barma V, Deweer B, Dürr A, Dodé C, Feingold J, Pillon B, Agid Y, Brice A, and Dubois B (1998). Are cognitive changes the first symptoms of Huntington's disease? A study of gene carriers. *Journal of Neurology, Neurosurgery and Psychiatry* **64**: 172–177.

Hamilton JM, Murphy C, and Paulsen JS (1999). Odor detection, learning and memory in Huntington's disease. *Journal of the International Neuropsychological Society* **5**: 609–615.

Hanes KR, Andrewes DG, and Pantelis C (1995). Cognitive flexibility and complex integration in Parkinson's disease, Huntington's disease and schizophrenia. *Journal of the International Neuropsychological Society* **1**: 545–553.

Hans MB and Gilmore TH (1968). Social aspects of Huntington's chorea. *British Journal of Psychiatry* **114**: 93–98.

Hayden MR, Ehrlich R, Parker H, and Ferera SJ (1980). Social perspectives in Huntington's chorea. *South African Medical Journal* **58**: 201–203.

Heathfield KWG (1967). Huntington's chorea: investigation into prevalence in N.E. Metropolitan Regional Hospital Board area. *Brain* **90**: 203–233.

Heindel WC, Butters N, and Salmon DP (1988). Impaired learning of a motor skill in patients with Huntington's disease. *Behavioural Neuroscience* **102**: 141–147.

—— Salmon DP, Shults CW, Walicke PA, and Butters N (1989). Neuropsychological evidence for multiple implicit memory systems: a comparison of Alzheimer's, Huntington's and Parkinson's disease patients. *Journal of Neuroscience* **9**: 582–587.

—— Salmon DP, and Butters N (1990). Pictorial priming and cued recall in Alzheimer's disease and Huntington's disease. *Brain and Cognition* **13**: 282–295.

—— Salmon DP, and Butters N (1991). The biasing of weight judgments in Alzheimer's disease and Huntington's disease: a priming or programming phenomenon. *Journal of Clinical and Experimental Neuropsychology* **13**: 189–203.

Hodges JR, Salmon DP, and Butters N (1991). The nature of the naming deficit in Alzheimer's and Huntington's disease. *Brain* **114**: 1547–1558.

Huntington G. (1872). On chorea. *The Medical and Surgical Reporter* **26**: 317–321.

Huntington's Disease Collaborative Research Group (1993). A novel gene containing a trinucleotide repeat that is expanded and unstable on Huntington's disease chromosomes. *Cell* **72**: 971–983.

Huntington Study Group (1996). Unified Huntington's disease rating scale: reliability and consistency. *Movement Disorders* **11**: 136–142.

Jacobs DH, Shuren J, and Heilman KM (1995). Impaired perception of facial identity and facial affect in Huntington's disease. *Neurology* **45**: 1217–1218.

Jahanshahi M, Brown RG, and Marsden CD (1993). A comparative study of simple and choice reaction time in Parkinson's, Huntington's and cerebellar disease. *Journal of Neurology, Neurosurgery and Psychiatry* **56**: 1169–1177.

Jason GW, Pajurkova EM, Suchowersky O, Hewitt J, Hilbert C, Reed J, and Hayden MR (1988). Presymptomatic neuropsychological impairment in Huntington's disease. *Archives of Neurology* **45**: 769–773.

Jensen P, Fenger K, Bolwig TG, and Sorensen SA (1998). Crime in Huntington's disease: a study of registered offences among patients, relatives and controls. *Journal of Neurology, Neurosurgery and Psychiatry* **65**: 467–471.

Josiassen RC, Curry LM, and Mancall EL (1983). Development of neuropsychological deficits in Huntington's disease. *Archives of Neurology* **40**: 791–796.

King M (1985). Alcohol abuse and Huntington's disease. *Psychological Medicine* **15**: 815–819.

Kirkwood SC, Siemers E, Stout JC, Hodes ME, Conneally PM, Christian JC, and Foroud T (1999). Longitudinal cognitive and motor changes among presymptomatic Huntington disease gene carriers. *Archives of Neurology* **56**: 563–568.

Knopman D and Nissen MJ (1991). Procedural learning is impaired in Huntington's disease: evidence from the serial reaction time task. *Neuropsychologia* **29**: 245–254.

Knowlton BJ, Squire LR, Paulsen JS, Swerdlow NR, Swenson M, and Butters N (1996). Dissociations within nondeclarative memory in Huntington's disease. *Neuropsychology* **10**: 538–548.

Lange KW, Sahakian BJ, Quinn NP, Marsden CD, and Robbins TW (1995). Comparison of executive and visuospatial memory function in Huntington's disease and dementia of Alzheimer type matched for degree of dementia. *Journal of Neurology, Neurosurgery and Psychiatry* **58**: 598–606.

Lawrence AD, Sahakian BJ, Hodges JR, Rosser AE, Lange KW, and Robbins TW (1996). Executive and mnemonic functions in early Huntington's disease. *Brain* **119**: 1633–1645.

—— Weeks RA, Brooks DJ, Andrews TC, Watkins LH, Harding AE, Robbins TW, and Sahakian BJ (1998a). The relationship between striatal dopamine receptor binding and cognitive performance in Huntington's disease. *Brain* **121**: 1343–1355.

—— Hodges JR, Rosser AE, Kershaw A, Ffrench-Constant C, Rubinsztein DC, Robbins TW, and Sahakian BJ (1998b). Evidence for specific cognitive deficits in preclinical Huntington's disease. *Brain* **121**: 1329–1341.

Leroi I and Michalon M (1998). Treatment of the psychiatric manifestations of Huntington's disease: a review of the literature. *Canadian Journal of Psychiatry* **43**: 933–940.

Lishman WA (1998). *Organic psychiatry. The psychological consequences of cerebral disorder*, 3rd edn. Oxford: Blackwell Science.

Lovestone S, Hodgson S, Sham P, Differ AM, and Levy R (1996). Familial psychiatric presentation of Huntington's disease. *Journal of Medical Genetics* **33**: **128–131.**

Lundervold AJ and Reinvang I (1995). Variability in cognitive function among persons at high genetic risk of Huntington's disease. *Acta Neurological Scandinavica* **91**: 462–469.

—— Reinvang I, and Lundervold A (1994). Characteristic patterns of verbal memory function in patients with Huntington's disease. *Scandinavian Journal of Psychology* **35**: 38–47.

MacMillan JC, Snell RG, Tyler A, Houlihan GD, Fenton I, Cheadle JP, Lazarou LP, Shaw DJ, and Harper PS (1993). Molecular analyses and clinical correlations of the Huntington's disease mutation. *Lancet* **342**: 954–958.

Mayberg HD, Starkstein SE, Peyser CE, Brandt J, Dannals RF, and Folstein SE (1992). Paralimbic frontal lobe hypometabolism in depression associated with Huntington's disease. *Neurology* **42**: 1791–1797.

Mayeux R, Stern Y, Herman A, Greenbaum L, and Fahn S (1986). Correlates of early disability in Huntington's disease. *Annals of Neurology* **20**: 727–731.

Mindham RHS, Steele C, Folstein MF, and Lucas J (1985). A comparison of the frequency of major affective disorder in Huntington's disease and Alzheimer's disease. *Journal of Neurology, Neurosurgery and Psychiatry* **48**: 1172–1174.

Minski L and Guttmann E (1938). Huntington's chorea: a study of 34 families. *Journal of Mental Science* **84**: 21–96.

Mohr E, Brouwers P, Claus JJ, Mann UM, Fedio P, and Chase TN (1991). Visuospatial cognition in Huntington's disease. *Movement Disorders* **6**: 127–132.

—— Claus JJ, and Brouwers P (1997). Basal ganglia disease and visuospatial cognition: are there disease-specific impairments? *Behavioural Neurology* **10**: 67–75.

Monsch AU, Bondi MW, Butters N, Paulsen JS, Salmon DP, Brugger P, and Swenson MR (1994). A comparison of category and letter fluency in Alzheimer's disease and Huntington's disease. *Neuropsychology* **8**: 25–30.

Morris M (1991). Psychiatric aspects of Huntington's disease. In PS Harper, ed. *Huntington's disease* (ed. P.S. Harper), pp 81–126. Philadelphia: W.B. Saunders.

Neary D, Snowden JS, Northen B, and Goulding PJ (1988). Dementia of frontal lobe type. *Journal of Neurology, Neurosurgery and Psychiatry* **51**: 353–361.

Nordin S, Paulsen JS, and Murphy C (1995). Sensory and memory-mediated olfactory dysfunction in Huntington's disease. *Journal of the International Neuropsychological Society* **1**: 281–290.

Oliver JE (1970). Huntington's chorea in Northamptonshire. *British Journal of Psychiatry* **116**: 241–253.

Paulsen JS, Butters N, Sadek JR, Johnson SA, Salmon DP, Swerdlow NR, and Swenson MR (1995a). Distinct cognitive profiles of cortical and subcortical dementia in advanced illness. *Neurology* **45**: 951–956.

—— Salmon DP, Monsch AU, Butters N, Swenson MR, and Bondi MW (1995b). Discrimination of cortical from subcortical dementias on the basis of memory and problem-solving tests. *Journal of Clinical Psychology* **51**: 48–58.

Pflanz S, Besson JAO, Ebmeier KP, and Simpson S (1991). The clinical manifestation of mental disorder in Huntington's disease: a retrospective case record study of disease progression. *Acta Psychiatrica Scandinavica* **83**: 53–60.

Pillon B, Dubois B, Ploska A, and Agid Y (1991). Severity and specificity of cognitive impairment in Alzheimer's, Huntington's, and Parkinson's diseases and progressive supranuclear palsy. *Neurology* **41**: 634–643.

—— Deweer B, Agid Y, and Dubois B (1993). Explicit memory in Alzheimer's, Huntington's and Parkinson's diseases. *Archives of Neurology* **50**: 374–379.

Podoll K, Caspary P, Lange HW, and Noth J (1988). Language functions in Huntington's disease. *Brain* **111**: 1475–1503.

Potegal M (1971). A note on spatial-motor deficits in patients with Huntington's disease: a test of a hypothesis. *Neuropsychologia* **9**: 233–235.

Ranen NG, Peyser CE, and Folstein SE (1993). *A physician's guide to the management of Huntington's disease*. New York: Huntington's Disease Society of America.

Rich JB, Troyer AK, Bylsma FW, and Brandt J (1999). Longitudinal analysis of phonemic clustering and switching during word list generation in Huntington's disease. *Neuropsychology* **13**: 525–531.

Robbins LN, Helzer JE, Croughan J, and Ratcliffe KS (1981). National Institute of Mental Health Diagnostic Interview Schedule. *Archives of General Psychiatry* **38**: 381–389.

—— Helzer JE, Weissman MM, Orvaschel H, Gruenberg E, Burke JD, and Regier DA (1984). Lifetime prevalence of specific psychiatric disorders in three sites. *Archives of General Psychiatry* **41**: 949–958.

Rohrer D, Salmon DP, Wixted JT, and Paulsen JS (1999). The disparate effects of Alzheimer's disease and Huntington's disease on semantic memory. *Neuropsychology* **13**: 381–388.

Rosenberg NK, Sorensen SA, and Christensen AL (1995). Neuropsychological characteristics of Huntington's disease carriers: a double blind study. *Journal of Medical Genetics* **32**: 600–604.

Rosser AE and Hodges JR (1994). Initial letter and semantic category fluency in Alzheimer's disease, Huntington's disease and progressive supranuclear palsy. *Journal of Neurology, Neurosurgery and Psychiatry* **57**: 1389–1394.

Rothlind JC, Bylsma FW, Peyser C, Folstein SE, and Brandt J (1993a). Cognitive and motor correlates of everyday functioning in early Huntington's disease. *Journal of Nervous Mental Disorders* **181**: 194–199.

—— Brandt J, Zee D, Codori AM, and Folstein S (1993b). Unimpaired verbal memory and oculomotor control in asymptomatic adults with the genetic marker for Huntington's disease. *Archives of Neurology* **50**: 799–802.

Rouleau I, Salmon DP, Butters N, Kennedy C, and McGuire K (1992). Quantitative and qualitative analyses in clock drawings in Alzheimer's and Huntington's disease. *Brain and Cognition* **18**: 70–87.

Saugstad L and Ødegård Ø (1986). Huntington's chorea in Norway. *Psychological Medicine* **16**: 39–48.

Schoenfeld M, Myers RH, Cupples LA, Berkman B, Sax DS, and Clark E (1984). Increased rates of suicide among patients with Huntington's disease. *Journal of Neurology, Neurosurgery and Psychiatry* **47**: 1283–1287.

Shoulson I. (1981). Huntington's disease: functional capacities in patients treated with neuroleptic and antidepressant drugs. *Neurology* **31**: 1333–1335.

—— and Fahn S (1979). Huntington's disease: clinical care and evaluation. *Neurology* **29**: 1–3.

Siemers E, Foroud T, Bill DJ, Sorbel J, Norton JA, Hodes ME, Niebler G, Conneally M, and Christian JC (1996). Motor changes in presymptomatic Huntington disease gene carriers. *Archives of Neurology* **53**: 487–492.

Snowden JS, Craufurd D, Griffiths HL, and Neary D (1998). Awareness of involuntary movements in Huntington's disease. *Archives of Neurology* **55**: 801–805.

Snowden J, Craufurd D, Griffiths H, Thompson J, and Neary D (2000). Longitudinal evaluation of cognitive disorder in Huntington's disease. *Journal of the International Neuropsychological Society* **6**: 33–44.

Snowden JS, Craufurd D, Thompson J, and Neary D (2002). Psychomotor, executive and memory function in preclinical Huntington's disease. *Journal of Clinical and Experimental Neuropsychology* **24**(2): 133–145.

Spitzer RL and Endicott J (1978). *Schedule for affective disorders and schizophrenia*. New York, NY: New York State Psychiatric Institute.

—— and Robbins E (1977). *Research Diagnostic Criteria (RDC). for a selected group of functional disorders*. New York, NY: New York State Psychiatric Institute.

Sprengelmeyer R, Lange H, and Homberg V (1995). The pattern of attentional deficits in Huntington's disease. *Brain* **118**: 145–152.

Sprengelmeyer R, Young AW, Calder AJ, Karnat A, lange H, Homberg V, Perrett DI, and Rowland D (1996). Loss of disgust. Perception of faces and emotions in Huntington's disease. *Brain* **119**: 1647–1665.

Starkstein SE, Brandt J, Bylsma F, Peyser C, Folstein M, and Folstein SE (1992). Neuropsychological correlates of brain atrophy in Huntington's disease: a magnetic resonance imaging study. *Neuroradiology* **34**: 487–489.

Strauss ME and Brandt J (1990). Are there neuropsychological manifestations of the gene for Huntington's disease in asymptomatic at-risk individuals? *Archives of Neurology* **7**: 905–908.

Thompson J, Snowden JS, Neary D, and Craufurd D (2002). Behavior in Huntington's disease. Dissociating cognitive and mood based changes. *Journal of Neuropsychiatry and Clinical Neurosciences* **14**: 37–43.

Tsuang D, DiGiacomo L, Lipe H, and Bird TD (1998). Familial aggregation of schizophrenia-like symptoms in Huntington's disease. *American Journal of Medical Genetics (Neuropsychiatric Genetics)* **81**: 323–327.

Watkins LH, Rogers RD, Lawrence AD, Sahakian BJ, Rosser AE, and Robbins TW (2000). Impaired planning but intact decision making in early Huntington's disease: implications for specific fronto-striatal pathology. *Neuropsychologia* **38**: 1112–1125.

Weigell-Weber M, Schmid W, and Spiegel R (1996). Psychiatric symptoms and CAG expansion in Huntington's disease. *American Journal of Medical Genetics* **67**: 53–57.

Weinberger DR, Berman KF, Iadarola M, Driesen N, and Zec RF (1988). Prefrontal cortical blood flow and cognitive function in Huntington's disease. *Journal of Neurology, Neurosurgery and Psychiatry* **51**: 94–104.

Wexler NS (1979). Genetic "Russian roulette": the experience of being at risk for Huntington's disease. In *Genetic counselling: psychological dimensions* (ed. S. Kessler), pp. 190–220. New York: Academic Press.

Willingham DB and Koroshetz WJ (1993). Evidence for dissociable motor skills in Huntington's disease patients. *Psychobiology* **21**: 173–182.

—— —— Peterson EW (1996). Motor skills have diverse neural bases: spared and impaired skill acquisition in Huntington's disease. *Neuropsychology* **10**: 315–321.

Wing JK, Cooper JE, and Sartorius N (1984). *Measurement and classification of psychiatric symptoms*. Cambridge: Cambridge University Press.

Zappacosta B, Monza D, Meoni C, Austoni L, Soliveri P, Gellera C, Alberti R, Mantero M, Penati G. Caraceni T, and Girotti F (1996). Psychiatric symptoms do not correlate with cognitive decline, motor symptoms or CAG repeat length in Huntington's disease. *Archives of Neurology* **53**: 493–497.

4 Imaging Huntington's disease

David J. Brooks and Thomasin Andrews

Introduction

Huntington's disease (HD) is an autosomal dominant condition characterized by the onset of a mixed movement disorder, usually in middle age. The most characteristic clinical feature of the movement disorder is the presence of chorea. However, reduced speed of movement is also evident, particularly when patients perform sequential or simultaneous tasks. Later in the condition extrapyramidal rigidity is a feature and young-onset cases often present with the akinetic rigid Westphal variant (Marshall and Shoulson 1997). The essential locomotor features of HD can be thought of as a failure to filter out unwanted movements combined with an inability to perform volitional movements efficiently.

The genetic basis of the disease is an expansion of a CAG trinucleotide repeat in the IT15 gene on chromosome 4 leading to a glutamine expansion in the huntingtin protein with the formation of cytoplasmic and nuclear aggregations (Davies *et al.* 1997; DiFiglia *et al.* 1997; Huntington's Disease Collaborative Research Group 1993). The relationship of aggregation to the disease is unclear, and the cause of neuronal dysfunction and death unknown. These topics are discussed in detail in Chapters 11–13. The pathology of HD targets the striatum with loss of dopamine D1- and D2-receptor expressing γ-aminobutyric acid (GABA)ergic medium spiny neurones (Augood *et al.* 1997). Preclinical HD shows the greatest predilection for D2- and adenosine A2A-bearing striatal neurones that project to external globus pallidum (GPe), while in the choreic form D1-bearing projections to substantia nigra pars reticulata (SNr) are also involved (Albin *et al.* 1990; Glass *et al.* 2000). The akinetic rigid variant targets D2-bearing striatal projections to GPe and D1-bearing striatal projections to internal globus pallidum (GPi) and SNr in an equal fashion. At end-stage, HD is associated with cortical atrophy. The global and molecular neuropathology is described in detail in Chapter 8. During the preclinical stage asymptomatic mutation carriers may exhibit early subtle motor and cognitive signs of disease though debate still remains over whether these are cortical or subcortical in origin (Brandt and Bylsma 1993; Lawrence *et al.* 1996).

There is little post-mortem data from preclinical or early HD, but a variety of brain imaging techniques have been used *in vivo* to study patients and asymptomatic mutation carriers. These studies have extended our understanding of the natural history and time course of the disease and clarified the functional anatomy underlying the various symptomatologies of HD. Additionally, they provide a measure of disease progression so that in future the efficacy of putative neuroprotective agents can be objectively assessed.

Structural imaging

A number of *in vivo* studies have employed computerized tomography (CT) and volumetric magnetic resonance imaging (MRI) to demonstrate caudate and putamen atrophy in patients with HD. Degree of caudate atrophy has been shown to correlate with disease duration (Kuhl *et al.* 1982; Oepen and Ostertag 1981; Starkstein *et al.* 1989), severity of dementia (Bamford *et al.* 1989; Sax *et al.* 1983; Starkstein *et al.* 1988, 1992), severity of movement disorder (Kuhl *et al.* 1982), impairment of eye movements (Starkstein *et al.* 1988), and total functional capacity (TFC) (Starkstein *et al.* 1988; Stober *et al.* 1984). In a longitudinal study, Bamford *et al.* (1995) reported that CT measures of caudate atrophy correlate poorly with neuropsychological deficits in a cohort of patients with advanced disease. In contrast, Starkstein *et al.* (1992), using MRI, found that a battery of neuropsychological tests correlated with caudate atrophy, frontal atrophy, and atrophy of the left sylvian cistern. Early studies of asymptomatic 'at-risk' subjects using linear measures of caudate size failed to show caudate atrophy (Mazziotta *et al.* 1987; Young *et al.* 1987). Aylward *et al.* (1994), using a more sensitive MR volumetric approach, found that asymptomatic at-risk subjects for HD had smaller basal ganglia structures than those of controls. A subsequent series revealed that putamen volume was the best predictor of DNA marker status (Aylward *et al.* 1996). Harris *et al.* (1996) compared MR volumetric and single-photon emission CT (SPECT) blood flow measures for a group of patients with mild to moderate HD and a group of healthy volunteers. Putamen volume was decreased by 54 per cent compared with only a 21 per cent decrease in caudate blood flow. Level of disability correlated best with putamen volume, while neuropsychological performance, rated on a battery of tests, correlated best with global atrophy as reflected by cerebrospinal fluid volume.

In a longitudinal series, Aylward and co-workers (1997) were able to demonstrate significant decreases in caudate, putamen, and total basal ganglia volumes in 23 HD patients over a mean of 20 months. Both age at clinical disease onset and length of trinucleotide repeat correlated with rate of basal ganglia volume change. In a follow-up report the same workers found that annual rates of caudate atrophy were 7.24, 4.90, and 2.43 per cent per annum, respectively, for patients with moderate, mild, or asymptomatic HD as rated with the Quantified Neurological Examination (QNE) (Aylward *et al.* 2000). These mean rates of progression of caudate volume loss were not significantly different between the three cohorts but, for the clinically affected patients, rate of caudate atrophy correlated with disease duration.

MRI volumetry has also been used to examine *in vivo* relative levels of cortical and subcortical degeneration in HD. While the most affected areas were invariably striatal structures, significant atrophy was also detected in the thalamus and in inferior cortical areas (orbitofrontal and temporo-occipital cortical regions), especially in mesial temporal lobe structures (Jernigan *et al.* 1991). A significant degree of white matter degeneration was also noted. While the established view is that cognitive deficits in early HD are primarily due to striatal pathology, volumetric evidence of limbic involvement and increased cerebrospinal fluid volume suggests that cortical dysfunction may also be a contributor towards mnestic and behavioural difficulties.

Functional imaging

Functional imaging provides a sensitive means of detecting and characterizing regional changes in brain metabolism and receptor binding in movement disorders. There are three main approaches to functional imaging: Positron emission tomography (PET) allows quantitative examination of regional cerebral blood flow (rCBF), glucose and oxygen metabolism (rCMRGlc, rCMRO$_2$, respectively), and brain pharmacology. SPECT gives semiquantitative estimates of rCBF and receptor binding. The bulk of reports concerning *in vivo* brain function in HD have, to date, concerned PET and so this chapter will concentrate on this technique but compare SPECT findings where relevant. There are two basic approaches to examining the changes in cerebral function that are associated with movement disorders. First, abnormalities in resting levels of regional cerebral metabolism, blood flow, and neuroreceptor binding can be examined. Second, either abnormal cortical and subcortical activity associated with involuntary movement *per se* can be studied or patients with movement disorders can be asked to perform motor tasks in order to reveal abnormalities in their patterns of cerebral activation.

Studies of resting cerebral metabolism

Levels of rCBF and rCMRGlu in a structure reflect integrated levels of synaptic activity (Lassen *et al.* 1978). In the first reported PET study in HD, Kuhl *et al.* (1982) used ^{18}F-2-fluoro-2-deoxyglucose (^{18}FDG) to demonstrate reduced striatal glucose metabolism in patients with early HD. Subsequently, Hayden and co-workers (1986) confirmed these findings and also showed that significant reductions in caudate glucose metabolism could be detected in patients with early HD when only minimal structural changes were visible on CT.

Severity of bradykinesia and rigidity and total functional capacity (TFC) have been reported to correlate best with caudate hypometabolism while severity of chorea, eye movement abnormalities, and motor function correlate with putamen hypometabolism (Young *et al.* 1986). As levels of caudate and putamen metabolism are intercorrelated in HD, however, it is probably not meaningful to try and ascribe individual locomotor deficits to one or other of these structures based on PET findings. Severity of dystonia was found to correlate with levels of thalamic hypermetabolism.

Subsequently, it was demonstrated that significantly reduced striatal glucose metabolism could be detected in up to 75 per cent of relatives at high risk for HD based on linkage analysis findings (Grafton *et al.* 1990; Hayden *et al.* 1987b; Kuwert *et al.* 1993). This was at a time before the IT15 gene had been identified. Grafton and colleagues (1990) were able to identify a subgroup of 'high-risk' subjects for HD who had reduced striatal metabolism in the absence of any soft symptoms or signs of disease. This clearly established that there is an identifiable period of time in which striatal degeneration is occurring in HD prior to the onset of clinical symptoms. In these studies PET was more sensitive than CT or the presence of early clinical signs for identifying subclinical disease activity; however, volumetric MRI has not, to date, been directly compared with FDG PET. Grafton *et al.* (1992a) then went on to demonstrate that subjects at high risk for HD who had significantly reduced striatal glucose metabolism at baseline showed an annual 3.1 and 1.9 per cent decline in their caudate and putamen glucose utilization, respectively, and an annual 3.6 per cent increase in their bicaudate ratio on CT.

^{18}FDG PET measures of cortical metabolism lie in the normal range in preclinical HD but advanced patients develop extensive cortical hypometabolism initially targeting prefrontal and inferior parietal areas (Kuwert *et al.* 1990). Whether the early cortical dysfunction is due to local pathology or to functional depression of cortical neurones secondary to striatal pathology remains unclear. Berent *et al.* (1988) reported that neuropsychological measures of verbal learning and memory correlated selectively with levels of caudate metabolism. Mayberg and colleagues (1992) found reduced anterior cingulate along with striatal metabolism in patients with early HD but orbitofrontal–inferior parietal cortex hypometabolism was only present in those patients with superadded clinical depression. In contrast, SPECT series have reported correlations between patient mini-mental state examination (MMSE) scores and mean cortical blood flow, particularly in frontotemporal and parietal cortices (Sax *et al.* 1996; Tanahashi *et al.* 1985). In one SPECT study it was noted that performance on specific tests of 'frontal lobe' function (Wisconsin Card Sorting Test (WCST) and Picture Arrangement) correlated most strongly with levels of caudate blood flow while recognition memory, language, and perceptual impairments correlated with cortical rather than striatal blood flow (Hasselbalch *et al.* 1992). Given these findings, it seems likely that cortical dysfunction does contribute towards the behavioural impairments present even in early HD.

Cerebral activation

Two activation studies with $H_2^{15}O$ PET have investigated changes in levels of rCBF during performance of a motor activation task. The first study (Weeks *et al.* 1997a) compared levels of rCBF during movement of a joystick in freely chosen directions when paced by a tone with levels when at rest. The second study (Bartenstein *et al.* 1997) used paced sequential finger opposition movements as its paradigm. Both these studies reported reduced striatal, mesial premotor, and dorsal prefrontal activation in HD with relative overactivity of lateral premotor and parietal areas. More recently, Deckel and co-workers (2000) used technetium-99m labelled hexamethyl propyleneamine oxime (^{99m}Tc-HMPAO) SPECT to measure rCBF while subjects solved a maze problem on a computer visual display unit (VDU) or studied a previously solved maze. When rCBF was normalized to global values, HD patients showed relatively reduced levels of striatal and orbitofrontal activity during maze-solving. Taken together, these three studies suggest that the functional effect of HD pathology is to reduce striatal, mesial premotor, and prefrontal activation due to loss of basal ganglia connections resulting in a compensatory recruitment of normally redundant cortical areas (parietal, insular) in order to facilitate task performance.

In a follow up study, Bartenstein and co-workers examined brain processing of vibrotactile stimulation to the index fingers in HD (Boecker *et al.* 1999). In the control cohort, brain activation was lateralized to the side opposite to the applied stimulus and included primary sensory cortex (S1), secondary sensory cortex (S2), globus pallidus, and ventrolateral thalamus. HD patients showed decreased activation of contralateral S2, parietal areas 39 and 40, and lingual gyrus, bilateral prefrontal cortex (Brodmann areas 8, 9, 10, and 44), S1, and the contralateral basal ganglia. There was a relatively enhanced aberrant activation of ipsilateral sensory cortical areas—caudal S1, S2, and insular cortex. These findings suggest that HD is not just a disorder of motor but also of sensory processing characterized by reduced contralateral and enhanced ipsilateral cortical and subcortical activation on passive sensory stimulation.

Weinberger *et al.* (1988) using SPECT studied cerebral activation in HD patients during performance of the WCST. The HD subjects showed impaired performance despite having normal baseline levels of resting cortical rCBF. Levels of prefrontal flow seen during the task correlated inversely with caudate volume. This finding suggests that: (1) impaired WCST performance relates to caudate rather than prefrontal pathology; (2) increased activation of an intact frontal cortex is required as a compensatory mechanism for caudate dysfunction. A second study from the same group supported these viewpoints. HD patients showed increased prefrontal and reduced parietal rCBF during WCST performance while patients with schizophrenia showed the reverse pattern (Goldberg *et al.* 1990).

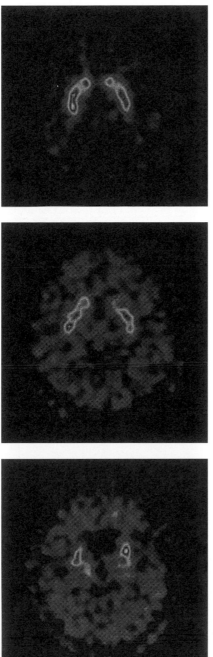

Normal
subject

Asymptomatic
HD gene carrier

Clinically affected
HD case

Fig. 4.1 ^{11}C-raclopride PET scans of dopamine D2 binding.

Postsynaptic dopamine receptor binding

Selective dopamine D1 and D2 receptor antagonists have been developed as PET and SPECT tracers to allow *in vivo* measurements of striatal dopamine binding in both clinically affected and asymptomatic HD mutation carriers. Dopamine receptor binding potentials (BPs)—the ratio of specific to nonspecific tracer volumes of distribution—provide a direct marker of basal ganglia function.

Severe loss of both striatal D1 and D2 receptor binding has been demonstrated in HD at post-mortem (Cross and Rossor 1983; Reisine *et al.* 1977) and *in vivo* using both PET and SPECT (see Fig. 4.1; Wong *et al.* 1985; Brandt *et al.* 1990; Ginovart *et al.* 1997; Hagglund *et al.* 1987; Ichise *et al.* 1993; Leenders *et al.* 1986; Sedvall *et al.* 1994). Clinically affected patients with HD show a parallel loss of striatal D1 and D2 dopamine receptor binding with mean binding potentials reduced by 60 per cent (range 40–80 per cent) (Turjanski *et al.* 1995). PET has also demonstrated that around 50 per cent of at-risk asymptomatic adult HD gene carriers have reduced striatal D1 and D2 receptor binding. These healthy, at-risk subjects were individually found to have binding potentials reduced up to 50 per cent below the population mean (Antonini *et al.* 1996; Hayden *et al.* 1987a; Weeks *et al.* 1996). When combined with Turjanski's observations, the above findings suggest that symptom onset in HD corresponds with a 30–50 per cent loss of striatal dopamine D1 and D2 receptor binding.

Using ^{11}C-SCH 23390 and ^{11}C-raclopride PET, Andrews *et al.* (1999) examined the correlation between motor and total functional scores rated with the unified HD rating scale (UHDRS) and levels of striatal D1 and D2 binding in HD gene carriers. Thirteen subjects were studied, nine of whom were asymptomatic of whom four had no signs on PET examination. There was a significant correlation between UHDRS motor and TFC scores and both striatal D1 and D2 binding in HD gene carriers (see Fig. 4.2). These workers concluded that

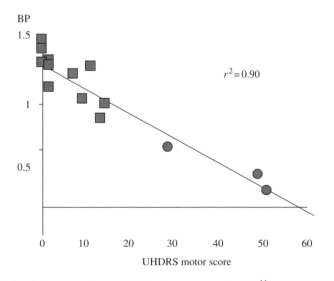

Fig. 4.2 A correlation between putamen D1 binding measured with ^{11}C-SCH23390 PET and motor UHDRS score in asymptomatic HD gene carriers (squares) and clinically affected individuals (circles). BP, D1 binding potential.

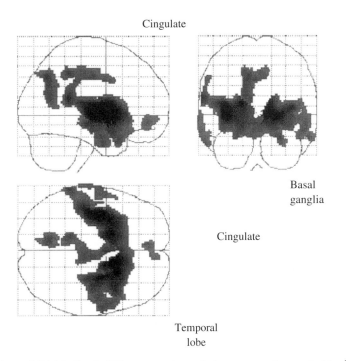

Fig. 4.3 Reductions of D1 binding in HD gene carriers relative to controls revealed by ^{11}C-SCH23390 PET and statistical parametric mapping ($p < 0.001$).

both PET measures of striatal dopamine binding and the UHDRS provide sensitive means of detecting the presence of early disease in asymptomatic HD gene carriers.

PET measures of caudate and putamen D1 and D2 receptor binding have been shown to correlate with performance on prefrontal tasks, such as Tower of London, spatial span, and letter fluency (Lawrence *et al.* 1998), and with performance on symbol digit modality and trail-making (Brandt *et al.* 1990) in clinically affected patients and asymptomatic mutation carriers, again suggesting a possible causative association between basal ganglia pathology and cognitive dysfunction.

Two series from the Karolinska Institute have reported reductions in cortical D1 dopamine binding in HD using ^{11}C-SCH23390 PET. Both used a region of interest approach; Sedvall *et al.* (1994) reported reduced D1 binding in frontal lobe and Ginovart *et al.* (1997) reported reduced binding in temporal lobe. Using statistical parametric mapping we have localized significant reductions in ^{11}C-SCH23390 binding in Huntington's disease patients relative to controls and asymptomatic mutation carriers in bilateral caudate and putamen, in prefrontal area 10, cingulate gyrus, precuneus, and temporal lobe regions (see Fig. 4.3). A covariate of interest analysis of ^{11}C-SCH23390 uptake found that D1 binding in both striatal and temporal lobe voxels correlated significantly with UHDRS cognitive scores.

Dopamine binding in HD and models of basal ganglia connectivity

In the Penney–Young model (Penney and Young 1986) chorea is hypothesized to result from early loss of enkephalin containing striatopallidal neurones from the indirect pathway. As these neurones preferentially express D2 sites (Gerfen 1992), it was predicted that patients with early choreic HD would show preferential loss of D2-bearing neurones while patients with akinetic rigid or advanced HD would show a nonselective loss of both D1- and D2-bearing neurones. Post-mortem autoradiographic studies, however, have demonstrated a similar loss of both D1 and D2 receptors in early HD. Striatal areas lose both D1 and D2 receptors, the former being more affected (Joyce *et al.* 1988; Richfield *et al.* 1991), while D1 receptors are decreased in GPi and SNr and D2 receptors are decreased in GPe as pathological stage increases (Augood *et al.* 1997; Richfield *et al.* 1991).

The relationship between striatal D1 and D2 receptor loss in HD patients and asymptomatic mutation carriers has been investigated *in vivo* using PET (Ginovart *et al.* 1997; Turjanski *et al.* 1995; Weeks *et al.* 1996) and has demonstrated *parallel* reductions of both D1 and D2 striatal binding at all stages of the disease, regardless of phenotype. Severity of rigidity, but not chorea, correlates with the extent of dopamine receptor loss (Turjanski *et al.* 1995). These studies, therefore, do not support a model in which D2-receptor-bearing neurones are preferentially targeted in early choreic HD.

In Folstein and Hedreen's model of chorea (Hedreen and Folstein 1995), degeneration of striosomal–nigral neurones causes disinhibition of nigrostriatal dopaminergic neurones, resulting in increased dopaminergic activity in the striatum. This would decrease the excitability of the (inhibitory) D2-receptor-bearing enkephalin-containing striatal neurones that project to GPe, resulting in increased thalamocortical output and chorea. Combined D1 and D2 receptor loss in early choreic HD would remain compatible with this model (with perhaps greater loss of D1 receptors from caudate) as the neurodegenerative process preferentially targets striosomal neurones in very early disease. However, this model also predicts that there should be increased levels of striatal dopamine, which has not been established.

PET studies of the integrity of the presynaptic nigrostriatal dopaminergic system in HD have been inconsistent in their findings. One *in vivo* case study reported normal ^{18}F-dopa uptake in a patient with markedly reduced D2 binding (Leenders *et al.* 1986); however, ^{18}F-dopa uptake reflects striatal dopa decarboxylase activity rather than dopamine levels. Ginovart *et al.* (1997) used ^{11}C-labelled beta-carbomethoxy-3 beta-(4-iodophenyltropane) (^{11}C-βCIT) PET to study dopamine transporter binding and reported reduced tracer uptake in caudate and putamen. The dopamine transporter is located presynaptically and transports dopamine from the synaptic cleft back into the presynaptic neurone. The uptake of ^{11}C-βCIT, however, is flow-dependent and so this finding may not selectively reflect decreased expression or availability of the dopamine transporter. Downregulation of striatal dopamine transporters, however, would be more in favour of decreased rather than increased dopamine levels, this being a mechanism to maintain synaptic transmitter levels.

Further studies are needed to determine the true status of the nigrostriatal dopaminergic system in HD. A better understanding of the distribution of receptors between the various subpopulations of striatal efferents with new, more specific ligands will enable us to untangle the pathological substrates of chorea, dystonia, bradykinesia, and rigidity in HD.

Objective measurement of HD progression

Grafton and co-workers (1992b) were the first to use PET to follow striatal function longitudinally in HD gene carriers. These workers reported that subjects at high risk for HD based on linkage analysis showed annual 3.1 and 1.9 per cent mean declines in caudate and putamen glucose utilization, respectively. As, however, [18]FDG uptake reflects both glial and neuronal metabolism, it is not a specific marker of striatal neuronal function in HD. Antonini and colleagues (1997) have reported serial ^{11}C-raclopride and [18]FDG PET findings in six asymptomatic HD carriers. They noted a mean annual 6.3 per cent reduction in striatal D2 binding and a 2.3 per cent reduction in glucose metabolism suggesting that dopamine binding may provide a more sensitive objective *in vivo* marker of HD progression. One of their five subjects showed no change in D2 binding suggesting that their disease was quiescent at the time of PET. More recently, with ^{11}C-raclopride PET, mean annual progression rates of 7.0 and 3.7 per cent for loss of striatal D2 binding in clinically affected and asymptomatic HD gene carriers, respectively, have been reported (Hussey *et al.* 1998).

Using serial ^{11}C-SCH 23390 and ^{11}C-raclopride PET, we have followed striatal dopamine D1 and D2 receptor binding over a mean of 40 months in 13 HD gene carriers (nine asymptomatic at baseline) and another three at-risk relatives (see Fig. 4.4; Andrews *et al.* 1999). Seven mutation negative relatives were also serially scanned as controls. The clinically affected subjects showed mean annual reductions of 5.0 and 3.0 per cent for striatal D1 and D2 binding, respectively, while asymptomatic gene carriers showed mean annual reductions of

Baseline study

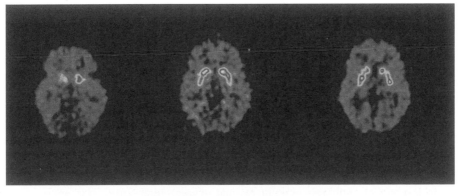

Follow-up study

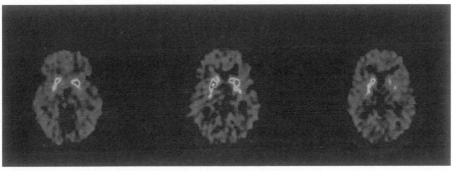

Fig. 4.4 Serial ^{11}C-SCH23390 PET studies in an asymptomatic HD gene mutation carrier 3 years apart. Loss of striatal and cortical D1 binding is evident in the second scans.

2.0 and 4.0 per cent, respectively. These reduction rates were significantly higher than those seen for the combined mutation negative and at-risk groups where no loss of dopamine binding was detected. Levels of striatal D1 and D2 binding were correlated cross-sectionally at baseline and at the follow-up in HD but annual rates of loss of D1 and D2 binding were not correlated. The rate of loss of striatal D2 binding correlated with CAG repeat length for the asymptomatic HD gene carrier cohort.

If the nine asymptomatic gene carriers were separated into subgroups with 'active' (>5 per cent total reduction) and 'inactive' disease, then the actively progressing subgroup (5 of 9) showed mean 4.4 and 6.4 per cent annual reductions in striatal D1 and D2 binding, respectively. This, along with Antonini *et al.*'s (1997) findings, suggests that PET can be used to detect those asymptomatic HD gene carriers where disease is active and who may be potential candidates for neuroprotective or restorative therapy. The results also confirm that HD may not become active until middle life. In support of this, one of our asymptomatic HD gene carriers with low striatal D1 and D2 binding (60 per cent of normal at baseline) became clinically affected over a 3-year follow-up period when their D1 and D2 binding fell to 58 and 51 per cent of normal, respectively.

It is difficult to assess the relative rates of progression of early and late disease based on reported PET findings. Our data and those of Antonini *et al.* (1998) suggest that asymptomatic gene carriers showing active loss of striatal dopamine binding disease may progress faster than clinically affected cases and that progression correlates with CAG repeat length. In favour of this viewpoint, post-mortem data (Augood *et al.* 1997) has shown D1 binding per surviving striatal neurone is markedly reduced in early disease but then may rise as subpopulations expressing D1 sites but unaffected by HD pathology survive. The PET data of Hussey *et al.* (1998) however, are more in favour of the converse: further longitudinal progression studies are required to clarify this issue.

Opioid and benzodiazepine binding

PET ligands binding to opioid and benzodiazepine receptors have also been used to investigate changes in brain neurochemistry in HD patients. Using ^{11}C-diprenorphine PET, Weeks and co-workers (1997b) found significantly reduced opioid receptor binding in the caudate and lentiform nuclei, midbrain, cingulate, and medial temporal cortex with increased binding in thalamus and prefrontal areas in patients with early HD. These findings confirm that HD is not simply a disorder of basal ganglia function. Striatal opioid receptor binding was less severely compromised than dopamine receptor binding at equivalent stages of disease suggesting, however, that this would prove to be a less sensitive marker of disease activity.

GABA is the main neurotransmitter in over 90 per cent of striatal neurones. Benzodiazepine (BDZ) antagonists bind to a modulatory site on the $GABA_A$ receptor complex. Using ^{11}C-flumazenil PET, Holthoff *et al.* (1993) found that HD patients with reduced striatal glucose metabolism showed a 20 per cent reduction in central BDZ binding in caudate but normal binding in the lentiform nucleus. As the lentiform nucleus signal includes contributions from both putamen and pallidum, these workers concluded that normal signal probably represented a combination of decreased putamen and increased pallidal signal, the latter occurring as a response to loss of GABA afferents. Kunig and colleagues (2000) have recently confirmed this finding and extended it by reporting an inverse correlation in HD between putamen D2 binding, measured with ^{11}C-raclopride PET, and ^{11}C-flumazenil uptake. They interpreted this as indicating a relative upregulation of putamen BDZ binding in HD.

PET can thus be used to determine the relative vulnerability of different populations of receptors and neuronal subtypes in HD.

Transplantation in HD

Experimental grafting of foetal mesencephalic cells into the striatum of adults with parkinsonism has been reported to produce significant clinical improvements in the majority of younger patients (Lindvall 1999). In parkinsonism the cell bodies of the degenerating neurones are in the substantia nigra and the striatum is their target tissue. The implanted cells are thought to produce their early clinical effects by secreting dopamine tonically into the striatum; however, it is thought that, later, the foetal mesencephalic cells differentiate, form connections, and come under physiological control.

For striatal cell grafts to be therapeutic in HD, the cells must send outputs to globus pallidum and substantia nigra, the target nuclei of the degenerating medium spiny striatal neurones, and form connections with glutamatergic cortical efferents and dopaminergic nigrostriatal afferents. Transplantation of embryonic striatal tissue into the degenerated striatum of rat and primate models of HD has been shown to be safe, and has demonstrated good graft survival with differentiation and integration of striatal grafts into host striatum (Brasted *et al.* 1999a,b). Small-animal ^{11}C-raclopride PET has been able to detect recovery of striatal dopamine D2 binding in rats and marmosets lesioned with ibotenic acid after implantation of foetal striatal, but not foetal cortical, tissue (Fricker *et al.* 1997; Kendall *et al.* 1998; Torres *et al.* 1995). In primate models, recovery of skilled motor and cognitive performance has been reported within 2 months of grafting, and improvements in dystonia scores within 4–5 months (Palfi *et al.* 1998). No improvement in cognitive or motor function was seen in three sham-operated monkey controls. Physiological, neurochemical, and anatomical studies have shown that a partial restoration of striatal input and output circuitry by implanted striatal neurones does occur, but the time course of this in primates and humans remains unclear.

Groups in the USA, France, and England have now begun clinical studies of the possible therapeutic effects of striatal allografts in patients with HD. Recently, Bachoud-Levi and co-workers (2000a,b) have reported the preliminary FDG PET findings for five HD patients implanted with striatal cells from 8–9 week gestation foetuses. Three of the subjects were felt to have improved over the course of 12 months in this series while two deteriorated. In the three who clinically improved it was possible to detect striatal graft function, as evidenced by loci of increased glucose utilization, but not in the two cases who subsequently showed deterioration.

Conclusions

1. PET measures of striatal D1 and D2 binding with ^{11}C-SCH23390 and ^{11}C-raclopride PET correlate well with UHDRS motor and functional scores.

2. ^{18}FDG, ^{11}C-SCH23390, and ^{11}C-raclopride PET can all be used to objectively measure the rate of loss of striatal metabolism and dopamine D1 and D2 receptor binding in asymptomatic and clinically affected adult HD mutation carriers. Additionally, serial ^{11}C-SCH23390 and ^{11}C-raclopride PET can identify a subset of asymptomatic mutation carriers who are actively progressing and who would be suitable for future trials of putative neuroprotective or restorative therapies.

3. Measures of dopamine binding appear to provide a more sensitive marker of disease activity than measures of glucose utilization, possibly because the latter also reflect glial activity.

4. Further large prospective studies are needed to further characterize the time course of the pathological process in presymptomatic and clinical disease, and to investigate the relationship between changes in regional striatal dopamine-receptor binding and the various symptomatologies of the disease.

5. Reductions in resting cortical blood flow and D1 binding can be demonstrated in both clinically affected and asymptomatic HD mutation carriers, particularly in prefrontal and temporal regions, and the anterior cingulate gyrus.

6. Levels of cortical function in HD correlate with performance on behavioural tasks suggesting that both striatal and cortical dysfunction contribute to cognitive status even in early disease.

7. During motor tasks, HD patients show reduced striatal, mesial premotor, and prefrontal activation but overactivate lateral parietal and premotor areas to compensate.

The first HD patients have now received foetal cell implants. In the future it is hoped that neural precursor cells propagated *in vitro* will replace primary foetal tissue in therapeutic neural transplantation. Research into other strategies including neurotrophic factors such as ciliary neurotrophic factor (CNTF), caspase inhibitors, and gene therapy may result in new treatments that either halt the onset of the disease or significantly slow its progression. In any future treatment trial, it will be necessary to have objective measures of disease progression to complement the semi-objective clinical assessment scales. ^{11}C-SCH23390 and ^{11}C-raclopride PET have been shown to provide reliable and objective biological measures of striatal dysfunction in HD.

References

Albin RL, Reiner A, Anderson KD, Penney JB, and Young AB (1990). Striatal and nigral neuron subpopulations in rigid Huntington's disease: implications for the functional anatomy of chorea and rigidity-akinesia. *Annals of Neurology* **27**: 357–365.

Andrews TC, Weeks RA, Turjanski N, *et al.* (1999). Huntington's disease progression PET and clinical observations. *Brain* **122**: 2353–2363.

Antonini A, Leenders KL, Spiegel R, *et al.* (1996). Striatal glucose metabolism and dopamine D-2 receptor binding in asymptomatic gene carriers and patients with Huntington's disease. *Brain* **119**: 2085–2095.

—— Feigin A, Dhawan V, and Eidelberg D (1997). PET studies of Huntington's disease rate of progression. *Neurology* **48** (suppl. 2): A120.

—— Eidelberg D (1998). [C-11]Raclopride-PET studies of the Huntington's disease rate of progression: relevance of the trinucleotide repeat length. *Annals of Neurology* **43**: 253–255.

Augood SJ, Faull RLM, and Emson PC (1997). Dopamine D-1 and D-2 receptor gene expression in the striatum in Huntington's disease. *Annals of Neurology* **42**: 215–221.

Aylward EH, Brandt J, Codori AM, Mangus RS, Barta PE, and Harris GJ (1994). Reduced basal ganglia volume associated with the gene for Huntington's disease in asymptomatic at-risk persons. *Neurology* **44**: 823–828.

Aylward EH, Codori AM, Barta PE, Pearlson GD, Harris GJ, and Brandt J (1996). Basal ganglia volume and proximity to onset in presymptomatic Huntington disease. *Archives of Neurology* **53**: 1293–1296.

—— Li Q, Stine OC, *et al.* (1997). Longitudinal change in basal ganglia volume in patients with Huntington's disease. *Neurology* **48**: 394–399.

—— Codori AM, Rosenblatt A, *et al.* (2000). Rate of caudate atrophy in presymptomatic and symptomatic stages of Huntington's disease. *Movement Disorders* **15**: 552–560.

Bachoud-Levi A, Remy P, Nguyen JP, *et al.* (2000a). Motor and cognitive improvements in patients with Huntington's disease after neural transplantation. *Lancet* **356**: 1975–1979.

Bachoud-Levi AC, Bourdet C, Brugieres P, *et al.* (2000b). Safety and tolerability assessment of intrastriatal neural allografts in five patients with Huntington's disease. *Experimental Neurology* **161**: 194–202.

Bamford KA, Caine ED, Kido DK, Plassche WM, and Shoulson I (1989). Clinical–pathologic correlation in Huntington's disease—a neuropsychological and computed tomography study. *Neurology* **39**: 796–801.

—— Cox C, and Shoulson I (1995). A prospective evaluation of cognitive decline in early Huntington's disease—functional and radiographic correlates. *Neurology* **45**: 1867–1873.

Bartenstein P, Weindl A, Spiegel S, *et al.* (1997). Central motor processing in Huntington's disease—a PET study. *Brain* **120**: 1553–1567.

Berent S, Giordani B, Lehtinen S, Markel D, Penney JB, Buchtel HA, and Starosta-Rubinstein S (1988). Positron emission tomographic scan investigations of Huntington's disease: cerebral metabolic correlates of cognitive function. *Annals of Neurology* **23**: 541–546.

Boecker H, Ceballos-Baumann A, Bartenstein P, *et al.* (1999). Sensory processing in Parkinson's and Huntington's disease—investigations with 3D H_2-O-15-PET. *Brain* **122**: 1651–1665.

Brandt J, Folstein SE, Wong DF, Links J, Dannals RF, McDonnell-Sill A, Starkstein S, Anders P, Strauss ME, Tune LE, *et al.* (1990). D2 receptors in Huntington's disease: positron emission tomography findings and clinical correlates. *Journal of Neuropsychiatry and Clinical Neuroscience* **2**: 20–7.

Brandt JA and Bylsma FW (1993). The dementia of Huntington's disease. In *Neuropsychology of Alzheimer's disease and other dementias* (ed. RW Parks, RF Zec, and RS Wilson), pp. 265–282. New York: OUP.

—— Watts C, Robbins TW, and Dunnett SB (1999a). Associative plasticity in striatal transplants. *Proceedings of the National Academy of Sciences, USA* **96**: 10524–10529.

Brasted PJ, Watts C, Torres EM, Robbins TW, and Dunnett SB (1999b). Behavioural recovery following striatal transplantation: effects of postoperative training and P-zone volume. *Experimental Brain Research* **128**: 535–538.

Cross A and Rossor M (1983). Dopamine D1 and D2 receptors in Huntington's disease. *European Journal of Pharmacology* **88**: 223–229.

Davies SW, Turmaine M, Cozens BA, DiFiglia M, Sharp AH, Ross CA, Scherzinger E, Wanker EE, Mangiarini L, and Bates GP (1997). Formation of neuronal intranuclear inclusions underlies the neurological dysfunction in mice transgenic for the HD mutation. *Cell* **90**: 537–548.

Deckel AW, Weiner R, Szigeti D, Clark V, and Vento J (2000). Altered patterns of regional cerebral blood flow in patients with Huntington's disease: a SPECT study during rest and cognitive or motor activation. *Journal of Nuclear Medicine* **41**: 773–780.

DiFiglia M, Sapp E, Chase KO, Davies SW, Bates GP, Vonsattel JP, and Aronin N (1997). Aggregation of huntingtin in neuronal intranuclear inclusions and dystrophic neurites in brain. *Science* **277**: 1990–1993.

Fricker RA, Torres EM, Hume SP, Myers R, Opacka-Juffrey J, Ashworth S, Brooks DJ, and Dunnett SB (1997). The effects of donor stage on the survival and function of embryonic striatal grafts in the adult rat brain. II. Correlation between positron emission tomography and reaching behaviour. *Neuroscience* **79**: 711–722.

Gerfen CR (1992). The neostriatal mosaic: multiple levels of compartmental organisation. *Trends in Neurosciences* **15**: 133–138.

Ginovart N, Lundin A, Farde L, *et al.* (1997). PET study of the pre- and post-synaptic dopaminergic markers for the neurodegenerative process in Huntington's disease. *Brain* **120**: 503–514.

Glass M, Dragunow M, and Faull RLM (2000). The pattern of neurodegeneration in Huntington's disease: a comparative study of cannabinoid, dopamine, adenosine and GABA(A) receptor alterations in the human basal ganglia in Huntington's disease. *Neuroscience* **97**: 505–519.

Goldberg TE, Berman KF, Mohr E, and Weinberger DR (1990). Regional cerebral blood flow and cognitive function in Huntington's disease and schizophrenia—a comparison of patients matched for performance on a prefrontal-type task. *Archives of Neurology* **47**: 418–422.

Grafton ST, Mazziotta JC, Pahl JJ, St George Hyslop P, Haines JL, Gusella J, Hoffman JM, Baxter LR, and Phelps ME (1992). Serial changes of glucose cerebral metabolism and caudate size in persons at risk for Huntington's disease. *Archives of Neurology* **49**: 1161–1167.

—— *et al.* (1990). A comparison of neurological, metabolic, structural, and genetic evaluations in persons at risk for Huntington's disease. *Annals of Neurology* **28**: 614–621.

Hagglund J, Aquilonius SM, Eckernas SA, Hartvig P, Lundquist H, Gullberg P, and Langstrom B (1987). Dopamine receptor properties in Parkinson's disease and Huntington's chorea evaluated by positron emission tomography using 11C-N-methyl-spiperone. *Acta Neurologica Scandinavica* **75**: 87–94.

Harris GJ, Aylward EH, Peyser CE, *et al.* (1996). Single photon emission computed tomographic blood flow and magnetic resonance volume imaging of basal ganglia in Huntington's disease. *Archives of Neurology* **53**: 316–324.

Hasselbalch SG, Oberg G, Sorensen SA, *et al.* (1992). Reduced regional cerebral blood flow in Huntington's disease studied by SPECT. *Journal of Neurology, Neurosurgery and Psychiatry* **55**: 1018–1023.

Hayden MR, Martin WRW, Stoessl AJ, Clark C, Hollenberg S, Adam MJ, Ammann W, and Harrop R (1986). Positron emission tomography in the early diagnosis of Huntington's disease. *Neurology* **36**: 888–894.

—— Hewitt J, Martin WRW, Clark C, and Amman A (1987a). Studies in persons at risk for Huntington's disease. *New England Journal of Medicine* **317**: 382–383.

—— Stoessl AJ, Clark C, Ammann W, and Martin WRW (1987b). The combined use of positron emission tomography and DNA polymorphisms for preclinical detection of Huntington's disease. *Neurology* **37**: 1441–1447.

Hedreen JC and Folstein SE (1995). Early loss of neostriatal striosome neurons in Huntington's disease. *Journal of Neuropathology and Experimental Neurology* **54**: 105–120.

Holthoff VA, Koeppe RA, Frey KA, Penney JB, Markel DS, Kuhl DE, and Young AB (1993). Positron emission tomography measures of benzodiazepine receptors in Huntington's disease. *Annals of Neurology* **34**: 76–81.

Huntington's Disease Collaborative Research Group (1993). A novel gene containing a trinucleotide repeat that is expanded and unstable on Huntington's disease chromosomes. *Cell* **72**: 971–983.

Hussey D, Stewart D, Houle S, and Guttman M (1998). [C-11] Raclopride striatal binding potential as a measure of Huntington's disease progression: implications for prospective neuroprotective studies. *Journal of Nuclear Medicine* **39**: 932.

Ichise M, Toyama H, Fornazzari L, Ballinger JR, and Kirsh JC (1993). Iodine-123-IBZM dopamine-D2 receptor and technetium-99m-HMPAO brain perfusion SPECT in the evaluation of patients with and subjects at risk for Huntington's disease. *Journal of Nuclear Medicine* **34**: 1274–1281.

Jernigan TL, Salmon DP, Butters N, and Hesselink JR (1991). Cerebral structure on MRI. 2. Specific changes in Alzheimer's and Huntington's diseases. *Biological Psychiatry* **29**: 68–81.

Joyce JN, Lexow N, Bird E, and Winokur A (1988). Organization of dopamine D1 and D2 receptors in human striatum—receptor autoradiographic studies in Huntington's disease and schizophrenia. *Synapse* **2**: 546–557.

Kendall AL, Rayment FD, Torres EM, Baker HF, Ridley RM, and Dunnett SB (1998). Functional integration of striatal allografts in a primate model of Huntington's disease. *Nat. Med.* **4**: 727–729.

Kuhl DE, Phelps ME, Markham CH, Metter EJ, Riege WH, and Winter EJ (1982). Cerebral metabolism and atrophy in Huntington's disease determined by 18FDG and computed tomographic scans. *Annals of Neurology* **12**: 425–434.

Kunig G, Leenders KL, Sanchez-Pernaute R, *et al.* (2000). Benzodiazepine receptor binding in Huntington's disease: [C-11]flumazenil uptake measured using positron emission tomography. *Annals of Neurology* **47**: 644–648.

Kuwert T, Lange HW, Langen KJ, Herzog H, Aulich A, and Feinendegen LE (1990). Cortical and subcortical glucose consumption measured by PET in patients with Huntington's disease. *Brain* **113**: 1405–1423.

———— Boecker H, Titz H, Herzog H, Aulich A, Wang BC, Nayak U, and Feinendegen LE (1993). Striatal glucose consumption in chorea-free subjects at risk of Huntington's disease. *Journal of Neurology* **241**: 31–36.

Lassen NA, Ingvar DH, and Skinhoj E (1978). Brain function and blood flow. *Scientific American* **239**: 50–59.

Lawrence AD, Sahakian BJ, Hodges JR, Rosser AE, Lange KW, and Robbins TW (1996). Executive and mnemonic functions in early Huntington's disease. *Brain* **119**: 1633–1645.

—— Weeks RA, Brooks DJ, *et al.* (1998). The relationship between striatal dopamine receptor binding and cognitive performance in Huntington's disease. *Brain* **121**: 1343–1355.

Leenders KL, Frackowiak RSJ, Quinn N, and Marsden CD (1986). Brain energy metabolism and dopaminergic function in Huntington's disease measured *in vivo* using positron emission tomography. *Movement Disorders* **1**: 69–77.

Lindvall O (1999). Cerebral implantation in movement disorders: state of the art. *Movement Disorders* **14**: 201–205.

Marshall FJ and Shoulson I (1997). Clinical features and treatment of Huntington's disease. In *Movement disorders: neurological principles and practice* (ed. RL Watts and WC Koller), pp. 491–502. New York: McGraw Hill.

Mayberg HS, Starkstein SE, Peyser CE, Brandt J, Dannals RF, and Folstein SE (1992). Paralimbic frontal-lobe hypometabolism in depression associated with Huntington's disease. *Neurology* **42**: 1791–1797.

Mazziotta JC, Phelps M, Pahl J, Baxter L, Riege W, Hoffman J, Huang S, Gusella J, and Hyslop PKDMC (1987). Glucose metabolism and DNA polymorphism studies in Huntington's disease (HD). *Journal of Nuclear Medicine* **28**: 655.

Oepen G and Ostertag C (1981). Diagnostic value of CT in patients with Huntington's chorea and their offspring. *Journal of Neurology* **225**: 189–196.

Palfi S, Conde F, Riche D, *et al.* (1998). Foetal striatal allografts reverse cognitive deficits in a primate model of Huntington's disease. *Nature Medicine* **4**: 963–966.

Penney JB Jr and Young AB (1986). Striatal inhomogeneities and basal ganglia function. *Movement Disorders* **1**: 3–15.

Reisine TD, Fields JZ, Stern LZ, Johnson PC, Bird ED, and Yamamura HI (1977). Alterations in dopaminergic receptors in Huntington's disease. *Life Sciences* **21**: 1123–1128.

Richfield EK, O'Brien CF, Eskin T, and Shoulson I (1991). Heterogeneous dopamine receptor changes in early and late Huntington's disease. *Neuroscience Letters* **132**: 121–126.

Sax DS, O'Donnell B, Butters N, Menzer L, Montgomery K, and Kayne HL (1983). Computed tomographic, neurologic, and neuropsychological correlates of Huntington's disease. *International Journal of Neuroscience* **18**: 21–36.

—— Powsner R, Kim A, *et al.* (1996). Evidence of cortical metabolic dysfunction in early Huntington's disease by single photon emission computed tomography. *Movement Disorders* **11**: 671–677.

Sedvall G, Karlsson P, Lundin A, Anvret M, Suhara T, Halldin C, *et al.* (1994). Dopamine D1 receptor numbers—a sensitive PET marker for early brain degeneration in Huntington's disease. *European Archives of Psychiatry and Clinical Neuroscience* **243**: 249–255.

Starkstein SE, Brandt J, Folstein S, *et al.* (1988). Neuropsychological and neuroradiological correlates in Huntington's disease. *Journal of Neurology, Neurosurgery and Psychiatry* **51**: 1259–1263.

—— Folstein SE, Brandt J, Pearlson GD, Mcdonnell A, and Folstein M (1989). Brain atrophy in Huntington's disease—a CT-scan study. *Neuroradiology* **31**: 156–159.

—— Brandt J, Bylsma F, Peyser C, Folstein M, and Folstein SE (1992). Neuropsychological correlates of brain atrophy in Huntington's disease—a magnetic resonance imaging study. *Neuroradiology* **34**: 487–489.

Stober T, Wussow W, and Schimrigk K (1984). Bicaudate diameter—the most specific and simple CT parameter in the diagnosis of Huntington's disease. *Neuroradiology* **26**: 25–28.

Tanahashi N, Meyer JS, Ishikawa Y, *et al.* (1985). Cerebral blood flow and cognitive testing correlate in Huntington's disease. *Archives of Neurology* **42**: 1169–1175.

Torres EM, Fricker RA, Hume SP, Myers R, Opacka-Juffry J, Ashworth S, Brooks DJ, and Dunnett SB (1995). Assessment of striatal graft viability in the rat *in vivo* using a small diameter PET scanner. *NeuroReport* **6**: 2017–2021.

Turjanski N, Weeks R, Dolan R, Harding AE, and Brooks DJ (1995). Striatal D_1 and D_2 receptor binding in patients with Huntington's disease and other choreas: a PET study. *Brain* **118**: 689–696.

Weeks RA, Piccini P, Harding AE, and Brooks DJ (1996). Striatal D_1 and D_2 dopamine receptor loss in asymptomatic mutation carriers of Huntington's disease. *Annals of Neurology* **40**: 49–54.

—— Ceballos-Baumann AO, Boecker H, Piccini P, Harding AE, and Brooks DJ (1997a). Cortical control of movement in Huntington's disease. A PET activation study. *Brain* **120**: 1569–1578.

—— Cunningham VJ, Piccini P, Waters S, Harding AE, and Brooks DJ (1997b). ^{11}C-diprenorphine binding in Huntington's disease: a comparison of region of interest analysis and statistical parametric mapping. *Journal of Cerebral Blood Flow Metabolism* **17**: 943–949.

Weinberger DR, Berman KF, Iadarola M, Driesen N, and Zec RF (1988). Prefrontal cortical blood flow and cognitive function in Huntington's disease. *Journal of Neurology, Neurosurgery and Psychiatry* **51**: 94–104.

Wong DF, Links JM, Wagner HNJ, Folstein SE, Suneja S, Dannals RF, Ravert HT, Wilson AA, Tune LE, Pearlson G, Folstein MF, Bice A, and Kuhar NJ (1985). Dopamine and serotonin receptors measured *in-vivo* in Huntington's disease with C-11 N-methylspiperone PET imaging. *Journal of Nuclear Medicine* **26**: P107.

Young AB, Penney JB, Starosta-Rubinstein S, Markel DS, Berent S, Giordani B, and Ehrenkaufer R (1986). PET scan investigations of Huntington's disease: cerebral metabolic correlates of neurological features and functional decline. *Annals of Neurology* **20**: 296–303.

—— —— Starosta-Rubinstein S, Markel D, Berent S, Rothley J, Betley A, and Hichwa R (1987). Normal caudate glucose metabolism in persons at-risk for Huntington's disease. *Archives of Neurology* **44**: 254–257.

Section 2   The genetics of Huntington's disease

5 Huntington's disease: genetic and molecular studies

Peter S. Harper and Lesley Jones

Introduction

Before the gene and mutation for Huntington's disease (HD) were identified in 1993, our understanding of the inheritance and other genetic aspects of the disorder was based principally on the results of family studies and other approaches of classical genetics. When the first edition of this book was published, in 1991, it was already clear that HD showed a number of puzzling and unusual features, but without direct knowledge of the gene and mutation these could not be explained, although speculation was possible.

Ten years later, we face a different problem. Our molecular understanding of HD and its mutational basis has so radically transformed our knowledge and interpretation of its genetics that it is impossible to discuss many areas meaningfully without already having outlined the molecular advances. The approach taken here is thus first to describe some of the classical genetic studies, together with aspects that have been relatively little changed by molecular developments; we then outline the work leading to isolation of the gene and the properties of the HD mutation, before returning to specific aspects of HD genetics, such as anticipation, parental origin effects, and apparently sporadic cases, where classical and molecular studies are inextricably linked. Finally, we address some of the important areas of molecular diagnosis in HD. The structure and function of the HD gene and its protein product are taken up in the following chapters.

Early genetic studies

The hereditary nature of HD has been clear since the earliest descriptions, as noted in the opening chapter of this book. Indeed, the term 'hereditary chorea' was commonly used in these descriptions to distinguish it from other forms of chorea. Mendel's work on the basic laws of inheritance was published in 1865, but had to wait until 1900 before its recognition; despite this, George Huntington's original 1872 description shows clearly how the disorder follows the pattern of dominant inheritance: 'One or more of the offspring almost invariably suffer from the disease, if they live to adult age. But if by any chance these children go through life without it, the thread is broken and the grandchildren and great-grandchildren of the original shakers may rest assured that they are free from the disease'.

In the early years of the twentieth century, following the rediscovery of Mendel's work, scientists were eager to find examples of Mendelian inheritance in human diseases. HD soon became accepted as such an example, and Jelliffe (1908) and Punnett (1908) both recognized this, as did Davenport in his early book (1911), which interestingly also suggested the possibility of Mendelian inheritance for other types of chorea. The specific and detailed study of New England HD families by Davenport and Muncey (1916) confirmed the view of HD as an autosomal dominant disorder. However, it was not until the systematic and quantitative analysis of Julia Bell (1934) that this conclusion was placed on firm and detailed foundations. Myrianthopoulos (1966) provided a useful account of the early genetic studies on HD, and Conneally (1984) produced an excellent review of the subject up to that time, including a detailed assessment of possible modifying factors.

In recent years, it has become clear that Mendelian inheritance may be much more variable than previously supposed, as a result of biological mechanisms such as DNA instability and genetic imprinting, and that even well-established Mendelian disorders can show significant departures from expected Mendelian ratios. HD has proved to be one such condition, so before describing the discrepancies and unusual aspects it is worth examining closely the evidence on which autosomal dominant inheritance is based, rather than simply assuming this as an accepted fact. Hopefully, this should also serve to introduce the reader unfamiliar with genetics to the simple but fundamental facts involved.

HD as a Mendelian disorder

The principal findings to be expected in a disorder showing autosomal dominant inheritance are summarized in Table 5.1, and Fig. 5.1 shows diagrammatically the pattern of segregation on which it is based. Equal sex incidence, equal transmission by both sexes, a 50 per cent proportion of affected offspring born to an affected parent, and lack of transmission by unaffected family members are all features that appear evident from any large HD pedigree, but unless these are analysed quantitatively a significant deviation can be missed.

The sex incidence of HD found in major studies has varied considerably but overall is close to the equality expected. Bell (1934) found a 53.5 per cent male incidence in a total of 956 cases, and Pearson *et al.* (1955) also showed a slight male excess (66 of 117), while Reed *et al.* (1958) found a deficiency of male cases (85 of 203). Data from the Wales register (Sarfarazi *et al.* 1987) for the South Wales area, where ascertainment was considered close to complete, showed 283 affected males and 284 affected females, as close to equality as it is possible to achieve. Another possible approach is to examine the sex ratio of affected individuals from sibships with an affected parent. Reed *et al.* (1958) found no significant difference from 50 per cent regardless of the age cut-off used.

When parental transmission of HD is examined, most studies again agree closely with the expected 50 per cent value. Bell (1934) found that 55.2 per cent of 744 cases originated from the father, although there was an excess of father–son transmissions (60.3 per cent), no such difference being seen when the disorder was maternally transmitted. The striking difference

Table 5.1 Criteria for autosomal dominant inheritance as applied to HD

Equal incidence in both sexes
Equal transmission by both sexes (but differential effect of sex of affected parent on age of onset)
50% of offspring of an affected person also become affected (but only by old age)
No transmission of the disorder by those offspring remaining free from HD

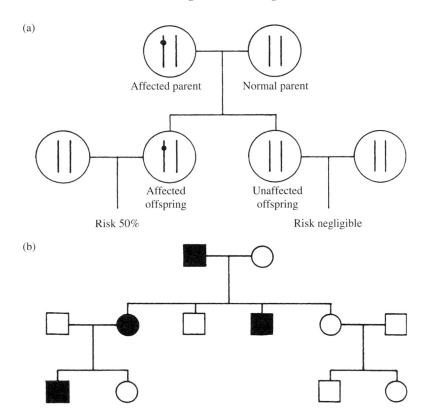

Fig. 5.1 Mendelian autosomal dominant inheritance in HD. (a) To show segregation pattern in offspring of affected and unaffected individuals. Affected individuals are normally heterozygotes, with a 50 per cent risk of transmitting the gene to offspring. (Note. For a late-onset disorder such as HD, 'affected' implies ultimately affected, not necessarily at the time of reproduction.) Those not inheriting the gene have a negligible chance of having affected offspring. (b) A schematic pedigree to show autosomal dominant transmission in HD. Transmission is by and to each sex equally, with an average 50 per cent of offspring of an affected person affected. Such an 'idealized' pedigree is rarely seen in practice.

that emerges when the data are divided by age of onset, especially the paternal transmission of juvenile cases, is discussed later in the chapter. The important point to be noted here is that there is no overall disturbance of the expected Mendelian ratio.

Testing the expected ratio of 50 per cent for the affected offspring of affected parents requires careful classification by age as well as the identification of the proband to minimize bias. Bell (1934) found a slight excess of affected offspring (55.6 per cent) in her collected data on 1162 offspring from 240 sibships. Any sibship containing unaffected members aged under 40 years was omitted. She felt that ascertainment bias towards sibships with multiple affected members was likely and explained the deviation from 50 per cent. These basic ratios deserve a careful reanalysis in the light of possible mechanisms, described later, such as meiotic drive, that might produce a genuine departure from the expected 50 per cent.

More detailed segregation analysis was done in the studies of Sjögren (1936), Panse (1942), Reed *et al.* (1958), and Stevens (1976), all of which gave values of close to 50 per cent,

Table 5.2 Percentage of affected among offspring of affected parents (sibships containing unaffected members aged under 40 years omitted)

Reference	% affected
Bell 1934	55.6
Sjögren 1936	43.0
Reed *et al.* 1958	52.5 (48.2*)
Stevens 1976	52.5

*Equivocal cases counted as normal.

although with some variation depending on the age criteria used. The data at the 40-year cut-off point, which allows comparison between all these early studies, are summarized in Table 5.2.

The fourth criterion for autosomal dominant inheritance (lack of transmission by an unaffected person) is also age-related, and is bound up with the subject's age at onset and penetrance of the gene, and is dealt with further in relation to genetic counselling in Chapter 7. Penetrance, the proportion of individuals carrying the abnormal gene who show signs of the disease, is clearly minimal in childhood and low in early adult life, but the number of cases who have had an affected parent and child, but themselves have remained unaffected while living to old age is essentially zero. It is actually very difficult to document such a case satisfactorily, but in practice the only 'skipped generations' seen are those where the intervening parent has died relatively young or has not been documented medically.

This complete penetrance of the HD gene in offspring of affected individuals needs to be contrasted with the existence of apparently healthy mutation carriers in the older generations, a topic discussed in the light of molecular developments later in the chapter when we consider genetic instability in relation to intermediate alleles and potential new mutations.

In summary, HD fulfils the basic criteria for a Mendelian autosomal dominant disorder, albeit one of great variability in age at onset. It is when we start to examine some of the detailed aspects that unexpected findings are encountered, findings that we can now, to a large extent, explain in terms of the unusual and unstable nature of the HD mutation.

The HD gene and mutation

Before we can go further in discussing some of the genetic aspects of HD, we have to describe the work that has led from the gene being an abstract concept to a specific entity, with a highly specific and unusual mutational defect. The research that resulted in the isolation of the gene for HD in 1993 represents a landmark in our understanding of the disorder, probably the single most important finding in the history of research into HD, as indicated in Chapter 1. The discovery brought to an end a long and sometimes frustrating search for the gene, involving an international collaboration that was perhaps unique in its scope and duration. It also opened the door to broader biological approaches to the disease that were impossible without knowledge of the specific gene involved.

In view of the critical importance of this work, it is appropriately described in a historical manner, since the new discoveries did not appear from nowhere, but grew in a systematic, if at times slow and not entirely predictable, manner from earlier studies. It is important not to forget these earlier steps, even if their significance has largely been superseded by the later work for which they provided essential foundations. HD, as it has been in so many other respects, was the prototype for comparable studies on numerous other genetic disorders.

The search for the HD gene

The HD gene was mapped in a classic study of its type which now forms part of the history of positional cloning (Huntington's Disease Collaborative Research Group 1993). Many of the techniques used commonly in mapping studies were developed on the HD project. Conceptually, this, like all gene-mapping projects, depended upon detecting genetic linkage. Genetic linkage—the co-inheritance of two genes, or genetically determined phenotypes, because of their physical proximity on chromosomes—had been recognized very early in the study of the genetics of simple organisms such as *Drosophila*. Linkage was first applied to the mapping of human disease genes in the 1970s using the then relatively few available genetic markers, such as blood groups. The first genetic studies searching for the location of the HD gene took place in the 1970s (Lindstrom *et al.* 1973; Brackenridge *et al.* 1978; Pericak-Vance *et al.* 1978; Hodge *et al.* 1980; Volkers *et al.* 1980) but a confirmed linkage finding was not published until 1983 (Gusella *et al.* 1983). The work leading up to this finding is described in detail in the previous edition of this book (Harper 1996a).

Apart from enabling the positional cloning of the HD gene, the linkage of the G8 marker to HD immediately had two other major implications. First, it allowed the possibility of presymptomatic testing of individuals at risk for HD, and prenatal diagnosis of at-risk pregnancies. These issues are discussed in Chapter 7. Second, it demonstrated that restriction fragment length polymorphism (RFLP) analysis could be used to locate a human disease gene of completely unknown function regardless of where it might be placed on the human genome. The advance was clearly of general importance for research on genetic disorders. It also captured the attention of some of the best minds in molecular biology and medical genetics, thus ensuring future progress both for HD research and more generally.

The work of Gusella and colleagues in 1983 placed the HD gene on the short (p) arm of chromosome 4, using a marker called G8 that mapped to the region. As a decision to try and map the HD gene had only been taken the year before by these workers, this was rapid progress, and thus encouraged the continued search for the gene itself. The original finding was confirmed and the further mapping facilitated by the availability of an extremely large HD kindred from Venezuela (Wexler *et al.* 1985). This and other large families with HD became the focus of an intense search for the gene, using linkage and linkage disequilibrium mapping to narrow down the area of interest. Crucially, two things allowed this mapping to proceed. First, technological advances in gene mapping gave more markers that could be used, with a greater coverage of the genome, and the analysis of these markers became much more tractable: these advances facilitated the gene mapping efforts in many inherited disorders. Second, more specific to HD research, much of this work was funded and facilitated by the Hereditary Disease Foundation, driven by Nancy Wexler and her father Milton Wexler. The fascinating story of the people and the research involved has been told by Alice Wexler (1995) in her book, *Mapping fate*.

Once a relatively circumscribed region of the genome had been defined—the critical region— the genes in the region were cloned, sequenced, and the HD population was investigated for possible mutations in these genes segregating with the disease. Fortunately, one further important clue to the nature of the gene in question was given by the earlier cloning of other disease-causing genes with a particular mutational type. Several genes with mutations that proved to be expansions in trinucleotide repeat sequences had been cloned in the early 1990s: Kennedy's disease (spinal and bulbar muscular atrophy, SBMA; LaSpada *et al.* 1991); fragile X syndrome (Oberlé *et al.* 1991); and myotonic dystrophy (Brook *et al.* 1992; Fu *et al.* 1992; Mahadevan *et al.* 1992). A search was thus instigated for genes in the critical region that contained trinucleotide repeat sequences and, indeed, several genes previously cloned in the region proved to contain such repeat sequences: these genes and their repeats were re-examined in the HD population. Several repeats were analysed that proved not to be expanded in HD and then a gene in the critical region, the inspiringly named 'interesting transcript 15' (IT15), proved to contain a CAG repeat in its first exon that was expanded in HD cases (Huntington's Disease Collaborative Research Group 1993). This landmark event was the successful end of a 10-year cloning effort, involving six research groups, four in the USA and two in the UK—a truly international collaboration. A personal view of these exciting events, which gives some of the less scientific details that inevitably fail to appear in the published papers, has been written by one of us (Harper 1993b).

The gene itself proved to contain 67 exons and encoded a very large 350 kDa protein, named huntingtin. The CAG repeat was translated to give a polyglutamine tract, which was expressed in the protein. More details of the transcript, the protein huntingtin, and its possible downstream effects are given in Chapters 11–13. It is of note that when the gene was cloned it had no identifying homologies in the databases and to a very large extent this remains true today—again, more details can be found in Chapter 12. Since the cloning of the HD gene, several other genes with expanded CAG repeats have been isolated. All lead to neurodegenerations, have similar sizes of disease-causing repeats, and lead to expanded glutamine tracts in their cognate proteins. The molecular and clinical characteristics of these polyglutamine diseases are compared with each other and with HD in Chapter 14.

The CAG repeat expansion

This section summarizes what we now know about the mutational defect in HD and how it relates to the phenotype of the disease. This and the following sections also cover some areas of the classical genetics of HD, such as new mutation, anticipation, and parental origin effects, where the discovery of the mutation has so radically changed our understanding that they can be meaningfully discussed only in the context of the molecular basis. Information about the mutation and its relationship to genetic and phenotypic aspects of HD initially grew at a remarkable speed, and provided answers to many of the previously puzzling aspects of the disorder. By September 1993, only 6 months after the initial report, a wealth of data was presented at the Boston meeting of the World Federation of Neurology HD Research Group, much of it summarized in a special issue of the *Journal of Medical Genetics* in December 1993.

The CAG repeat: the normal and expanded range

The original *Cell* publication had shown that all patients with HD studied had a CAG repeat number clearly greater than that in the normal population (Huntington's Disease Collaborative Research Group 1993), and subsequent studies defined the normal and abnormal ranges more accurately. Three such studies were soon published in *Nature Genetics* (Snell *et al.* 1993b;

Duyao *et al.* 1993; Andrew *et al.* 1993a), followed by a large number of studies from different populations over the following year. Figure 5.2 shows the data from several of these based on European HD families, but the distributions in the other studies are remarkably similar. It can be seen that the HD and normal ranges have quite distinct peaks (at 40 and 16 repeats, respectively), but that the tails of the two curves approach each other closely. We now know that there is a narrow region of overlap, even though few individuals are represented in this borderline region. Not surprisingly, the greater the number of individuals studied, the closer the two ranges come together. It is now clear that there is no absolute separation—a conclusion of great practical importance when the information is being used diagnostically, as well as being of likely significance in terms of the relationship between size of expansion and disease pathogenesis, both topics discussed later.

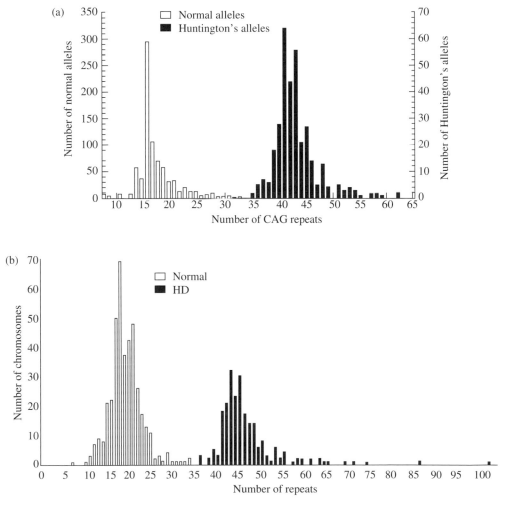

Fig. 5.2 (*Cont.*)

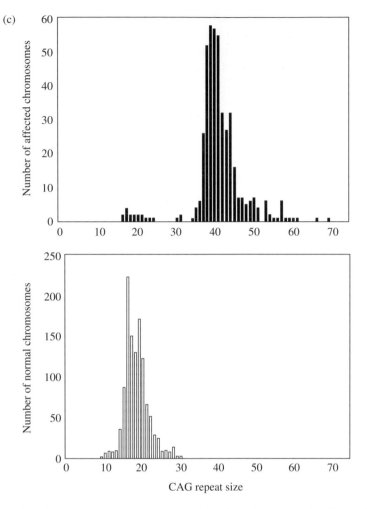

Fig. 5.2 Ranges of CAG repeat number in normal individuals and patients with HD in different HK populations, showing the close approximation of normal and HD ranges. (a) Scotland (from Barron *et al.* 1993). (b) Northwest England (from Craufurd and Dodge 1993, by courtesy of the authors). (c) Wales (from Snell *et al.* 1993). In this series individuals considered to have HD but with clearly normal results have not been excluded (see text).

Together with the population and family studies of the HD mutation, a series of papers appeared giving improved or simplified methods of analysis. The most significant finding in relation to this was that another (CCG) repeat existed immediately 3′ to the CAG repeat, which was variable in the normal population (7–12 repeats) and could thus confuse the sizing of the CAG repeats close to the borderline of normal and abnormal (Rubinsztein *et al.* 1993; Andrew *et al.* 1994a; Barron *et al.* 1994). This repeat was included in most of the original studies, something that should be borne in mind when comparing different series. This and other technical factors, along with the extensive experience gained internationally over the past 8 years, has resulted in adjustment of what should be considered the normal, abnormal, and intermediate ranges (ACMG/ASHG 1998), though this in part relates to definitions rather than actual change. Interestingly, the CCG polymorphism is not randomly distributed in patients with HD, who have a higher frequency of large CCG alleles than the general population, a finding of significance in relation to the possible origins of the HD mutation, as discussed in Chapter 6. There are also reports of a polymorphism at the 3′ end of the CAG repeat. This usually has a CAACAG sequence (both CAA and CAG encode glutamine) but, in a few people, the CAA codon does not occur and thus primers that overlap with this end of the repeat will fail to amplify. This rare polymorphism may lead to an erroneous diagnostic result (Gellera *et al.* 1996).

Figure 5.2(c) also illustrates another finding common to all the major mutation studies, although excluded in some of the figures: a small number of patients with HD show a completely normal result. This interesting group is considered in more detail later, but for the present it suffices to emphasize that most have proved to be the result of sample mix-up, misdiagnosis, or to be atypical in some way (MacMillan *et al.* 1993a; Andrew *et al.* 1994b; Kremer *et al.* 1994), so that the CAG expansion can be considered as accounting for the mutation in over 99 per cent of patients with true HD. Reviews of the mutational and related molecular data on HD have been provided by Gusella *et al.* (1993), Harper (1993a, 1996), Albin and Tagle (1995), Gusella and MacDonald (1994), and Goldberg *et al.* (1994).

Sensitivity and specificity of the HD mutation

HD and other disorders resulting from expanded trinucleotide repeats are highly unusual among genetic disorders in showing a single mutation underlying almost all cases of the disease. For most Mendelian disorders, for instance in Duchenne muscular dystrophy, a wide variety of mutations is seen, often involving different mechanisms such as deletion and duplication as well as single nucleotide polymorphisms (SNPs). Phenotypic differences observed in these diseases can often be related to the extent, nature, or site of mutation. Even for diseases where one common mutation accounts for most cases (for example, cystic fibrosis), a range of other, rarer, mutations usually occurs. The finding of a single mutational mechanism underlying a disorder such as HD is thus of both theoretical and practical significance and deserves close examination.

First, a closer look is needed at the small proportion of cases considered clinically to have HD, but showing no mutational defect (studies of isolated cases or those referred for diagnosis are dealt with later). The study of Andrew *et al.* (1994b) provides the largest series, although the data were obtained from diagnostic samples in the Canadian HD prediction consortium, and so are likely to be less uniform in terms of clinical validation than in a number of the earlier studies (for example, Snell *et al.* 1993). It has already been noted that sample mix-up or misclassification was the most common cause for apparent absence of mutation in both this series and that of MacMillan *et al.* (1993a) but, even among the remaining few with no mutation, most were clinically atypical when the records were reassessed. In this category the related neurodegenerative disorder dentatorubro-pallidoluysian atrophy (DRPLA) has proved to be the most frequently confused condition. Not only are the clinical features similar in some cases (see Chapter 2), but DRPLA is also due to a trinucleotide repeat expansion, as discussed in Chapter 14. A number of other rare genetic diseases that have been confused at times with HD are mentioned below.

Until the availability of a specific mutation test, neuropathology was the accepted gold standard for the firm diagnosis of HD, with well-defined qualitative and quantitative criteria established. Both classical and molecular neuropathology are covered in detail in Chapter 8. The existence of stored samples of brain from large series of well-characterized cases has given the opportunity for comparison of the molecular and neuropathological diagnosis (Xuereb *et al.* 1996). As can been seen from Table 5.3, the agreement is remarkably good, with virtually all cases showing typical neuropathology also having the HD mutation present. DRPLA would have been excluded by its different neuropathology (see Chapter 14).

Most studies of the HD mutation have been based on specific populations but, as these have accumulated from a wide variety of countries, it has become clear that the expanded CAG repeat is the underlying mutation in all populations studied. This has considerable epidemiological significance for our understanding of the origin and spread of HD, as is discussed in the next chapter, where these studies are referenced. It also has practical significance, because it means that, unlike the situation for many genetic disorders, analysis of the expanded repeat can be used in diagnosis and prediction universally, throughout the world, without the need for modification on account of particular local mutational distributions. In addition to the specific studies in different countries, Kremer *et al.* (1994) have reported the geographical origins of an extensive series of 1000 patients with HD, originating from 43 different population groups and including all major races. All were found to show the expansion, with a comparable range of repeat numbers, confirming the universality of the HD mutation.

It can thus be concluded that the overwhelming majority—possibly all—HD cases result from the same mutational mechanism of trinucleotide repeat expansion and that, where the mutation is not found, the most likely explanation is either some form of sampling or clinical error, or an alternative diagnosis (such as DRPLA) if the features are not typical for HD. The neuropathologists come out of the analysis with considerable credit, and careful neuropathological study remains of practical importance, particularly in the interpretation of past cases where material is no longer available for molecular analysis.

Turning to specificity, it is important to know whether the HD mutation could underlie clinical disorders currently thought to be different from HD, a topic discussed more fully in Chapter 2. Broadly, the conclusion to be reached is that the mutation appears to be as specific as it is sensitive. The single family originally diagnosed (and reported) as having benign hereditary chorea but showing the HD mutation should be noted (MacMillan *et al.* 1993b); typical features were present in some but not all members and this illustrates how slow in progression HD may be in some cases. No series of chorea as a whole has yet been reported, but the absence of the mutation in some cases diagnosed as senile chorea is significant (Shinotoh

Table 5.3 Correlation of molecular and neuropathological abnormality in HD (grade 0 cases excluded)*

HD mutation	Neuropathological changes typical of HD	
	Yes	No
Present	153	0
Absent	4	11

*Taken from Xuereb *et al.* (1996).

et al. 1994). Also of importance is the lack of the HD mutation in large series of patients with schizophrenia (Kremer *et al.* 1994; Rubinzstein *et al.* 1994; St Clair 1994). Of the 349 patients in these three series, only one showed a possible expansion; the borderline value of 36 repeats and the normal striatal pathology in this patient make it likely that the molecular and clinical findings were unrelated. The specificity of the HD mutation is further confirmed by its absence in a series of 75 demented elderly patients (Norbury *et al.* 1995) and in a group of 88 patients with Alzheimer's disease (Kremer *et al.* 1994).

Clinical correlates of CAG repeat size

One of the key consequences of genetic instability in HD and other trinucleotide repeat disorders is that different individuals carrying the mutation will have different degrees of expansion in the CAG repeat sequence. The broad definition and extent of the abnormal range has been discussed above; the problems associated with the borderline range of 'intermediate alleles' are considered later in this chapter and in Chapter 7. Here we examine the relationships of CAG repeat numbers in the abnormal range with clinical and pathological features of the disease. A large amount of information is now available on this topic, not only for HD, but for other trinucleotide disorders and this is summarized in Table 5.4. It will be seen that the extent of the repeat sequence is of considerable importance in relation to the phenotype, but that it is far from being the exclusive determinant.

Age of onset

This was the first and most obvious factor to study, because of its availability in most cases and its numerical nature, but all clinicians involved with HD will be aware of the difficulty in defining it precisely (see Chapter 2) and the potential for bias. However, these factors are considerably outweighed by the volume of data.

A strong inverse correlation between repeat number and age at onset was apparent from the initial studies (Andrew *et al.* 1993a; Duyao *et al.* 1993; MacMillan *et al.* 1993a; Snell *et al.* 1993) and this was supported by numerous further studies in a wide range of populations (Norremolle *et al.* 1993; Zuhlke *et al.* 1993a; Claes *et al.* 1995). Figure 5.3 shows the relationship for the Welsh HD population. The CAG repeat length appears to account for 47–73 per cent of the variance in age of onset in studies of various HD populations (Craufurd and Dodge 1993; Ranen *et al.* 1995; Brinkman *et al.* 1997; Squitieri *et al.* 2000; Rosenblatt *et al.* 2001),

Table 5.4 Genotype–phenotype correlations in HD

Phenotype characteristic	Degree of correlation
Age at onset	Clear inverse correlation, especially for juvenile cases with large repeat numbers
Rate of progression of disease	Correlation probably absent or weak
Psychiatric features	Little evidence for correlation with repeat number, but correlation within families
Neuropathological/imaging changes	Strong correlation with degree of atrophy, cell loss, and inclusion load

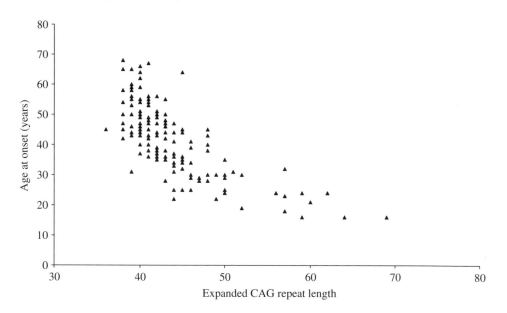

Fig. 5.3 Data from the Welsh HD population showing the inverse correlation of CAG repeat length with age of onset.

although it was estimated to account for only 7 per cent of this variance in late-onset cases (Goldberg *et al.* 1993).

When the data are looked at in more detail, a range of onset can be established for each specific repeat number. Brinkman *et al.* (1997), have done this for a large series of 1049 individuals, allowing cumulative probability curves for age at onset to be derived. However, it is important to note the considerable variation for each repeat number. For example, with a repeat number of 41 ($n = 98$), onset ranged from 35 to 75 years, with a cumulative probability of 0.38 by age 50 (95 per cent confidence intervals 0.48–0.26) and 0.88 by age 65 (0.94–0.76). Also the strength of the correlation varies considerably in different parts of the range, being greatest for the largest repeats, which are frequently associated with juvenile onset of disease, and weakest in the lower part of the abnormal range, corresponding to the vast majority of adult-onset HD cases.

Telenius *et al.* (1993) studied 42 juvenile cases and found a strong correlation of 0.86 for this group, suggesting that CAG repeat number was the main determinant for juvenile onset. A few cases with exceptionally large repeats, estimated at up to 250 have been reported (Nance *et al.* 1999). A comparable relationship is also seen with juvenile onset of other CAG repeat disorders, such as DRPLA and the spinocerebellar ataxias (see Chapter 14). These expansions are an order of magnitude less, though, than those that may be seen in the trinucleotide repeat diseases where the repeat sequence is not translated in the protein, such as fragile X syndrome, Friedreich's ataxia, and myotonic dystrophy. In myotonic dystrophy repeat lengths of up to 5000 have been detected (Harper 2001). Repeats of this size encoding polyglutamine do not occur because of the extreme selection pressure against them; once a polyglutamine repeat has reached >60, juvenile onset of HD will militate against these repeats being transmitted to give yet further expansion.

Those HD patients with late onset have a correspondingly lesser correlation with repeat number. Kremer *et al.* (1993) found that this contributed only 7 per cent of the variance in patients with onset over 50, while there was no significant correlation for onset over the age of 60 years. James *et al.* (1994) found repeat numbers of only 38–39 in a series of 10 patients with onset in the range 60–77 years. Siesling *et al.* (2000) found patients with positive family history had higher CAG repeat lengths and younger age of onset than those with suspect family history, probably due to ascertainment bias and the mildness and greater likelihood of clinical confusion surrounding late-onset HD. The study of Almqvist *et al.* (2001) suggests a similar trend, as it detected a much higher rate of late-onset HD than previously reported: 17.7 per cent of their serially diagnosed cases in British Colombia. This is almost certainly because the diagnostic test was used to distinguish HD from the more common late-onset neurodegenerations such as Alzheimer's disease and parkinsonism, both of which can resemble HD in the elderly. These findings are important as they have implications for succeeding generations of the families involved. These elderly onset patients merge imperceptibly with the intermediate allele range described more fully below.

Clinical symptoms

Juvenile HD patients have a different onset and course of disease from those of the great majority of HD patients with midlife onset. Their distinguishing symptoms are described fully in Chapter 2, but the main features are the presence of rigidity rather than chorea, dystonia, and an early and rapid cognitive decline. Their symptoms therefore correlate with repeat length but it is difficult to separate this from the correlation with age at onset. This is discussed further in Chapter 2.

A specific study of cognitive abnormalities by Jason *et al.* (1997) showed some correlation with repeat number, but this was largely removed when other related factors such as age at onset and disease duration were allowed for. Two reports have demonstrated that some changes in motor and cognitive function in presymptomatic gene carriers can be correlated to their CAG repeat length (Foroud *et al.* 1995; Siemers *et al.* 1996). This indicates that CAG length may influence very early changes.

The clinical features of adult-onset HD seem to have little relationship to CAG repeat number. In particular, no evidence for CAG repeat length influencing whether HD patients have predominantly psychiatric symptoms has emerged. MacMillan *et al.* (1993a) found no difference in repeat number when a series of 149 patients was grouped as having either predominantly neurological or predominantly psychiatric clinical features; a comparable result was found by Claes *et al.* (1995) in 59 patients, and similar conclusions were reached by two more detailed studies. Weigell-Weber *et al.* (1996), in a series of 71 patients, examined personality change, depression, psychosis, and nonspecific psychiatric features, and found no relationship to repeat number in any of the groups. A similar though smaller study by Zappacosta *et al.* (1996) also failed to show any relationship between CAG number and psychiatric symptoms, including depression and cognitive involvement.

Thus the conclusion has to be that the CAG repeat number plays little or no role in the important determination of whether or not HD patients develop prominent psychiatric features, nor in what these features may be. It possibly plays a role in the presymptomatic development of motor features but this is likely to be related to age of onset. However, the psychiatric symptoms of HD do tend to cluster in families, implying that other familial factors apart from the

HD repeat influence the specific symptoms of the disease (Lovestone *et al.* 1996; Tsuang *et al.* 1998, 2000). This topic is discussed below in the section 'Genetic modifiers of HD'.

Progression

In contrast to the clear relationship between CAG repeat number and age of disease onset, there is little evidence for a similar correlation with rate of disease progression. A potentially confounding factor in assessing these studies is the varying evidence from different series as to whether age at onset and disease progression are themselves related.

Neither Kieburtz *et al.* (1994) nor Ashizawa *et al.* (1994) found any evidence of correlation between repeat number and rate of deterioration in serially assessed American patients, both studies showing the correlation with age at onset discussed above. However, a study of Russian patients by Illiaroshkin *et al.* (1994) did show a significantly more rapid decline, both neurological and psychiatric, with larger repeat numbers. Brandt *et al.* (1996) studied this in the Venezuela population, in which a relationship between age at onset and rate of decline had previously been documented, and found no correlation between repeat number and rate of decline once age at onset had been eliminated as a variable. They also pointed out that Illarioshkin *et al.* had not assessed their patients serially, but had measured decline indirectly from a combination of severity and disease duration.

Taking the evidence as a whole, CAG repeat number does not seem to be an important factor in disease progression, a conclusion that is not only of practical importance in giving prognosis for affected or presymptomatic individuals, but is also relevant to our understanding of how the CAG, or rather the polyglutamine repeat it gives rise to, is involved in disease pathogenesis.

Pathology

Attempts to relate the degree of molecular defect to neuropathological abnormalities have in the past produced rather varying results. Neal *et al.* (1994) could find no correlation between CAG number and specific neuropathological features, while Sieradzan *et al.* (1999) likewise found no relationship to degree of atrophy in various parts of the brain. However, Furtado *et al.* (1996) did show correlation of repeat number and cell loss in caudate and putamen, even after allowing for two severely affected juvenile cases. More recent data from Wales also indicate a significant correlation (Fig. 5.4).

The largest study to date, that of Penney *et al.* (1997), demonstrated a clear relationship of CAG repeat length with severity of pathology in a series of 89 HD brains. The correlation was linear between striatal atrophy divided by age at death and CAG repeat number, with an intercept at 35.5 CAG. This study predicts that the pathological process begins at birth and develops linearly over time. This fits in well with the one-hit hypothesis of HD and other neurodegenerations (Clarke *et al.* 2000). This suggests that the death of any neurone is a random event; the risk of death of any neurone is constant over time and independent of the death of other neurones. The one hit may be the crossing of a threshold involving many processes or the single hit implied in the name. In HD it has been suggested that nucleation of huntingtin polyglutamine tracts, the starting point that would presumably lead eventually to microscopically visible aggregate formation, is just such a random event (Perutz and Windle 2001).

Becher *et al.* (1998) showed a correlation of CAG repeat number and density of intranuclear inclusions in striatum and cortex in 20 patients, although Sieradzan *et al.* (1999) found significant

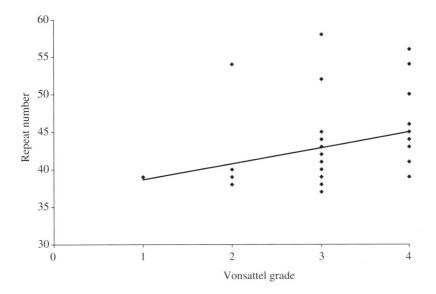

Fig. 5.4 Correlation of pathological Vonsattel grade with CAG repeat number, taken from the Welsh cohort. Thirty-seven brains were analysed in this study and there is a significant correlation between expansion size of CAG and pathological severity even in this relatively small sample ($p=0.037$).

correlation only with inclusion numbers in cortex and not in striatum. Butterworth *et al.* (1998) showed a correlation of CAG repeat length with degree of striatal DNA fragmentation in 27 HD brains. *In vitro* studies (see Chapters 11 and 12) are also now demonstrating a relationship between CAG repeat number and formation of protein aggregates.

Several studies of different brain imaging approaches have been reported and all suggest a correlation of severity with CAG repeat number. Culjkovic *et al.* (1999) found a greater degree of caudate atrophy by CT scanning with increased repeat number in 11 patients, while Antonini *et al.* (1998), in a study of 10 affected and 8 presymptomatic patients using PET scanning, found a relationship with loss of striatal dopamine-2 receptors. The loss of dopamine D2 receptors may reflect the loss of the medium spiny neurones from the caudate (see Chapter 8). This evidence, along with the pathological evidence of correlation of repeat length with grade of atrophy at death, supports the hypothesis that pathological severity is related to CAG length. Jenkins *et al.* (1998) using nuclear magnetic resonance (NMR) spectroscopy analysis of striatal energy metabolism, likewise found a correlation with CAG repeat number. The last two reports both integrated their data to indicate a more rapid decline with increasing CAG numbers, but since this was based on indirect estimates rather than serial studies there remain the same reservations as there were for the study of Illiaroshkin *et al.* (1994).

In conclusion, the number of repeats possessed by an HD mutation carrier is strongly correlated with age at onset of disease, especially for large repeat expansions. It is also correlated with severity of brain pathology, but not with the development of psychiatric features or rate of decline. The very fact that age at onset and disease duration are themselves such strong determinants for the nature and course of the disease makes it difficult to exclude a minor independent role for CAG repeat number, but it is clear that most of its influence is likely to result from its primary effect on age at onset.

Parental origin and juvenile HD

The two most puzzling features to arise from family studies of HD in the premolecular era were, first, the finding that most juvenile and early-onset cases of HD were paternally transmitted and, second, that there appeared to be 'anticipation', that is, progressively earlier onset in successive generations, in male-transmitted cases. Until recently, these observations were entirely unexplained, although there were plenty of hypotheses. Now they cannot only be largely explained, but can also be seen as part of the same phenomenon of genetic instability of the trinucleotide repeat mutation, and to share these features with other disorders showing a similar mutational mechanism. It is therefore worth examining closely how our knowledge of this area has evolved.

Paternal inheritance of juvenile HD

The first suggestion that childhood or juvenile HD was usually transmitted by an affected father came from Bruyn (1968). Bruyn's collected data on transmission of the juvenile form was confused by his finding that there was also an excess of female juvenile cases, something not confirmed in later studies. It was the study of Merrit *et al.* (1969) that showed clearly that paternal transmission was a genuine biological phenomenon. They reported seven families containing 14 affected children and reviewed previous literature on a further 110 siblings with HD of onset at age under 21 years. The sex incidence of the affected children was approximately equal (70 male, 64 female) but there was a striking excess of affected fathers (84, compared with 22 mothers).

Confirmation came from the pooled experience of the World Federation of Neurology (WFN) research group on HD (Barbeau 1970), which found 26 of 33 juvenile cases (under 20 years) to be paternally transmitted, only six maternally. Since then the finding has been observed in HD populations worldwide, including Venezuela and the mixed-race population of South Africa (Hayden 1979).

A more detailed analysis of the situation showed two points of practical importance. First, there is no absolute demarcation between the transmission of 'juvenile' and 'adult' cases. Myers *et al.* (1983) showed that the proportion of male-transmitted cases fell steadily when cases were grouped as juvenile, early, adult, and late-onset. Second, for the extremely rare instances of HD beginning before 10 years of age, there is exclusive paternal transmission (Clarke and Bundey 1990; Went *et al.* 1983), an observation of considerable significance when a young child in a HD family develops a neurological illness. As already discussed in Chapter 2, the clinical presentation in this age group is often most atypical, so that the parental transmission may be a major factor in supporting the diagnosis or in making it less likely. In view of the close correspondence between juvenile onset and the rigid form of HD, it is not surprising that the predominantly paternal transmission was found to apply to the latter group also.

The observation and confirmation of this striking sex-related effect made investigators reassess the earlier data to see whether it had been overlooked, and also to look in more detail at the overall and unselected data for HD populations to see how far the findings might be relevant to adult and late-onset HD. The data of Myers *et al.* (1983) showed a deficiency of paternal transmission in their late-onset group (onset at 50–70 years), with 29 per cent having an affected father and 71 per cent an affected mother, contrasting markedly with values of 91 and 9 per cent, respectively, for the parental origin of their juvenile cases.

Bird *et al.* (1974) analysed age at death in parent–offspring pairs and showed a marked reduction in age at death in the offspring when the father was the affected parent (9.73 years) compared with little difference when the mother was affected (2.04 years). They obtained similar results from analysing previous data in the literature. Interestingly, the overall younger age at death in offspring compared with parent had already been noted by Penrose (1948) in his re-analysis of Bell's (1934) data, but the significance of the difference between maternal and paternal transmission had not been appreciated. Thus, use of age at death as opposed to onset can be queried in these studies, but it is certainly more definitive when older data are being considered, while no marked effect of age at onset on survival has been shown in any of the major studies when bias is allowed for, so that the conclusions regarding age at onset and age at death are probably comparable.

Stevens (1976) examined age at onset in relation to parental transmission in his UK data and found a reduction in age at onset with paternal transmission, although this was significant only for male cases. Newcombe *et al.* (1981), using data from the South Wales study, analysed differences in age at onset by a log rank method, as well as by previous methods, and confirmed an overall correlation between paternal transmission and reduced age at onset. Both this study and that of Stevens also made the interesting observation that, when data were available for three generations, the group with earliest onset was that in which transmission was grandfather–father–offspring. This finding is now clearly explicable in terms of instability of the mutation.

The largest data set available, the US Huntington's Roster, was analysed for effects of parental transmission by Conneally (1984) and Boehnke *et al.* (1983), with further detailed analyses by Farrer and Conneally (1985) and Ridley *et al.* (1988, 1991). The age-at-onset curve in this material was clearly different for offspring of affected fathers and mothers across a wide age range (Fig. 5.5). As in other studies this was principally due to an 8-year reduction in age at onset of paternally transmitted cases, offspring of affected mothers showing little reduction (Table 5.5). Even after excluding juvenile cases, there was still a 5.6-year reduction in the age at onset of paternally transmitted cases.

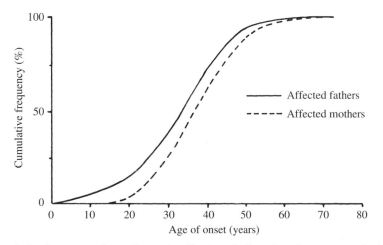

Fig. 5.5 Cumulative frequency of age of onset in offspring of affected mothers compared with offspring of affected fathers. HD Roster data (from Conneally 1984 with kind permission of the author).

Table 5.5 Age at onset and death in HD. Differences between parent and child

Study	Father–child	Mother–child
Boehnke *et al.* 1983	8.06+11.27 (*n*=276)	1.41+7.62 (*n*=281)
Bird *et al.* 1974	9.73+1.92 (*n*=70)	2.04+0.93 (*n*=52)
Previous literature analysed by Bird *et al.* 1974	9.67+1.14 (*n*=114)	3.01+1.52 (*n*=55)
Ridley *et al.* 1988	6.73 (skewed)	1.35+8.49 (*n*=899)

The independence of the effects of parental transmission from the racial genetic background of the population has been shown by the finding of Folstein *et al.* (1987) that the reduced age at onset in offspring of affected fathers was found equally among Blacks and Whites in the Maryland (USA) population, as well as in South African mixed-race families, as already mentioned.

Anticipation

Although the concept of anticipation is an old one, the disorder for which most evidence existed has been myotonic dystrophy (Fleischer 1918), and for many years it was around this condition that debate revolved as to whether anticipation even existed as a true biological phenomenon (Penrose 1948; Höweler *et al.* 1989; Harper *et al.* 1992). By the time myotonic dystrophy was recognized as due to an unstable trinucleotide repeat in late 1991, it was already clear that anticipation also existed in HD (Ridley *et al.* 1988, 1991), providing a clear parallel between the two disorders and prompting an intensive (and eventually successful) search for a comparable repeat sequence in HD.

The studies of Ridley *et al.* were based on the extensive 'HD roster' US database, and allowed anticipation to be clearly documented through three generations, but only in the male line, as noted above. They were able to show that juvenile cases occurred particularly in male-transmitted cases that had themselves presented with early onset, with no such comparable effect in the offspring of early-onset affected females.

Molecular basis of anticipation and parental origin effects

Identification of the HD mutation provided an immediate resolution for many of these observations; again, this was helped by the parallel with myotonic dystrophy for which comparable issues had been worked through during the previous year (Harley *et al.* 1992; Harper 1996b). The correlation of age at onset with extent of mutational defect, already discussed, was the first important fact, with juvenile and other early-onset cases showing the largest expansions in the gene. Next, two-generation data (harder to obtain than for myotonic dystrophy) showed clearly that the anticipation seen in individual families and overall was closely paralleled by an increased number of CAG repeats (Andrew *et al.* 1993a; Duyao *et al.* 1993; HD Collaborative Research Group 1993). The parental origin differences could also be explained by the molecular data, with the greatest increase in repeat number being seen in male transmissions, although, interestingly, some tendency to increase was also seen in female transmissions.

Quantitative studies have confirmed that both the anticipation and the parent-of-origin differences are mediated principally through the number of CAG repeats. In a series of 254 parent–child pairs with HD (Kremer *et al.* 1995), expansion was seen in 70 per cent of meioses. Although small increases in repeat number (up to seven repeats) were seen in transmission by both sexes (47.1 per cent of males and 37.8 per cent of females), large increases (more than seven repeats) were seen almost exclusively in the offspring of males (21.0 versus 0.7 per cent in the offspring of females). The largest increases were particularly likely to occur in individuals who themselves had the largest expansions (Trottier *et al.* 1994; Ranen *et al.* 1995), confirming a size-dependent instability in this group, which is also seen in myotonic dystrophy (Harley *et al.* 1993; Lavedan *et al.* 1993).

The extreme effect of this process is seen in patients with juvenile HD, who have the largest expansions, which are predominantly paternally transmitted (Telenius *et al.* 1993). The lesser instability of female meioses means that it is rare for a female transmission to increase sufficiently to cause such a case, in the same way as it is rare for female intermediate allele carriers to have clinically affected offspring.

As yet, we know little about why where should be such a marked sex difference in the expansion of the CAG repeat, but evidence has come from analysis of sperm from males affected with HD (Andrew *et al.* 1993a; HD Collaborative Research Group 1993; MacDonald *et al.* 1993). The main finding from these studies is that the mean repeat number in sperm is greater than that seen in blood from the same individual, but also that there is a much greater range of repeat numbers. Analysis of single sperm (Leeflang *et al.* 1995; Chong *et al.* 1997) gives a clearer picture of the distribution of sperm with different repeat numbers generated at male meiosis, confirming a high frequency (>90 per cent) of increased repeat number for alleles already in the normal range, while for an intermediate allele carrier this figure was still over 50 per cent, with 8 per cent in the clinically significant range. As yet, comparable data are not available for females, but these results strongly suggest that the main cause of male anticipation and paternal transmission of juvenile HD lies in the genetic instability of the repeat during spermatogenesis, rather than in subsequent somatic instability during embryonic development.

Before leaving the area of intergenerational changes, it should be noted that the HD mutation may decrease, as well as increase in extent, as is to be expected for a dynamic mutation, and as has been well documented in myotonic dystrophy (Abeliovich *et al.* 1993; Brunner *et al.* 1993). In the study of Kremer *et al.* (1995) a modest decrease of between 1 and 4 in repeat number was seen in 18 per cent of transmissions, although larger decreases were not observed. Decreases were also observed in the single-sperm study of Leeflang *et al.* (1995). This should be borne in mind when an 'intermediate' allele is observed during predictive testing for a person whose affected parent may have a repeat number at the lower end of the HD range.

New mutations and intermediate alleles

This is a topic where our understanding has been so totally changed by new knowledge that not only the facts but our entire concept of the 'new mutation' is now radically different from that which we had before the gene was isolated. Seen with the advantage of hindsight, it is clear that early work studying possible new mutations was searching for something that did not exist. Now we recognize that mutation in HD is a progressive rather than a discontinuous process.

The early studies on mutation in HD concentrated on identifying isolated HD cases and estimating their frequency. All the major surveys of HD reported such isolated cases as accounting for only a small proportion of the total. Shaw and Caro (1982) combined data from a number of studies and estimated that isolated cases represented only 2 per cent, at most, of all cases, or 5 per cent of all families. These values fell to 0.04 and 0.1 per cent, respectively, when applying more rigorous criteria. In the South Wales study (Walker *et al.* 1983) no case could seriously be considered as representing a new mutation among 418 patients from 101 kindreds. The same was true for several of the other major studies, including that of Reed and Neel (1959), which found 36 'isolated' cases among 801 studied (196 kindreds), and that of Wendt and Drohm (1972) in Germany, which found no likely mutation among 1032 cases studied. As Shaw and Caro (1982) stated of their own cases: 'all peter out through lack of information rather than definite knowledge of the origin of the disease through mutation'.

The early estimates all had a number of serious problems. Many clinicians were reluctant to accept an isolated case as HD without full neuropathology, while a considerable number of such cases now diagnosed as HD through molecular analysis would not have been recognized. Geneticists also ruled out as new mutations cases that could be linked through previous generations, even though these ancestors appeared to have remained free from HD. It is not surprising that the subject stayed confused until the specific mutation was identified, although all were agreed that the great majority of patients with HD (over 95 per cent) received the disease from a parent who was affected, or who might have been had they lived long enough.

From the moment when the HD mutation was recognized as a trinucleotide repeat, possible new mutation cases were re-evaluated. The original *Cell* publication (HD Collaborative Research Group 1993) documented two families considered to represent new mutations and showed that in each case the father carried an allele in the range intermediate between normal and HD. These 'intermediate alleles' have proved to be a topic of considerable significance, both theoretical and practical (see Chapter 7), not only for HD but also for other trinucleotide repeat disorders whose basis is genetic instability. The initial step in the recognition and characterization of intermediate alleles was the study of apparently sporadic cases and their parents. As mentioned, this was already documented in the original HD Collaborative Research Group (1993) publication, but larger series of sporadic cases proved in most clinically typical cases to show the HD mutation (MacMillan *et al.* 1993a; Davis *et al.* 1994; Mandich *et al.* 1996).

When parents of such cases were studied (Goldberg *et al.* 1993; Myers *et al.* 1993), it became clear that, while the clinical phenotype of HD might arise *de novo* and thus be considered as a new mutation, the molecular defect did not, with one parent invariably showing an expanded allele, usually in the 30–38 repeat range, but not associated with evidence of clinical disease, even at an advanced age. In all six cases in the series of Goldberg *et al.* where parental origin could be determined, the father was the one with the intermediate allele, a finding confirmed in subsequent series, though occasional instances of maternal intermediate alleles leading to clinical HD in the next generation have been recorded (Sanchez *et al.* 1997; Laccone and Christian 2000). It is now clear that a predominantly, though not exclusively paternal origin of disease in the first clinically manifesting generation is a feature of trinucleotide disorders in general, including myotonic dystrophy (Lopez de Munain *et al.* 1995; Harper 2001). The wider aspects of parental origin effects have been discussed in an earlier section of this chapter.

A recent study of all patients referred to the Canadian British Columbia genetics clinic for HD tests has shed light on the incidence of HD in the absence of a family history of the disease (Almquist *et al.* 2001). A small proportion of these cases appear to be genuinely isolated, although it was difficult to be precise about family history in many cases. Even so, the rate observed in this series, at around 8 per cent, was similar to that previously reported, for instance, in the Leiden series, at 6.3 per cent (Siesling *et al.* 2000). 205 patients were referred to the British Columbia clinic over a 7 year period from 1993 with suspected symptomatic HD. Of the 89 patients with no family history of HD, 34 had a repeat expansion of 36 CAG or greater, in the HD range. Fifteen of the 34 reported some family history of a disorder including involuntary movements and/or dementia, and some of these relatives had had a diagnosis of parkinsonism or Alzheimer's disease. In the 19 patients with no clear family history only one could unequivocally be proven to be clinically *de novo*, with an expansion from a paternal allele of 33 CAG, and one had a repeat expanded from a non-penetrant 39 CAG repeat in the father. The rest had incomplete family histories or one or both parents had died before the age of 60, so no assessment of likely intermediate alleles could be carried out. Thus, although the apparent proportion of isolated cases in this study is 8 per cent, there is a substantial proportion of unknown and unknowable situations.

The recognition of intermediate allele carriers has led to an assessment of penetrance of the HD phenotype in this borderline repeat range. Although early case reports may have been affected by technical problems in giving an exact and reproducible repeat number, a multi-centre study (Rubinsztein *et al.* 1996) re-analysed 178 individuals with a CAG repeat in the 30–39 range in a single laboratory and estimated the penetrance of the HD phenotype at different points in this range. Clearly, age is a critical factor in interpreting this, but the finding of six clinically normal individuals aged 75 to over 90 in the 36–39 repeat range is a clear indication of incomplete penetrance in this range, while no individuals with 35 repeats or less were found to have HD. On the basis of this and subsequent studies, risk estimates have been developed for use in genetic counselling and presymptomatic testing (see Chapter 7) that estimate the likelihood of an individual with a particular repeat number developing HD.

Late-onset HD, as noted above, has been proven in some centres to be confused with other late-onset neurodegenerations, such as Alzheimer's disease and parkinsonism (Almqvist *et al.* 2001). Now that an unequivocal test can discriminate HD in the elderly, estimates can be made for the rate of mutations expanded into the disease-causing range appearing in the population. Falush *et al.* (2000) used the nearly 2000 individuals with repeat lengths greater than or equal to 36 in the University of British Columbia HD series and also used the data for CAG lengths in sperm generated by Leeflang *et al.* (1999) to estimate mutational parameters. They found that penetrance at repeat lengths of up to 41 CAG was not complete and that the new mutation rate would be around 10 per cent of currently known cases in each generation. These figures seem high, but, until we have many more years of HD data with CAG repeat length, the true figures will remain unknown. Indeed, as only patients displaying clinical symptoms that make the clinician suspect HD or those with a family history generally undergo testing, the true pattern of population distribution of the HD repeat may remain unclear.

A related genetic counselling issue is how great is the risk for the offspring of an intermediate allele carrier having an expansion in the clinically significant range? An important observation in this respect was the finding of Goldberg *et al.* (1995), using analysis of blood and sperm, that instability was greater when the intermediate allele occurred in a family with HD than when it occurred in the general population. None of 62 meioses from the general population intermediate alleles increased to 36 or more repeats, a finding of some practical significance since around 2 per cent of the population was estimated to carry an allele in the 29–35 range. A related observation is that of McNeil *et al.* (1997) who showed that distant collateral branches of an HD family had a lower chance of an intermediate allele producing clinical HD. Those differences also support the involvement of other genetic loci in the instability process, which is discussed below. However, a further study, using single-sperm analysis (Chong *et al.* 1997), has shown that the risk for such general population intermediate allele carriers could be significant, possibly as high as 6 per cent for a clinically significant expansion, while the comparable risk for offspring of a male carrier from an HD family may be at least 10 per cent.

The factors involved in the generation of intermediate alleles and in their expansion into the HD range are clearly part of the broader mechanisms responsible for genetic instability and are discussed later in this chapter. It is relevant to note, though, that the study of Chong *et al.* showed that the DNA sequence surrounding the CAG appeared to have an important effect. In particular, the lack of interruption between the CAG repeat and an adjacent CCG repeat favoured instability.

Origins of the HD mutation

It is now clear that, while a small proportion of HD cases may behave clinically as new mutations, in terms of having no clinically affected parents or other ancestors, none of these cases are truly *de novo* in the molecular sense, as all have a parent in the intermediate allele range as described above. What remains much less clear is how individuals with such intermediate alleles originate from the general population and how many generations need to elapse before instability sufficient to result in HD occurs. The mechanisms involved in the generation of instability are clearly highly relevant to this and are discussed below, while the population aspects are intimately related to the geographical studies of prevalence and related factors, and are discussed more fully in Chapter 6—under the topic of molecular epidemiology.

HD homozygotes

Almost all the genes for HD, as for other rare dominantly inherited disorders, are present in heterozygotes, who also possess a normal allele at this locus. For the gene to occur in the homozygous state requires one of several exceedingly rare events to occur. An individual inheriting the HD gene could undergo a new mutation at the normal allele (a vanishingly rare event given the rarity of mutation in HD). A person could receive two copies of the HD gene from the affected parent and no normal gene from the healthy parent (this 'uniparental disomy' has been recorded for cystic fibrosis and may occur more commonly than previously recognized). Or, least unlikely, both parents might possess the HD gene, in which case there would be a one in four chance that any child would receive a 'double dose'. Such homozygosity for other dominantly inherited disorders has been much more severe than in the heterozygous state, often being fatal in early life. Achondroplasia, hereditary haemorrhagic telangiectasia, and familial hypercholesterolaemia are examples of this. Any homozygote for HD might therefore have been expected to show a severe and distinctive neurological disorder or, alternatively, the homozygous state might be so lethal as to appear as an excess of spontaneous abortions or stillbirths, or as a deficiency in the observed number of affected offspring.

Several instances of possible homozygosity for HD have been reported over the years; Hindringer (1935) reported a consanguineous marriage in a family from southern Germany where the two affected parents had five children, three with typical HD, one unaffected, and one infant death. Eldridge *et al.* (1973) described an American family where both parents in a first-cousin marriage were affected (details on the father were scanty). The affected son had typical HD with onset aged 34 years; one of the two sibs had died in infancy, the other from a war injury. Both families were small and the information incomplete, so that no firm conclusions could be drawn other than to say that no unusual neurological features were observed among affected offspring. Most of our important information on homozygosity has come from the Venezuelan isolate with HD, already described, where the combination of high HD prevalence and extreme isolation produced several instances where both parents were affected.

A detailed report on the largest of these sibships has appeared (Wexler *et al.* 1987), with further details after isolation of the HD gene (Huntingtons Disease Collaborative Research Group 1993). The value of this study is not only that the sibship is extremely large (14 sibs) and both parents living, but that molecular studies of linked markers, and now of the mutation, made it possible to identify with high probability which individuals were homozygous for the HD gene quite independently of their clinical status. Four of the 14 sibs proved to be homozygous for the high-risk genotype, a proportion consistent with Mendelian segregation and making prenatal lethality improbable. Nor did any members of the sibship show unusual clinical features that would not have been expected in heterozygotes in this population. At the time of the first study (1986) the offspring were relatively young (16–42 years) and only minor neurological signs were present; subsequent follow-up confirmed definite HD in at least one of the four probable homozygotes, but still did not show any distinguishing clinical features from those in heterozygotes. Analysis of the mutation itself confirmed the original assessment of homozygosity (Huntingtons Disease Collaborative Research Group 1993), as shown in Fig. 5.6.

In a separate study Myers *et al.* (1989) analysed four possible homozygotes from three New England families where both parents were affected. One of these showed a 95 per cent chance of being homozygous on molecular testing, but clinical features and age at onset were

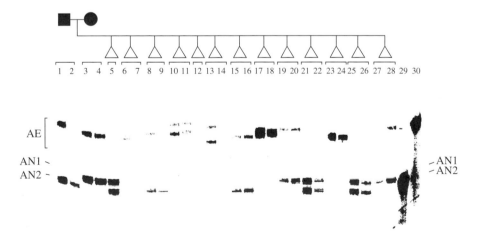

Fig. 5.6 Homozygosity for the HD mutation in part of the large Venezuelan kindred with two affected parents. Some individuals can be seen to have two abnormal alleles (AN) (identities altered to preserve confidentiality). (From HD Collaborative Research Group (1993), courtesy of James Gusella, Marcy MacDonald, and Cell Press.)

comparable to those of affected heterozygotes in the family. A further report (Durr *et al.* 1999) has shown a homozygous patient with 42 and 46 repeats whose presentation was similar to that of a sib with 48 and 17 repeats. However, the small number of reports does not rule out a small difference between homozygote and heterozygote, as pointed out by Narain *et al.* (1999), though a major difference is unlikely. It must not be forgotten that homozygosity by common descent may be producing recessive effects at other loci.

The effect of homozygosity can also be examined in transgenic mice with the human mutation knocked into their *Hdh* gene, that is, with the human expansion inserted into the endogenous mouse HD gene. Here, there are differences between *Hdh* knock-in homozygotes and heterozygotes with the same CAG repeat length. These differences manifest in the earlier age of onset of behavioural phenotypes and pathology, including inclusion formation. The differences appear to be in timing, not in phenotype. For instance, in mice with 150 CAG repeats, onset of behavioural abnormalities was 60 weeks in heterozygotes and 25 weeks in homozygotes (Lin *et al.* 2000) and similar results are seen for timing of pathological changes in other knock-in models (Wheeler *et al.* 1999). Reports on duration of phenotype and age at death are not yet available for these mice. However, the mice represent a much more uniform genetic background on which to analyse these differences and they carry very long repeats. Given that a large proportion of variation in age of onset is accounted for by repeat length in the juvenile cases, which these mice parallel much better than they do the adult cases, it is perhaps unsurprising that human homozygotes for repeats in the adult-onset range show no apparent adverse effect due to homozygosity.

So, in the human population the homozygote for HD is little or no more severely affected than the heterozygote, at least when the same mutation is inherited by common descent. This situation, unlike that so far encountered for some other dominantly inherited disorders, has considerable implications for our understanding of HD. It provides some evidence for the view that HD is not the result of loss of function of the normal HD gene, a view also supported by the absence of HD in chromosomal deletions of the region, such as Wolf–Hirschhorn syndrome, and by the evidence for direct involvement of the polyglutamine repeat in pathogenesis. However, in the more uniform genetic background of a mouse carrying a very expanded repeat that leads to a phenotype including a movement disorder, carrying two copies of the gene certainly does decrease the age of onset of that phenotype. This cannot be related directly to the human situation where a homozygote carrying two extremely long repeats is very unlikely to arise, as such large expansions occur through the male line only and in any case would give rise to such early onset as to render anyone carrying even one copy of such long repeats unlikely to have children. Thus, there may be an effect in humans homozygous for HD but it is either overwhelmed by other variables or undetectable because of the inevitably small sample size.

There are also practical genetic consequences for HD homozygotes, as illustrated in Fig. 5.7. The parents of an HD homozygote will have a three in four chance of an offspring with HD (one of whom will on average be homozygous) and a one in four chance of a normal homozygous offspring. For the children of an HD homozygote all would be expected to develop HD, even though the other parent will remain healthy, because all will inevitably receive one HD gene from the homozygous HD parent.

With predictive testing widespread, it now sometimes happens that an individual appears to possess two alleles in the HD range even though the disorder is known in only one side of the family. Possibilities to consider in this difficult situation are unsuspected consanguinity

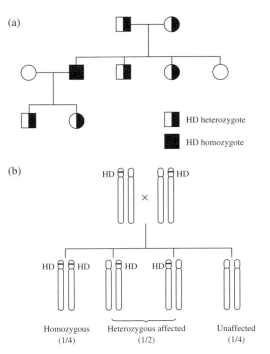

(a)

HD heterozygote

HD homozygote

(b)

Fig. 5.7 Homozygosity for HD. (a) Pedigree. (b) Diagram to show segregation of chromosomes. When both parents are affected, the chance of an offspring being homozygous for the HD gene is one in four (sex is not important). All offspring of a homozygous affected person would be heterozygous for HD (i.e. affected).

(including incest), as well as true HD on the other side of the family. The relative stability of intermediate alleles in the general population, already noted, is important for risk estimates when one of the alleles is in this range, as discussed in Chapter 7.

Twins

The study of monozygous (identical) twin pairs provides an opportunity for assessing the role of environmental factors in the onset and clinical phenotype of HD. In the context of a dynamic trinucleotide repeat expansion it also now allows evaluation of the extent to which somatic genetic instability, particularly in early embryonic development, may be important. So far, direct molecular studies on such twin pairs are limited, but the early genetic data are worth careful examination as they give clear indications as to what may be expected from molecular studies.

Many of the early twin studies in HD did not document zygosity accurately, but Table 5.6 summarizes the data on those where monozygosity seems likely; the remaining early pairs are reviewed by Myrianthopoulos and Rowley (1960). The principal feature to emerge from these studies is the similarity between the co-twins, especially regarding age at onset. There are no reports of complete discordance, that is, of the co-twin remaining healthy after a considerable interval. Although some pairs have varied in clinical presentation, such as that of Oepen (1973), where one had mainly rigidity and the other choreic movements, the overall impression is one of close similarity. This suggests that purely environmental influences are likely to be relatively small, and that the same may be true for somatic instability of the CAG repeat

Table 5.6 Monozygotic twin pairs with HD studied before identification of the HD mutation

Reference	Sex	Evidence for zygosity	Age at onset	Clinical notes
Rosanoff and Handy 1935	F	Appearance only	35/35	
Entres 1921	F		41/41	Died at 54 and 56 years
	M		45/45	Died at 64 and 65 years
Parker 1958	M		42/42	Died 3 months apart
Myrianthopoulos and Rowley 1960	F	Blood groups, dermatoglyphs	22/22	Similar course; mental deterioration mild in one
Schiottz-Christensen 1969	F		24/24	
Oepen 1973	F	Blood groups, skin grafts	22/25	Similar; slight differences on detailed psychological test
Husquinet *et al.* 1973	F	Blood group, dermatoglyphs		Both severe psychiatric symptoms, slight chorea worsened by L-dopa
Bird and Omenn 1975	F	Blood groups, RBC enzymes	Both mid-20s	Chorea marked in one, minimal in the other
Bachman *et al.* 1977	F	HLA and blood groups	5/5	Both with rigidity and dementia

during early development. In this respect HD may differ from other trinucleotide repeat disorders such as myotonic dystrophy and fragile X syndrome, where the extent of expansion and instability is much greater, and where somatic and possibly developmental variation are also more prominent.

Direct analysis of the HD mutation has been undertaken on a series of four monozygotic twin pairs (MacDonald *et al.* 1993), whose onset was within 3 years of each other for members of the pair. The repeat number was also identical for the members of all four pairs, strongly supporting the determination of the repeat number in gametogenesis, rather than in development. By contrast, a further pair with identical repeat number reported by Georgiou *et al.* (1999) showed considerable clinical differences in motor and psychological features, though age at onset was similar (early 30s).

Identical twins also pose a special problem for presymptomatic testing, since an adverse result in one automatically confirms that the co-twin also has the HD gene. In such a situation, testing would seem unwise unless both twins were requesting it.

Genetic modifiers of HD

The finding that the CAG repeat in the HD gene accounted for part of the variation in age of onset of HD drew attention to factors that might account for the rest of this variation, especially in the common adult-onset form of the disease where people with the same repeat length may have very different ages of onset (see the section on 'Age of onset'). The possibility that other genetic loci might be involved in the presentation of HD had actually been recognized for a long time before the cloning of the gene in 1993. Bell (1934) carried out the first systematic analysis of data in the literature and gave an accurate distribution of age at onset and death, but also an analysis of variance. Bell found that there was a high correlation in age of onset between parent and child (0.54) and sibs (0.64), which pointed very clearly to a genetic basis for the age of onset of HD. Analysis of Bell's data led Haldane (1941) to conclude that most of this variation was the result of modifying genes.

Later work by Farrer *et al.* (1984) and Farrer and Conneally (1985) used the American HD roster to provide convincing evidence that genetic factors were important in determining age at onset and age at death in HD. They detected the correlations observed by Bell but also found an equally strong correlation with age at death of the normal—non-HD—parent, as well as between HD and normal sibs and parents with HD and their normal children. There was no correlation of age at death between patients with HD and their spouses, making environmental effects unlikely. This provides conclusive evidence that age at onset and death are not solely determined by the HD gene itself. Farrer *et al.* (1984) proposed that normal ageing genes expressed in the basal ganglia might be involved, and that these would not be allelic with the HD gene as they were also inherited by sibs discordant for HD.

Thus, well before the discovery of the HD mutation, it was already clear that not all genetic variation in HD could be attributed to the HD locus itself. A series of studies of the correlation between CAG repeat length, age of onset, and other phenotypic features have confirmed this. As mentioned above, the CAG repeat length appears to account for 47–73 per cent of the variance in age of onset in studies of various HD populations (Craufurd *et al.* 1995; Ranen *et al.* 1995; Brinkman *et al.* 1997; Squitieri *et al.* 2000; Rosenblatt *et al.* 2001). Ranen *et al.* (1995) further concluded that that 16 per cent of the residual variance in age of onset was accounted for by the parent's age of onset. A recent study examining the relative influences of CAG repeat length and family background on age of onset of motor symptoms has concluded that, although CAG length accounts for the largest proportion of the variance, 11–19 per cent of the additional variance was accounted for by the sibship to which the person belonged (Rosenblatt *et al.* 2001).

In addition, there have been a number of studies that have examined how specific symptoms are inherited in HD families. Lovestone *et al.* (1996) reported a family in which the initial presentation of HD was with a severe psychiatric syndrome, and where several other family members had psychosis, which led them to believe that a familial factor was influencing the presentation of the disease. Tsuang *et al.* (1998) examined two families where schizophrenia-like symptoms segregated with HD and then went on to study psychosis in a larger cohort of 22 HD patients showing psychosis and 22 patients without psychosis (Tsuang *et al.* 2000). The main conclusion was that HD patients with psychosis were significantly more likely to have a first-degree relative with psychosis than those who presented with HD without psychosis. This segregation of psychotic symptoms with HD held true in 8 of 9 families in this study. Thus this finding confirms the earlier studies that implicated family background as important in disease symptoms, and indicates that other genetic factors may influence particular phenotypes in HD.

Given the evidence for other genetic influences, past and present, it is unsurprising that various groups have examined variations in genes that were thought to be important in HD for association with the disease, mainly using age at onset as a correlate in analyses. Age at onset, as has already been mentioned, is relatively easily ascertained on a large number of affected people, is quantitative, and is known to reflect residual genetic variation in HD patients unaccounted for by CAG repeat length. Thus, a few studies of possible modifying genes have been reported, using age of onset as a correlate for genetic analysis.

The purpose of such studies is primarily to use genetics to decide whether pathways and proteins suggested to be important in HD are actually involved in the pathogenic process in such a way as to influence age of onset or other measurable clinical parameters. Genes that influence age at onset are likely to be important in early pathogenic events, subsequent to the repeat expansion being translated into polyglutamine in huntingtin. Thus, such studies have the potential to discriminate between the numerous pathogenic mechanisms proposed as contributing to HD. Genes that are candidates for such studies include: (1) genes known to influence normal human ageing; (2) genes encoding proteins known to interact with huntingtin; (3) genes encoding proteins involved in pathways suggested to be important in HD pathogenesis, such as cell death, protein degradation, transcription, neurotransmitter receptor signalling, and vesicle recycling; (4) genes encoding proteins with glutamine tracts; and (5) genes predisposing to DNA repeat instability, particularly repeat expansion. The reason genes encoding proteins containing polyglutamine tracts are attractive as candidate modifiers is that glutamine tracts bind to each other and many proteins, particularly transcription factors, contain them; it has been suggested that polyglutamine tracts bind together through a polar zipper mechanism (Perutz *et al.* 1994). Alterations in proteins containing these tracts might alter their binding to huntingtin and mediate downstream cellular effects. TATA-binding protein (TBP) for instance, with a polymorphic repeat varying from 25 to 42 glutamines is found in the intranuclear inclusions of HD and other trinucleotide repeat diseases, presumably bound through the proteins' respective glutamine tracts.

Three genetic modifiers of the HD gene have been reported, each probably accounting for only a small proportion of the variance in age of onset of HD. A noncoding TAA repeat polymorphism in the 3' UTR of the kainate receptor (GluR6) gene was reported to account for varying amounts of the residual age at onset variation in HD (Rubinsztein *et al.* 1997; MacDonald *et al.* 1999). The kainate receptor can mediate excitotoxicity in the brain and thus coding alterations in the gene, in linkage disequilibrium with this marker, might lead to altered activity, giving increased or decreased risk for excitotoxic damage subsequent to the damage caused by the glutamine expansion; this belongs to the third category above. *APOE* genotype had a small but significant effect with the ε2ε3 genotype associated with an earlier onset in males than females (Kehoe *et al.* 1999). This study also found an effect of the normal HD allele on age at onset, a result reported previously from an overlapping cohort (Snell *et al.* 1993) but not replicated in other studies. The population in this study, from South Wales in the UK, may have given this result because it is genetically more homogeneous than other populations analysed in this way. *APOE* genotype is the only robust genetic risk factor associated with late-onset Alzheimer's disease (Hardy 1997), where it does have an influence on age at onset, and may influence the age of onset in other neurodegenerative diseases, thus falling into the first category mentioned above. The final genetic variation detected as influencing age of onset in HD is a length polymorphism in a polyglutamine tract encoded in the CA150 gene, a transcription factor of unknown function, which interacts directly with huntingtin. Length changes in the tract correlate with age of onset of disease. This modifying gene falls into both categories (2) and (4) above.

These studies will undoubtedly be extended in the coming years as more candidates are proposed and as our knowledge of all aspects of HD increases. They are now much easier to carry out technically with high throughput methods. The availability of the full human genome sequence, along with increasing numbers of variants within the genome now deposited in public databases, will make this effort feasible, where previously it was not an achievable possibility. Gene expression and proteomic studies using human and transgenic mouse samples, currently underway in various centres, will also, undoubtedly, throw up a large number of new candidates with possible involvement in HD pathogenesis. Genetics will be one way to separate those genes that encode proteins likely to be involved in primary pathogenic events from those, the large majority, that have downstream effects. A genetic linkage study is also taking place examining HD sib-pairs with known ages of onset and repeat lengths to detect genomic regions likely to carry modifying genes in a classic sib-pair linkage study design, which involves the collaboration of a number of large centres. Thus the era of genetic analysis in HD is not over, and genetics still has the potential to shed light on the underlying pathogenic mechanisms of HD.

Mosaicism in HD

In other trinucleotide repeat disorders, notably fragile X syndrome and myotonic dystrophy, where the repeat lengths reach much greater values than in HD, there is considerable evidence of genetic instability affecting somatic tissues as well as the germline. This is often evident in the expanded repeat being seen as a poorly defined band, or even a smear, on a Southern blot or polymerase chain reaction (PCR) preparation, while differences between tissues such as muscle and blood may be seen (Ashizawa *et al.* 1993). Some patients with fragile X syndrome may even show discrete mosaicism, with distinct cell lines of widely differing repeat number.

The range of expansion seen in the HD repeat is much less than that for these other disorders, so it is not surprising that somatic instability seems to be of only minor significance. The strongest evidence that this can occur, at least during early development, comes from the analysis of monozygotic twin pairs, which provide a valuable natural experiment, as discussed below. MacDonald *et al.* (1993) showed no clear difference in repeat number between fresh blood and lymphoblastoid lines set up many years before. Nor were there differences between blood and brain repeat number in 19 patients, nor any other detectable tissue difference. Likewise, Zuhlke *et al.* (1993b) found no evidence of somatic instability in a wide range of tissues, including different areas of the brain, while De Rooij *et al.* (1995) found only minimal differences within the brain. However, Telenius *et al.* (1994) and Aronin *et al.* (1995) did observe tissue mosaicism in the brain, especially in the basal ganglia and cerebral cortex, and most marked in juvenile-onset cases. A further finding suggesting some somatic instability was the observation in two juvenile cases of a reduced repeat number in the cerebellum, a finding of possible significance in relation to the unusual clinical features of this form. Ansved *et al.* (1998) showed no increase in repeat number of HD muscle in comparison to blood, whereas this was observed in Kennedy's disease (and is more strikingly seen in myotonic dystrophy: Ashizawa *et al.* 1994).

Somatic mosaicism is also observed, rarely, in lymphocytes taken for DNA analysis. This could potentially complicate the molecular diagnostics in presymptomatic cases. We have seen one such case where a man whose father had died with a clinical diagnosis of HD came to clinic for presymptomatic testing. The normal procedures for presymptomatic testing were followed and the DNA extracted from blood gave one normal and, unusually, two abnormal, alleles. These were a main band at 37 CAG and a fainter band at 42 CAG (Fig. 5.8). The result was consistent in three independent DNA samples including one collected a number of years earlier as part of a research project. The conclusion is that two populations of lymphocytes exist, one with a 37 CAG expansion and one with a 42 CAG expansion, most probably arising

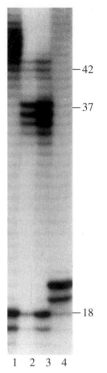

Fig. 5.8 Genetic mosaicism in DNA from blood in an HD case. The CAG repeat was amplified using a PCR that excluded the CCG repeat (Barron *et al.* 1994). Lane 1 shows a positive control with a normal allele of 18 repeats and an affected allele of 46 repeats. Lanes 2 and 3 show independent DNA samples amplified from the index case, demonstrating the mosaicism: one normal allele of 18 repeats and two expanded alleles of 37 and 42 repeats. Lane 4 shows a juvenile-onset case with an expanded repeat size outside the known range, with a trinucleotide background signal facilitating the sizing of the repeats.

as a result of two distinct cell lineages from an early developmental stage. This unusual situation has not been reported before in HD but has occurred in other trinucleotide repeat disorders (Hellenbroich *et al.* 2001; Martorell *et al.* 2000). The father in this case was symptomatic at death at 45 years and almost certainly had a full mutation. Neither the proband's brother nor his children had an expanded repeat in the HD gene.

Recent studies in HD transgenic mice have also demonstrated varying levels of germline and somatic mosaicism. Several HD transgenic mouse lines have demonstrated germline instability of the repeat, particularly in paternal transmission, as in human HD; this is discussed in Chapter 13. This observed germline instability is generally assumed to be related to DNA replication errors, such as slippage, but somatic mosaicism observed in terminally differentiated cells in many triplet repeat diseases is almost certainly caused by the operation of other processes on the DNA; these may include alteration in chromatin structure and repair. The notable report of reduced CAG repeat instability in R6/1 mouse brain and other tissues in the absence of the *Msh2* mismatch repair gene implicates DNA repair in the mechanism of somatic instability (Kovtun and McMurray 2001).

Somatic instability has generally been found to be greatest in the striatum in human HD and in a number of mouse models (Telenius *et al.* 1993; Aronin *et al.* 1995; Mangiarini *et al.* 1997; Wheeler *et al.* 1999; Manley *et al.* 1999). The most dramatic report in transgenic mice is that of Kennedy and Shelbourne (2000) who used small pool PCR in their aged mice with expanded CAGs knocked into the mouse *Hdh* gene. They found huge instability, particularly in the striatum of the transgenic mice. The small pool PCR technique allows the DNA of a very limited number of cells to be analysed and thus, if long repeats are present, they are more likely to be amplified than if a larger sample is taken, where preferential amplification of shorter alleles will disguise the presence of any long alleles in the original sample. It has been suggested that this amplification in the striatum could be the basis for the initial degeneration of this brain region in HD. If this is the case then factors disposing to somatic expansion would be expected to have a role in controlling the age of onset of HD.

Molecular mechanisms of repeat expansion

One of the questions that arises from a study of HD and other diseases caused by trinucleotide and other repeat expansions is the molecular mechanism by which those expansions occurred in the first place. There have been various studies that have attempted to address this question both by looking at repeats in populations and estimating how they may have evolved, and by examining size changes in repeats in various experimental systems. Much of the epidemiological evidence is given in Chapter 6 and will only be referred to here, but experiments and observations in bacteria, yeast, cell culture, and mice have revealed possible mutational mechanisms.

DNA undergoes a number of processes during which size changes in repeats could possibly occur. These include replication, recombination, transcription, and repair. *In vitro* studies have shown that triplet repeats can adopt a number of unusual structures including hairpins, quadruplexes, slipped structures, and non-B DNA helices. In yeast and *E. coli* orientation-dependent expansions or contractions occur depending on which repeat is on the leading or lagging strand at replication and these are almost certainly due to hairpin structures forming in the single-stranded sections of the DNA (Kang *et al.* 1995; Maurer *et al.* 1996). In meiotic recombination in yeast single-stranded CNG repeats were also found to form hairpin structures (Moore *et al.* 1999) and instability was also associated with double-strand break formation and repair in the repeats, which gave both expansions and contractions of repeats. Further evidence suggests that really large expansions occurring in the germline might be due to gene conversions (Jakupciak and Wells 2000). Clearly, recombination occurs mainly in germ cells and replication only in dividing cells, so these mechanisms can account for germline instability and some somatic instability, but not that in postmitotic, terminally differentiated cells.

Most of the cells affected in HD, however, are postmitotic. If instability is also occurring in these cells, and the evidence above indicates that it is, then length change is likely only to occur during repair or transcription. As mentioned above, the best evidence for the mechanism of this instability is that the HD transgenic R6/1 models, when crossed with $Msh2^{-/-}$ mice, have no expansion of the HD mutation in germ cells, compared with HD/$Msh2^{+/+}$ mice which do (Kovtun and McMurray 2001). As the mice had similar sperm counts and thus no evidence for loss of recombination, this almost certainly reflects a loss of gap repair function.

The CAG repeat in the HD gene is an example of a microsatellite, a DNA sequence of di-, tri-, or tetranucleotide repeats that may be polymorphic; these sequences are widely used as markers in genomic linkage and association studies. They are recognized as having a relatively high mutation rate giving length changes, which makes them informative markers in linkage studies as they have a high rate of heterozygosity. The rate of germline mutations in human tetranucleotide markers was examined as part of a genome screen and found to be 1.8×10^{-3} per allele transmission (Xu *et al.* 2000). There is no reason to expect a fundamental difference between tri- and tetranucleotide markers in mutation rates. There were three times as many size changes on paternal rather than maternal transmission, although expansions and contractions were equally common in either case. Eighty-five per cent of the transmissions involved a change in size of one repeat unit and expansions to more than 50 units very rarely occurred. The overall rates of expansion and contraction were equal. The most interesting finding was that there was an equilibrium length for such repeats, so small repeats tended to expand but larger repeats to contract so that an equilibrium size was reached where expansion balanced contraction. Xu *et al.* (2000) suggested that this observation would be better explained by a defect in a repair mechanism rather than DNA strand slippage, in agreement with Kovtun and McMurray (2001).

The exact mechanism for expansion that renders alleles in the normal range likely to expand into the intermediate range, and alleles in the intermediate range likely to expand into the disease range is not clear. It is, however, important to note that there does seem to be a progression of increasing repeat sizes in the intermediate and adult-onset range, with few large changes, and it may be that some changes in DNA repair or other mechanisms underlie the observation of Goldberg *et al.* (1995) that intermediate alleles in an HD family are more likely to expand into the disease range than those in the general population. Such defects may have allowed such alleles to expand in the first place. The clarification of the mechanisms underlying instability is, however, most likely to come from further studies of the larger repeat expansions, those of myotonic dystrophy, fragile X syndrome, and Friedreich's ataxia.

Molecular diagnostics

Until the HD mutation was identified, it was impossible to use molecular techniques in diagnosis of the disorder, although linkage analysis had made prediction feasible within a family. The advent of a direct molecular test, with a remarkable degree of both sensitivity and specificity, as seen above, has revolutionized both diagnosis and prediction in HD. Molecular analysis has already become an integral part of diagnosis, and the implications are covered in this section. The topic of presymptomatic testing is dealt with in Chapter 7 and the issues involved and clinical approaches differ widely from those in diagnosis, even though the same technology is used in the testing process.

HD provides a striking example of the speed (quite possibly too hasty) at which new genetic developments can be incorporated into clinical practice. Within days of the original *Cell* publication on the HD gene (Huntingtons Disease Collaborative Research Group 1993), laboratories worldwide were analysing their own series of research samples, while within a few months the techniques were put into service use, both in diagnosis and presymptomatic testing. An important aid in this was the improvement of methods for analysis of the mutation; PCR conditions were adapted (Goldberg *et al.* 1993; Riess *et al.* 1993; Warner *et al.* 1993) and a nonradioactive method devised (Valdes *et al.* 1993). Further adaptations have been suggested by Williams *et al.* (1999) and Bruland *et al.* (1999). The adjacent CCG repeat was recognized and alterations were made to exclude it (Rubinsztein *et al.* 1993; Andrew *et al.* 1994a; Barron *et al.* 1994), as already described. As a result, analysis of the HD mutation has become a relatively straightforward technique that can be used by any experienced diagnostic molecular laboratory. Quality control schemes have now been set up in the UK (Stenhouse and Middleton-Price 1996) and Europe-wide (Losekoot *et al.* 1999). It is clear that there remains room for improvement since the latter study showed a 1.3 per cent rate of misdiagnosis. In the USA, laboratory guidelines have also been produced (ACMG/ASHG 1998), giving not only recommended laboratory procedures but also interpretation of the ranges of results, including intermediate alleles (see Chapters 7 and 15). The different repeat number groups defined in these guidelines are complex and not all would agree that they are the most appropriate, especially in relation to presymptomatic testing. It is also of considerable concern that a survey of US laboratories (Wertz and Reilly 1997) showed that over half the laboratories had no defined policy on testing healthy children for HD, and that 22 per cent had performed testing on healthy children below the age of 12 years, usually at parental request.

It has already been noted that apparent false-negative results in HD are more likely to be due to sampling or other errors than to true absence of the mutation (Andrew *et al.* 1994b). Two other laboratory sources of confusion should be mentioned at this stage. The first is the possibility that an unusually large expansion might fail to amplify with PCR, and thus be missed. This is a major consideration in myotonic dystrophy, where expansions may be of several thousand copies. In HD the range is much less, with even juvenile cases rarely exceeding 100 repeats. Thus the chance of missing an abnormality for this reason is very small and the necessity for undertaking Southern analysis to detect a large expansion is largely confined to cases where juvenile HD is suspected. Nance *et al.* (1999) have discussed the complex laboratory and clinical issues involved in the investigation of suspected juvenile HD in relation to an exceptionally large expansion of 250 repeats. They emphasize the need for the use of modified PCR as well as Southern analysis, and stress also the importance of close cooperation between the molecular laboratory and clinicians involved in planning coordinated investigation. A second possibility for only one allele being detected and HD being missed is the existence of a rare polymorphism affecting one of the PCR primer-annealing sites (Cross *et al.* 1994). Again, this can be resolved by Southern analysis, so most diagnostic laboratories prefer to use this or some other form of back-up test if only one allele is identified on the primary test, even though most such cases will be homozygotes for a common normal allele.

Defining the borderline of the normal and abnormal ranges has received considerable attention since it became clear that they were so close as to give the possibility of overlap. Fortunately, the steep curves of both normal and HD distributions, and the wide separation of the peaks, means that results in the borderline range account for only a small proportion (2–3 per cent) of the total, but it is essential that a clear policy is available for anticipating and handling them, as discussed further in Chapter 7. Assuming that a method is used that excludes the CCG repeat, there is now general agreement that a result of 39 repeats or more in a clinically symptomatic individual is likely to indicate HD. No unequivocal results in this range have been reported in the normal population, though penetrance may be less than complete for 39 repeats. Likewise, a result of 34 or less is almost certainly normal in terms of clinical disease, though not in terms of consequences for the next generation. Although a few results in this range were reported in the early HD series, none has been encountered subsequently or confirmed by newer techniques. Thus the problem lies with the very small number of results lying in the 34–38 repeat range, although many diagnostic laboratories have the policy of repeating all in the range 31–39, to allow for any PCR error or difficulty in reading through stutter bands. Rubinzstein *et al.* (1996) have produced a combined analysis of samples and data from different centres falling in this borderline range. Of 178 individuals with a repeat number of 30–40, 7 affected individuals had 36 repeats, while 6 healthy elderly individuals were found with 36–39 repeats. The implications of this study in relation to the general topic of intermediate alleles are further discussed in Chapter 7.

When such an intermediate result is found in a clinically abnormal individual, there are several approaches to resolving uncertainty. First, the test should be repeated, using a second sample if necessary. Second, if a family history of HD exists, then samples from parents should be taken where possible, to determine whether the borderline result has been transmitted from the HD or unaffected side of the family. In a number of cases it has turned out that the smaller allele has come from the affected parent, allowing a confident prediction of normality, whereas if a borderline result is also present in the affected parent and is the allele that has been transmitted, it is more likely to be associated with the disease. If the result is confirmed as being in the equivocal range, its interpretation will depend on the diagnostic context. Thus it will be unlikely to be relevant if the clinical situation is suspected juvenile HD, but more likely to be so if the picture is of mild disease in later life. The particular problems posed by the finding of intermediate alleles in the relatives of an isolated case of HD are discussed in more detail in Chapter 7.

Turning to the clinical aspects of diagnostic testing, the initial research studies involved isolated cases considered with varying degrees of certainty to be HD. MacMillan *et al.* (1993a) reported 98 cases of suspected HD with no validated family history: 93 of these showed the HD mutation, with a repeat number distribution identical to that of familial cases. Of the five not showing the mutation, two were clinically atypical. This high frequency of the HD mutation in part reflects the fact that these patients had formed part of a population survey of HD and that most with uncertain diagnosis had already been excluded. Davis *et al.* (1994), based in a specialist neurological centre, analysed 44 sporadic cases and found the mutation in 25 of 28 with clinically typical features, but in only 5 of 16 where the diagnosis was classically doubtful.

Both these studies were retrospective, but a subsequent series of consecutive patients with samples referred by neurologists as suspected HD showed 53 per cent to have the mutation (MacMillan *et al.* 1995).

It is thus clear that molecular analysis is of considerable value in confirming whether an apparently sporadic case of what appears to be typical HD is actually this disorder, as well as providing confirmation in cases where either the whole family or one particular individual is atypical. The occurrence of possible HD at the extremes of life has been particularly difficult and mutational analysis will certainly help in the diagnosis of possible juvenile HD and in distinguishing HD of late onset from other causes of senile chorea. The family originally diagnosed as benign hereditary chorea (MacMillan *et al.* 1993b) shows how this usually distinct condition can also be confused. The recent studies from Netherlands (Siesling *et al.* 2000) and Vancouver (Almqvist *et al.* 2001) have shown how elderly cases without a clear family history are considerably more frequent than previously recognized.

As diagnostic testing for HD becomes more widespread and routine, there are dangers that it could be used inappropriately. The first consideration applies when testing is undertaken in an isolated case where neither patient nor family members are aware of the possibility of the condition being genetic. It is essential that those undertaking the test make it clear in advance that the result might have genetic implications to the family as a whole, as well as clinical implications. It is especially important to clarify this in advance when the patient is unable to give consent, whether on account of dementia or psychiatric illness. A second consideration, even more important, applies in a situation where a family history of HD exists, but the symptoms are not typical. This is not diagnostic testing but presymptomatic prediction, and in such a situation careful consideration should be given to whether the individual should be handled through a protocol appropriate for presymptomatic testing (see Chapter 7) or indeed whether testing is appropriate at all. If the mutation is indeed detected in such a person (usually at 50 per cent risk), there is no guarantee that its presence is necessarily related to the symptoms that the patient has, and an unwanted and potentially harmful predictive test result may have been generated inadvertently. The dangers of this have already been pointed out in relation to juvenile HD, and we have encountered the problem in relation to psychiatric indications for molecular testing, a topic discussed more fully in Chapter 3.

Disorders mimicking HD

There are a number of diseases that can be clinically misdiagnosed as HD. A more detailed discussion of the symptoms that may lead to confusion and the characteristics that can be used to achieve a differential diagnosis is given in Chapter 2. The most common confusion is probably with the related polyglutamine disease DRPLA, as mentioned above. Late-onset HD seems to have been confused with parkinsonism or Alzheimer's disease in some cases with no family history in British Columbia (Almqvist *et al.* 2001). In the analyses of the HD repeat after the gene was cloned every study observed a low rate of clinical cases of HD with no expansions. Some of these cases were probably sample mix-ups as mentioned above, but some were noted to be clinically atypical. So it seems that there is a group of rare cases, which may or may not show atypical symptoms, that are not due to an expansion in the HD gene (Vuillaume *et al.* 2000).

Some of these disorders are rare autosomal dominant diseases that look like HD and some of these have now had genes associated with them. An HD-like disease in a single pedigree was mapped to chromosome 20p12, the site of the prion protein PrP gene, and found to segregate with a 192 nucleotide insertion in the PrP gene, encoding eight octapeptide repeats. This disease was called HD-like 1 (HDL1). In this context it is of interest that a case of variant Creutzfeldt–Jacob disease (vCJD) has been found to carry an HD intermediate allele, which raises the possibility that having an HD repeat in the intermediate range might influence the risk of developing vCJD (Harper *et al.* 2001) though this will need confirming. Margolis *et al.* (2001) reported an HD-like disease (HDL2) with very similar symptoms and pathology to HD, almost certainly associated with an expanded polyglutamine tract, as an antibody that detects only expanded polyglutamine-containing inclusions found such inclusions in post-mortem brain from a member of this family. The gene involved is junctophilin-3 (Holmes *et al.* 2001). Finally, a late-onset basal ganglia disease first detected in families in the north of England was associated with an insertion in the ferritin light-chain gene (Curtis *et al.* 2001). The symptoms are variable but include a movement disorder, although unlike in HD cognitive function is generally preserved. The same mutation was detected in five apparently unrelated people with the disease. Histochemistry detected abnormal aggregates of ferritin and iron in the brain and the authors have called the disease neuroferritinopathy.

Thus a number of rare genetic diseases have been confused with HD but, as discussed above, most clinically diagnosed HD turns out to be due to the CAG expansion in the HD gene. There remains a subset of such familial diseases that have as yet no gene associated with them (Vuillaume *et al.* 2000) but, given appropriate family structures, the increased power of genome mapping studies may locate these genes, though it remains possible that some will prove to be nongenetic, that is, true 'phenocopies'. It may also be that finding the causes of these very rare diseases might shed light on the pathogenetic mechanisms of HD.

Conclusions

The genetics of HD has moved a long way in a very short time. From the recognition of the cardinal features of the disease by Huntington in 1872 to finding a linkage in the genome in 1983 took over a century. From there it took a decade to find the gene, and many of the genetic characteristics, such as the correlation with age of onset of disease, were then clarified very quickly. Now we are at the stage where genetics has provided the tool—the gene and its mutation—for us to study the pathological mechanisms of disease in many different model systems. We can also use genetics to help us refine our ideas about the pathogenetic mechanisms of HD. Genetic research in HD has been hugely illuminating, as the later chapters in this book will reveal.

References

ACMG/ASHG (1998). ACMG/ASHG statement. Laboratory guidelines for Huntington disease genetic testing. The American College of Medical Genetics/American Society of Human Genetics Huntington Disease Genetic Testing Working Group. *Am. J. Hum. Genet.* **62** (5), 1243–1247.

Abbott, M.H., Folstein, S.E., and Abbey, H. (1987). Psychiatric manifestations of homocystinuria due to cystathionine beta-synthase deficiency: prevalence, natural history, and relationship to neurologic impairment and vitamin B6-responsiveness. *Am. J. Med. Genet.* **26**, 959–969.

Abeliovich, D., Lerer, I., Pashut-Lavon, I., Shmueli, E., Raas-Rothschild, A., and Frydman, M. (1993). Negative expansion of the myotonic dystrophy unstable sequence. *Am. J. Hum. Genet.* **52**, 1175–1181.

Albin, R.L. and Tagle, D.A. (1995). Genetics and molecular biology of Huntington's disease [see comments]. *Trends Neurosci.* **18**, 11–14.

Almqvist, E., Elterman, D., MacLeod, P., and Hayden, M. (2001). High incidence rate and absent family histories in one quarter of patients newly diagnosed with Huntington disease in British Columbia. *Clin. Genet.* **60**, 198–205.

Andrew, S.E., Goldberg, Y.P., Kremer, B., Telenius, H., Theilmann, J., Adam, S., Starr, E., Squitieri, F., Lin, B., and Kalchman, M.A. (1993a). The relationship between trinucleotide (CAG). repeat length and clinical features of Huntington's disease [see comments]. *Nat. Genet.* **4**, 398–403.

Andrew, S., Theilmann, J., Almqvist, E., Norremolle, A., Lucotte, G., Anvret, M., Sorensen, S.A., Turpin, J.C., and Hayden, M.R. (1993b). DNA analysis of distinct populations suggests multiple origins for the mutation causing Huntington disease. *Clin. Genet.* **43**, 286–294.

—— Goldberg, Y.P., Theilmann, J., Zeisler, J., and Hayden, M.R. (1994a). A CCG repeat polymorphism adjacent to the CAG repeat in the Huntington disease gene: implications for diagnostic accuracy and predictive testing. *Hum. Mol. Genet.* **3**, 65–67.

Andrew, S.E., Goldberg, Y.P., Kremer, B., Squitieri, F., Theilmann, J., Zeisler, J., Telenius, H., Adam, S., Almquist, E., and Anvret, M. (1994b). Huntington disease without CAG expansion: phenocopies or errors in assignment? *Am. J. Hum. Genet.* **54**, 852–863.

Ansved, T., Lundin, A., and Anvret, M. (1998). Larger CAG expansions in skeletal muscle compared with lymphocytes in Kennedy disease but not in Huntington disease. *Neurology* **51**, 1442–1444.

Antonini, A., Leenders, K.L., and Eidelberg, D. (1998). [11C]raclopride-PET studies of the Huntington's disease rate of progression: relevance of the trinucleotide repeat length. *Ann. Neurol.* **43**, 253–255.

Aronin, N., Chase, K., Young, C., Sapp, E., Schwarz, C., Matta, N., Kornreich, R., Landwehrmeyer, B., Bird, E., and Beal, M.F. (1995). CAG expansion affects the expression of mutant Huntingtin in the Huntington's disease brain. *Neuron* **15**, 1193–1201.

Ashizawa, T., Dubel, J.R., and Harati, Y. (1993). Somatic instability of CTG repeat in myotonic dystrophy. *Neurology* **43**, 2674–2678.

Ashizawa, T., Wong, L.J., Richards, C.S., Caskey, C.T., and Jankovic, J. (1994). CAG repeat size and clinical presentation in Huntington's disease. *Neurology* **44**, 1137–1143.

Bachman, D., Butler, I., and McKhann, G. (1977). The long term treatment of juvenile Huntington's chorea with dipropylacetic acid. *Neurology* **27**, 193–197.

Barbeau, A. (1970). Parental ascent in the juvenile form of Huntington's chorea. *Lancet* **2**, 937.

Barron, L.H., Rae, A., Holloway, S., Brock, D.J., and Warner, J.P. (1994). A single allele from the polymorphic CCG rich sequence immediately 3' to the unstable CAG trinucleotide in the IT15 cDNA shows almost complete disequilibrium with Huntington's disease chromosomes in the Scottish population. *Hum. Mol. Genet.* **3**, 173–175.

Becher, M.W., Kotzuk, J.A., Sharp, A.H., Davies, S.W., Bates, G.P., Price, D.L., and Ross, C.A. (1998). Intranuclear neuronal inclusions in Huntington's disease and dentatorubral and pallidoluysian atrophy: correlation between the density of inclusions and IT15 CAG triplet repeat length. *Neurobiol. Dis.* **4**, 387–397.

Bell, J. (1934). In *Treasury of human inheritance* (ed. R.A. Fisher), pp. 1–67. Cambridge University Press: Cambridge.

Bird, E.D., Caro, A.J., and Pilling, J.B. (1974). A sex related factor in the inheritance of Huntington's chorea. *Ann. Hum. Genet.* **37**, 255–260.

Bird, T.D. and Ommen, G.S. (1975). Monozygotic twins with Huntington's chorea in a family expressing the rigid variant. *Neurology* **25**, 1126–1129.

Boehnke, M., Conneally, P.M., and Lange, K. (1983). Two models for a maternal factor in the inheritance of Huntington disease. *Am. J. Hum. Genet.* **35**, 845–860.

Brackenridge, C.J., Case, J., Chin, E., Prospect, D.N., Teltscher, B., and Wallace D.C. (1978). A linkage study of the loci for Huntington's disease and some common polymorphic markers. *Ann. Hum. Genet.* **48**, 203–211.

Brandt, J., Bylsma, F.W., Gross, R., Stine, O.C., Ranen, N., and Ross, C.A. (1996). Trinucleotide repeat length and clinical progression in Huntington's disease. *Neurology* **46**, 527–531.

Brinkman, R.R., Mezei, M.M., Theilmann, J., Almqvist, E., and Hayden, M.R. (1997). The likelihood of being affected with Huntington disease by a particular age, for a specific CAG size. *Am. J. Hum. Genet.* **60**, 1202–1210.

Brook, J.D., McCurrach, M.E., Harley, H.G., Buckler, A.J., Church, D., Aburatani, H., Hunter, K., Stanton, V.P., Thirion, J.P., and Hudson, T. (1992). Molecular basis of myotonic dystrophy: expansion of a trinucleotide (CTG). repeat at the 3' end of a transcript encoding a protein kinase family member. *Cell* **68**, 799–808.

Bruland, O., Almqvist, E.W., Goldberg, Y.P., Boman, H., Hayden, M.R., and Knappskog, P.M. (1999). Accurate determination of the number of CAG repeats in the Huntington disease gene using a sequence-specific internal DNA standard. *Clin. Genet.* **55**, 198–202.

Brunner, H.G., Jansen, G., Nillesen, W., Nelen, M.R., de Die, C.E., Howeler, C.J., van Oost, B.A., Wieringa, B., Ropers, H.H., and Smeets, H.J. (1993). Brief report: reverse mutation in myotonic dystrophy. *New Engl. J. Med.* **328**, 476–480.

Bruyn, G.W. (1968). Huntington's chorea: historical, clinical and laboratory synopsis. In *Handbook of neurology* (ed. P.J. Vinken and G.W. Bruyn), pp. 298–378. North Holland, Amsterdam.

Butterworth, N.J., Williams, L., Bullock, J.Y., Love, D.R., Faull, R.L., and Dragunow, M. (1998). Trinucleotide (CAG). repeat length is positively correlated with the degree of DNA fragmentation in Huntington's disease striatum. *Neuroscience* **87**, 49–53.

Chong, S.S., Almqvist, E., Telenius, H., LaTray, L., Nichol, K., Bourdelat-Parks, B., Goldberg, Y.P., Haddad, B.R., Richards, F., Sillence, D., Greenberg, C.R., Ives, E., Van den Engh, G., Hughes, M.R., and Hayden, M.R. (1997). Contribution of DNA sequence and CAG size to mutation frequencies of intermediate alleles for Huntington disease: evidence from single sperm analyses. *Hum. Mol. Genet.* **6**, 301–309.

Claes, S., Van Zand, K., Legius, E., Dom, R., Malfroid, M., Baro, F., Godderis, J., and Cassiman, J.J. (1995). Correlations between triplet repeat expansion and clinical features in Huntington's disease [see comments]. *Arch. Neurol.* **52**, 749–753.

Clarke, D.J. and Bundey, S. (1990). Very early onset Huntington's disease: genetic mechanism and risk to siblings. *Clin. Genet.* **38**, 180–186.

Clarke, G., Collins, R.A., Leavitt, B.R., Andrews, D.F., Hayden, M.R., Lumsden, C.J., and McInnes, R.R. (2000). A one-hit model of cell death in inherited neuronal degenerations. *Nature* **406**, 195–199.

Conneally, P.M. (1984). Huntington disease: genetics and epidemiology. *Am. J. Hum. Genet.* **36**, 506–526.

Craufurd, D. and Dodge, A. (1993). Mutation size and age at onset in Huntington's disease. *J. Med. Genet.* **30**, 1008–1011.

Cross, G., Pitt, T., Sharif, A., Bates, G., and Lehrach, H. (1994). False-negative result for Huntington's disease mutation. *Lancet* **343**, 1232.

Culjkovic, B., Stojkovic, O., Vojvodic, N., Svetel, M., Rakic, L., Romac, S., and Kostic, V. (1999). Correlation between triplet repeat expansion and computed tomography measures of caudate nuclei atrophy in Huntington's disease. *J Neurol.* **246**, 1090–1093.

Curtis, A.R., Fey, C., Morris, C.M., Bindoff, L.A., Ince, P.G., Chinnery, P.F., Coulthard, A., Jackson, M.J., Jackson, A.P., McHale, D.P., Hay, D., Barker, W.A., Markham, A.F., Bates, D., Curtis, A., and Burn, J. (2001). Mutation in the gene encoding ferritin light polypeptide causes dominant adult-onset basal ganglia disease. *Nat. Genet.* **28**, 350–354.

Davenport, C.B. (1911). *Heredity in relation to eugenics.* Holt, reissued Arno Press (1972), New York.

Davenport, C.B. and Muncey, M.D. (1916). Huntington's chorea in relation to heredity and insanity. *Am. J. Insanity* **73**, 195–220.

Davis, M.B., Bateman, D., Quinn, N.P., Marsden, C.D., and Harding, A.E. (1994). Mutation analysis in patients with possible but apparently sporadic Huntington's disease. *Lancet* **344**, 714–717.

De Rooij, K.E., De Koning Gans, P.A., Roos, R.A., Van Ommen, G.J., and den Dunnen, J.T. (1995). Somatic expansion of the (CAG)n repeat in Huntington disease brains. *Hum. Genet.* **95**, 270–274.

Durr, A., Hahn-Barma, V., Brice, A., Pecheux, C., Dode, C., and Feingold, J. (1999). Homozygosity in Huntington's disease. *J. Med. Genet.* **36**, 172–173.

Duyao, M., Ambrose, C., Myers, R., Novelletto, A., Persichetti, F., Frontali, M., Folstein, S., Ross, C., Franz, M., and Abbott, M. (1993). Trinucleotide repeat length instability and age of onset in Huntington's disease [see comments]. *Nat. Genet.* **4**, 387–392.

Eldridge, R., O'Meara, K., Chase, T., and Donnelly, E.F. (1973). Offspring of consanguineous parents with Huntington's chorea. In *Huntington's chorea* (ed. A. Barbeau, T.N. Chase, and G.W. Paulson), pp. 1872–1972. Raven Press, New York.

Entres, J.L. (1921). *Zur Klinik und Vererbung der Huntingtonschen Chorea*, Monographien aus des Gesamtgebiete der Neurologie und Psychiatrie, no. 27. Springer, Berlin.

Falush, D., Almqvist, E.W., Brinkmann, R.R., Iwasa, Y., and Hayden, M.R. (2000). Measurement of mutational flow implies both a high new-mutation rate for Huntington disease and substantial under-ascertainment of late-onset cases. *Am. J. Hum. Genet.* **68**, 373–385.

Farrer, L.A. and Conneally, P.M. (1985). A genetic model for age at onset in Huntington disease. *Am. J. Hum. Genet.* **37**, 350–357.

—— —— Yu, P.L. (1984). The natural history of Huntington disease: possible role of "aging genes". *Am. J. Med. Genet.* **18**, 115–123.

Fleischer, B. (1918). Uber myotonische Dystrophie mit Rataract. *Von Graefes Arch. Klin. Exp. Opthalmol.* **96**, 91–133.

Folstein, S.E., Chase, G.A., Wahl, W.E., McDonnell, A.M., and Folstein, M.F. (1987). Huntington's disease in Maryland: clinical aspects of racial variation. *Am. J. Hum. Genet.* **41**, 168–179.

Foroud, T., Siemers, E., Kleindorfer, D., Bill, D.J., Hodes, M.E., Norton, J.A., Conneally, P.M., and Christian, J.C. (1995). Cognitive scores in carriers of Huntington's disease gene compared to noncarriers. *Ann. Neurol.* **37**, 657–664.

Fu, Y.H., Pizzuti, A., Fenwick, R.G., Jr., King, J., Rajnarayan, S., Dunne, P.W., Dubel, J., Nasser, G.A., Ashizawa, T., and de Jong, P. (1992). An unstable triplet repeat in a gene related to myotonic muscular dystrophy. *Science* **255**, 1256–1258.

Furtado, S., Suchowersky, O., Rewcastle, B., Graham, L., Klimek, M.L., and Garber, A. (1996). Relationship between trinucleotide repeats and neuropathological changes in Huntington's disease. *Ann. Neurol.* **39**, 132–136.

Gellera, C., Meoni, C., Castellotti, B., Zappacosta, B., Girotti, F., Taroni, F., and DiDonato, S. (1996). Errors in Huntington disease diagnostic test caused by trinucleotide deletion in the IT15 gene. *Am. J. Hum. Genet.* **59**, 475–477.

Georgiou, N., Bradshaw, J.L., Chiu, E., Tudor, A., O'Gorman, L., and Phillips, J.G. (1999). Differential clinical and motor control function in a pair of monozygotic twins with Huntington's disease. *Mov. Dis.* **14**, 320–325.

Goldberg, Y.P., Kremer, B., Andrew, S.E., Theilmann, J., Graham, R.K., Squitieri, F., Telenius, H., Adam, S., Sajoo, A., and Starr, E. (1993). Molecular analysis of new mutations for Huntington's disease: intermediate alleles and sex of origin effects [see comments]. *Nat. Genet.* **5**, 174–179.

—— Telenius, H., and Hayden, M.R. (1994). The molecular genetics of Huntington's disease. *Curr. Opin. Neurol.* **7**, 325–332.

—— McMurray, C.T., Zeisler, J., Almqvist, E., Sillence, D., Richards, F., Gacy, A.M., Buchanan, J., Telenius, H., and Hayden, M.R. (1995). Increased instability of intermediate alleles in families with sporadic Huntington disease compared to similar sized intermediate alleles in the general population. *Hum. Mol. Genet.* **4**, 1911–1918.

Gusella, J.F. and MacDonald, M.E. (1994). Huntington's disease and repeating trinucleotides. *New Engl. J. Med.* **330**, 1450–1451.

—— Wexler, N.S., Conneally, P.M., Naylor, S.L., Anderson, M.A., Tanzi, R.E., Watkins, P.C., Ottina, K., Wallace, M.R., and Sakaguchi, A.Y. (1983). A polymorphic DNA marker genetically linked to Huntington's disease. *Nature* **306**, 234–238.

—— MacDonald, M.E., Ambrose, C.M., and Duyao, M.P. (1993). Molecular genetics of Huntington's disease. *Arch. Neurol.* **50**, 1157–1163.

Haldane J.B.S. (1941). The relative importance of principal and modifying genes in determining some human diseases. *J. Genet.* **41**, 149–157.

Hardy, J. (1997). Amyloid, the presenilins and Alzheimer's disease [see comments]. *Trends. Neurosci.* **20**, 154–159.

Harley, H.G., Brook, J.D., Rundle, S.A., Crow, S., Reardon, W., Buckler, A.J., Harper, P.S., Housman, D.E., and Shaw, D.J. (1992). Expansion of an unstable DNA region and phenotypic variation in myotonic dystrophy. *Nature* **355**, 545–546.

—— Rundle, S.A., MacMillan, J.C., Myring, J., Brook, J.D., Crow, S., Reardon, W., Fenton, I., Shaw, D.J., and Harper, P.S. (1993). Size of the unstable CTG repeat sequence in relation to phenotype and parental transmission in myotonic dystrophy. *Am. J. Hum. Genet.* **52**, 1164–1174.

Harper, P.S. (1993a). Clinical consequences of isolating the gene for Huntington's disease [editorial]. *Br. Med. J.* **307**, 397–398.

—— (1993b). The gene for Huntington's disease—a personal view. *MRC News* **6**, 38–40.

—— (ed.) (1996a). *Huntington's disease*, 2nd edn. W.B. Saunders, London.

Harper, P.S. (1996b). New genes for old diseases: the molecular basis of myotonic dystrophy and Huntington's disease. The Lumleian Lecture 1995. *J. R. Coll. Physicians, Lond.* **30**, 221–231.

—— (2001). *Myotonic dystrophy*. W.B. Saunders, London.

Harper, P.S., Harley, H.G., Reardon, W., and Shaw, D.J. (1992). Anticipation in myotonic dystrophy: new light on an old problem. *Am. J. Hum. Genet.* **51**, 10–16.

—— Evans, R., Elliston, L., Ironside, J.W., Jones, A.L., and Lazarou, L.P. (2001). Huntington's disease intermediate allele and new variant CJD [abstract]. *Am. J. Hum. Genet.* **69** (4), 547.

Hayden, M.R. (1979). Huntington's chorea in South Africa. Thesis, University of Cape Town.

Hellenbroich, Y., Schwinger, E., and Zuhlke, C. (2001). Limited somatic mosaicism for Friedreich's ataxia GAA triplet repeat expansions identified by small pool PCR in blood leukocytes. *Acta Neurol. Scand.* **103**, 188–192.

Hindringer, P. (1935). Eine neue Chorea-Huntington-sippe. Thesis [Quoted by Eldridge *et al.* 1973].

Hodge, S.E., Spence, M.A., Crandall, B.F., Sparkes, R.S., Sparkes, M.C., Crist, M., and Tideman, S. (1980). Huntington disease: linkage analysis with age-of-onset corrections. *Am. J. Med. Genet.* **5**, 247–254.

Holmes, S.E., O'Hearn, E., Rosenblatt, A., Callahan, C., Hwang, H.S., Ingersoll-Ashworth, R.G., Fleisher, A., Stevanin, G., Brice, A., Potter, N.T., Ross, C.A., and Margolis, R.L. (2001). A repeat expansion in the gene encoding junctophilin-3 is associated with Huntington disease-like 2. *Nat. Genet.* **29**, 377–378.

Höweler, C.J., Busch, H.F., Geraedts, J.P., Niermeijer, M.F., and Staal, A. (1989). Anticipation in myotonic dystrophy: fact or fiction? *Brain* **112**, 779–797.

Huntington's Disease Collaborative Research Group (1993). A novel gene containing a trinucleotide repeat that is expanded and unstable on Huntington's disease chromosomes. The Huntington's Disease Collaborative Research Group [see comments]. *Cell* **72**, 971–983.

Huntington, G. (1872). On chorea. *Med. Surg. Rep.* **26**, 320–321.

Husquinet, H., Franck, G., and Vranckx, C. (1973). Detection of future cases of Huntington's chorea by the L-dopa load test: experiment with two monozygotic twins. In *Huntington's chorea* (ed. A. Barbeau, T.N. Chase, and G.W. Paulson), pp. 301–310. Raven Press, New York.

Illarioshkin, S.N., Igarashi, S., Onodera, O., Markova, E.D., Nikolskaya, N.N., Tanaka, H., Chabrashwili, T.Z., Insarova, N.G., Endo, K., and Ivanova-Smolenskaya, I.A. (1994). Trinucleotide repeat length and rate of progression of Huntington's disease. *Ann. Neurol.* **36**, 630–635.

Jakupciak, J.P. and Wells, R.S. (2000). Gene conversion (recombination) mediates expansions of CTGCAG repeats. *J. Biol. Chem.* **275** (51), 40003–40013.

James, C.M., Houlihan, G.D., Snell, R.G., Cheadle, J.P., and Harper, P.S. (1994). Late-onset Huntington's disease: a clinical and molecular study. *Age Ageing* **23**, 445–448.

Jason, G.W., Suchowersky, O., Pajurkova, E.M., Graham, L., Klimek, M.L., Garber, A.T., and Poirier-Heine, D. (1997). Cognitive manifestations of Huntington disease in relation to genetic structure and clinical onset. *Arch. Neurol.* **54**, 1081–1088.

Jelliffe, S.E. (1908). A contribution to the history of Huntington's disease; a preliminary report. *Neurographs* **1**, 114–124.

Jenkins, B.G., Rosas, H.D., Chen, Y.C., Makabe, T., Myers, R., MacDonald, M., Rosen, B.R., Beal, M.F., and Koroshetz, W.J. (1998). ^{1}H NMR spectroscopy studies of Huntington's disease: correlations with CAG repeat numbers. *Neurology* **50**, 1357–1365.

Kang, S., Jaworski, A., Ohshima, K., and Wells, R.D. (1995). Expansion and deletion of CTG repeats from human disease genes are determined by the direction of replication in *E. coli. Nat. Genet.* **10**, 213–218.

Kehoe, P., Krawczak, M., Harper, P.S., Owen, M.J., and Jones, A.L. (1999). Age of onset in Huntington disease: sex specific influence of apolipoprotein E genotype and normal CAG repeat length. *J. Med. Genet.* **36**, 108–111.

Kennedy, L. and Shelbourne, P.F. (2000). Dramatic mutation instability in HD mouse striatum: does polyglutamine load contribute to cell-specific vulnerability in Huntington's disease? *Hum. Mol. Genet.* **9**, 2539–2544.

Kieburtz, K., MacDonald, M., Shih, C., Feigin, A., Steinberg, K., Bordwell, K., Zimmerman, C., Srinidhi, J., Sotack, J., and Gusella, J. (1994). Trinucleotide repeat length and progression of illness in Huntington's disease. *J. Med. Genet.* **31**, 872–874.

Kovtun, I.V. and McMurray, C.T. (2001). Trinucleotide expansion in haploid germ cells by gap repair. *Nat. Genet.* **27**, 407–411.

Kremer, B., Squitieri, F., Telenius, H., Andrew, S.E., Theilmann, J., Spence, N., Goldberg, Y.P., and Hayden, M.R. (1993). Molecular analysis of late onset Huntington's disease. *J. Med. Genet.* **30**, 991–995.

—— Goldberg, P., Andrew, S.E., Theilmann, J., Telenius, H., Zeisler, J., Squitieri, F., Lin, B., Bassett, A., and Almqvist, E. (1994). A worldwide study of the Huntington's disease mutation. The sensitivity and specificity of measuring CAG repeats [see comments]. *New Engl. J. Med.* **330**, 1401–1406.

Kremer, B., Almqvist, E., Theilmann, J., Spence, N., Telenius, H., Goldberg, Y.P., and Hayden, M.R. (1995). Sex-dependent mechanisms for expansions and contractions of the CAG repeat on affected Huntington disease chromosomes. *Am. J. Hum. Genet.* **57**, 343–350.

Laccone, F. and Christian, W. (2000). A recurrent expansion of a maternal allele with 36 CAG repeats causes Huntington disease in two sisters. *Am. J Hum. Genet.* **66**, 1145–1148.

La Spada, A.R., Wilson, E.M., Lubahn, D.B., Harding, A.E., and Fischbeck, K.H. (1991). Androgen receptor gene mutations in X-linked spinal and bulbar muscular atrophy. *Nature* **352**, 77–79.

Lavedan, C., Hofmann-Radvanyi, H., Shelbourne, P., Rabes, J.P., Duros, C., Savoy, D., Dehaupas, I., Luce, S., Johnson, K., and Junien, C. (1993). Myotonic dystrophy: size- and sex-dependent dynamics of CTG meiotic instability, and somatic mosaicism. *Am. J. Hum. Genet.* **52**, 875–883.

Leeflang, E.P., Zhang, L., Tavare, S., Hubert, R., Srinidhi, J., MacDonald, M.E., Myers, R.H., de Young, M., Wexler, N.S., and Gusella, J.F. (1995). Single sperm analysis of the trinucleotide repeats in the Huntington's disease gene: quantification of the mutation frequency spectrum. *Hum. Mol. Genet.* **4**, 1519–1526.

—— Tavare, S., Marjoram, P., Neal, C.O., Srinidhi, J., MacFarlane, H., MacDonald, M.E., Gusella, J.F., de Young, M., Wexler, N.S., and Arnheim, N. (1999). Analysis of germline mutation spectra at the Huntington's disease locus supports a mitotic mutation mechanism. *Hum. Mol. Genet.* **8**, 173–183.

Lin, C.H., Tallaksen-Greene, S., Chien, W.M., Cearky, J.A., Jackson, W.S., Crouse, A.B., Ren, S., Li, X.J., Albin, R.L., and Detloff, P.J. (2001). Neurological abnormalities in a knock-in mouse model of Huntingtons disease. *Hum. Mol. Genet.* **10** (2), 137–144.

Lindstrom, J.A., Bias, W.B., Schimke, R.N., *et al.* (1973). Genetic linkage in Huntington's chorea. *Advan. Neurol.* **1**, 203–208.

Lose Koot, M., Bakker, B., Laccone, F., Stenhouse, S., and Elles, R. (1999). A European pilot quality assessment scheme for molecular diagnosis of Huntingtons disease. *Eur. J. Hum. Genet.* **7** (2), 217–222.

Lopez de Munain, A., Cobo, A.M., Poza, J.J., Navarrete, D., Martorell, L., Palau, F., Emparanza, J.I., and Baiget, M. (1995). Influence of the sex of the transmitting grandparent in congenital myotonic dystrophy. *J. Med. Genet.* **32**, 689–691.

Lovestone, S., Hodgson, S., Sham, P., Differ, A.M., and Levy, R. (1996). Familial psychiatric presentation of Huntington's disease. *J. Med. Genet.* **33**, 128–131.

MacDonald, M.E., Barnes, G., Srinidhi, J., Duyao, M.P., Ambrose, C.M., Myers, R.H., Gray, J., Conneally, P.M., Young, A., and Penney, J. (1993). Gametic but not somatic instability of CAG repeat length in Huntington's disease. *J. Med. Genet.* **30**, 982–986.

—— Vonsattel, J.P., Shrinidhi, J., Couropmitree, N.N., Cupples, L.A., Bird, E.D., Gusella, J.F., and Myers, R.H. (1999). Evidence for the GluR6 gene associated with younger onset age of Huntington's disease. *Neurology* **53**, 1330–1332.

MacMillan, J.C., Snell, R.G., Tyler, A., Houlihan, G.D., Fenton, I., Cheadle, J.P., Lazarou, L.P., Shaw, D.J., and Harper, P.S. (1993a). Molecular analysis and clinical correlations of the Huntington's disease mutation [see comments]. *Lancet* **342**, 954–958.

—— Morrison, P.J., Nevin, N.C., Shaw, D.J., Harper, P.S., Quarrell, O.W., and Snell, R.G. (1993b). Identification of an expanded CAG repeat in the Huntington's disease gene (IT15) in a family reported to have benign hereditary chorea. *J. Med. Genet.* **30**, 1012–1013.

MacMillan, J.C., Davies, P., and Harper, P.S. (1995). Molecular diagnostic analysis for Huntington's disease: a prospective evaluation. *J. Neurol. Neurosurg. Psychiatry* **58**, 496–498.

Mahadevan, M., Tsilfidis, C., Sabourin, L., Shutler, G., Amemiya, C., Jansen, G., Neville, C., Narang, M., Barcelo, J., and O'Hoy, K. (1992). Myotonic dystrophy mutation: an unstable CTG repeat in the 3′ untranslated region of the gene. *Science* **255**, 1253–1255.

Mandich, P., Di Maria, E., Bellone, E., Ajmar, F., and Abbruzzese, G. (1996). Molecular analysis of the IT15 gene in patients with apparently 'sporadic' Huntington's disease. *Eur. Neurol.* **36**, 348–352.

Mangiarini, L., Sathasivam, K., Mahal, A., Mott, R., Seller, M., and Bates, G.P. (1997). Instability of highly expanded CAG repeats in mice transgenic for the Huntington's disease mutation [see comments]. *Nat. Genet.* **15**, 197–200.

Manley, K., Shirley, T.L., Flaherty, L., and Messer, A. (1999). Msh2 deficiency prevents *in vivo* somatic instability of the CAG repeat in Huntington disease transgenic mice. *Nat. Genet.* **23**, 471–473.

Margolis, R.L., O'Hearn, E., Rosenblatt, A., Willour, V., Holmes, S.E., Franz, M.L., Callahan, C., Hwang, H.S., Troncoso, J.C., and Ross, C.A. (2001). A disorder similar to Huntington's disease is associated with a novel CAG repeat expansion. *Ann. Neurol.* **50**, 373–380.

Martorell, L., Monckton, D.G., Gamez, J., and Baiget, M. (2000). Complex patterns of male germline instability and somatic mosaicism in myotonic dystrophy type 1. *Eur. J. Hum. Genet.* **8**, 423–430.

Maurer, D.J., O'Callaghan, B.L., and Livingston, D.M. (1996). Orientation dependence of trinucleotide CAG repeat instability in *Saccharomyces cerevisiae*. *Mol. Cell Biol.* **16**, 6617–6622.

McNeil, S.M., Novelletto, A., Srinidhi, J., Barnes, G., Kornbluth, I., Altherr, M.R., Wasmuth, J.J., Gusella, J.F., MacDonald, M.E., and Myers, R.H. (1997). Reduced penetrance of the Huntington's disease mutation. *Hum. Mol. Genet.* **6**, 775–779.

Merrit, A.D., Conneally, P.M., Rahman, N.F., and Drew, A.L. (1969). Juvenile Huntington's chorea. In *Progress in neurogenetics* (ed. A. Barbeau and J.R. Brunnette), pp. 645–650. Excerpta Medica Foundation, Amsterdam.

Moore, H., Greenwell, P.W., Liu, C.P., Arnheim, N., and Petes, T.D. (1999). Triplet repeats form secondary structures that escape DNA repair in yeast. *Proc. Natl. Acad. Sci., USA* **96**, 1504–1509.

Myers, R.H., Goldman, D., Bird, E.D., Sax, D.S., Merril, C.R., Schoenfeld, M., and Wolf, P.A. (1983). Maternal transmission in Huntington's disease. *Lancet* **1**, 208–210.

—— Leavitt, J., Farrer, L.A., Jagadeesh, J., McFarlane, H., Mastromauro, C.A., Mark, R.J., and Gusella, J.F. (1989). Homozygote for Huntington disease. *Am. J. Hum. Genet.* **45**, 615–618.

—— MacDonald, M.E., Koroshetz, W.J., Duyao, M.P., Ambrose, C.M., Taylor, S.A., Barnes, G., Srinidhi, J., Lin, C.S., and Whaley, W.L. (1993). *De novo* expansion of a (CAG)n repeat in sporadic Huntington's disease [see comments]. *Nat. Genet.* **5**, 168–173.

Myrianthopoulos, N.C. (1966). Huntington's chorea. *J. Med. Genet.* **3**, 298–314.

—— and Rowley, P.T. (1960). Monozygotic twins concordant for Huntington's disease. *Neurology* **10**, 506–511.

Nance, M.A., Mathias-Hagen, V., Breningstall, G., Wick, M.J., and McGlennen, R.C. (1999). Analysis of a very large trinucleotide repeat in a patient with juvenile Huntington's disease. *Neurology* **52**, 392–394.

Narain, Y., Wyttenbach, A., Rankin, J., Furlong, R.A., and Rubinsztein, D.C. (1999). A molecular investigation of true dominance in Huntington's disease. *J. Med. Genet.* **36**, 739–746.

Neal, J.W., Fenton, I., MacMillan, J.C., *et al.* (1994). A study comparing mutation triplet repeat size and phenotypes in patients with Huntington's disease. *Neurodegeneration* **3**, 73–77.

Newcombe, R.G., Walker, D.A., and Harper, P.S. (1981). Factors influencing age at onset and duration of survival in Huntington's chorea. *Ann. Hum. Genet.* **45**, 387–396.

Norbury, G.G., Hindley, N.J., Jobst, K.A., *et al.* (1995). Late-onset Huntington's disease as a cause of dementia: where should the clinician's index of suspicion lie? *16th International Meeting of the World Federatin of Neurology Research Group on Huntington's Disease* [abstract].

Nossemolle, A., Riess, O., Epplen, J.T., Fenger, K., Hashclt, L., and Sorensen, S.A. (1993). Trinucleotide repeat elongation in the huntingtin gene in Huntington disease patients from 71 Danish families. *Hum. Mol. Genet.* **2** (9), 1475–1476.

Oberle, I., Rousseau, F., Heitz, D., Kretz, C., Devys, D., Hanauer, A., Boue, J., Bertheas, M.F., and Mandel, J.L. (1991). Instability of a 550-base pair DNA segment and abnormal methylation in fragile X syndrome. *Science* **252**, 1097–1102.

Oepen, H. (1973). Discordant features of monozygotic twin markers with Huntington's chorea. In *Advances in neurology* (ed. A. Barbeau, T.N. Chase, and G.W. Paulson), pp. 199–201. Raven Press, New York.

Panse, F. (1942). *Die Erbchorea; eine klinische-genetische Studie*. Thieme, Leipzig.

Parker, N. (1958). Observations on Huntington's chorea based on a Queensland survey. *Med. J. Australia* **45**, 351–359.

Pearson, J.S., Peterson, M.C., Lazarte, J.A., Blodgett, H.E., and Kley, I.B. (1955). An educational approach to the social problem of Huntington's chorea. *Proc. Mayo Clin.* **30**, 349–357.

Penney, J.B. Jr, Vonsattel, J.P., MacDonald, M.E., Gusella, J.F., and Myers, R.H. (1997). CAG repeat number governs the development rate of pathology in Huntington's disease [see comments]. *Ann. Neurol.* **41**, 689–692.

Penrose, L.S. (1948). The problem of anticipation in pedigrees of dystrophia myotonica. *Ann. Eugenics* **14**, 125–132.

Pericak-Vance, M.A., Conneally, P.M., Merritt, A.D., Roos, R., Norton, J.A. Jr, and Vance, J.M. (1978). Genetic linkage studies in Huntington disease. *Cytogenet. Cell Genet.* **22**, 640–645.

Perutz, M.F. and Windle, A.H. (2001). Cause of neural death in neurodegenerative diseases attributable to expansion of glutamine repeats. *Nature* **412**, 143–144.

—— Johnson, T., Suzuki, M., and Finch, J.T. (1994). Glutamine repeats as polar zippers: their possible role in inherited neurodegenerative diseases. *Proc. Natl. Acad. Sci., USA* **91**, 5355–5358.

Punnett, R.C. (1908). Mendelian inheritance in man. *Proc. R. Soc. Med.* **1**, 135–168.

Ranen, N.G., Stine, O.C., Abbott, M.H., Sherr, M., Codori, A.M., Franz, M.L., Chao, N.I., Chung, A.S., Pleasant, N., and Callahan, C. (1995). Anticipation and instability of IT-15 (CAG)*n* repeats in parent–offspring pairs with Huntington disease. *Am. J. Hum. Genet.* **57**, 593–602.

Reed, T.E. and Neel, J.V. (1959). Huntington's chorea in Michigan. 2: Selection and mutation. *Am. J. Hum. Genet.* **11**, 107–136.

Reed, T.W., Chandler, J.H., Hughes, E.M., and Davidson, R.T. (1958). Huntington's chorea in Michigan. 1: Demography and genetics. *Am. J. Hum. Genet.* **10**, 201–225.

Ridley, R.M., Frith, C.D., Crow, T.J., and Conneally, P.M. (1988). Anticipation in Huntington's disease is inherited through the male line but may originate in the female. *J. Med. Genet.* **25**, 589–595.

—— Farrer, L.A., and Conneally, P.M. (1991). Patterns of inheritance of the symptoms of Huntington's disease suggestive of an effect of genomic imprinting. *J. Med. Genet.* **28**, 224–231.

Riess, O., Noerremoelle, A., Soerensen, S.A., *et al.* (1993). Improved PCR conditions for the stretch of (CAG)*n* repeats causing Huntington's disease. *Hum. Mol. Genet.* **2**, 637.

Rosanoff, A.J. and Handy, L.M. (1935). Huntington's chorea in twins. *Arch. Neurol. Psychiatry* **33**, 839–841.

Rosenblatt, A., Brinkman, R.R., Liang, K.Y., Almqvist, E.W., Margolis, R.L., Huang, C.Y., Sherr, M., Franz, M.L., Abbott, M.H., Hayden, M.R., and Ross, C.A. (2001). Familial influence on age of onset among siblings with Huntington disease. *Am. J. Med. Genet.* **105**, 399–403.

Rubinsztein, D.C., Barton, D.E., Davison, B.C., and Ferguson-Smith, M.A. (1993). Analysis of the huntingtin gene reveals a trinucleotide-length polymorphism in the region of the gene that contains two CCG-rich stretches and a correlation between decreased age of onset of Huntington's disease and CAG repeat number. *Hum. Mol. Genet.* **2**, 1713–1715.

—— Leggo, J., Goodburn, S., Crow, T.J., Lofthouse, R., DeLisi, L.E., Barton, D.E., and Ferguson-Smith, M.A. (1994). Study of the Huntington's disease (HD) gene CAG repeats in schizophrenic patients shows overlap of the normal and HD affected ranges but absence of correlation with schizophrenia. *J. Med. Genet.* **31**, 690–693.

—— —— Coles, R., Almqvist, E., Biancalana, V., Cassiman, J.J., Chotai, K., Connarty, M., Crauford, D., Curtis, A., Curtis, D., Davidson, M.J., Differ, A.M., Dode, C., Dodge, A., Frontali, M., Ranen, N.G., Stine, O.C., Sherr, M., Abbott, M.H., Franz, M.L., Graham, C.A., Harper, P.S., Hedreen, J.C., and Hayden, M.R. (1996). Phenotypic characterization of individuals with 30–40 CAG repeats in the Huntington disease (HD) gene reveals HD cases with 36 repeats and apparently normal elderly individuals with 36–39 repeats. *Am. J. Hum. Genet.* **59**, 16–22.

—— —— Chiano, M., Dodge, A., Norbury, G., Rosser, E., and Craufurd, D. (1997). Genotypes at the GluR6 kainate receptor locus are associated with variation in the age of onset of Huntington disease. *Proc. Natl. Acad. Sci., USA* **94**, 3872–3876.

Sanchez, A., Mila, M., Castellvi-Bel, S., Rosich, M., Jimenez, D., Badenas, C., and Estivill, X. (1997). Maternal transmission in sporadic Huntington's disease. *J. Neurol. Neurosurg. Psychiatry* **62**, 535–537.

Sarfarazi, M., Quarrell, O.W., Wolak, G., and Harper, P.S. (1987). An integrated microcomputer system to maintain a genetic register for Huntington disease. *Am. J. Med. Genet.* **28**, 999–1006.

Shaw, M. and Caro, A. (1982). The mutation rate to Huntington's chorea. *J. Med. Genet.* **19**, 161–167.

Shinotoh, H., Calne, D.B., Snow, B., Hayward, M., Kremer, B., Theilmann, J., and Hayden, M.R. (1994). Normal CAG repeat length in the Huntington's disease gene in senile chorea. *Neurology* **44**, 2183–2184.

Siemers, E., Foroud, T., Bill, D.J., Sorbel, J., Norton, J.A., Jr., Hodes, M.E., Niebler, G., Conneally, P.M., and Christian, J.C. (1996). Motor changes in presymptomatic Huntington disease gene carriers. *Arch. Neurol.* **53**, 487–492.

Sieradzan, K.A. and Mann, D.M. (1998). On the pathological progression of Huntington's disease [letter; comment]. *Ann. Neurol.* **44**, 148–149.

—— Mechan, A.O., Jones, L., Wanker, E.E., Nukina, N., and Mann, D.M. (1999). Huntington's disease intranuclear inclusions contain truncated, ubiquitinated huntingtin protein. *Exp. Neurol.* **156**, 92–99.

Siesling, S., Vegter-van de Vlis, M., Losekoot, M., Belfroid, R.D., Maat-Kievit, J.A., Kremer, H.P., and Roos, R.A. (2000). Family history and DNA analysis in patients with suspected Huntington's disease. *J. Neurol. Neurosurg. Psychiatry* **69**, 54–59.

Sjögren, T. (1936). Verlungsmedizinische Untersuchungen über Huntington's Chorea in einer scwedischen Bauernpopulation. *Z. Menschliche Vererbungs Konstitutionlehre* **19**, 131–165.

Snell, R.G., MacMillan, J.C., Cheadle, J.P., Fenton, I., Lazarou, L.P., Davies, P., MacDonald, M.E., Gusella, J.F., Harper, P.S., and Shaw, D.J. (1993). Relationship between trinucleotide repeat expansion and phenotypic variation in Huntington's disease [see comments]. *Nat. Genet.* **4**, 393–397.

Squitieri, F., Sabbadini, G., Mandich, P., Gellera, C., Di Maria, E., Bellone, E., Castellotti, B., Nargi, E., de Grazia, U., Frontali, M., and Novelletto, A. (2000). Family and molecular data for a fine analysis of age at onset in Huntington disease. *Am. J. Med. Genet.* **95**, 366–373.

St.Clair, D. (1994). Expanded CAG trinucleotide repeat of Huntington's disease gene in a patient with schizophrenia and normal striatal histology [letter]. *J. Med. Genet.* **31**, 658–659.

Stenhouse, S.A.R. and Middleton-Price, H. (1996). Quality assurance in molecular diagnosis: the UK experience. In *Molecular diagnosis of genetic diseases* (ed. R. Elles), pp. 341–352. Humana Press, Totowa, New Jersey.

Stevens, D.L. (1976). Huntington's chorea: a demographic genetic and clinical study. Thesis, University of London.

Telenius, H., Kremer, H.P., Theilmann, J., Andrew, S.E., Almqvist, E., Anvret, M., Greenberg, C., Greenberg, J., Lucotte, G., and Squitieri, F. (1993). Molecular analysis of juvenile Huntington disease: the major influence on (CAG)*n* repeat length is the sex of the affected parent. *Hum. Mol. Genet.* **2**, 1535–1540.

—— Kremer, B., Goldberg, Y.P., Theilmann, J., Andrew, S.E., Zeisler, J., Adam, S., Greenberg, C., Ives, E.J., and Clarke, L.A. (1994). Somatic and gonadal mosaicism of the Huntington disease gene CAG repeat in brain and sperm [published erratum appears in *Nat. Genet.* 1994 May; **7** (1), 113]. *Nat. Genet.* **6**, 409–414.

Trottier, Y., Biancalana, V., and Mandel, J.L. (1994). Instability of CAG repeats in Huntington's disease: relation to parental transmission and age of onset. *J. Med. Genet.* **31**, 377–382.

Tsuang, D., DiGiacomo, L., Lipe, H., and Bird, T.D. (1998). Familial aggregation of schizophrenia-like symptoms in Huntington's disease. *Am. J. Med. Genet.* **81**, 323–327.

—— Almqvist, E.W., Lipe, H., Strgar, F., DiGiacomo, L., Hoff, D., Eugenio, C., Hayden, M.R., and Bird, T.D. (2000). Familial aggregation of psychotic symptoms in Huntington's disease. *Am. J. Psychiatry* **157**, 1955–1959.

Valdes, A.M., Slatkin, M., and Freimer, N.B. (1993). Allele frequencies at microsatellite loci: the stepwise mutation model revisited. *Genetics* **133**, 737–749.

Volkers, W.S., Went, L.N., Vegter-van der Vlis, M., Harper, P.S., and Caro, A. (1980). Genetic linkage studies in Huntington's chorea. *Ann. Hum. Genet.* **44**, 75–79.

Vuillaume, I., Meynieu, P., Schraen-Maschke, S., Destee, A., and Sablonniere, B. (2000). Absence of unidentified CAG repeat expansion in patients with Huntington's disease-like phenotype. *J. Neurol. Neurosurg. Psychiatry* **68**, 672–675.

Walker, D.A., Harper, P.S., Newcombe, R.G., and Davies, K. (1983). Huntington's chorea in South Wales: mutation, fertility and genetic fitness. *J. Med. Genet.* **20**, 12–17.

Warner, J.P., Barron, L.H., and Brock, D.J. (1993). A new polymerase chain reaction (PCR) assay for the trinucleotide repeat that is unstable and expanded on Huntington's disease chromosomes. *Mol. Cell Probes* **7**, 235–239.

Weigell-Weber, M., Schmid, W., and Spiegel, R. (1996). Psychiatric symptoms and CAG expansion in Huntington's disease. *Am. J. Med. Genet.* **67**, 53–57.

Wendt, G.G. and Drohm, D. (1972). *Die Huntingtonsche Chorea. Eine Populationsgenetische Studie.* Thieme, Stuttgart.

Went, L.N., Vegter-van der Vlis, M., Bruyn, G.W., and Volkers, W.S. (1983). Huntington's chorea in the Netherlands. The problem of genetic heterogeneity. *Ann. Hum. Genet.* **47**, 205–214.

Wertz, D.C. and Reilly, P.R. (1997). Laboratory policies and practices for the genetic testing of children: a survey of the Helix network. *Am. J. Hum. Genet.* **61**, 1163–1168.

Wexler, A. (1995). *Mapping fate: a memoir of family, risk and genetics research.* University of California Press, Los Angeles.

Wexler, N.S., Conneally, P.M., Housman, D., and Gusella, J.F. (1985). A DNA polymorphism for Huntington's disease marks the future. *Arch. Neurol.* **42**, 20–24.

—— Young, A.B., Tanzi, R.E., Travers, H., Starosta-Rubinstein, S., Penney, J.B., Snodgrass, S.R., Shoulson, I., Gomez, F., and Ramos Arroyo, M.A. (1987). Homozygotes for Huntington's disease. *Nature* **326**, 194–197.

Wheeler, V.C., Auerbach, W., White, J.K., Srinidhi, J., Auerbach, A., Ryan, A., Duyao, M.P., Vrbanac, V., Weaver, M., Gusella, J.F., Joyner, A.L., and MacDonald, M.E. (1999). Length-dependent gametic CAG repeat instability in the Huntington's disease knock-in mouse. *Hum. Mol. Genet.* **8**, 115–122.

Williams, L.C., Hegde, M.R., Herrera, G., Stapleton, P.M., and Love, D.R. (1999). Comparative semi-automated analysis of (CAG) repeats in the Huntington disease gene: use of internal standards. *Mol. Cell Probes* **13**, 283–289.

Xu, X., Peng, M., and Fang, Z. (2000). The direction of microsatellite mutations is dependent upon allele length. *Nat. Genet.* **24**, 396–399.

Xuereb, J.H., MacMillan, J.C., Snell, R., Davies, P., and Harper, P.S. (1996). Neuropathological diagnosis and CAG repeat expansion in Huntington's disease. *J. Neurol. Neurosurg. Psychiatry* **60**, 78–81.

Zappacosta, B., Monza, D., Meoni, C., Austoni, L., Soliveri, P., Gellera, C., Alberti, R., Mantero, M., Penati, G., Caraceni, T., and Girotti, F. (1996). Psychiatric symptoms do not correlate with cognitive decline, motor symptoms, or CAG repeat length in Huntington's disease. *Arch. Neurol.* **53**, 493–497.

Zuhlke, C., Riess, O., Schroder, K., Siedlaczck, I., Epplen, J.T., Engel, W., and Thies, U. (1993a). Expansion of the (CAG)n repeat causing Huntington's disease in 352 patients of German origin. *Hum. Mol. Genet.* **2**, 1467–1469.

Zuhlke, C., Riess, O., Bockel, B., Lange, H., and Thies, U. (1993b). Mitotic stability and meiotic variability of the (CAG)n repeat in the Huntington disease gene. *Hum. Mol. Genet.* **2**, 2063–2067.

6   The epidemiology of Huntington's disease

Peter S. Harper

Until now this book has concentrated on the effects of Huntington's disease (HD), whether clinical or pathological, on the individual, but HD now requires to be placed in its population context. Questions that arise are: how common is the disorder? is it increasing or declining? what geographical variations are there, and how can these be accounted for? Accurate population data are clearly essential for the planning of services for patients and families, as well as for the interpretation of preventive measures, and it is for the collection and analysis of these data that we look to the disciplines of epidemiology and genetics. Much of the information in this chapter comes from an earlier review by the author (Harper 1992) but, as with all aspects of HD research, any interpretation and conclusions now need to be reassessed in the light of our new knowledge of the molecular basis of HD. (For this reason a short section on molecular epidemiology has been added, although fuller details are reserved for Chapter 5.)

Epidemiology, evolving out of the study of infective diseases, has now assumed a major role in the study of chronic disorders whose causation is complex and usually poorly understood. Multiple sclerosis, motor neurone disease, and stroke are examples of major neurological disorders where the epidemiological approach has played an important part in determining hypotheses about causation of these diseases, as well as simply documenting their frequency and variation. For HD the situation is rather different. We know that, as a Mendelian disorder, there is a specific gene determining it; the route to understanding the pathogenesis of the disease is thus principally molecular, not epidemiological. Likewise, the most satisfactory guide to frequency of the disorder is careful study of complete families rather than surveys restricted to primary cases, while those at risk for the disease are also mostly family members, rather than the population at large. For all these reasons most of the data discussed in this chapter have been obtained not by classical epidemiological methods but by means of family surveys. The methods of traditional epidemiology appear cumbersome and rather inadequate when applied to HD, as is clearly seen in the papers by epidemiologists in the early Centennial volume on HD (Schoenberg 1979; Kurtzke 1979; Hogg et al. 1979). Before the detailed situation is described, the different general approaches are outlined below.

Family studies

Systematic family studies have provided the great majority of existing population data for HD. Their success has usually resulted from the fact that they have been carried out by an experienced and dedicated worker or small team, based in the area under study and making up in tenacity and determination what may have been lacking in scientific skills. The sheer effort and detective work involved in tracing families from old and fragmentary records rarely receive a mention in the published results; nor too do the discomforts and even hazards of the work, not to mention the numerous fruitless visits that end in finding someone 'not at home'. The combined experiences of those involved in HD family surveys would make the basis of a series of fascinating novels—but, sadly, can be pursued no further here!

Returning to the scientific aspects, any family study will be meaningless in epidemiological terms unless it is systematic and complete. This essentially means that a point prevalence study is being aimed at, with the following criteria well defined from the outset.

1. The geographical area must be well defined (usually corresponding to some administrative or political boundary). The area must be sufficiently large to avoid bias from a particularly large kindred, but sufficiently small to allow complete coverage of all of it by the investigator (500 000 to 5 million probably represents outer limits for population size). All parts of the area should ideally be covered with equal thoroughness.

2. As many separate methods of ascertainment should be used as possible, for example, general and psychiatric hospital records; letters to family doctors, neurologists, and other clinicians; existing genetics records; death certificates. If multiple ascertainment is frequent this is usually an indication that ascertainment is not going to be seriously deficient.

3. Intensive search for secondary cases is essential. In HD, more than in most genetic disorders, all investigators are struck by the number of new affected patients discovered through a detailed and systematic family survey, often as the result of a home visit, whose existence was totally unsuspected, and who would not have been included in any survey limited to primary cases. The thoroughness of this aspect will probably be the largest single factor in determining prevalence.

4. Any study must be continued over a considerable period of time. Three years is probably a minimum, five preferable, but even then new families will be found to appear in areas where one was confident one had achieved total ascertainment. It is even better to repeat the survey after an interval; this usually produces a significant increase in prevalence.

5. A prevalence date should be chosen that is sufficiently remote (5–10 years) from the time of study to allow existing cases to be recognized and diagnosed but not to have died and been forgotten.

6. Now that molecular prediction and diagnosis are possible, it is essential to avoid including healthy mutation carriers as 'cases', while the effects of detecting isolated cases that might not have been clearly identified clinically as HD, must also be considered.

When all these factors have been worked out, it remains to determine how many HD patients were alive and resident in the area on the prevalence date chosen, and to compare this with the total population of the area at the same date.

The author's original South Wales study (Walker *et al.* 1981) shows how this can be done. The fact that it predates molecular studies does not make it less useful though it may have to be modified in the light of these, as discussed below. It was carried out over a period of almost 5 years (1973–8), with a prevalence date of 25/26 April 1971, corresponding to the decennial census. The area chosen (industrial South Wales) was compact, had well defined boundaries, and had a total population on the prevalence date of 1 720 901, giving a resulting prevalence estimate of 7.61 per 100 000. It should be noted that, when re-analysed 10 years later, taking a prevalence date of 1981, the prevalence was found to be higher at 8.85 per 100 000 (Quarrell

Table 6.1 Prevalence estimates of HD in South Wales

	Walker *et al.* (1981)	Quarrell *et al.* (1988)
Prevalence date	April 1971	April 1981
Census population	1 720 000	1 728 000
Number living affected	131	153
Prevalence (per 100 000)	7.61	8.85

et al. 1987). Table 6.1 summarizes some of the epidemiological aspects of the South Wales study.

Once the prevalence rate is accurately determined, one can also work out the heterozygote frequency for the disorder and the estimated absolute number of gene carriers in the population, as described later.

Molecular diagnosis and prevalence estimates

Molecular analysis for the HD mutation is now part of medical practice, not only in the confirmation of a clinical diagnosis, but also in patients who would not otherwise have been firmly diagnosed as having HD. A particular group relevant to this is that of elderly patients, often without a family history. Two studies have recently assessed the impact of molecular diagnosis on prevalence and both suggest a considerable increase over earlier estimates is likely. Siesling *et al.* (2000) in the Netherlands, analysing data from the well documented Leiden HD roster, found a prevalence 14 per cent higher than previously, mainly due to recognition of cases without a known family history. Almqvist *et al.* (2001) reported a survey from British Columbia and found an additional 24 per cent of cases; there were also a few who did not show the mutation.

The use of molecular analysis must clearly be taken into account in any future prevalence studies, especially if they are being compared with older data from the same region. It will be essential to record whether molecular analysis was comprehensive for the area under study and to categorize separately any individuals detected by presymptomatic testing. Otherwise the estimate will become one related to heterozygote frequency (see below) rather than of disease prevalence.

General surveys of neurological diseases

It is clearly important to be able to compare the frequency of HD with that of other neurological disorders, and a comparative epidemiological study of the major causes of neurological disability might be considered a suitable way to approach this, especially where medical diagnostic records are accurate. Unfortunately, this does not work well in practice and such estimates are likely to be inaccurate. Thus Kurland (1958) studying a variety of neurological and neuromuscular disorders in Rochester, New York estimated a prevalence of 6.7 per 100 000, but this was based on only two cases. The reaction of any HD investigator would have been to visit these two personally, in the anticipation of finding several more unsuspected cases among relatives. As a result of a series of separate studies, data now exist for

Table 6.2 Prevalence of inherited neurological disorder in South Wales*

Disorder	No of living affected	Prevalence (per 100 000)
Huntington's disease	79	8.4
Neurofibromatosis (type 1)	125	13.3
Tuberous sclerosis	13	1.4
Hereditary spastic paraplegia	30	3.2
Charcot-Marie-Tooth disease	116	12.3
Myotonic dystrophy	65	6.9
Duchenne muscular dystrophy	40	8.8[†]
Becker muscular dystrophy	23	2.4[†]
Facioscapulohumeral muscular dystrophy	27	2.9

*Based on 1988 (June) total population, for mid and south Glamorgan, of 939 300.
Data by courtesy of Dr John MacMillan (MacMillan and Harper 1991).
[†]Prevalence for males only.

South Wales for a number of different inherited neurological disorders, based on extensive family surveys. While these estimates may well differ considerably from those of other areas, they are valuable for comparing the different disorders and are given in Table 6.2.

Analysis of death rate

The use of statutory information on causes of death derived from death certificates is subject to a number of disadvantages, notably that HD may not appear on the death certificate, either because the immediate cause of death was something else, or because the physician filling in the certificate may have wished to protect the family from the adverse effects of HD being officially recognized as the cause. A further difficulty is that HD did not have a specific international code until 1968 (ICD 331.0, hereditary chorea). For the subsequent 10 years this category reflects HD accurately, since other causes of hereditary chorea are very rare, but, unfortunately, a further charge in 1979 relegated HD to a subset (333.4) so that the three-figure code (often the only one complete) now again contains other major diseases besides HD. Despite these problems, however, information on death rates is available from all areas without the need for special surveys or systems of collection. It is also likely to be comparable between regions in a way that individual surveys may not be. For this reason the study of Hogg *et al.* (1979) of death rate data for the USA is important. Based on the data of 1968–74, the study showed a remarkably uniform pattern of mortality from HD, with an age-adjusted death rate ranging only between 0.96 and 1.35 per million. These data are considered further in relation to specific surveys in the USA but, while they are certainly an underestimate, they provide a valuable baseline. A more recent study in the USA by Lanska *et al.* (1988) has analysed the mortality from HD when this is given as a subsidiary condition rather than the main cause of death. This considerably increased the recognized mortality rate by around 8 per cent over the values previously found by Hogg *et al.* Comparable data for the European countries are also available. Table 6.3 summarizes some of these.

Death certificates can also be used longitudinally to follow any possible increase or decrease in HD. Caro (1977) noted a marked increase between 1959 and 1974, and that

Table 6.3 Approximate average annual HD death rates per million population by sex and country (from Kurtzke 1979)

Country	Period	Male	Female
US total	1968–74	1.1 (1.0–1.1)*	1.2 (1.1–1.3)
US white	1968–74	1.2 (1.1–1.2)	1.3 (1.2–1.4)
US non-white	1968–74	0.4 (0.3–0.6)	0.4 (0.3–0.5)
Sweden	1969–74	1.7 (1.2–2.3)	1.7 (1.2–2.3)
Denmark	1951–68	1.4 (1.1–1.9)	1.4 (1.1–1.9)
Denmark	1969–75	1.8 (1.2–2.6)	1.9 (1.3–2.7)
England and Wales[†]	1960–73	1.5 (1.4–1.6)	1.6 (1.5–1.7)
Japan	1969–75	01. (0.1–0.1)	0.2 (0.1–0.2)

*Values in parentheses are 95% confidence intervals.
[†]Cod 331 total.

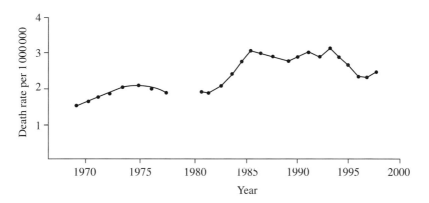

Fig. 6.1 Death rate from HD in England and Wales, 1968–99. Three-year moving averages based on data of Table 6.4, kindly provided by the UK Office of National Statistics. Note that the discontinuity produced by the changes in ICD coding in 1978 does not appear to have altered the rate.

some increase was still present when the data were corrected for inaccuracy of certification, something that he had found to improve over this period. The same trend was noted and discussed by the Office of Health Economics report on HD (1980). Figure 6.1 and Table 6.4 show these data extended up to the present time. The mortality rate is still considerably less than to be expected from the prevalence data shown in the detailed surveys. Broadly, these data agree with the trend in different prevalence surveys carried out at different times in showing that both prevalence and mortality from recognized HD have increased. However, it would seem unwise to assume that any true major recent changes in mortality can be inferred from these figures.

It is worth noting here that mortality data are of little use in monitoring changes resulting from genetic counselling and presymptomatic testing since death rates reflect births occurring on average 50 years later. Hence the importance of birth rate data based on those known to be at risk, which will give a more sensitive indication of any recent changes. Any changes in

Table 6.4 Deaths from HD in England and Wales, 1968–99 (data kindly supplied by The Office of National Statistics)*

Year	No. of deaths	Population (× 10³)	Rate (per 1 000 000 population)
1968	71	48 593.0	1.5
1969	71	48 826.8	1.5
1970	78	48 891.1	1.6
1971	89	49 152.0	1.8
1972	99	49 327.1	2.0
1973	82	49 459.0	1.7
1974	111	49 467.9	2.2
1975	85	49 469.8	1.7
1976	96	49 459.2	1.9
1977	106	49 440.4	2.1
1978	71	49 442.5	1.4
1979	92	49 508.2	1.9
1980	82	49 603.0	1.7
1981	89	49 634.3	1.8
1982	96	49 601.4	1.9
1983	109	49 653.7	2.2
1984	142	49 763.6	2.9
1985	155	49 923.5	3.1
1986	151	50 075.4	3.0
1987	137	50 242.9	2.7
1988	127	50 393.0	2.5
1989	152	50 678.0	3.0
1990	143	50 869.5	2.8
1991	154	51 099.5	3.0
1992	136	51 276.9	2.7
1993	108	51 439.2	3.5
1994	106	51 620.5	2.1
1995	114	51 820.2	2.2
1996	129	52 010.2	2.5
1997	121	52 211.2	2.3
1998	113	52 427.9	2.2
1999	136	52 689.9	2.6

*1968–78: Hereditary chorea (ICD 331.1); 1979–present: Huntington's chorea (ICD 333.4).

death rate are likely to indicate factors operating half a century ago and may be very different to those that are occurring at present.

HD in different countries

Variation in the frequency of HD between countries has long been recognized, as outlined in Chapter 1. Early studies in North America stressed the common ancestry of most cases from a small number of founding immigrants, and the gene was thought to have come principally from England. It soon became clear, however, that this was an oversimplification, and a broader 'northern European' origin of the gene became accepted. It is only recently that surveys based on adequate ascertainment have been available from a wider range of countries, and these are still far from complete. This section attempts to record the existing data as fully as possible and to plot them visually in the hope that more accurate comparative analysis will soon be possible. This has now become of particular importance in view of the realization that prevalence differences may relate to variation in the normal distribution of trinucleotide repeat length polymorphisms in different populations (see below).

United States of America

In looking at the detailed distribution of HD throughout the world it is appropriate to begin with the USA. Following George Huntington's description of the disorder, attention initially focused on its occurrence in New England and its British origin (Jelliffe 1908). Much has been written of the supposed descent of most New England cases from three original migrants from East Anglia. As discussed in Chapter 1, most of this is likely to be inaccurate or erroneous. The extensive data of Davenport and Muncey (1916) likewise deal mainly with the New England families and must be regarded more as a compilation than a survey, though one of considerable historical significance.

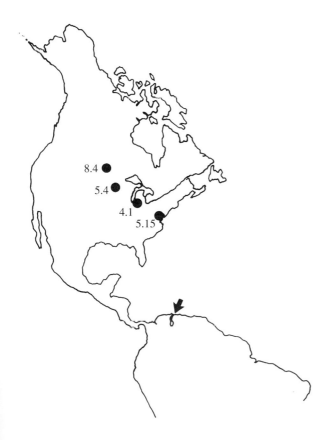

Fig. 6.2 North American prevalence estimates for HD (see Table 6.5 for details). The number of detailed population studies has been few in comparison with Europe. The Venezuelan focus of HD is arrowed.

The first critical and detailed analysis was that of Reed and colleagues in Michigan (Reed *et al.* 1958; Reed and Neel 1959). Their prevalence rate of 4.2 per 100 000 is likely to be an underestimate since ascertainment was based mainly on hospitals, but it represents a landmark in careful design of the study. Reed *et al.* studied the origin of their 124 kindreds and found that over half (73) could not be traced back to a progenitor outside the USA. Those that could were almost equally divided between three groups, Britain, Germany, and other various European countries. An even greater predominance of German origin was found by Falstein and Stone (1939) in Iowa, with German origin kindreds accounting for 27 of the 62 kindreds of known origin, while Britain and Ireland had contributed only nine.

The various prevalence estimates for different regional studies in North America are summarized in Table 6.5. Much the most detailed of these is the Maryland study of Folstein *et al.* (1987), which used intensive ascertainment from multiple sources and which undertook a detailed family analysis and search for secondary cases. Folstein's monograph (1989) gives a full description of the methods used in this valuable study and gives practical information on guidelines to follow in undertaking work of this type. The overall prevalence estimate of 5.15 per 100 000 is likely to be the closest available to the true figure and the only one providing an accurate estimate for the Black American population, a topic discussed below.

The US Huntington's roster, a record of HD families, primarily for research purposes, from all parts of the country (Conneally 1984; Gersting *et al.* 1984), has already been described in Chapter 1. While it cannot be used for prevalence data and could be biased in some respects (for example, towards the recording of large kindreds), its size and scope have made it an invaluable resource in providing large samples for quantitative analysis on a variety of genetic and other topics.

A number of other American studies for which prevalence estimates are frequently cited are too incomplete to be of serious use. Thus, the survey of Korenyi and Whittier (1977) in New York City and Long Island was simply based on estimating the number of children of patients recorded in hospital notes and assuming that half would be affected. The estimate of Myrianthopoulos (1973) for HD in New York Jews was based on the 70 Jewish families who

Table 6.5 Prevalence studies of HD: North America

Reference	Prevalence year	Region	Number affected	Population	Prevalence (per 100 000)
Reed *et al.* 1958	1940	Michigan	203	4 932 562	4.1(overall) 4.2 (Whites) 1.5 (Blacks)
Shokeir 1975		Manitoba and Saskatchewan	162	1 926 942	8.4
Pearson *et al.* 1955	1955	Minnesota	117	3 174 000	5.43
Folstein *et al.* 1987	1980	Maryland	217	4 217 000	5.15 (overall) 4.94 (Whites) 6.37 (Blacks)
Kokmen *et al.* 1994	1960 1990	Minnesota	—	—	6.3 1.9
Almqvist *et al.* 2001	1993–2000	British Columbia	205	—	0.69 (annual incidence)

were members of the lay society. This certainly suggests that the disorder is not uncommon in Jews, but cannot be taken as a specific prevalence estimate. Kurland's (1958) estimate of 6.7 per 100 000 for Rochester, Minnesota was based on only two cases. A further small Minnesota study of Olmstead County (Kokmen *et al.* 1994) showed a comparable prevalence for the year 1960 (6.0/100 000 for females, 6.6 for males), but for 1990 the corresponding figures were only 1.8 and 2.0. The extremely wide confidence intervals again emphasize the limitations of small population studies. Thus the USA remains remarkably understudied in terms of detailed prevalence, when compared with Europe.

The population mobility seen in many parts of the USA makes it less easy to use regional genetic registers as a means of estimating and monitoring the prevalence of HD. It is thus difficult to draw conclusions as to whether the differences between the various prevalence estimates are real or simply reflect the methods of the different studies. An indication that differences are probably not great comes from the death certificate data, which, as discussed earlier, has the advantages of being systematically and uniformly collected in all states, even though it is likely to be a considerable underestimate of the true incidence of HD. When states are grouped as major census regions the highest age-adjusted death rate (1.36 per 10^6) is in the north-central and western regions and the lowest in the southern region (0.96 per 10^6), a difference that is extremely small (Hogg *et al.* 1979).

Canada

Canada has produced some remarkable concentrations of genetic disorders, especially among its isolated French-Canadian populations. Myotonic dystrophy, oculopharyngeal muscular dystrophy, and tyrosinaemia are striking examples which have been well documented. HD, by contrast, appears to be principally of English origin and does not show a restricted geographical distribution, though the first Canadian report (MacKay 1904) was of a French-Canadian family from Quebec.

Clarke and McArthur (1924) reported a large southern Ontario family with HD, of English origin, while further four-generation Ontario cases were reported subsequently and reviewed by Archibald (1938). Barbeau and Fullum (1962) undertook a major systematic study of HD in Canada, documenting no fewer than 820 cases from 104 families. Of these families, 75 could be traced to an origin outside Canada, 55 coming from Britain and Ireland, the USA contributing only 9, while 4 were from Germany and only 3 from France. Barbeau *et al.* (1964) were able to trace 123 French-Canadian cases to a single common ancestor who came from France to Montreal in 1645. The only other significant HD focus of probable French origin is that in Nova Scotia, originally reported by Hattie in 1909 and reassessed by Winsor and Welch (1973). This group originated from eastern France and came to Canada via the USA.

Barbeau and Fullum did not attempt a prevalence estimate, but Shokeir (1975) surveyed the Prairie provinces of Saskatchewan and Manitoba and found the remarkably high prevalence of 8.4 per 100 000. Like several other investigators he found an increased fertility both compared with the general population and with unaffected sibs. There is no note as to the origin of the families in this study.

British Columbia was found by Hall and Te-Juceto (1983) to have 386 affected individuals from 121 kindreds. It has since become a major centre for HD research and has also taken a major initiative in establishing a coordinated nationwide predictive testing programme, allowing valuable combined data to be obtained on this difficult topic, as well as ensuring equitable delivery of the service to the population as a whole. Almqvist *et al.* (2001) have recently reassessed the British Columbia frequency in the light of molecular diagnosis, finding an incidence of 6.9 per million per year. Twenty-four per cent of cases had no known previous family history and might not have been included in studies prior to molecular analysis.

South America

The remarkable Venezuelan isolate and its contribution to HD research in general has already been mentioned in Chapters 1 and 5. Over 100 individuals are affected, with large families producing a particularly high number at risk among young people, some with both parents affected. The clinical aspects have been documented by Young *et al.* (1986) and Penney *et al.* (1990), and the probable homozygotes by Wexler *et al.* (1987).

The affected families are located in a number of villages at the edge of Lake Maracaibo, some very isolated (Figs 6.3 and 6.4). The combination of geographical and social isolation produced by fear of the disease has reduced intermarriage with the surrounding communities and has resulted in extreme poverty and lack of medical facilities. While genealogical tracing has inter-connected the different branches and identified a common ancestor living around 1830, it is still not certain whether the disorder has a European origin and, if so, from what country it came.

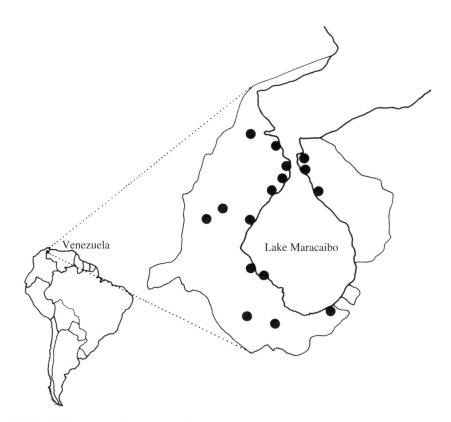

Fig. 6.3 HD in Venezuela. Occurrence of HD in communities around Lake Maracaibo, Venezuela (based on the US Congressional Report 1977).

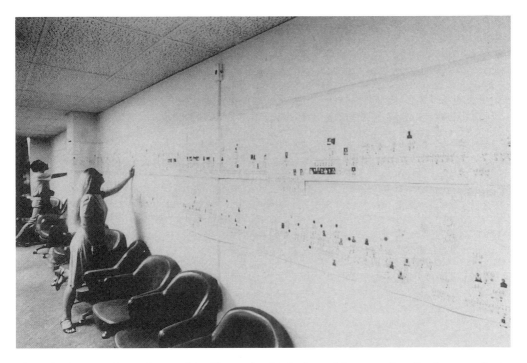

Fig. 6.4 The extensive pedigree of the Venezuelan kindred, requiring several walls of a room for its display (courtesy pf Dr Nancy Wexler).

In epidemiological terms there is much to be learned from this unique community, which should progressively emerge from longitudinal studies still in progress . It is already clear that the pattern of decline seen in the disease is comparable to that elsewhere despite the adverse socio-economic situation and absence of drug treatment (Young *et al.* 1986; Penney *et al.* 1990), while the likely homozygotes have so far shown no clinical differences from heterozygotes (Wexler *et al.* 1987; Huntington's Disease Collaborative Research Group 1993). The community illustrates the rapid expansion of a dominantly inherited genetic disorder that can occur when the gene is introduced into a population with a high natural rate of increase. It also shows how social acceptance of a disorder such as HD may paradoxically be better achieved in a relatively simple community with a high frequency of the condition. It will be of great interest to see whether changes in community attitudes will result in uptake of predictive and prenatal testing and what changes these developments will in turn produce in the population.

In other parts of South and Latin America, a further focus of high prevalence has been reported from Peru and a survey carried out in Chile (Cruz-Coke 1987) as well as cases from the Caribbean (Beaubrun 1962). The long-standing recognition of the disorder is shown by reports from Cuba and Brazil that date back to 1890 and 1891, respectively (Arostegui 1890; Couto 1891).

Britain

In the UK HD has been studied more intensively than in any other part of the world, with systematic prevalence studies in no fewer than 15 different regions, in addition to less complete reports. In general, the more recent studies have shown a higher prevalence than the earlier ones and are likely to be closer to full ascertainment, especially those based outside major conurbations where population mobility is greater. From the data given in Table 6.6 and Fig. 6.5, no obvious pattern emerges to suggest a single focus of the disease, with high prevalence seen in regions as far apart as Wales and north-east Scotland, while populations of Celtic and Saxon origin likewise do not differ appreciably. Northern Ireland has been thoroughly studied (Morrison *et al.* 1995), but data for the Republic of Ireland are incomplete (Morrison 1995), apart from the localized area of Donegal, where the prevalence was shown to have declined from 4.6 to 1.6 per 100 000 over the 30-year period to 1991 (Morrison and Nevin 1993), in association with marked immigration and population decline in this small (*c.*150 000) population. In some studies it is possible to break down the overall prevalence estimate into figures for particular districts, as shown in the data for Wales given in Fig. 6.5. This relatively uniform pattern is now recognized to be the case for most of Europe.

Table 6.6 Prevalence estimates for HD in the UK

Study	Prevalence year	Region	Map no.	Number affected	Population	Prevalence ($\times 10^{-5}$)
Bickford and Ellison 1953	1950	Cornwall	1	19	340 941	5.57
Pleydell 1954	1954	Northamptonshire	2–5	13	263 000	5.0
Pleydell 1955	1954	Northamptonshire		17	263 000	6.5
Reid 1960	1954	Northamptonshire		19	263 000	7.2
Oliver 1970	1968	Northamptonshire		27	428 000	6.3
Heathfield 1967	1965	Essex	6	81	3 271 000	2.5
Cameron and Venters 1967		S.E. Scotland	7	154	1 163 877	7.2
Bolt 1970	1968	W. Scotland	8	30	2 959 600	5.2
Heathfield and MacKenzie 1971		Bedfordshire	9	30	427 970	7.5
Glendinning 1975	1965	Somerset	10	33	632 000	5.5
Stevens 1976	1966	Leeds and Yorkshire	11	133	3 190 000	4.17
Caro 1977	1971	E Anglia	12	54	584 415	9.24
Harper *et al.* 1979	1971	S Wales	13	131	1 720 901	7.61
Simpson and Johnston 1989	1984	Grampian, NE Scot	14	47	462 891	9.95
Quarrell *et al.* 1988	1981	N. Wales	15	34	621 000	5.5
Quarrell *et al.* 1988	1981	S. Wales	16	153	1 728 000	8.85
Nevin and Morrison 1990*	1975	N. Ireland	17	93	1 536 000	6.05
Dennis 1990*	1987	Wessex	18	92	2 457 473	3.74
Garrett 1990*	1987	Devon	19	46	1 010 000	4.6
Garrett 1990*	1987	Cornwall	20	22	453 100	4.9
Shiwach 1994	1985	Oxford Health Reg.	2–5	138	2 437 300	5.7
Morrison *et al.* 1995	1991	N. Ireland	17	101	1 569 971	6.4

*Personal communication based on genetic registers; underascertainment of varying degree likely. The author is grateful for permission to quote these unpublished data.

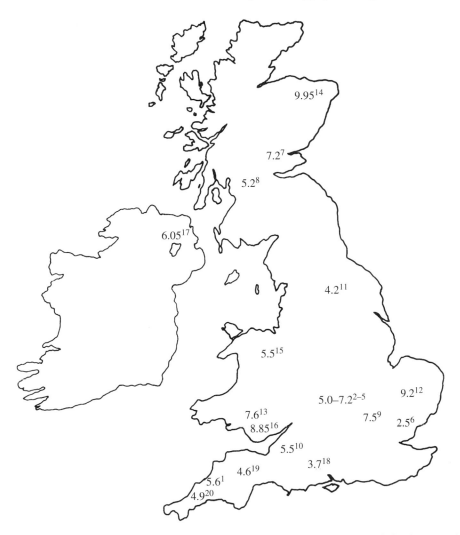

Fig. 6.5 HD in Britain. The map shows the result of prevalence studies based on defined geographical regions (see Table 6.6 for details). The superscript numbers refer to the published sources given in the table.

Britain has been the origin of HD in numerous populations around the world, including the USA, Canada, Australia, and South Africa—in fact everywhere that there was substantial British colonization. Almost all of this migration has occurred during the past 300 years, much during the past century, so that it has often been possible to document the likely gene carriers who founded the new populations, and their area of origin in the UK. Not all of this research has been accurate, as witnessed by the overelaboration of the history of the New England families derived from East Anglia. These were erroneously interpreted by Vessie (1932), Critchley (1934), and others as documented by Caro (1979) and Caro and Haines (1975) (see Chapter 1). So far it has not been possible to prove common descent between these distant HD populations and living HD patients in Britain. Molecular analysis will probably not help in this, given the single mutational mechanism underlying essentially all cases and the existence of several haplotypes in most large populations.

Although population mobility continually militates against the complete ascertainment of HD, the well developed and regionally based medical genetics services in the UK have resulted in a series of systematically maintained genetic registers for the disorder. Thus a steady approach towards total ascertainment of patients and those at risk is likely that will allow not only more complete data on prevalence in different parts of the country, but also the monitoring of any trends resulting from genetic counselling and the application of predictive testing.

Germany

The shadow of the Nazi era still lies heavily on all aspects of work on HD in Germany. The study of Panse (1942) in the Rhineland region, following on the early work of Entres (1921) was one of the first and most thorough analyses of the genetic aspects, and his prevalence estimate of 3.1 per 100 000 is probably more accurate than that of later studies, agreeing closely with the estimate of Wendt and Drohm (1972) for the Kassel region in 1939. The association of Panse's work with the abuses of the Third Reich was documented in the previous edition of this book (Harper1996, Chapter 11) and by Harper (1992). The principal later study was that of Wendt *et al.* (1959, 1960, 1961) brought together in a detailed monograph by Wendt and Drohm (1972). An attempt was made to ascertain all families in West Germany and detailed tables of prevalence are given for different regions. The overall prevalence for 1950 of 2 per 100 000 is likely to be an underestimate compared with the more intensive surveys in specific regions, particularly since the authors state that the work had to be curtailed owing to cessation of funding. Reluctance of families to cooperate on account of past experiences could also have hindered ascertainment, though the Nazi policy of compulsory sterilization and killing of affected patients could have contributed to the lower post-war estimates. A later study in Franconia (Przuntek and Steigerwald 1987) has given a higher value of close to 5 per 100 000. A German origin is likely for a significant number of the HD families in North America, as already mentioned, and this also applies to other populations that received large-scale German immigration such as Australia.

Not surprisingly, there remains extreme sensitivity in Germany to such topics as genetic registers and presymptomatic testing for HD, an attitude that applies generally to new developments in genetics. The uptake of presymptomatic testing in Germany is markedly less than in neighbouring countries (Yapidzakis *et al.* 2002).

Other European countries

Data available from specific studies are shown in Table 6.7 and Fig. 6.6. Although it was thought in the past that the disorder is more frequent in northern than in southern Europe, it seems that the difference may well be slight—if it exists at all. Southern European countries such as Italy and Greece are well represented in the origins of migrant HD families in Australia and North America. Apart from a few older studies (for example, Belgium) where ascertainment has almost certainly been incomplete, most specific prevalence estimates are in the 3–5 per 100 000 range, suggesting a relatively uniform frequency over a wide part of Europe. This distribution has considerable implications for the origins of HD, as discussed later. A notable exception to the European pattern of HD (as for most genetic disorders) could

Table 6.7 Prevalence estimates for HD in Europe (excluding the UK)

Country	Map no.	Reference	Prevalence (per 100 000)
Belgium	1	Husquinet 1970	1.63
Finland	2	Palo *et al.* 1987	0.5
France			
Northern	3	Petit 1970	4.0
Haute Vienne	4	Leger 1974	4.8
Germany			
Rhineland	5	Panse 1942	3.2
Kassel	6	Wendt and Drohm 1972	3.2
Federal Republic	—	Wendt and Drohm 1972	3.2
Franconia	7	Przuntek and Steigerwald 1987	4.8
Iceland	8	Gudmundsson 1969	2.7
Italy			
Lazio	9	Frontali *et al.* 1990	2.56
Emilia	10	Mainini *et al.* 1982	4.8
Liguria	11	Roccatagliata and Albano 1976	4.5
Toscana	12	Arena *et al.* 1979	2.34
Florence		Groppi *et al.* 1986	4.1
Malta	13	Cassar 1967	7.8
Norway	14	Saugstad and Odegard 1986	6.7
Poland	15	Cendrowski 1964	4.8
Sweden	16	Mattsson 1974	4.7
Switzerland	17	Zolliker 1989	3.8–4.8
Yugoslavia			
Rijeka district	18	Sepcic *et al.* 1989	4.46

be Finland (Palo *et al.* 1987), whose exceptionally low prevalence of 0.5 per 100 000 in this study is comparable to that of Japan, though even here recent molecular analysis has shown more than one DNA haplotype associated with the disease (Ikonen *et al.* 1990). However, more recent studies, based on extended family analysis, now suggest that the prevalence may be comparable to that of other European populations, though most families showed haplotypes suggestive of foreign origin (Ikonen *et al.* 1992).

Asia

There is a lack of detailed prevalence studies from any Asian country, but it cannot be assumed from this that HD is absent or even rare. In India there has been a series of case and family reports, principally from Punjab and other parts of north India (Chhutani 1957; Singh *et al.* 1959; Khosla and Arora 1973). One of the Caribbean families of Beaubrun (1962) originated from Madras. Further data have been provided by Shiwach and Lindenbaum (1990) who undertook a detailed survey of immigrants from the Indian subcontinent to Britain. They found 22 cases among an immigrant population of 1.26 million, giving an age-adjusted prevalence estimate of 1.75 per 100 000. Bearing in mind possible restrictions of immigration and likely underascertainment, this suggests that the true prevalence may well approach the European level.

HD in Chinese patients has been described principally outside mainland China itself, from Hong Kong (Singer 1962), where a prevalence estimate of 0.37 per 100 000 (Leung *et al.* 1992;

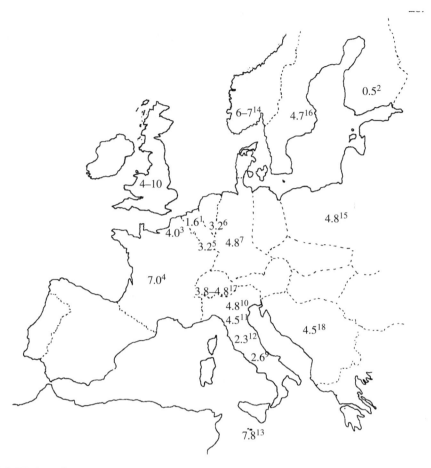

Fig. 6.6 HD in various European countries (see Table 6.7 for details). The superscript numbers refer to the published sources given in the table. It can be seen that there is a high prevalence rate for HD in most European countries where it has been studied intensively; Finland is a possible exception (but see text).

Chang *et al.* 1994) must be considered provisional, Taiwan (Tsuang 1969), and Singapore (Tay 1970; Wong *et al.* 1993). Several reports have confirmed the mutational basis as a CAG expansion (Chan *et al.* 1995; Soong and Wang 1995; Zeng *et al.* 1995). It is well recognized in mainland China (Lo 1990, personal communication) but no prevalence estimate exists. There are case reports from Thailand (Phanthumchinda and Locharernkul 1992) and Malaysia (Lee *et al.* 1994). In Soviet Central Asia a study by Kozlova *et al.* (1986) reported a high frequency in the Shamkhor region of Azerbaijan, but again without a specific prevalence estimate.

On the western margin of Asia, Bayulkem and Turek (1961) recorded 35 cases of HD in Turkey between 1947 and 1959, and found them to be evenly distributed over the country. More recently, a number of Arab families have been reported from Saudi Arabia, probably of indigenous origin in at least some cases, and showing the expected mutational defect (Scrimgeour *et al.* 1994; Bohlega *et al.* 1995).

Australia

Australia has been the site of a series of prevalence studies in different states, as well as of more general HD research. The surveys in Victoria (Brothers and Meadows 1955; Brothers 1964) and Queensland (Parker 1958; Wallace and Parker 1973) have confirmed HD as a major problem in these populations.

The origins and spread of HD in Australia provide a parallel to those that occurred in North America a century or more before. Rapid spread in an expanding population has occurred, with a mainly but not exclusively British origin (Gale and Bennett 1969). The only documented cases in Aborigines have also had a European origin (Hahn 1990, personal communication). Interestingly, and perhaps relevant in view of previous suggestions of criminality in association with the disorder, no association has been found between HD in Australian families and an ancestor having been 'transported' from Britain for criminal offences.

Table 6.8 and Fig. 6.7 summarize the data for Australia, New Zealand, and other Pacific regions. A central register has in the past recorded all cases in Australia (Chiu and Teltscher 1978) but the specific prevalence studies in Queensland and Victoria still probably represent the most accurate estimates for the Australian mainland; individual states are now maintaining their own registers.

The island of Tasmania has long been recognized as an unusual focus of HD. In 1949 Brothers reported an exceptionally large kindred on the island, derived from a single ancestor whose origin was Somerset, England. Forty years later, a thorough study was undertaken by Pridmore (1990a–c), who established a genetic register and analysed a number of genetic aspects. The recent situation can be summarized as follows. The kindred reported by Brothers is still responsible for most cases of HD on the island; as of 1990 it had produced 198 affected individuals, 40 still living, together with 731 relatives with a risk greater than 10 per cent. This kindred shows an unusually high mean age at onset (48.6 years) and death (62.9 years), though several juvenile cases have occurred. The usual trinucleotide repeat expansion has been documented in it (Pridmore *et al.* 1995) It is interesting that a study by Glendinning (1975) in Somerset, the county of origin of this family, has also documented a large late-onset

Table 6.8 HD in Australia and Asia

Country	Study	Prevalence (per 100 000)
Tasmania	Brothers 1949; Conneally 1984	17.4
Tasmania	Pridmore 1990c	12.1
Victoria	Brothers 1964	4.58
Queensland	Parker 1958	2.3
Queensland	Wallace and Parker 1973	6.3
New Zealand	Lintott 1990, personal communication	5.7
Japan	Kishimoto *et al.* 1957	0.38
	Narabayashi 1973	0.45
	Kanazawa 1983	0.11
	Nakashima *et al.* 1996	0.65
	Adachi and Nakashima 1999	0.72
Indian subcontinent (UK immigrants)	Shiwach and Lindenbaum 1990	1.75
Hong Kong Chinese	Leung *et al.* 1992	0.37

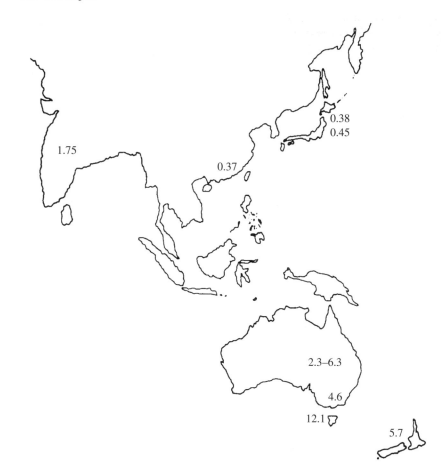

Fig. 6.7 HD in Asia and Australasia (see Table 6.8 for details). Note the exceptionally low prevalence for Japan. The estimate for India is based on a study of immigrants in the UK.

kindred. Documentation of a common origin would be of interest and possibly of importance in helping to define the genetic factors influencing stability of the mutation.

While a small number of unrelated HD cases have been recognized in Tasmania, the overall data are still dominated by the one large kindred. Pridmore has shown that fertility is increased over the general population and that unaffected sibs show diminished fertility, as discussed in Chapter 5. The current prevalence estimate is 12.1 per 100 000, less than the earlier value of 17.4 per 100 000 based on Brothers' figures, but still much higher than in most populations.

The Pacific islands

HD has been found to occur in New Guinea and some of the smaller island groups of the Pacific and would appear to antedate any European settlement there (Hetherington and Wechsler 1942; Scrimgeour 1980, 1982). The interesting and plausible suggestion has been made that the gene could have been introduced by the crews of visiting whaling ships from North America, which were active in the sperm whale fishery in the first half of the 19th century. Scrimgeour (1983) searched the records of whaling voyages and found that a number of surnames of crew members were surnames present in known HD families from New England recorded in the Davenport and Muncey (1916) archives, University of Minnesota. While no direct link has been proved, the predominance of New Englanders in the whaling industry and their frequent sexual relations with islanders make this a reasonable hypothesis for these small populations, where genetic drift could have subsequently increased the gene frequency in some cases. Molecular haplotype studies could provide further evidence.

Japan

The remarkably low prevalence of HD in Japan is of great interest in relation to the possible origins of the disorder and the relationship to the population distribution of trinucleotide repeat polymorphisms. Whereas for many parts of the world this could be attributed to lack of ascertainment, this is certainly not so for Japan, where well developed neurological services and extensive neurological and neuropathological research would undoubtedly have identified most cases. Narabayashi (1973) reviewed the considerable number of population studies on HD (over 40) from Japan, while it is of interest that some allied disorders such as chorea–acanthocytosis and DRPLA (see Chapter 2) appear to be unusually frequent.

Kishimoto *et al.* (1957) undertook a prevalence study of HD in Aichi prefecture and obtained a prevalence of 0.38 per 100 000. An updated estimate of 0.45 per 100 000 was given by Narabayashi (1973). These values are one-tenth the prevalence in most European origin populations. A further estimate was made by Kanazawa (1983) in Ibaraki prefecture, which gave an even lower prevalence (0.11 per 100 000); only three living cases (one doubtful) could be identified in a population of 2 638 280. Kanazawa pointed out that Kishimoto's original study was done in the part of Japan known to contain HD families, so it seems likely that HD is indeed exceptionally rare, though widely scattered.

Two more recent studies have confirmed the low prevalence of HD in Japan. Nakashima *et al.* (1996) found a prevalence of 0.65/100 000 (10 cases) in the San-in area, while Adachi and Nakashima (1999) reported a prevalence of 0.72/100 000 for western Japan (including the San-in area). These studies included mutation and haplotype analysis and it should be noted that one of the 10 San-in cases did not show a CAG expansion, so should now perhaps not strictly be classified as HD.

There is no evidence for foreign admixture in the Japanese cases, but the reason for the low prevalence is of great interest in relation to the difference between Japanese and Caucasian populations for normal frequencies of alleles at a number of different trinucleotide repeat loci, including those for HD, DRPLA, and myotonic dystrophy (see Chapter 5).

Africa

The frequency of HD in African populations has become a topic of great interest since it was realized that there are marked normal population differences between the major ethnic groups, not only for HD but for other trinucleotide repeat disorders, as discussed in the section 'The molecular epidemiology of HD'.

South Africa

The occurrence and origins of HD in South Africa have been documented in considerable detail, thanks largely to the work of Hayden (Hayden 1979, 1981; Hayden *et al.* 1980a,b).

Table 6.9 Prevalence of HD in South Africa (based on Hayden 1979)

	Number	Population	Prevalence (per 100 000)
White	97	4 367 000	2.22
Mixed race (coloured)	53	2 432 000	2.17
Black	3	16 647 000	0.01

Following an earlier study of Klintworth (1962), Hayden set out to document all cases of HD in the republic, work that provided the foundations of his subsequent monograph (1981) and for continued research on HD after leaving South Africa for Canada.

Hayden was able to document 481 cases of HD in South Africa and the most striking feature of his study was the relative rarity of the disorder among the Black population, only 11 cases, three still living, being recorded. There were also no cases of Asian origin. By contrast, the disorder was relatively common in both White South Africans and in those of mixed race (coloured), giving the prevalence estimates shown in Table 6.9. Since Hayden's study a report of eight further cases from four families of Black South Africans has appeared (Joubert and Botha 1988), but there is little doubt that the difference is a real one, even though exaggerated by differential ascertainment as discussed below.

Initially, there were thought to be 134 separate kindreds of HD in South Africa, but careful genealogical study progressively reduced this to 74. All the main founding European groups were represented and of particular interest was the demonstration by Hayden (1979) that some of the largest family groups could be linked with ancestors from Holland who also have HD descendants living there today. One such group, traced over 14 generations to the seventeenth century, links together 50 present families containing over 200 individuals, representing three-quarters of all HD patients of Afrikaner origin. A British origin was found for 15 kindreds, while smaller numbers have had their origin in Germany, Lithuania (a Jewish kindred), and France (via Mauritius). A definite origin could not be assigned to most of the mixed-race families, but the frequency similar to that of the White population supports a largely European origin.

Detailed study of the South African patients showed clinical and genetic features essentially similar to those of HD elsewhere, except for a somewhat earlier onset and death especially in the mixed-race cases, a finding that could reflect the action of modifying genes as discussed in Chapter 5. Juvenile cases also showed a shorter duration of the illness, again differing from most other studies, but this estimate excluded living cases and is thus an underestimate. More recently, four African-origin families from South Africa were reported as showing the CAG expansion, but without detailed haplotype information (Silber *et al.* 1998).

Mauritius

This small island population, 2000 kilometres east of South Africa, provides a good example of the 'founder effect'. A single kindred of French origin has produced 6 affected individuals and 60 at risk, giving a prevalence in the White population of 48 per 100 000 (Hayden 1979). Some members of the kindred have since migrated to smaller islands and to mainland South Africa. While not of general significance, this illustrates the practical importance of 'micro-epidemiology' to the provision of health services in a community.

Other African populations and American Blacks

Outside South Africa, there have been only isolated reports from other Black African countries, including Uganda (Hutton 1956), Kenya (Harries 1973), Nigeria (Osuntoken 1973), and Ghana (Haddock 1973). This case material is summarized by Hayden (1979), Wright *et al.* (1981), and Folstein *et al.* (1987). More recent reports include a six-generation family from Togo (Grunitzky *et al.* 1995) and a study of three families from Zimbabwe (Scrimgeour *et al.* 1992) from which the authors tentatively estimated a prevalence of 0.5–1 per 100 000. This material does not allow any general conclusion to be drawn other than that HD exists in most African countries, but appears to be uncommon. None of these cases outside South Africa have been restudied with molecular analysis so far.

Information on American Blacks is available from several studies, but the completeness of ascertainment can again be questioned in most of these, while the small numbers of Blacks in each survey make accurate estimates impossible. Thus Reed *et al.* (1958) found a frequency in Blacks of around one-third of that in the White population, but this was based on only three cases, a number not significantly different from that of eight expected on the basis of an equal prevalence in the races. Wright *et al.* (1981) in South Carolina, specifically studied HD in Blacks and found a prevalence of 0.97 per 100 000, but again this was based on only nine patients.

The overall death rate data reported by Hogg *et al.* (1979) are of interest in comparing the frequency in the races in America, since these are standardized across the entire country. These show very small numbers of deaths recorded for Blacks from HD in most states. The authors were reluctant to draw any firm conclusions on prevalence from the data.

Perhaps the most interesting study comparing HD in American Blacks and Whites is that of Folstein *et al.* (1987) in Maryland. They found, after intensive attempts to ascertain all cases in the state, that the prevalence in Blacks was at least equal to that in Whites (6.37 compared with 4.94 per 100 000). Interestingly, this similar value is also seen in the death rates for the state given by Hogg *et al.* The Maryland study made the important point that most cases in Blacks were not ascertained through the usual survey methods and would have been missed in many studies. Almost half the cases of HD in Blacks were only ascertained by direct study of family members. Folstein *et al.* made a detailed clinical comparison between HD in Black and White patients and found an earlier onset in Blacks, as had Hayden (1979) previously. There was more severe bradykinesia, more frequent involvement of eye movements, and less severe psychiatric illness. Paternal transmission of early cases was found in both races, while the duration of disease was similar. Because the primary mutational defect is now known to be the same in both, the different genetic background against which the same mutation is acting is likely to be responsible.

It has previously been assumed that most HD in American Blacks is the result of admixture with Caucasian genes, but Folstein *et al.* could trace such an origin in only one of 23 cases. It thus seems likely that HD in American Blacks is longstanding in Black populations, may well be more frequent than is recognized at present, and could at least in part be of African origin. As already mentioned, the question is now of considerable interest in relation to the normal population distribution of trinucleotide repeat numbers at the HD locus. It has also proved of importance in other trinucleotide repeat disorders such as myotonic dystrophy, which is virtually absent in sub-Saharan Africa, (Goldman *et al.* 1996) and where the only documented case (Dada 1973) has proved to show a different haplotype from others worldwide (Krahe *et al.* 1995).

Migration and spread of the HD mutation

The history of the spread of HD in different countries of the world is essentially that of the population movements of their inhabitants. Until now most attention has focused on the origins of the disorder in recently settled countries, but it is equally important to examine the migration patterns in countries where population is long established and, at first sight, more stable.

A very recent finding that may necessitate reassessment of the earlier evidence for HD in African origin families is that of Holmes *et al.* (2001) who have found a novel trinucleotide repeat expansion (HD-L2) in a series of HD-like patients, all of African descent.

HD is frequent in all those countries derived from European settlement in the past three centuries, including the USA, Canada, Australia, and South Africa. The situation for those countries colonized by Spain and Portugal, notably South and Central America, is less clear, partly because accurate prevalence data are not available, possibly also because the immigrants to these countries did not replace the indigenous population genetically to the extent of the first group.

A number of surveys have recorded the origins of the HD families studied, usually in terms of the earliest traceable ancestor. The early American surveys mentioned earlier in the chapter are especially interesting in this respect. The studies of Falstein and Stone (1939) in Illinois and of Marx (1973) in Minnesota both show a predominantly German origin, this being three times more common than a British origin, while in the Michigan study of Reed *et al.* (1958) the two origins were equal. A Scandinavian origin was frequent in the Minnesota study, reflecting the origins of this population. In all these surveys, around half of the families could not be traced back to outside the USA. The Australian population studies show a similarly wide range of origins, showing that multiple introductions of the disorder have occurred in all those countries whose population has been derived from relatively recent immigration.

Equally important is the evidence these studies provide for internal migration. In both America and Australia an origin from other states in the same country is more prominent than origin from a foreign country and reflects, in America especially, the successive waves of settlement involving those already in the country. There is much less evidence regarding migration patterns for those populations generally regarded as stable. The studies in Belgium (Husquinet 1970) and Yorkshire, England (Stevens 1976) show that, while 'foreign' immigration is much less than for the recently settled countries, internal migration is still significant, accounting for around 40 per cent of original ancestors. The South Wales study (Walker 1979) showed similar results, with only 4 per cent of kindreds derived from outside Britain but 43 per cent from outside Wales.

The South Wales study analysed the topic of migration in considerable detail and attempted to compare the findings for HD families with the general population in the area, which underwent considerable population expansion in the century 1820–1920 due to the Industrial Revolution. Of the 100 kindreds for which the earliest ancestor had a known origin, 46 came from the study area of industrial South Wales, 11 from other counties of Wales, while 18 were from the adjacent area of south-west England. By contrast, the general population of industrial South Wales received only half as many immigrants from south-west England as from the rest of Wales at this time so that in terms relative to overall migration there has been a contribution of HD ancestors from south-west England four times that from the rest of Wales.

Table 6.10 Local concentrations of HD due to large individual kindreds

Region	Reference
Lake Maracaibo, Venezuela	Avila-Giron 1973
Tasmania, Australia	Brothers 1949; Pridmore 1990c
Moray Firth, Scotland	Lyon 1962
Gwent, South Wales	Walker *et al*. 1981
Northern Sweden	Sjögren 1936

While it is important to trace the origins of ancestors, it is the migration in each generation that is more relevant to such activities as the maintaining of registers. When the South Wales data were analysed in this way, only 43 of 412 affected individuals were born outside Wales. Emigration as well as immigration can be studied. Seventy-seven per cent of South Wales born patients and 79 per cent of their first-degree relatives at risk were found to have remained in the area, while 8 and 13 per cent, respectively, had migrated out of Wales. For a genetic register it is these relatives at risk that are of particular importance. A loss of around 20 per cent per generation is considerable, but for many populations a much higher proportion could be expected.

The final level at which migration in HD can be analysed is the level of the individual kindred. Since such kindreds will inevitably be extensive, and represent a selected one or few out of many in a region, it is unwise to generalize from them, but their study is of considerable significance to their immediate locality, as indicated earlier in this chapter. The Venezuelan isolate, much the largest of such kindreds, has already been described, but one of the large South Wales families, descended from a single immigrant from outside Wales, is an example of how static such a kindred may be, once it has established itself in a locality. Of the 55 known affected and 177 at-risk descendants, only 24 had moved further than a 10-kilometre distance from the original point of settlement 120 years ago.

Table 6.10 lists some of the well documented concentrations of HD in particular populations that are either known or suspected to be derived from a single founding ancestor. As already mentioned, these local foci of HD can cause a considerable burden for the overall health of the community, especially when the population is isolated and without medical facilities. Now that it is clear from studies worldwide that virtually all cases result from the same mutational mechanism, measures such as presymptomatic or prenatal testing will be considerably easier to offer, although the social attitudes in the population will be the determining factor as to whether such tests prove to be acceptable and to have any effect on long-term prevalence.

Heterozygote and gene frequency

The prevalence of HD and its variation in different populations have been discussed fully above, but a note is required here regarding the frequency of heterozygotes for HD and of the mutation itself. For many genetic disorders these three factors will differ widely from each other. Thus for a common autosomal recessive condition, such as cystic fibrosis, where most of the abnormal genes are present in heterozygotes, the heterozygote frequency is around 100-fold greater than the frequency of the disease (1 in 20–25 compared with 1 in 1600–2000).

For an X-linked recessive disorder such as Duchenne muscular dystrophy, the heterozygous state will be confined to females, themselves essentially unaffected. However, for a rare, fully penetrant, autosomal dominant disorder, where the homozygotes are negligible in frequency and essentially all genes for the disorder are present in heterozygotes, who will show the condition, the disease frequency and heterozygote frequency should be the same.

The reason that this is not the case in HD is the feature that underlies most of the problems in its genetics. Although essentially fully penetrant by old age (see Chapter 5 for discussion of intermediate alleles), most heterozygotes for the HD mutation will be symptomless for most (in some cases all) of their life. Thus only a proportion of heterozygotes in a population will be recognized as being affected at any one time, even though almost all (apart from those with intermediate alleles) will develop the disease if they live long enough. The heterozygote frequency can thus be regarded as equivalent to the birth incidence of those expected to be affected in future—clearly an important figure to be able to measure directly. However, even now that molecular developments have made this technically feasible, there would be strong ethical contraindication to any population survey for the mutation in early life. Even 'anonymous' studies could be open to abuse unless all identification were removed and destroyed prior to the analysis. We thus have to rely on indirect estimates based both on the prevalence, which will be dependent on the particular population studied, and the curve of age at onset, which has proved to be remarkably similar across a wide range of populations.

It can justifiably be asked whether these approaches, devised before the HD mutation was characterized, are still valid now that we know that individuals exist with intermediate alleles whose offspring may be at risk for HD. At present it seems likely that the situation is little changed by this, provided one bears in mind that the results of estimates refer to HD heterozygotes with a repeat number in the 'definite HD range' and do not include those in the 'intermediate allele' category. For the practical purpose of estimating the number of future cases, it is the former that provides the information needed.

Several methods are available for estimating heterozygote frequency using prevalence data; these have been well discussed by Stevens (1973, 1976), Walker *et al.* (1981), and Newcombe (1981) and the formulae are given in these papers. Since the results closely parallel the prevalence estimates for a population, no comprehensive list is given here, but Table 6.11 shows, as an example, the South Wales heterozygote frequency (Walker *et al.* 1981), estimated using a variety of methods. It can be seen that, apart from method 1, based on crude prior risks and not recommended, the others give a reasonably comparable frequency. Method 2, originally

Table 6.11 Heterozygote frequency for HD. Estimates using different methods, based on the South Wales data of Walker *et al.* (1981)

Population studied	1 720 901
No. of affected living	131
Prevalence	7.61 per 100 000
Estimate of heterozygote frequency (see text for details)	
1	34.9
2	17.2
3	24.9–26.8
4	15.8–19.1
5	20.2

used by Reed *et al.* (1958) and corresponding to method A of Stevens (1973), utilizes the age-at-onset distribution uncorrected, while method 3 (method B of Stevens) derives age-dependent risks for each individual and was used first by Reed and Neel (1959). Method 4 (Stevens method C) introduces an allowance for age at onset in a particular parent, while the age-at-onset curve is adjusted to account for individuals likely to be unascertained because they have yet to develop the disorder (Newcombe 1981).

Regardless of the method used, the main question those studying HD wish to know is: how much greater is the heterozygote frequency (representing birth incidence) than the prevalence? Fortunately, there is close agreement on this between studies. The analysis of Walker *et al.* (1981) gave a value of 2.6, agreeing closely with those of 2.4–2.7 from other studies.

In summary, it is reasonable to take as a rough guide for heterozygote frequency a value of 2.5 times the prevalence estimate. To put the figures for heterozygote frequency in a different way, there are likely to be 150 asymptomatic gene carriers for every 100 affected individuals. The gene frequency will simply be half the heterozygote frequency, since everyone has two alleles at each locus. Conneally (1984) has shown that the number of individuals at risk for HD in a population (including only first-degree relatives) is around five times the number of affected, that is, twice the heterozygote frequency. This is to be expected as for every symptomless or affected gene carrier there will be one sib who has not inherited the HD gene.

Fertility and genetic fitness

All genetic disorders are subject to a balance between genes that enter a population by new mutation and migration, and those genes lost through early mortality or failure to reproduce. If we are to understand why a disorder such as HD is more common in some populations than in others, whether there has been in the past or still is an increase or decrease in the frequency, and whether genetic counselling or other newly introduced measures are altering the previous state, we must first understand as fully and accurately as possible the factors involved in this delicate balance. The actual mechanisms involved are discussed in Chapter 5.

Unfortunately, for those undertaking such studies, the balance is not a static one, but is likely to vary with time and with the population involved. We also need not only accurate and unbiased data from HD families, but equivalent information from the normal population, which may not be available in comparable form. It is thus not surprising that our information on this subject, while extensive, is variable and at times contradictory, but it is worth making a critical evaluation of it here. All of these data were collected before the HD mutation was identified. The recent suggestion, based on its unstable nature, that HD might actually be increasing in frequency over the centuries (Rubinsztein *et al.* 1994) and the quantitative analysis of population flow between different repeat numbers (Falush *et al.* 2001) make these data on fertility still of relevance.

Before proceeding further it is important to clarify definitions that may be confusing to the nongeneticist. By 'fertility' is meant the mean number of offspring born to an individual with the condition under study. In making an estimate for a disorder such as HD, only live births are generally included, and data are often restricted to those considered likely to have completed their families (for example, those aged over 45 years). It is important to include individuals who have never married and to avoid biases such as overascertainment of large families and combining data from widely different dates.

Genetic fitness differs from fertility in considering the reproduction of those possessing the HD gene rather than those who are or later become affected. Until now it has not been possible to estimate genetic fitness directly, but it can be derived from estimates of fertility in the same way as can the heterozygote frequency from estimates of prevalence. Since almost all HD genes are present in heterozygotes, who will eventually develop the disorder if they live long enough, it matters little whether fitness or fertility is used as the measure, provided like is compared with like. Finally, while fitness is a relative measure, using genetically normal relatives (usually sibs) as a comparison, fertility estimates may be relative or absolute, these latter using appropriate normal population data as the control group.

The results of the main studies on fertility and fitness in HD are summarized in Table 6.12. It can be seen that they vary considerably and that, taking a value of 1.0 as 'normal', some show a reduction, some are close to normal, and others are actually increased. However, all are agreed on one point: compared with most serious genetic disorders the values are high, supporting the basic clinical observation that most patients reproduce and that onset of the disorder is commonly after a family has been completed.

It is worth examining in more detail some of the individual studies and asking why they should differ so considerably in some of their conclusions. The first major study was that of Reed and Neel (1959), based on a survey in Michigan, USA, and a model of thoroughness and for reported detailed data. The most striking finding was reduced fertility and fitness of male HD affected individuals compared with females, and compared with either sex in the general population. This was partly due to a higher proportion of male patients who never married (26 per cent versus 8 per cent of females). When unaffected sibs were used as comparison, however, the reduction in male genetic fitness was much less, while female choreics were significantly more fit than their unaffected sibs.

Table 6.12 Fertility and genetic fitness in HD

	Fertility			Fitness		
	Overall	Male	Female	Overall	Male	Female
Studies showing decrease						
Kishimoto *et al.* 1959	—	—	—	0.65	0.61	0.68
Reed and Neel 1959	0.82	0.66	0.98	1.03	0.82	1.25
Stine and Smith 1990		(coefficient of selection 0.36)				
Studies showing increase						
Marx 1973	1.16	0.95	1.40	—	0.99	1.39
Shokeir 1975	1.14	—	—	1.38	—	—
Stevens 1976	1.36	1.09	1.61	1.39	1.03	1.52
Walker 1979	1.25–1.34	1.43–1.55	1.0–1.30	1.46	1.66	1.29
Walker *et al.* (1983)*						
Studies showing close to normal level						
Wendt and Drohm 1972	0.95	0.93	0.96	0.96	0.93	1.03
Wallace and Parker 1973	1.0	0.88	1.13	1.28	1.11	1.52
Mattsson 1974	—	—	—	0.97	0.87	1.07
Mastromauro *et al.* (1989)	—	1.05	1.07	—	1.01	0.98

*General population estimates divided by decades of birth.

Taking the sexes together, there was no difference between affected and unaffected. Reed and Neel's (1959) other major finding was that unaffected sibs also showed reduced fertility in comparison with the general population. They suggested that this might reflect a general deterrence from reproduction by those at risk, affecting equally those with and without the HD gene. However, it could be that their general population data, although carefully chosen, were inappropriate, as most later studies have shown no marked differences between unaffected sibs and population data. Thus it remains open whether their study should be interpreted as showing a reduced fertility (most marked in males) based on the absolute data, or a near-normal fertility (somewhat increased in females) based on the comparisons with sibs.

One other early study, that of Kishimoto *et al*. (1957, 1959), also showed a reduced fertility; cousins were used for comparison but no detailed data were given. Given the much rarer prevalence of HD in Japan and the different social structures, a more detailed study is needed. A third and more recent study, which appears to show reduced genetic fitness in HD, used an entirely different approach. Stine and Smith (1990) analysed HD in the Afrikaner population of South Africa. Based on the proportion of current patients with HD whose descent could be traced or original founders of the population, they estimated that this was less than would have been predicted from the known expansion of the Afrikaner population as a whole, suggesting some selective disadvantage to the HD gene. By contrast, no significant disadvantage was found for another autosomal dominant disorder common in the population, porphyria variegata.

The series of papers showing an apparent increase in fertility and fitness now requires examination. Two are from North America (Marx 1973; Shokeir 1975) and two from the UK (Stevens 1976; Walker *et al*. 1983). An increased fitness for the HD gene should imply some selective biological advantage, and would be highly unusual for a dominantly inherited genetic disorder. If this situation were maintained, a gradual replacement of the normal allele by the HD allele could be expected, a somewhat implausible situation, although raised again more recently (Rubinsztein *et al*. 1994) in light of the unstable nature of the mutation.

Criticisms of these findings have included bias from large families, where affected members are likely to have reproduced preferentially, the inappropriate use of unaffected sibs as controls, and inclusion of older data where non-reproducing affected patients may be underrepresented. While these are valid points, it is difficult to explain the finding of increased fertility as entirely due to bias. Thus, in the study of Walker *et al*. (1983), the control values of normal sibs, normal second-degree relatives, and general population data were all closely comparable, while the ascertainment was close to complete, at least for recent cases. This study did not show the sex differences for marriage and reproduction found by Reed and Neel (1959), nor was there any difference in the data for patients whose main clinical features were psychiatric compared with those whose presentation was principally neurological. There were no detectable differences in the pattern of family building and no evidence of clustering of births in the years preceding onset that might have suggested an effect of behavioural changes in this period.

Several studies have shown no clear difference in fertility and fitness estimates between HD and normal individuals. These include two European reports (Wendt and Drohm 1972; Mattsson 1974), one from Australia (Wallace and Parker 1973), and one from North America (Mastromauro *et al*. 1989). The Australian study did, however, show a lowered male reproductive rate due to failure to marry. Wallace (1976) has discussed the various social reasons that could underlie this. The most recent study, that of Mastromauro *et al*. (1989), found no differences between unaffected sibs and the general population. This may well be the last such study to be performed before population dynamics are altered by the widespread use of presymptomatic testing for the gene.

Taking all these studies together, a reasonable conclusion is that the HD mutation has little if any biological disadvantage, but neither is there definite evidence of any specific factors on which to base a possible reproductive advantage. It seems quite possible that, during a century where the normal family size has declined dramatically, and which has seen striking population increases associated with migration, the balance may have varied from time to time and from place to place as to whether the HD mutation has had a slight relative advantage or disadvantage. These same variations have made it impossible to provide entirely satisfactory matching normal data; but despite these drawbacks the various studies will be of long-term value in allowing comparison with future changes resulting from genetic prediction. It can certainly be concluded that the HD mutation is unlikely to decline or die out spontaneously. Whether any true tendency for its frequency to increase as a result of genetic instability exists, as suggested by Rubinsztein *et al.* (1994), remains to be proven.

The molecular epidemiology of HD

Almost all the population studies of HD cited in this chapter were carried out before the 1993 discovery of its genetic and mutational basis. This discovery in no way invalidates the data, but it does have a profound effect on its interpretation. Even before the identification of the HD gene, genetic linkage data had shown that only a single major genetic locus was involved (Gusella *et al.* 1983; Conneally *et al.* 1989). The recognition of specific haplotypes made it unlikely that HD had a single origin worldwide, though it was considered that the number of different mutations was small.

At this time, the concept of mutation in HD was that expected for most Mendelian disorders: a number of specific and differing changes in the gene affecting its function, probably mainly point mutations as there was a complete absence of visible chromosome abnormality associated with the disease. A situation comparable to that seen in cystic fibrosis might have been predicted, with one frequent mutation and a number of rare ones. Such a situation would have allowed studies of the different mutational patterns in different populations, possibly showing broad geographical trends and correlations with prevalence. Such studies have proved of great interest in relation to the spread of other genetic disorders, such as phenylketonuria, cystic fibrosis, and haemoglobinopathies. Where apparently identical mutations have been found in widely separate populations, haplotype studies have in some cases been able to resolve the question of whether they had a common descent or not, as with the inherited amyloid mutations in Portugal and Scandinavia.

Once HD was recognized as being due to an expanded and unstable trinucleotide (CAG) sequence, a radically different concept of mutation was required, necessitating a reassessment of our views on the origins of HD and its prevalence in different populations. The molecular details and patterns of genetic transmission of this mutation are discussed in Chapter 5, but the significance for epidemiological studies and concepts needs consideration here.

The first point of relevance is that essentially all cases of HD worldwide are due to the same mutational mechanism and show an identical, although variable in extent, CAG repeat expansion. This has a great practical advantage in allowing molecular testing anywhere in the world, but it also means that there is no immediate way of using the mutation itself to determine origin.

What is clear now is that all overt cases of HD ultimately have an ancestral origin from healthy individuals who carry an 'intermediate allele', with a repeat number in between the normal range and that causing disease. This means that there is no longer any need to search for or to postulate affected individuals as the ancestors who may have introduced the gene. Since all populations contain a small proportion of individuals with repeat numbers in or approaching this range, it is also much more likely that cases of HD in a stably populated country will have an indigenous origin from such individuals, with gradual increase over many generations until the clinically significant range is reached. Of course, migration cannot be dismissed, especially for small populations and where there is historical evidence, but there is no longer any necessity for such migration to have occurred in the explanation of the overall distribution of HD.

The normal CAG range and population frequency of HD

The extensive migrations of recent centuries can, as shown above, account for much of the variation in prevalence between different regions and even countries. This variation can be considerable when the additional factors of genetic drift and founder effect have been operating, especially for small, isolated, or rapidly increasing populations.

It is likely, however, that these variations are based on more fundamental differences between the major ethnic groups and that these may be related to the normal population variation at the HD locus. It is already clear that the prevalence of HD in Japan (and possibly in other, less well documented East Asian countries) is an order of magnitude less than for Caucasian populations. A low prevalence also seems likely in sub-Saharan Africa, though the higher prevalence in American Blacks may argue against this.

Evidence is now becoming available from studies of the normal range of CAG repeats in different populations that supports the view that population prevalence of HD may relate to the frequency of alleles in the higher normal range, these acting as a source over many generations of still higher repeat number alleles that become significantly unstable and lead ultimately to the range of repeat number producing clinical HD (see Chapter 5). Although most initial reports designed to distinguish the normal and HD repeat ranges have been insufficient in number to give conclusive information, a number of studies have now specifically examined the normal population distributions, in some cases comparing several different trinucleotide repeat loci, notably those for DRPLA and myotonic dystrophy as well as HD.

The main conclusions that can be drawn from these studies (Rubinzstein *et al.* 1994; Watkins *et al.* 1995) are that the normal distribution of HD CAG repeat alleles in Caucasians shows a larger proportion of higher repeat number alleles compared with that in either Asian or African populations, supporting the hypothesis that the frequency of HD is related to the frequency of such normal alleles. Further support comes from the finding that for DRPLA, a disorder particularly frequent in Japan, Japanese and other Asian populations show a greater proportion of higher repeat number normal alleles (Watkins *et al.* 1995; Deka *et al.* 1995). Likewise, the studies of myotonic dystrophy, virtually absent in sub-Saharan Africa, show the same relationship with normal variation at the locus, with a deficiency of high repeat number alleles in African populations (Goldman *et al.* 1996).

A separate approach to the distant origins of HD in different populations comes from the study of detailed genetic haplotypes. Variation in and around the HD gene allows a composite genetic profile to be built up that can identify mutations with a common origin, even though the actual HD mutation is identical worldwide. Particularly useful for this are the CCG repeat adjacent to the CAG expansion and the glutamic acid polymorphism Δ 2642 (Almqvist *et al.* 1995). Differences in haplotype can be used to distinguish lineages of more recent origin as well as differences between major ethnic groups. The main conclusion to be drawn is that most populations, even individual countries such as Sweden (Almqvist *et al.* 1994), show several haplotypes, indicating that HD has arisen repeatedly on different genetic backgrounds (Andrew *et al.* 1993; Squitieri *et al.* 1994), rather than resulting from a unique ancestral event as appears to be the case in myotonic dystrophy. The possible role of these polymorphisms as modifiers of the HD phenotype is addressed in Chapter 5.

In summarizing our understanding of the epidemiology of HD in the light of molecular advances, the following points now seem clear, at least in principle, if not in detail.

1. At a local or small population level, the prevalence of HD is greatly dependent on such local factors as presence of one or a few unusually large kindreds, and on population movements in the area.

2. At the level of larger populations (that is, over 5 million) or specific countries the prevalence is relatively uniform within a major ethnic group (at least for Caucasian populations) and such differences that are observed are as likely to result from variable ascertainment as from true differences. Populations with rapid recent expansion from a few founders may be exceptions. At this level haplotype data suggest multiple origins of the disorder and even rigorous ascertainment will not be complete on account of the continuing emergence of new cases from healthy parents carrying intermediate alleles.

3. Variations in the normal distribution of CAG repeat lengths are likely to affect only differences between the major ethnic groupings, rather than being responsible for differences within such groups. It seems likely that such CAG repeat length differences underlie the 10-fold prevalence difference between Japan and Caucasian populations, and possibly the less securely documented low prevalence in other East Asian and African countries.

Population effects of genetic testing

A final relevant question is whether the use of molecular analysis as a criterion for diagnosis of HD is likely to have a major effect on prevalence estimates. Almost all the data given in this chapter are based on studies prior to identification of the mutation. The two recent studies from Japan both confirmed the previous low estimates, while a study from Northern Ireland (Morrison and Nevin 1993) showed a prevalence only slightly higher than a study of the same population 6 years before, though the actual prevalence dates used were separated by 26 years.

One difference that is likely to result from the use of molecular diagnosis is in the age of onset distribution of the disorder. Mutation analysis has allowed the recognition of HD in elderly individuals, often without a clear family history of the disorder, who would often not have been diagnosed on clinical grounds during their lifetime, and thus would not have been represented in earlier studies.

It is still too early to assess any effects on prevalence of prenatal diagnosis or of family limitation associated with genetic counselling, though some approximate information on births at risk can be obtained from the prospective use of genetic registers. Again, the previously unsuspected existence of cases with onset in old age, together with transmission of the disorder by individuals with intermediate alleles will result in a considerable number of individuals among their descendants already born with the mutation, before there is any recognition of the existence of HD in the kindred. The observation from the UK Huntington's Prediction Consortium that only around 15 per cent of those at high risk undergo predictive testing (Harper *et al.* 2000), while the use of prenatal diagnosis is extremely low (Simpson and Harper 2001), suggests that the use of molecular techniques is not likely to have major short-term effects on the prevalence of either the mutation or the clinical disorder.

If the possibility that a tendency may exist towards intergenerational expansion of CAG repeats in the upper normal range is added to all these variables (Rubinsztein *et al.* 1994), it can be seen that the prediction of future trends in the prevalence of HD and of the underlying subclinical but unstable mutations is extremely uncertain. Nevertheless, our knowledge of the mutational basis of HD has provided an explanation for at least some of the major population differences, as well as resolving many of the previously puzzling genetic features of the disorder, which were the subject of the last chapter.

References

Adachi Y and Nakashima K (1999) Population genetic study of Huntington's disease-prevalence and founder's effect in the San-in area, western Japan. *Nippon Rinsho—Japanese Journal of Clinical Medicine* **57** (4):900–904.

Almqvist E, Andre S, Theilmann J, Goldberg P, Zeisler J, Drugge U, Grandell U, Tapper-Persson M, Winblad B, Hayden M *et al.* (1994) Geographical distribution of haplotypes in Swedish families with Huntington's disease. *Human Genetics* **94** (2):124–128.

—— Spence N, Nichol K, Andrew SE, Vesa J, Peltonen L, Anvret M, Goto J, Kanazawa I, Goldberg YP *et al.* (1995) Ancestral differences in the distribution of the delta 2642 glutamic acid polymorphism is associated with varying CAG repeat lengths on normal chromosomes: insights into the genetic evolution of Huntington disease. *Human Molecular Genetics* **42** (2):207–214.

Almqvist EEW, Elterman DS, MacLeod PM and Hayden MR (2001) High incidence rate and absent family histories in one quarter of patients newly diagnosed with Huntington disease in British Columbia. *Clinical Genetics* **60**:198–205.

Andrew S, Theilmann J, Almqvist E, Norremolle A, Lucotte G, Anvret M, Sorensen SA, Turpin JC and Hayden MR (1993) DNA analysis of distinct populations suggests multiple origins for the mutation causing Huntington disease. *Clinical Genetics* **43** (6):286–294.

Archibald CH (1938) Huntington's chorea in Canada. *National Health Review* **6**:19–21.

Arena R, Nuti M and Iudice A (1979) Rilievi epidemiologici della corea di Huntington nella Toscanna nord-occidentale. *Atti 5 Riun Limpe* 123–133.

Arostegui G (1890) De la corea cronica progressiva. *Crónica Médico-quirúrgica Habana* **16**:74.

Avila Giron R (1973) Medical and social aspects of Huntington's chorea in the State of Zulia, Venezuela. In: *Advances in Neurology*, Vol. 1 (eds A Barbeau, TN Chase and GW Paulson), pp. 261–266. New York: Raven Press.

Barbeau A and Fullum G (1962) Origin and migration of Huntington's chorea in Canada: preliminary report. *Canadian Medical Association Journal* **87**:1242–1243.

—— Witeux C, Trudeau JG and Fullum G (1964) La chorée de Huntington chez les canadiens français: étude préliminaire. *Union Medicale du Canada* **93**:1178–1182.

Bayulkem F and Turek I (1961) Huntington's chorea in Turkey. *Psychiatric Quarterly* **35**:358–360.

Beaubrun MH (1962) Huntington's chorea in Trinidad. *Caribbean Medical Journal* **24**:45–50.

Bickford JAR and Ellison RM (1953) High incidence of Huntington's chorea in the Duchy of Cornwall. *Journal of Mental Science* **99**:291–294.

Bohlega S, McLean D, Omer S *et al.* (1995) Huntington's disease in Saudi Arabia. *Journal of Medical Genetics* **32**:325.

Bolt JMW (1970) Huntington's chorea in the west of Scotland. *British Journal of Psychiatry* **116**:259–270.

Brothers CRD (1949) The history and incidence of Huntington's chorea in Tasmania. *Proceedings of the Royal Australian College of Physicians* **4**:48–50.

—— (1964) Huntington's chorea in Victoria and Tasmania. *Journal of the Neurological Sciences* **i**:405–420.

—— Meadows AW (1955) An investigation of Huntington's chorea. *Victoria Journal of Medical Science* **101**:548–563.

Cameron D and Venters GA (1967) Some problems in Huntington's chorea. *Scottish Medical Journal* **12**:152–156.

Caro AJ (1977) *Huntington's Chorea; A Clinical Problem in East Anglia*. PhD thesis, University of East Anglia.

—— Haines S (1975) The history of Huntington's chorea. *Update* **11**:91–95.

Cassar P (1967) Huntington's chorea with special reference to its incidence in Malta. *St Luke's Hospital Gazette* June, pp. 3–13.

Cendrowski W (1964) Some remarks on the geography of Huntington's chorea. *Neurology Minneapolis* **14**:839–843.

Chan V, Yu YL, Chan TP, Yip B, Chang CM, Wong MT, Chan YW and Chan TK (1995) DNA analysis of Huntington's disease in southern Chinese. *Journal of Medical Genetics* **32** (2):120–124.

Chang CM, Yu YL, Fong KY, Wong MT, Chan YW, Ng TH, Leung CM and Chan V (1994) Huntington's disease in Hong Kong Chinese: epidemiology and clinical picture. *Clinical and Experimental Neurology* **31**:43–51.

Chhutani PN (1957) Huntington's chorea in India. *Journal of the Indian Medical Association* **29**:156–157.

Chiu E and Teltscher B (1978) Huntington's disease: the establishment of a national register. *Medical Journal of Australia* **2**:394–396.

Clarke CK and MacArthur JW (1924) Four generations of hereditary chorea. *Journal of Heredity* **15**:303–306.

Conneally PM (1984) Huntington's disease: genetics and epidemiology. *American Journal of Human Genetics* **36**:506–526.

—— Haines J, Tanzi R *et al.* (1989) No evidence of linkage heterogeneity between Huntington disease (HD) and G8 (D4310). *Genomics* **5**, 304–308.

Couto M (1891) Da corea de Huntington. *Brasil-Médico* **5**:341–344.

Craufurd D and Tyler A (1992) Predictive testing for Huntington's disease: protocol of the UK Huntington's Prediction Consortium. *Journal of Medical Genetics* **29**:915–918.

Critchley M (1934) Huntington's chorea and East Anglia. *Journal of State Medicine* **42**:575–587.

Cruz-Coke R (1987) Epidemiologica genetica de Corea de Huntington en Chile. *Review of Medicine Chile* **115**:483–485.

Dada TO (1973) Dystrophia myotonica in a Nigerian family. *East African Medical Journal* **50**:213–227.

Davenport CB and Muncey EB (1916) Huntington's chorea in relation to heredity and eugenics. *Eugenics Record Office Bulletin* **17**:195–222.

Deka R, Miki T, Yin SJ *et al.* (1995) Normal CAG repeat variation at the DRPLA locus in world populations. *American Journal of Human Genetics* **57**:508–511.

Entres JL (1921) *Zur Klinik und Vererbung der Huntington'schen Chorea. Monographien des Gesamtgebietes der Neurologie und Psychiatrie*, Vol. 27. Berlin: Springer.

European Community Huntington's Disease Collaborative Study Group (1993) Ethical and social issues in presymptomatic testing for Huntington's disease. *Journal of Medical Genetics* **30**:1028–1035.

Falstein EI and Stone H (1939) Huntington's chorea as a psychiatric and social problem in Illinois. *Illinois Medical Journal* **75**:164–168.

Falush D, Almqvist EW, Brinkmann RR, Iwasa Y and Hayden MR (2001) Measurement of mutational flow implies both a high new-mutation rate for Huntington disease and substantial underascertainment of late-onset cases. *American Journal of Human Genetics* **68**:373–385.

Folstein SE (1989) *Huntington's disease: a disorder of families.* Baltimore, MA: Johns Hopkins Press.

—— Chase GA, Wahl WE, McDonnell AM and Folstein MF (1987) Huntington's disease in Maryland: clinical aspects of racial variation. *American Journal of Human Genetics* **41**:168–179.

Frontali M, Malaspina P, Rossi C *et al.* (1990) Epidemiological and linkage studies on Huntington's disease in Italy. *Human Genetics* **85**:165–170.

Gale F and Bennett JH (1969) Huntington's chorea in a South Australian community of aboriginal descent. *Medical Journal of Australia* **2**:482–484.

Gersting JM, Conneally PM and Yount EA (1984) Huntington's disease research roster data base support with MEGADATS-3m. *Journal of Medical Systems Supplement* **8**:163–172.

Glendinning N (1975) *A study in Huntington's chorea.* MD thesis, University of London.

Goldman A, Ramsay M and Jenkins T (1996) Ethnicity and myotonic dystrophy: a possible explanation for its absence in sub-Saharan Africa. *Annals of Human Genetics* **60**:57–65.

Groppi C, Barontini F, Braco L, Sita D, Inzitari D, Amadulli L and Fratiglioni L (1986) Huntington's chorea: a prevalence study in the Florence area. *Acta Psychiatrica Scandinavica* **74**:266–268.

Grunitzky EK, Gnamey DR, Nonon SA and Balogou A (1995) Huntington disease in a large family in southern Togo. *Annales de Medecine Interne* **146** (8):581–583.

Gudmundsson KR (1969) Prevalence and occurrence of some rare neurological diseases in Iceland. *Acta Neurologica Scandinavica* **45**:114–118.

Gusella JF, Wexler NS, Conneally PM *et al.* (1983) A polymorphic DNA marker genetically linked to Huntington's disease. *Nature* **306**:234–238.

Haddock RDW (1973) Neurological disorders in Ghana. In: *Tropical Neurology* (ed. JD Spillane), pp. 143–160. Oxford: Oxford University Press.

Hall JG and Te-Juceto L (1983) Association between age of onset and paternal inheritance in Huntington's chorea. *American Journal of Medical Genetics* **16**:289–290.

Harper PS (1976) Genetic variation in Wales. *Journal of the Royal College of Physicians of London* **10**:321–332.

—— (1978) Benign hereditary chorea, clinical and genetic aspects. *Clinical Genetics* **13**:85–95.

—— (1986) The prevention of Huntington's chorea. The Milroy Lecture 1985. *Journal of the Royal College of Physicians of London* **20**:7–14.

—— (1992) The epidemiology of Huntington's disease. *Human Genetics* **89**:365–376.

—— (ed.) (1996) *Huntington's disease*, 2nd edn. London: W.B. Saunders.

—— (1996) New genes for old diseases: the molecular basis of myotonic dystrophy and Huntington's disease. *Journal of the Royal College of Physicians* **30**:221–231.

—— and Sarfarazi M (1985) Genetic prediction and family structure in Huntington's chorea. *British Medical Journal* **290**:1929–1931.

—— and Sunderland E (1984) *Population and genetic studies in Wales.* Cardiff: University of Wales Press.

—— Walker DA, Tyler A, Newcombe RG and Davies K (1979) Huntington's chorea. The basis for long-term prevention. *Lancet* **ii**:346–349.

Harper PS, Tyler A, Smith S, Jones P, Newcombe R and McBroom V (1981) Decline in the predicted incidence of Huntington's chorea associated with systematic genetic counselling and family support. *Lancet* **ii**:411–413.

—— —— Smith S, Jones P, Newcombe RG and McBroom V (1982) A genetic register for Huntington's chorea in South Wales. *Journal of Medical Genetics* **19**:241–245.

—— Youngman S, Anderson MA *et al.* (1985) Genetic linkage between Huntington's disease and the DNA polymorphism G8 in South Wales families. *Journal of Medical Genetics* **22**:447–450.

—— Quarrell WJ and Youngman S (1988) Huntington's disease: prediction and prevention. *Philosophical Transactions of the Royal Society. London* **319**:285–298.

—— Lim C, Craufurd D, on behalf of the UK Huntington's Disease Prediction Consortium (2000) Ten years of presymptomatic testing for Huntington's disease: the experience of the UK Huntington's Disease Prediction Consortium. *Journal of Medical Genetics* **37** (8):567–571.

Harries JR (1973) Neurological disorders in Kenya. In: *Tropical neurology* (ed. JD Spillane), pp. 207–222. Oxford: Oxford University Press.

Hattie WH (1909) Huntington's chorea. *Proceedings of the American Medical–Psychological Association* **16**:171–176.

Hayden MR (1979) *Huntington's Chorea in South Africa*. PhD thesis, University of Cape Town.

—— (1981) *Huntington's Chorea*. Berlin: Springer.

—— Hopkins HC, Macrae M and Beighton PH (1980a) The origin of Huntington's chorea in the Afrikaner population of South Africa. *South Africa Medical Journal* **58**:197–200.

—— MacGregor JM and Beighton PH (1980b) The prevalence of Huntington's chorea in South Africa. *South Africa Medical Journal* **58**:193–196.

Heathfield KWG (1967) Huntington's chorea: investigation into the prevalence of disease in the area covered by the North East Metropolitan Board. *Brain* **90**:203–232.

—— MacKenzie ICK (1971) Huntington's chorea in Bedfordshire. *Guys Hospital Reports* **120**:295–310.

Hetherington HB and Wechsler Z (1942) Huntington's chorea in a native Melanesian family of the British Solomon Islands. *Medical Journal of Australia* **1**:599–600.

Hogg JE, Massey EW and Schoenberg BS (1979) Mortality from Huntington's disease in the United States. *Advances in Neurology* **23**:27–33.

Huntington's Disease Collaborative Research Group (1993) A novel gene containing a trinucleotide repeat that is expanded and unstable in Huntington's disease chromosomes. *Cell* **72**:971–983.

Husquinet H (1970) La chorée de Huntington dans les 4 provinces Belges. In: *Comptes rendues 67 ième Congres Psychiatrie et Neurologie, langue francais* (ed. P Warot), pp. 1079–1118. Paris: Masson.

Hutton PW (1956) Neurological disease in Uganda. *East African Medical Journal* **33**:209–223.

Ikonen E, Palo J and Ott J (1990) Huntington's disease in Finland: linkage disequilibrium of chromosome 4RFLP haplotypes and exclusion of a tight linkage between the disease and D4S43 locus. *American Journal of Human Genetics* **46**:5–11.

Ikonen E, Ignatius J, Norio R *et al.* (1992) Huntington disease in Finland: a molecular and genealogical study. *Human Genetics* **89**:275–280.

Jelliffe SE (1908) A contribution to the history of Huntington's chorea: a preliminary report. *Neurographs* **1**:116–124.

Joubert J and Botha MC (1988) Huntington's disease in South African blacks: a report of 8 cases. *South Africa Medical Journal* **73**:489–494.

Kanazawa I (1983) *Prevalence Rate of Huntington's Disease in Ibaraki Prefecture*. Annual report of research committee of CNS degenerative diseases, Ministry of Health and Welfare of Japan, pp. 151–156.

Khosla SN and Arora BS (1973) Huntington's chorea—a clinical study. *Journal of the Association of Physicians of India* **21**:247–250.

Kishimoto K, Nakamura M and Sotokawa Y (1957) Population genetics study—Huntington's chorea in Japan. *Annual Report, Research Institute of Environmental Medicine* **9**:195–211.

Kishimoto K, Nakamura M and Sotokawa Y (1959) On population genetics of Huntington's chorea in Japan. In: *International Congress of Neurological Science* (ed L. Van Bogaert and J Radermecker), Vol. 4, pp. 217–226. London: Pergamon Press.

Klintworth GK (1962) Huntington's chorea in South Africa: a preliminary communication drawing attention to its frequent occurrence. *South African Medical Journal* **36**:896–898.

Kokmen E, Ozekmekci FS, Beard CM, O'Brien PC and Kurland LT (1994) Incidence and prevalence of Huntington's disease in Olmstead County, Minnesota (1950 through 1989) *Archives of Neurology* **51** (7):696–698.

Korenyi C and Whittier JR (1977) Huntington's disease (chorea) in New York State. *New York State Journal of Medicine* **77**:44–45.

Kozlova SI, Dadali EL, Prytkov AN *et al.* (1986) Population, demographic and clinical–genetic studies of the Huntington disease in an Azerbaijan local region. *Genetika* **22**:2534–2539.

Krahe R, Eckhart M, Ogunniyi AO *et al.* (1995) *De novo* myotonic dystrophy mutation in a Nigerian kindred. *American Journal of Human Genetics* **56**:1067–1074.

Kurland LT (1958) Descriptive epidemiology of selected neurologic and myopathic disorders with particular reference to a survey in Rochester, Minnesota. *Journal of Chronic Disorders* **8**:378–418.

Kurtzke JF (1979) Huntington's disease: mortality and morbidity data from outside the United States. *Advances in Neurology* **23**:13–25.

Lanska DJ, Levine L, Lanska MJ and Schoenberg BS (1988) Huntington's disease mortality in the United States. *Neurology* **38**:769–772.

Lee MK, Ng WK and Jeyakumar D (1994) Huntington disease: report of first case documented in Malaysia. *Medical Journal of Malaysia* **49** (3):297–300.

Leger JM, Ranouil R and Vallat JN (1974) Huntington's chorea in Limousin: statistical and clinical study. *Revue Medicale de Limoges* **5**:147–153.

Leung CM, Chan YW, Chan CM *et al.* (1992) Huntington's disease in Chinese: a hypothesis of its origin. *Journal of Neurology, Neurosurgery and Psychiatry* **55**:681–684.

Lyon RL (1962) Huntington's chorea in the Moray Firth area. *British Medical Journal* **i**:1301–1306.

MacKay M (1904) Hereditary chorea in eighteen members of a family, with a report of three cases. *Medical News* **85**:496–499.

MacMillan J and Harper PS (1991) Single-gene neurological disorders in South Wales: an epidemiological study. *Annals of Neurology* **30**:411–414.

MacMillan JC, Snell RG, Houlihan GD *et al.* (1993) Molecular analysis and clinical correlations of the Huntington's disease mutation. *Lancet* **342**:954–958.

Mainini P, Lucci B, Guidetti D and Casoli C (1982) Prevalenzia della mallattia di Huntington nelle Provincie di Reggio Emilia e Parma.

Marx RN (1973) Huntington's chorea in Minnesota. *Advances in Neurology* **1**:237–243.

Mastromauro CA, Meissen GJ, Cupples LA, Berkman B and Myers RH (1989) Estimation of fertility and fitness in Huntington's disease in New England. *American Journal of Medical Genetics* **33**:248–254.

Mattsson B (1974) Huntington's chorea in Sweden. 1. Prevalence and genetic data. *Acta Psychiatrica Scandinavica. Supplementum* **255**:211–255.

Morris M, Tyler A and Harper PS (1988) Adoption and genetic prediction for Huntington's disease. *Lancet* **ii**:1069–1070.

—— Tyler A, Lazarou L, Meredith L and Harper PS (1989) Problems in genetic prediction for Huntington's disease. *Lancet* **ii**:601–603.

Morrison PJ, Johnston WP and Nevin NC (1995) The epidemiology of Huntington's disease in Northern Ireland *Journal of Medical Genetics* **32**:524–530.

—— Nevin NC (1993) Huntington disease in County Donegal: epidemiological trends over four decades *Ulster Medical Journal* **62** (2):141–144.

Myrianthopoulos NC (1973) Huntington's chorea: the genetic problems five years later. *Advances in Neurology* **1**:150–152.

Nakashima K, Watanabe Y, Kusumi M, Nanba E, Maeoka Y, Igo M, Irie H, Ishino H, Fujimoto A, Kobayashi S *et al.* (1995) Prevalence and founder effect of Huntington's disease in the San-in area of Japan (1995). *Rinsho Shinkeigaku—Clinical Neurology* **35** (12):1532–1534.

—— Watanabe Y, Kusumi M, Nanba E, Maeoka Y, Nakagawa M, Igo M, Irie H, Ishino H, Fujimoto A, Goto J and Takahashi K (1996) Epidemiological and genetic studies of Huntington's disease in the San-in area of Japan. *Neuroepidemiology* **15** (3):126–131.

Narabayashi H (1973) Huntington's chorea in Japan: review of the literature. *Advances in Neurology* **1**:253–259.

Newcombe RG, Walker DA and Harper PS (1981) Factors influencing age at onset and duration of survival in Huntington's chorea. *Annals of Human Genetics* **45**:387–396.

Office of Health Economics (1980) Huntington's chorea. Publication 67, pp. 1–35. London: OHE.

Oliver JE (1970) Huntington's chorea in Northamptonshire. *British Journal of Psychiatry* **116**:241–253.

Osuntoken BO (1973) Neurological disorders in Nigeria. In: *Tropical neurology* (ed. JD Spillane), pp. 161–190. Oxford: Oxford University Press.

Palo J, Somer H, Ikonen E, Karila L and Peltonen L (1987) Low prevalence of Huntington's disease in Finland. *Lancet* **ii**:805–806.

Panse F (1942) *Die Erbchorea: eine klinische-genetische Studie.* Leipzig: Thieme.

Parker N (1958) Observation on Huntington's chorea based on a Queensland survey. *Medical Journal of Australia* **45**:351–359.

Pearson JS, Petersen MC, Lazarte JA, Blodgett HE and Kley IB (1955) An educational approach to the social problem of Huntington's chorea. *Proceedings of the Mayo Clinic* **30**:349–357.

Penney JB, Young AB and Shoulson I (1990) Huntington's disease in Venezuela: 7 years of follow-up on symptomatic and asymptomatic individuals. *Movement Disorders* **5**:93–99.

Petit H (1970) La maladie de Huntington. In: *Comptes rendues 67 ième Congres Psychiatrie et Neurologie, langue francais* (ed. P Warot), pp. 901–1058. Paris: Masson.

Phanthumchinda K and Locharernkul C (1992) Huntington's disease in Thailand: a case report. *Journal of the Medical Association of Thailand* **75**:123–126.

Pleydell MJ (1954) Huntington's chorea in Northamptonshire. *British Medical Journal* **ii**:1121–1128.

—— (1955) Huntington's chorea in Northamptonshire. *British Medical Journal* **ii**:889.

Pridmore SA (1990a) Age of onset of Huntington's disease in Tasmania. *Medical Journal of Australia* **153**:135–137.

—— (1990b) Age of death and duration in Huntington's disease in Tasmania. *Medical Journal of Australia* **153**:137–139.

—— (1990c) The prevalence of Huntington's disease in Tasmania. *Medical Journal of Australia* **153**:133–134.

—— Cook A, McCormick G *et al.* (1995) Trinucleotide expansion in Tasmanian HD families. *Australian and New Zealand Journal of Psychiatry* **29**:157.

Przuntek H and Steigerwald A (1987) Epidemiologische untersuchung zur Huntington'schen Erkrankung in Einzugsgebiet der Würzburger Neurologischen Universitätesklinik Unterbesanderer Beruiksichtigung der Untefrankischen raumes. *Nervenarzt* **58**:424–427.

Quarrell OWJ, Tyler A, Cole G and Harper PS (1986) The problem of isolated cases of Huntington's disease in South Wales. *Clinical Genetics* **30**:331–337.

—— Meredith AL, Tyler A *et al.* (1987) Exclusion testing for Huntington's disease in pregnancy with closely linked DNA markers. *Lancet* **i**:1281–1283.

—— Tyler A, Jones MP, Nordin M and Harper PS (1988) Population studies of Huntington's disease in Wales. *Clinical Genetics* **33**:189–195.

Reed TE and Neel JV (1959) Huntington's chorea in Michigan. II. Selection and mutation. *American Journal of Human Genetics* **11**:107–136.

Reed TW, Chandler JH, Hughes EM and Davidson RT (1958) Huntington's chorea in Michigan. I. Demography and genetics. *American Journal of Human Genetics* **10**:201–225.

Reid JJ (1960) Huntington's chorea in Northamptonshire. *British Medical Journal* **ii**:650.

Roccatagliata G and Albano C (1976) Storia naturale della corea di Huntington. *Rivista di Neurologia* **46**:297–332.

Rubinsztein DC, Amos W, Leggo J, Goodburn S, Ramesar RS, Old J, Bontrop R, McMahon R, Barton DE and Ferguson-Smith MA (1994) Mutational bias provides a model for the evolution of Huntington's disease and predicts a general increase in disease prevalence *Nature Genetics* **7** (4):525–530.

Sarfarazi M, Wolak G, Quarrell O and Harper PS (1987) An integrated microcomputer system to maintain a genetic register for Huntington's disease. *American Journal of Medical Genetics* **28**:999–1006.

Saugstad L and Odegard O (1986) Huntington's chorea in Norway. *Psychological Medicine* **16**:39–48.

Schoenberg BS (1979) Epidemiologic approach to Huntington's disease. *Advances in Neurology* **23**:1–11.

Scrimgeour EM (1980) Huntington's disease in two New Britain families. *Journal of Medical Genetics* **17**:197–202.

Scrimgeour EM (1982) Huntington's chorea in Papua. *Papua New Guinea Medical Journal* **25**:12–15.

—— (1983) Possible introduction of Huntington's chorea into Pacific Islands by New England whalemen. *American Journal of Medical Genetics* **15**:607–613.

—— Tahoon SA and Zawawi TH (1994) Huntington's disease in two unrelated Arab kindreds and in an Afghani family in Saudi Arabia. *Journal of Medical Genetics* **31**:819–820.

Sepic J, Antonelli L, Sepic-Grahovac D and Materljan E (1989) Epidemiology of Huntington's disease in Rijeka district Yugoslavia. *Neuroepidemiology* **8**:105–108.

Shiwach RS (1994) Prevalence of Huntington's disease in the Oxford region. *British Journal of Psychiatry* **165**:414–415.

—— Lindenbaum RH (1990) Prevalence of Huntington's disease among UK immigrants from the Indian subcontinent. *British Journal of Psychiatry* **157**:598–599.

Shokeir MHK (1975) Investigations on Huntington's disease in the Canadian prairies. I. Prevalence. *Clinical Genetics* **7**:345–348.

Simpson SA and Johnston AW (1989). The prevalence and patterns of care of Huntington's chorea in Grampian. *British Journal of Psychiatry* **155**:799–804.

Singer K (1962) Huntington's chorea in the Chinese. *British Medical Journal* **ii**:1311–1312.

Singh A, Singh S and Jolly SS (1959) Huntington's chorea: a report of 4 new pedigrees from Punjab. *Neurology (Bombay)* **7**:7–8.

Sjögren T (1936) Vererbungsmedizinische Untersuchungen über Huntingtons chorea in einer schwedischen Bauernpopulation. *Vererb-Konstit-Lehre* **19**:131–165.

Snell RG, Lazarou L, Youngman S *et al.* (1989) Linkage disequilibrium Huntington's disease: an improved localisation for the gene. *Journal of Medical Genetics* **26**:673–675.

—— MacMillan JC, Cheadle JP *et al.* (1993) Relationship between trinucleotide repeat expansion and phenotypic variation in Huntington's disease. *Nature Genetics* **4**:393–397.

Soong BW and Wang JT (1995) A study on Huntington's disease associated trinucleotide repeat within the Chinese population. *Proceedings of the National Science Council, Republic of China—Part B, Life Sciences* **19** (3):137–142.

Spillane J and Phillips R (1937) Huntington's chorea in south Wales. *Quarterly Journal of Medicine* **6**:403–425.

Squitieri F, Andrew SE, Goldberg YP, Kremer B, Spence N, Zeisler J, Nichol K, Theilmann J, Greenberg J, Goto J *et al.* (1994) DNA haplotype analysis of Huntington disease reveals clues to the origins and mechanisms of CAG expansion and reasons for geographic variations of prevalence. *Human Molecular Genetics* **3** (12):2103–2114.

Stevens DL (1973) The classification of variants of Huntington's chorea. *Advances in Neurology* **1**:57–64.

Stevens DL (1976) *Huntington's chorea: a demographic, genetic and clinical study.* MD thesis, University of London.

Stine OC and Smith KD (1990) The estimation of selection coefficient in Afrikaners: Huntington's disease, porphyria variegats, and lipoid proteinosis. *American Journal of Human Genetics* **46**:452–458.

Tay CH (1970) Huntington's chorea: report of a Chinese family in Singapore. *Journal of Medical Genetics* **7**:41–43.

Tsuang M-T (1969) Case report. Huntington's chorea in a Chinese family. *Journal of Medical Genetics* **6**:354–356.

Tyler A (1982) *The social, personal and economic burden of Huntington's chorea in South Wales*. MSc thesis, University of Wales.

—— Harper PS (1983) Attitudes of subjects at risk and their relatives towards genetic counselling in Huntington's chorea. *Journal of Medical Genetics* **20**:179–188.

—— Ball D and Craufurd D (1992) Presymptomatic testing for Huntington's disease in the UK. *British Medical Journal* **304**:1593–1596.

—— Harper PS, Walker DA, Davis K and Newcombe RG (1982) The socioeconomic burden of Huntington's chorea. *Journal of Biosocial Science* **14**:379–389.

—— Harper PS, Davis K and Newcombe R (1983) Family breakdown and stress in Huntington's chorea. *Journal of Biosocial Sciences* **15**:127–138.

—— Quarrell OWJ, Lazarou, LP, Meredith AL and Harper PS (1990) Exclusion testing in pregnancy for Huntington's disease. *Journal of Medical Genetics* **27**:488–495.

United States Congress Commission (1977) Report: *Commission for the Control of Huntington's Disease and its Consequences*. Washington: US Department of Health, Education and Welfare.

Vessie PR (1932) On the transmission of Huntington's chorea for 300 years—the Bures family group. *Journal of Nervous and Mental Disease* **76**:553–573.

Volkers WV, Went LN, Vegter-Vlis M, Harper PS and Caro A (1980) Genetic linkage studies in Huntington's chorea. *Annals of Human Genetics* **44**:75–80.

Walker DA (1979) *Huntington's chorea in South Wales*. MD thesis, University of Liverpool.

—— Harper PS, Wells CEC, Tyler A, Davies K and Newcombe RG (1981) Huntington's chorea in South Wales: a genetic and epidemiological study. *Clinical Genetics* **19**:213–221.

—— —— Newcombe RG and Davis K (1983) Huntington's chorea in South Wales. Mutation, fertility and genetic fitness. *Journal of Medical Genetics* **20**:12–17.

Wallace DC (1976) The social effect of Huntington's chorea on reproductive fitness. *Annals of Human Genetics* **39**:375–379.

—— and Parker N (1973) Huntington's chorea in Queensland: the most recent story. *Advances in Neurology* **1**:223–236.

Watkins WS, Bamshad M and Jorde LB (1995) Population genetics of trinucleotide repeat polymorphisms *Human Molecular Genetics* **4** (9):1485–1491.

Wendt GG and Drohm D (1972) *Die Huntingtonsche Chorea. Eine populations genetische Studie*. Stuttgart: Thieme.

—— Landzettel I and Unterreiner I (1959) Das Erkrankungsalter bei der Huntingtonschen Chorea. *Acta Genetica (Basel)* **9**:18–32.

—— Landzettel I and Solth K (1960) Krankheitsdauer und Lebenserwartung bei der Huntingtonschen Chorea. *Archiv für Psychiatrie and Nerven Krankheiten* **201**:298–312.

—— Solth K and Landzettel I (1961) Kinderzahl, Erkrankungsalter and Sterbealter bei der Huntingtonschen Chorea. *Anthropologischer Anzeiger* **24**:299–309.

Wexler NS, Young AB and Tanzi RE (1987) Homozygotes for Huntington's disease. *Nature* **326**:194–197.

Winsor EJ and Welch JP (1973) Huntington's chorea in Nova Scotia. *Medical Bulletin* **52**:108–109.

Wong MC, Ng IS and Lim SH (1993) Huntington's disease in five siblings. *Annals of the Academy of Medicine, Singapore* **22**:428–430.

Wood J, MacMillan JC, Thomas P *et al.* (1995) Characterising the Huntington's disease gene product. *Biochemical Society Transactions* **23**:595S.

—— —— Harper PS *et al.* (1996) Partial characterisation of murine huntingtin in human, mouse and rat brain. *Human and Molecular Genetics* **5**:481–487.

Wright HM, Still CN and Abramson RK (1981) Huntington's disease in black kindreds in South Carolina. *Archives of Neurology* **38**:412–414.

Young AB, Shoulson I and Penney JB (1986) Huntington's disease in Venezuela: neurologic features and functional decline. *Neurology* **36**:244–249.

Youngman S, (1989) *Studies on Huntington's disease using recombinant DNA techniques* PhD thesis, University of Wales.

—— Sarfarazi M, Quarrell OWJ *et al.* (1986) Studies of a DNA marker (G8) genetically linked to Huntington's disease in British families. *Human Genetics* **73**:333–339.

—— Shaw DJ, Gusella JF *et al.* (1988) A DNA probe D5 (D4S90) mapping to human chromosome 4p16.3. *Nucleic Acids Research* **16**:1648.

—— Sarfarazi M, Bucan M *et al.* (1989) A new DNA marker (D4S90) is located terminally on the short arm of chromosome 4, close to the Huntington disease gene. *Genomics* **5**:802–809.

Zeng Y, Chen M and Mao Y (1995) Molecular diagnosis of Huntington's disease: an analysis of two large families. *Chung-Hua i Hsueh Tsa Chih [Chinese Medical Journal]* **75** (11):689–693, 711–712.

Zolliker A (1949) Die Chorea Huntington in der Schweiz. *Schweiz Archiv für Neurologie und Psychiatrie* **64**:448–459.

7 Genetic counselling and presymptomatic testing

Aad Tibben

Introduction

Most families with Huntington's disease (HD) have lived for many generations with the awareness that nothing can be done to cure this devastating disease. The tragedy of HD has evoked feelings of hopelessness in family members, their friends and social contacts, and healthcare-givers, resulting in a lack of understanding and withdrawal of the support that is so much needed. Families have had to struggle to avoid ending up on the periphery of society. Over the last few decades, medical and pharmacological research has provided only palliative treatment for the characteristic movement and mood disorders. The care for patients has often been inappropriate, through lack of knowledge amongst both families and professional health carers. Children of affected patients could do nothing but wait to see whether the disease would also strike them. Some could cope and live with this threat. Others feared the onset of early signs of the disease, a fear that increased as the expected age of onset came within sight. Even in old age, individuals at risk could never be certain that they had escaped the disease. Barbara Vine (1989), in her book *The house of stairs*, has put into concise words the experience of someone at risk.

It is inescapable always the feeling that this may be it, this time it is no ordinary tiredness but the early warning itself, and the usual unease touched me, the usual quiver of panic. I am not old enough yet to be out of danger, I am still within the limit. But oh, what a bore it all is, how dreary and repetitive and simply boring after all these years, yet how can something be a bore and a terror at one and the same time? I have told no one, ever, but Bell and Cosette. Well, Cosette knew already, naturally she did. Does Bell remember? When she saw me at the station did she remember then and wonder if it had caught me yet or passed me by and left me safe?

In the 1970s, patient organizations in many countries were established that provided a great support for many families. Given the specific needs of HD patients, in a few countries, such as Australia, the United Kingdom, and the Netherlands, special care units were established for patients in the later stages of the disease. Although there were improvements in care, a cure was and remains in the future. With this in mind, it is understandable that the HD community experienced the discovery, in 1983, of a genetic marker that localized the HD gene to chromosome 4 as a great breakthrough (Gusella *et al.* 1983). This finding provided a vision of a better future and the hope that perhaps even a cure might eventually be a reality became stronger.

The discovery paved the way for presymptomatic testing, which was experienced by part of the HD community as a blessing, a herald of better times in which the disease could be controlled, cured, and prevented. The test provided the opportunity to relieve the uncertainty, to have prenatal tests in order to ensure that children would be free from the disorder, and to make informed plans for the future with respect to marriage, education, career, and financial provision. Even testing embryos prior to implantation has become possible, providing couples with the opportunity to have a pregnancy without the burden of termination after an unfavourable prenatal test result. In 2000 the first report of cell therapy and neuronal transplantation was published (Bachoud-Levi *et al.* 2000). Hoping was no longer an illusion but had become a reality.

The spectacular advances in genetics—opening up the possibility of relieving the anguish of being at risk—also presented a novel situation in medicine. The possibility of presymptomatic testing for HD heralded a new era in which presymptomatic testing for disorders with onset later in life would become available for many other—more or less rare—hereditary diseases with Mendelian transmission. Moreover, an increasing knowledge of genetic factors in combination with environmental influences would inevitably open up new perspectives for medicine. Individuals could now be better informed as to their future health and the risk factors that might threaten their future. HD had the dubious honour of becoming the paradigm that would provide the knowledge and experience for the establishment of presymptomatic testing programmes for other diseases. This development has not only affected the medical field, but has had far-reaching consequences, making presymptomatic testing an issue that has also had impacts on social, political, and economic issues. Presymptomatic testing programmes were also the prelude to the developments promised by the Human Genome Project. HD has thus been an important model that has guided the establishment of many other testing programmes.

With the possibility of presymptomatic testing, serious concerns were raised about the psychological consequences of test results, with the possibility of an increase in death by suicide among identified carriers of the gene. Suicide has long been recognized as a risk in families at risk for HD. Farrer reported a fourfold increase in the suicide rate among people affected compared with the rate of the general Caucasian population in the USA, though other studies have found a lower frequency (see Chapter 3). Attitudinal surveys of individuals at risk suggest that between 11 and 33 per cent have considered suicide a possible response in the future (Farrer 1986). These data highlighted the need for research to identify predictors of adjustment problems, such as depression and suicidal intentions, in those who would go on to request presymptomatic testing. Worldwide, a number of groups have monitored the attitudes of individuals at risk prior to the availability of the test.

Between 40 and 79 per cent of the individuals at risk reported an intention to take the test (Meiser and Dunn 2000). Interest in testing was found to be negatively associated with being married, and positively correlated with the number of affected relatives and earlier parental age of onset of HD. The reasons most commonly given for desiring a test in these surveys were wishing for certainty, relieving uncertainty, planning for the future, planning a family, and the need to inform children.

In this chapter, we will refer to the guidelines of the International Huntington Association (IHA) and World Federation of Neurology (WFN) Research Group on HD. They are widely used as a frame of reference for counsellors and other professionals involved in presymptomatic, prenatal, and confirmatory testing for HD (IHA/WFN 1994). It should be noted that the guidelines are a reflection of a year-long discussion between professionals and people from international lay organizations. They should be considered as giving assistance in administering the genetic test for HD and in protecting the well-being of those who choose to be tested and others who are involved in the testing process. These guidelines are still very valuable and practical, although, as time passes, they may need some amendments in the light of new insights and experiences. Many study groups have contributed extensively to refining the guidelines by providing, in addition to discussion, their data, clinical experiences, and case reports. The guidelines ought not to be used as a straitjacket but as a framework of recommended procedure for careful testing. Following the guidelines also provides a safety net that comforts the test candidate and his or her companion in the presymptomatic testing process.

Now, 15 years after its introduction, HD presymptomatic testing is relatively free from serious laboratory-related problems or uncertainties. Most of the difficulties encountered relate to the counselling and human aspects of the testing process. Therefore, pre- and post-test counselling ought to be incorporated in any programme of presymptomatic testing for HD along with the other preliminary sessions detailed herein.

Early approaches to prediction

Presymptomatic testing for HD is associated nowadays with linkage and molecular analysis. Yet, before the era of DNA-technology attempts were made to detect asymptomatic individuals who would eventually develop HD. The need for such tests has been recognized for even longer. Bell (1934) stated the situation clearly:

The almost continuous anxiety of unaffected members of these families over so long a period must be a great strain and handicap, even if they remain free from disquieting symptoms; it is thus of urgent importance that some means should be sought by which immunity of an individual could be predicted early in life, both from the point of view or relief to those who carry no liability to the disease and as an indication to others that they should abstain from parenthood. No facts in the clinical histories of patients provide definite guidance in this matter prior to the onset of symptoms, but the development of the science of genetics may at some future data enable us to obtain information concerning the inherent characteristics in such cases.

Early presymptomatic tests, such as detection of eye movement disorder or tremor and neuropsychological testing, attempted to demonstrate a difference between patients with HD and normal controls and then to ascertain what proportion of those at risk had the abnormality in question. Despite an ingenious variety of such tests, most of them had serious methodological shortcomings, such as small sample numbers, failure of the test to divide the at-risk group into two roughly equal proportions, and contradictory results if the tests were combined. The greatest methodological problem has been the lack of prospective follow-up, which was performed in only three studies (Chandler 1966; Lyle and Gottesman 1977; Klawans *et al.* 1980).

In retrospect, it is probably fortunate that none of these tests were sufficiently encouraging to result in widespread use, since little thought seems to have been given to what individuals might have been told about the result of such a test. The early approaches used for presymptomatic testing were fully discussed in the first edition of this book (Harper 1991). Perry (1981) made a point that remains extremely valid, at least with respect to research data.

While reviewing research proposals dealing with presymptomatic tests for Huntington's chorea I have been struck with the cavalier attitude of some investigators towards the use of the data they hope to generate. I suggest that pending development of an effective form of treatment, scientists who perform preclinical tests on persons at risk should ensure that the results of individual tests are not made available to those tested.

Fortunately, an accurate presymptomatic test for HD is now available, which has rarely been used in inappropriate ways. Professionals involved in other disorders have learned much in this respect from HD and from Perry's remarks. However, some cautionary comments must still be made. The technically simple mutation test might result in inadequate or absent counselling and support. Furthermore, there is the risk of abuse from inadvertent or inappropriate testing of research or other samples.

Genetic counselling and presymptomatic testing

Genetic counselling has been perhaps the most important way of assisting families with HD in managing the consequences of the disease, and in helping individuals at-risk to find creative solutions for their problems. The increased awareness of the genetic aspects of HD and genetics in general, together with the more widespread availability of genetic centres, have contributed to a more appropriate approach for those who ask for assistance in making important life decisions. Clinicians involved with families with HD may prefer to refer their patients to a clinical genetics centre to address the genetic questions. The way such questions are dealt with can have a profound impact on the attitude of individuals at risk, their partners and children, and on other relatives. Before the availability of presymptomatic testing, general counselling about the genetics of HD was the most important issue that led individuals at risk to visit the genetic counsellor. Currently, people often apply for general genetic counselling when they have only recently first learned of HD in their family, although many of them come with the intention of discussing presymptomatic or prenatal testing. Most people seen for genetic counselling with respect to HD are the asymptomatic children of an affected patient, seeking reassurance for themselves and their (future) children.

The situation in which applicants for genetic counselling already show subtle or suspicious clinical features is discussed in the section 'Neurological and psychological examination'. Before the availability of molecular tests, the diagnosis was based on positive family history and clinical features. In those patients where the diagnosis could not be made conclusively, uncertainties remained for offspring and other relatives. These people were referred to a genetics centre for more accurate risk estimations. Now that molecular tests are available for other specialists (neurologists, psychiatrists) to confirm or exclude the diagnosis in marginally affected patients, these individuals are less likely to be referred to a genetics centre.

The diagnostic difficulties in HD have thus been largely solved. In those cases where a diagnosis of HD is not confirmed, and where there are indications of heredity, individuals may be referred to a genetic centre for estimation of genetic risk.

Because most people asking for genetic counselling intend to take presymptomatic testing, the remainder of this chapter will focus on presymptomatic and prenatal testing. Yet it must be recognized that sometimes people apply for testing because they are of the opinion that a test result might solve their psychological problems. Experienced genetic counsellors know that alternative strategies for coping with personal risks and, subsequently, life decisions, might be preferable in some cases. It is, therefore important to present the general principles of genetic counselling, pedigree analysis, and risk estimation.

General principles of counselling

The American Society of Human Genetics has defined genetic counselling as a communication process that deals with the human problems associated with the occurrence or risk of occurrence of a genetic disorder in a family. This process involves an attempt by one or more appropriately trained persons to help the individual or family: (1) to comprehend the medical facts including the diagnosis, probable course of the disorder, and the available management; (2) to appreciate the way heredity contributes to the disorder and the risk of recurrence in specified relatives; (3) to understand the alternatives for dealing with the risk of recurrence; (4) to choose a course of action that seems to them appropriate in view of their risk, their family goals, and their ethical and religious standards and to act in accordance with that decision; and (5) to make the best possible adjustment to the disorder in an affected family member and/or to the risk of recurrence of that disorder (American Society of Human Genetics 1975). The definition emphasizes the two-way nature of the interaction between the test candidate and the counsellor. Moreover, counselling is considered as a process, taking place over a period of time. This process allows the assimilation of the potentially distressing information regarding diagnosis, prognosis, risk, emotional reactions, family dynamics, etc. The counselling process allows attention to the autonomous decisions taken by the test candidate. The appropriateness of the decisions can be discussed and weighed extensively. This all requires 'appropriately trained persons', which implies special knowledge and skills distinct from those needed in other medical and counselling interactions (Platt-Walker 1998).

Individuals at risk for HD often come for genetic counselling to discuss aspects of the disorder with which they find it difficult to deal. Exploring with them their experiences, emotional responses, goals, cultural and religious beliefs, financial and social resources, family and interpersonal dynamics, and coping styles has become an integral part of the counselling process. Many individuals at risk, with life-long experience of HD, are not fully aware of how the disorder has influenced their psychological make-up (Duisterhof and Tibben 2000). An experienced counsellor must be able to recognize and bring forth these responses. He or she can identify normal and maladjusted responses, reassure candidates that their reactions are normal, prepare them for the near future, new issues, and emotions that may come up, and help them to mobilize the resources needed to encourage coping and adjustment.

A central assumption of genetic counselling has been the non-directive approach. This assumption is often misunderstood in the sense that non-directiveness does not mean that the counsellor should never express his or her personal views, opinions, or feelings (Kessler *et al.* 1984; Djurdjinovic 1998). An individual at-risk can expect that the counsellor will provide some guidance when needed, to enable them to proceed in their own process of consideration. However, in order not to be coercive, the counsellor must possess a level of introspection and awareness of his or her own personal feelings and interests. The lack of treatment options and future perspectives may facilitate the psychological defences of professional persons such as denial and displacement of responsibility. HD families can be threatening to those professionals who have difficulties in working with conditions that cannot be cured. Although most professionals involved with management of the disorder are protected from the difficult and unsettling task of providing genetic counselling to healthy relatives at risk, this may prevent care-givers from establishing a relationship that is characterized by confidentiality, respect for autonomy, and empathy (Martindale 1987) Continuing education and an increase in awareness of the psychodynamics involved may lead to creative and constructive thinking about the current deficiencies in care and counselling services provided for HD families.

Pedigree analysis

The pedigree is the diagram that records the family history information, the tool for converting information provided by the client and/or obtained from the medical records into a standardized format. The construction of a pedigree is a very powerful instrument that allows confirmation of the autosomal dominant inheritance expected for HD, but also provides insight into those branches of the family that might benefit from counselling in the future. It can be considered as the cornerstone of good medical practice in genetic counselling, and is an incomparable opportunity to develop a working alliance with the test candidate that facilitates trust (Djurdjinovic 1998). Moreover, the joint construction with the person asking for counselling gives detailed information on who might be affected or of those who are suspected of developing early signs. Finally, drawing the pedigree gives access to the psychological dynamics and social relationships in the family, often over more than two generations. Intimate details and information about family events such as death and loss, divorce, separation, hospital admissions, suicides, behavioural problems, sexual abuse, alcohol abuse, denial of symptoms, etc. may be obtained. The process of pedigree construction gives insight into the medical, emotional, and social impact of HD for the family over the generations. Myths developed by the family may be revealed. In cases where the diagnosis has already been confirmed—clinically and by DNA analysis—in another member of the family, drawing a pedigree is still an important tool in counselling as it is a critical instrument for establishing a productive relationship with the person who comes for counselling.

Assessments about family stress and coping strategies can be made while investigating the family history. The test candidate and family may appear anxious and feel guilty when identifying members of the family as affected with HD. Counsellors should therefore be aware that medical information may not be accurate on older generations, or on living persons. Sometimes the counsellor must actively search for clues that indicate the possible onset of symptoms in family members. Discussing this information provides an opportunity to make observations about the test candidate and his or her partner that may eventually help the counsellor to become familiar with the family background. The interaction between the test candidate and their partner also gives information about family dynamics.

It should be borne in mind that, during the phase of collecting the family information, it is important to understand the test candidate's perception of the problem or reason for wishing the presymptomatic test, before setting the agenda for the remainder of the consultation. The most important reasons for wishing to learn about the genetic status are unbearable anxiety or uncertainty, the need to gain certainty, to plan a family, and to inform adolescent or adult children. It is difficult to think of other reasons that override the risks of an unfavourable test result. The counsellor may find it difficult to understand profoundly the reasons given by the test candidate, which might be an indication that underlying, conscious or unconscious motives may be present. An often-encountered feature is that adult children wish to relieve the guilt feelings in their parents, or individuals at risk need to reassure their partners.

Many textbooks on genetic counselling provide concise information on how to draw pedigrees, how to collect medical information on family history, and how to use a pedigree with respect to the psychosocial aspects of obtaining a family history. With care and practice it should not be difficult to construct a working pedigree in a reasonably short time that does not require redrawing later to look respectable.

It needs to be emphasized that a pedigree represents a valuable, confidential, and highly sensitive document. It should not be left lying around, photocopied unnecessarily, or sent to colleagues other than professionals who will respect it similarly (after informed consent has been received). Genetic centres have various policies regarding the pedigrees. Some centres add the pedigrees to the patient's hospital file or keep the pedigree in the family genetic file with a copy of relevant correspondence in the hospital notes. Others have a separate file that is not accessible for other hospital departments. If a pedigree and medical information about a person at risk asking for genetic counselling is already available because a family member had counselling in the past, then it is still valuable to draw a joint pedigree. If an existing pedigree is used, then any confidential data should be removed. For reasons of confidentiality the person at risk should not be informed of the medical information that is covered by the full pedigree. In addition, it should not be forgotten that such a policy is reassuring for the person at risk who learns that their information will be kept secret from other family members who come for counselling. '*Under no circumstances shall any member of the counselling team or the technical staff communicate information concerning the test or its results to third parties without the written permission of the applicant*' (International Guidelines, 4.2).

If the person involved in genetic counselling is also participating in HD research, then a clear method of separating service from research must be decided upon, so that research workers do not have inappropriate access to counselling data. Such a separation may not always be necessary, but it must be carefully considered, especially if research data are likely to be made available to other centres.

Worldwide local genetic registers for HD have been established that allow the study of important issues such as sex-related effects and age-at-onset correlation (Conneally 1984; Gersting *et al.* 1984; Quarrell *et al.* 1988; Harper 1996; Hille *et al.* 1999). A register, or 'roster', allows an approximate estimate of the numbers of family members at risk if one knows the numbers that are affected in an area (Conneally 1984). Individuals with HD are symptomatic for about one-third of their lives, meaning that there will be about twice as many asymptomatic gene carriers in the population as affected individuals (see Chapter 6). Those with the gene, whether symptomatic or not, will, on average, have an equivalent number of sibs who are not carrying the gene but who cannot be distinguished, so that the total number of first-degree relatives at risk will be around five times the number of affected individuals. In the previous edition of this book (Harper 1996) the Wales register was described, as an example. It should be emphasized that confidentiality is the cornerstone of any genetic register and particularly so for such a sensitive disorder as HD.

Risk estimation

A clear pattern of autosomal dominant inheritance in an HD pedigree allows an easy and clear estimation of basic risk for the children of affected persons. In essence, all patients with HD are heterozygous for the HD gene, having one normal as well as one abnormal copy. In practice, each child of an affected patient has an equal chance of inheriting the normal or abnormal gene, which means a risk of one-half or 50 per cent, regardless of the sex of the parent or

Table 7.1 Risk for a healthy individual at 50% prior risk of HD carrying the HD gene at different ages. Based on the life-table analysis of South Wales data (from Harper and Newcombe 1992)

Age (years)	Probability of an HD mutation (%)
20	49.6
22.5	49.3
25	49
27.5	48.4
30	47.6
32.5	46.6
35	45.5
37.5	44.2
40	42.5
42.5	40.3
45	37.8
47.5	34.8
50	31.5
52.5	27.8
55	24.8
57.5	22.1
60	22.1
62.5	18.7
65	12.8
67.5	10.8
70	6.2
72.5	4.6

child. In reality, the actual risk given may differ considerably from this and will be critically dependent on the age of the person concerned. Offspring of an individual with a mutant allele have a 50 per cent chance of inheriting the disease-causing mutation at conception. The probability that an asymptomatic person at risk has a disease-causing mutation remains close to 50 per cent during childhood and young adulthood, but gradually decreases with increasing age (Harper and Newcombe 1992) (Table 7.1). At 55 years of age there is still a 25 per cent empirical risk for an at-risk person with an affected parent to be a carrier of the gene.

In practice the risk does not decline significantly from the initial 50 per cent until after 30 years of age (except for siblings of a juvenile HD patient). Consequently, the children of a parent with HD wishing to make reproductive decisions will have to make these before there is any useful alteration in their own risk status. The risk curve is therefore most useful in older age groups, where the question is often at what age one can be reasonably sure of having escaped the disease. It turns out that the risk is present for significantly longer than many members in a family expect, reflecting the higher than previously recognized frequency of the disorder in old age. It is possible that the curve could be unduly cautious in this respect, because it is based on age at definite onset, something that will certainly be several years away, at least in an individual who is found to be totally normal on coming for genetic counselling.

Some people from large families with a considerable number of patients over two generations or more refer to the age of onset in their affected relatives. On the one hand, there is the
hope of later onset when the affected relatives became ill at an older age; on the other, despair
when the mean age of onset seems to be younger. In a number of studies it was demonstrated
that the range of variation was great within families, which can now be partly explained by the
instability of the mutation. The only situation that allows a departure from the general age
curve is when a sibling has already developed juvenile HD. Hayden *et al.* (1985) showed that
no siblings of juvenile cases developed HD after the age of 45 years; at the age of 30 and
40 years the risks were 33 and 5 per cent, respectively, compared with 43 and 30 per cent
for families in general (see Fig. 7.1). Clarke and Bundey (1990)) found comparable data for
siblings at risk where the age of onset in the affected child was under 10 years.

Second-degree relatives, with an affected grandparent, are often seen for genetic counselling, as they may be planning marriage or a family when their healthy parent is still at an
age of significant risk. Such individuals are still often given the simpler risk figure of 25 per
cent, based on half their parent's prior risk. In fact their risk will invariably be much less than
this, the actual figure depending not so much on their own age but on that of their parent.
Figure 7.2 shows the curves for such individuals where the child is between 20 and 40 years
younger than the parent at risk. In practice the risk for any grandchild less than 30 years is
close to half the parent's age-adjusted risk.

In keeping with the other CAG repeat expansion disorders, HD shows an inverse relationship between repeat size and the age of onset (see Chapters 5 and 14). The CAG repeat
accounts for approximately 50 to 77 per cent of the variation in the age of onset (Andrew *et al.*
1993; Duyao *et al.* 1993; Snell *et al.* 1993; Trottier *et al.* 1994; Lucotte *et al.* 1995; Brinkman
et al. 1997; Vuillaume *et al.* 1998). In a recent Canadian study (Brinkman *et al.* 1997), age-
dependent likelihood of onset curves were proposed that differed significantly for each CAG
repeat length in the 39 to 50 range (see Table 7.2). In a Dutch study (Maat-Kievit 2001),
the median age at onset for each repeat size is about 10 years later than the Canadian study

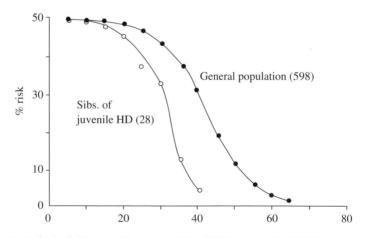

Fig. 7.1 Risk curves for individuals at 50 per cent risk of HD based on the US Huntington disease roster
(redrawn with permission for Hayden *et al.* 1985). Note the more rapid decline of risk in sibs of juvenile
cases, based on the observed age of onset in this group. The curves are based on uncorrected age at
onset, not a life-table approach.

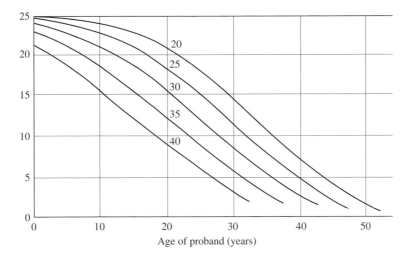

Fig 7.2 Risk curves for second-degree relatives. This series of curves shows the decline risk of carrying the HD gene with age for a proband who is the grandchild of a patient with HD and who has an unaffected living parent. The different curves correspond to the age of the intervening parent at risk at the time the proband was born.

Table 7.2 Observed age of onset versus CAG repeat size

CAG repeat size	Age at onset (years): Canadian study*		Age at onset (years): Dutch study[†]	
	Median value	Range[‡]	Median value	Range[‡]
39	66	59–72		
40* (≤40)[†]	59	56–61*	68	55–81#
41	54	52–56	65	58–72
42	49	48–50	64	60–68
43	44	42–45	60	56–64
44	42	40–43	55	52–58
45	37	36–39	50	47–53
46	36	35–37	45	43–47
47	33	31–35	41	39–43
48	32	30–34	37	35–39
49	28	25–32	38	36–40
50	27	24–30	34	30–38
51	33	27–39		
52	29	19–29		
≥53	23	20–26		

*Brinkman *et al.* (1997).
[†]Maat-Kievit *et al.* (2001).
[‡]95 per cent confidence intervals.

(Table 7.2). This difference might be explained by the differences in ascertainment especially regarding the inclusion of older patients without a clear family history.

The general policy in testing programmes is not to communicate the repeat length unless applicants ask for it. However, identified carriers do sometimes ask for the precise repeat length, in which case the details of the test results should not be withheld. Therefore, information concerning the age-dependent likelihood of being affected may be useful, but should be carefully handled in presymptomatic counselling sessions, especially since the confidence limits in the usual presymptomatic testing range are relatively wide.

The test candidate

Many people at risk for HD will ask for presymptomatic testing when visiting a genetics centre. 'What made you consider the presymptomatic test?' is an opening question that gives a first impression of the test candidate. When answering, the candidate gives a personal story that provides the counsellor with the opportunity to understand and appreciate who the test candidate is. Often, test candidates are very determined and hardly willing to go through the process of consideration again. A counsellor—sometimes serving as the devil's advocate—may encounter some resistance as they explore the motives for the test. This is understandable. The decision to take the test has been considered by most candidates for a long time. The advantages and disadvantages have been weighed up extensively and, once the decision to attend the genetic centre has been made, no counsellor ought to shake that decision. The counsellor might adopt the role of the devil's advocate if he or she believes that the test candidate might need extra confirmation of their decision.

The most important reason given for learning about one's personal risk is the need to obtain certainty or to relieve uncertainty. People at risk may have lived for many years with the threat of a devastating disorder that has ruined their life. They may have lived balanced between hope and fear, and based their life prospects upon the expectation that the disease will eventually take hold. The psychological make-up of individuals at risk can be profoundly influenced by this fear. Another reason for wanting the test may be the wish to start a family without the risk of passing the HD gene on to the next generation. Although this reason seems straightforward, it is often fraught with problems. One of the complexities is the ability to come up to the expectations of the partner with respect to starting a family. A situation regularly encountered occurs when an individual at risk presents with possible signs of the disease. Sometimes they are aware of these and fearful of a confirmation; in other instances the person is not aware of any alterations in their behaviour or physical condition. Some people fear the first signs of the disease and wish to use the process of learning about their genetic status as the first stage in the process of accommodating the cruel reality. In these cases people may visit the genetics centre because they know that they will receive as much time and careful attention as they may need.

The partner

For many partners of at-risk individuals, the future has been or becomes overshadowed by the disease, if not in the at-risk spouse, then perhaps in a close relative. In general there is a difference, both with the at-risk individual and their partner, between those who did not know about HD when the relationship started and those who were fully aware of HD from the beginning of the partnership. In between, are those individuals at risk who informed their partner about HD only when the relationship was beyond the point of no return. When applying for the test, '*the participant should be encouraged to select a companion to accompany him or her throughout all stages of the testing process: the pre-test stage, the taking of the test, the delivery of results, and the post-test stage*' (International Guidelines, 3). The companion is often the spouse/partner, a friend, a social worker, or any individual who has the confidence of the participant. In any case, it should be discussed whether the chosen companion is the most appropriate in the circumstances. Sometimes, a close relative from the HD side of the family accompanies the test candidate. This needs careful consideration. When it is the unaffected parent, it might be extremely helpful for the test candidate, provided the parent is able to provide unconditional support if the test result is unfavourable, and to express their relief when the result is normal. However, if the parent is still extremely burdened by their lifelong experiences of HD and unable to meet their child's needs, then such companionship may need to be discouraged.

Clinical experience has shown that the impact of the testing experience appears to be most intense for those support persons who are at-risk offspring of probands. Investigation of the meaning of the companion for the individual at risk is important in the very early stage of the first counselling session. 'What is your opinion about a presymptomatic test, and how do you feel about being involved?' might be an opening question for the partner before explaining the testing protocol and setting the agenda for the first session. Williams *et al.* (2000b) found that accompanying persons identified aspects of the protocol that did not fit their needs. They perceived the testing process as extending into subsequent care-giving responsibilities when the test was positive, and were uninformed regarding specific care-giving issues for family members with the gene mutation. Investigation of the needs of accompanying persons may allow more focused counselling of support persons during presymptomatic genetic HD testing.

'*The counselling unit should plan with the participant a follow-up protocol that provides for support during the pre- and post-test stages regardless of whether the participant chooses a companion*' (International Guidelines, 3.1). If individuals at risk do not bring a companion with them, this could reflect a lack of good friends to rely on, it could be an indication of underestimation of the implications of presymptomatic testing, or it may mirror their personal way of dealing with uncertainties and life issues.

The presymptomatic testing protocol

As the availability of DNA analysis for the HD gene was set to become a reality, the Committee of the IHA and the Working Group on HD of the WFN gave consideration to the manner in which these tests should be carried out (IHA/WFN 1994). The guidelines for protocols were first published in 1989 when the presymptomatic test made use of linkage analysis. After identification of the HD-gene in 1993, the guidelines were adjusted and then published in 1994. In general, the guidelines recommend that individuals at risk who participate in presymptomatic testing programmes are seen for two to four counselling sessions, spread over a 3-month period, before disclosure of the test results. Presymptomatic testing requires informed consent by the individual at risk, and the provision of psychological support. If the test is abnormal, counselling must be available for the family and others involved. The starting point is that presymptomatic tests should be offered only to individuals at risk who have had the appropriate counselling, are fully informed, and wish to proceed.

Although it is recommended that psychosocial support should be available close to the individual's community, the policy of many specialized genetic centres initially was to centralize the offer of presymptomatic testing and the additional psychosocial support, thereby gaining experience of psychosocial consequences that could be accompanied by psychological follow-up studies. Psychological pre- and post-test follow-up were offered on a research basis, by requesting informed consent from presymptomatic test participants. Information on the availability of the presymptomatic testing reached risk-carriers through the Newsletters of the HD Society, the general practitioner, neurologist, clinical genetics service, relatives, or the public networks. Pretest written information was provided in several centres. General information was mailed to all 50 per cent risk-carriers in one group (Quaid and Wesson 1995). The Vancouver Group mailed a description of the research project to all families on the HD registry, requesting them to contact the researcher (Fox *et al.* 1989). The follow-up studies have resulted in many publications on the effects of presymptomatic testing, as will be reviewed in the section 'Fifteen years experience'. The counselling process has certainly benefited from these studies. In those cases, where specialists less knowledgeable about the issues regarding presymptomatic testing offered the test, the lay organizations may have played an important role in providing information. The IHA has emphasized that, if no local lay organization is available, the specific centre should contact the IHA for further information (www.huntington-assoc.com).

Genetic centres providing the presymptomatic test have been committed to the use of the international guidelines, as has been confirmed at the biannual meetings of the Working Group on HD of the WFN and the IHA. Admittedly, after 10 years, testing centres have developed their own local protocols and guidelines, based on experience and local or national rules, but they have in common the requirement for multiple interviews before a test result is disclosed. The number and complexity varies, partly due to the number of associated psychological and other evaluations, but the basic structure involves at least the series shown in Table 7.3.

Table 7.3 Presymptomatic testing programme for HD

Interview one
    Sociodemographic details
    Confirmation of family and clinical data
    Assessment of impact of HD and test results
    Assessment of knowledge of HD and presymptomatic testing
    Reasons for requesting prediction
    Neurological examination*
Interview two
    Assessment of psychological, personality, and social resources (using standardized instruments*)
    Further counselling and discussion of disclosure session
    Nomination of professional support
    Signing of consent form
    Final blood sample
Interview three
    Disclosure of test results
Formal follow-up
    2 days–1 week (telephone)
    3 months
    12 months

*Genetic centres differ in the application of neurological examination and psychological assessment.

Collecting information on HD

Individuals at risk have often already made their decision regarding presymptomatic testing when they apply to the genetics centre. They are sure that HD is running in their family, that the diagnosis is confirmed, and probably that other relatives have had the test previously. Yet, '*It is important to verify that the diagnosis of HD in the family of the individual is correct* (International Guidelines, 6.1), and '*the possible need for DNA from one other affected family member and the possible problems arising from this*' (International Guidelines 5.2.2). The genetic counsellor may encounter some resistance when discussing the need for confirmation of the diagnosis before the test can be carried out. The individual at risk may experience this requirement as a delay to the test result, an unnecessary intervention in their personal process. As will be discussed later, there are several important laboratory issues that need specific consideration in relation to presymptomatic testing, and that may cause serious problems if ignored. A test candidate, having eventually decided to have a test, may not be interested in the whys and wherefores of these issues. The counsellor's communication skills are needed to both appreciate the test candidate's feelings and pass on caution if the laboratory issues are not adequately met. In some cases there is no living affected family member, or no affected relative willing to participate. Particularly sensitive is the situation where the individual at risk knows a relative, who may be unaware of or unwilling to acknowledge his or her symptoms, and who might be asked to contribute a blood sample. Approaching such a relative can be considered as an invasion of privacy, as a violation of the psychological defences against the threat of the disease. The counsellor should help the test candidate in deciding the best way to handle such a situation. '*Neither the counselling centre nor the test laboratory should establish direct contact with a relative whose DNA may be needed for the purpose of the test without permission of the applicant. All precautions should be taken when approaching such a relative*' (International Guidelines, 4.1).

Although test candidates are not always aware of it, identification of HD disease status (by family history, pathology, and DNA data) of relatives in a family is of paramount importance. Family members who may have had physical or mental complaints that went unnoticed because they were not hospitalized, under medical surveillance, or were misdiagnosed should be re-evaluated.

Sometimes it is necessary to perform additional investigations (for example, DNA analysis, neurological/psychiatric examination) in the parent without a family history, for interpretation of an intermediate or reduced penetrance allele found in the applicant. Medical records of at least one affected family member should always be obtained for confirmation of the diagnosis. If the test candidate has had neurological investigations, the records may be useful to further explore the motives for molecular testing.

The presymptomatic testing procedure involves the ongoing process of the assessment of the test candidate's beliefs about causation, and of emotional, experiential, social, educational, and cultural issues that may affect his or her perception of the information that is given in the course of the testing process.

Another central belief of genetic counselling is the conviction that asking for presymptomatic testing should be entirely voluntary. Many candidates at risk, however, do not feel as free as we would like to think they are. Individuals at risk can be referred for presymptomatic testing by other care-givers. Some individuals feel obliged to have the test before they feel free to start a relationship or a family. Sometimes there is explicit or implicit pressure from employers or insurance companies to have more precise risk estimations. A personal sense of right and wrong may also weigh heavily on their free choice. It is unrealistic therefore, to assume that individuals at risk can make voluntary decisions about using presymptomatic testing, based solely on their preferences, personal goals, and moral views (Baker *et al.* 1998).

Counsellors use their clinical judgement to decide what information is most likely to be important and helpful in a test candidate's adjustment to a test result.

Recommendations have also been made that the individuals at risk who proceed to testing should be given support and followed-up subsequent to the test. Although there is general agreement about the implementation of protocols in presymptomatic testing, the actual services offered may differ due to lack of health service resources or time on the part of the counsellor.

In general, testing protocols allow several visits for individuals at risk and are based on non-directive counselling. Participants are free to withdraw from the programme at any stage, and no pressure is applied to encourage them to continue if they do not wish to undertake the test.

Presymptomatic testing and the laboratory

The characteristics of the HD mutation, described in Chapter 5, form the basis for the confirmation of the HD diagnosis in individuals with clinical signs or those suspected to be affected. The highly specific and sensitive nature of the test makes it equally powerful in detection of the asymptomatic individual at risk. As a single type of mutation is responsible for all cases of HD, this means that the test can be applied in a standardized manner worldwide. There are several important laboratory issues that need specific consideration in relation to presymptomatic testing and that may cause serious problems if ignored. These include:

1. The type of sample. Blood is almost invariably used, although the relative lack of somatic variation would probably allow an accurate result from other tissues.

2. Duplicate samples. It is common to use two samples for mutation testing. The possibility of a sample switch, although very small, must be prevented. Some centres even collect the samples on separate occasions.

3. Methods of analysis. Initial polymerase chain reaction (PCR) methods included the adjacent CCG repeat, but current techniques are now largely standardized between laboratories and stringent quality control measures have been set up (see Chapter 5).

4. Diagnostic issues. Wherever possible a sample from the closest affected relative should be analysed, in addition to checking the clinical and (where available) neuropathological diagnosis. In the absence of such a sample, a normal test result needs to be interpreted with caution, although the strong correlation between the presence of the mutation and a firm clinical or neuropathological diagnosis of HD makes it unlikely that an error would result if these features were typical.

5. Results in the 'borderline' range (see also the section 'Exclusion testing by linkage'). The great majority of results will fall in a clearly interpretable range, either 40 or more repeats, giving an abnormal result, or fewer than 27 repeats if normal.

In general, HD presymptomatic testing is now relatively free from serious laboratory-related problems or uncertainties, but it remains important to explain to those who wish to take the test that no test is perfect and that there remains a small chance that the result will be inconclusive. Fourteen laboratories from 12 different countries participated in a European pilot quality assessment scheme for molecular diagnosis of HD. The laboratories analysed five cases, provided together with mock clinical information, and returned the reports in their normal laboratory format within a fixed period. The rate of misdiagnosis was 1/78 (1.3 per cent), but it is likely that it could be greater than this for less experienced laboratories. Most of the difficulties encountered today relate to the counselling and human aspects of the testing process (Losekoot *et al.* 1999).

'*The laboratory performing the test should not communicate the final results to the counselling team until very close to the time such results are to be revealed to the participant*' (International Guidelines, 4.1). Although the aim is to protect the participant from the possibility of counselling bias at any time, this point needs consideration. Some centres schedule an appointment for disclosing the test results with the provision that the results are available. If not, they will be told that the disclosure is delayed. Other centres will send an invitation to the tested person to receive their result. Individuals, from whom blood is taken for the test, may contact the centre or specific counsellor to ask whether the results are already available. If the specific counsellor has learned the outcome, he or she may inadvertently communicate the results. Even if they do not know the outcome, test candidates may interpret the nonverbal signs in terms of the test result. In my opinion, an experienced counsellor should keep the results secret as a precaution, for reasons of privacy, from anyone not involved in the testing procedure. But the counsellor must have the opportunity to digest the test result first, before communicating it to the test candidate. 'You never get used to telling people that they will get HD', said an experienced geneticist involved from the very beginning of presymptomatic testing.

The expanded allele

Initially, explanations of the mode of inheritance of HD and the estimation of basic risks for the children of affected individuals were quite simple, and identification of the mutation in the HD gene made presymptomatic testing technically simpler, more reliable, and available to everyone at risk. According to the International Guidelines, '*the limitations of the test (error rate, the possibility of an uninformative test, and so forth), should be addressed in the testing programme*' (International Guidelines 5.2.3), and '*Much more information will be needed about the implications of the number of repeats*' (International Guidelines 5.2.4).

Initially, counselling seemed much easier as a test candidate only learned about whether they carried the mutation or not. However, more data on the additional implications of the repeat size have made testing and counselling more complicated. We address this issue extensively in this section and the interpretation of any result in the context of presymptomatic testing may differ considerably from that when the test is used in clinical diagnosis (Chapter 5).

The wild-type allele of HD has six to 35 copies but affected subjects have between 36 and 121 repeats (Kremer *et al.* 1994; Rubinsztein *et al.* 1996). The HD and normal range have quite distinct peaks but the tails of both curves are close to or overlapping each other. There is no gap between normal and disease ranges in HD and reduced penetrance is found in the lower end of the disease range. The normal repeat segregates stably as a polymorphic locus, but the disease repeat size tends to fluctuate, mainly increasing but occasionally decreasing in successive generations (Andrew *et al.* 1997). This is the molecular basis of the observed anticipation in HD and is discussed in Chapter 5. The limits of the CAG repeat size in the HD gene have been redefined, based on the total number of normal and symptomatic individuals assessed (ACMG/ASHG 1998).

A *normal repeat*, with fewer than 27 CAGs, has never been associated with an HD phenotype, nor has it shown instability resulting in an HD allele in offspring (Duyao *et al.* 1993; Benjamin *et al.* 1994). Although the *intermediate repeat*, with 27 to 35 repeats, has not been associated with a HD phenotype, it has demonstrated instability and is found in 1.5 to 1.9 per cent of the general population (Goldberg *et al.* 1995). For offspring of an intermediate allele carrier, there is a risk of inheriting more than 36 repeats and a small risk that transmission might result in a HD allele with or without penetrance (Goldberg *et al.* 1993; Myers *et al.* 1993). The risk of expansion depends on the sex of the transmitting person, the repeat size, the level of mosaicism in sperm, whether the intermediate allele is on an HD haplotype, whether it has been identified in a new mutation family or in the general population, and other, as yet unknown factors (Zuhlke *et al.* 1993; Kremer *et al.* 1995; Leeflang *et al.* 1995). Risk estimates for expansion of an intermediate allele to 36 or more repeats in the offspring of male carriers vary between 2 and 10 per cent (Goldberg *et al.* 1993; Chong *et al.* 1997).

Expansions of intermediate alleles to 36 or more repeats in female carriers of intermediate alleles have not been reported and their risk seems to be much smaller than for male carriers (≤ 1 per cent). Expansions of intermediate alleles into the pathological range have also been described in Friedreich's ataxia, myotonic dystrophy, SCA7, and fragile-X syndrome (Imbert *et al.* 1993; Montermini *et al.* 1997; Murray *et al.* 1997; Stevanin *et al.* 1998). Repeat lengths of 36–39 CAGs have been associated with clinically and pathologically confirmed HD, although not in all cases, and it seems, therefore, that repeats in this size range are not always fully penetrant. Across this repeat range (36–39), increasing penetrance is possibly associated with increasing repeat length (Legius *et al.* 1994; Brinkman *et al.* 1997; McNeil *et al.* 1997; Rubinsztein *et al.* 1996). Penetrance of 36 to 39 repeat alleles may be higher in persons from confirmed HD kindreds than those from collateral branches of new mutations.

Higher repeat sizes are associated with a younger age at onset (Duyao *et al.* 1993; Andrew *et al.* 1993; Snell *et al.* 1993; Brinkman *et al.* 1997). This evolving knowledge about genotype–phenotype correlation in HD has made genetic counselling in a small, but substantial number of cases more complicated. Moreover, unexpected test results might lead to specific psychosocial problems such as feelings of guilt and reproach, and uncertainties about the risk of HD for test candidates, their children, and relatives. In the Dutch programme, certain types of specific cases have been encountered in the testing programme, reflecting different categories of subjects with repeats between 27 and 39. The categories can be discriminated through family structure, test results, the context of testing, and the clinical status of the test candidate. Each case has its own counselling issues (see Fig. 7.3).

Category 1   *Symptomatic test candidates inheriting a reduced penetrance allele on the HD haplotype.* A man requested testing for HD because he wished to inform his daughter about her chances of inheriting HD as she had entered adulthood (Fig. 7.3, case 1). His mother had died at the age of 53 years, having possibly had HD-related symptoms. Neuropathological study of her brain did not confirm HD, nor did later re-evaluation when her brother, with onset of HD at 43 years and a reduced penetrance repeat (39), died at the age of 56. His maternal grandparents and father had died young of unrelated causes. The man carried

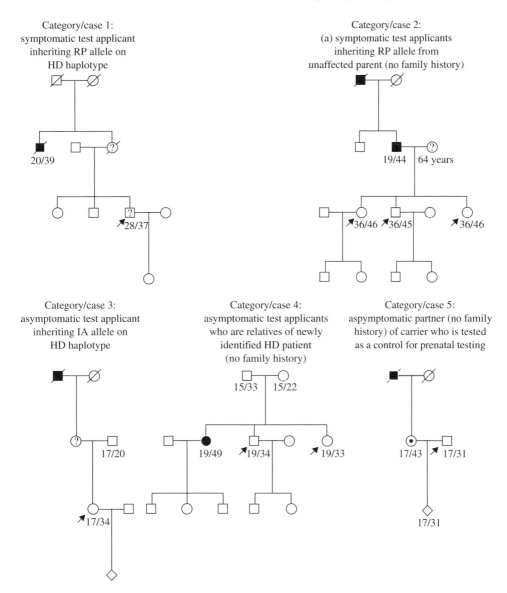

Fig. 7.3 Pedigrees of test applicants for HD in the five different categories of subjects with 27–39 repeats. (The numbers in the pedigrees refer to the CAG repeat sizes in the HD gene.)

alleles of 28 and 37 repeats. It was concluded that the man had a risk of developing HD with the possibility of reduced penetrance, and that his daughter had a 50 per cent risk of inheriting the reduced penetrance allele, which had an additional risk of expanding to an allele with an increased penetrance.

Category 2 *Asymptomatic test candidates inheriting an intermediate or reduced penetrance allele from unaffected parent (no family history).* Three siblings applied for presymptomatic testing to relieve uncertainty about their genetic status (Fig. 7.3, case 2). Their father and dead grandfather were diagnosed with HD. Because of a poor relationship, the sibs did not discuss the test with their mother who showed psychiatric symptoms, but no chorea and had no known family history of HD. All three applicants had one allele well within the affected range together with a reduced penetrance allele (36 repeats). This indicated that the mother might be affected, but she refused either a neurological assessment or DNA analysis. The sibs realized that the risk for their present and future children might be higher than 50 per cent. The two applicants who already had families decided to refrain from having further children. The one without children is considering prenatal diagnosis, accepting a foetus with 36 repeats, hoping for the possibility of reduced penetrance. The applicants might be homozygotes, which appears not to affect the clinical features or age at onset of HD to a significant extent (see Chapter 5). The relatives from the 'unaffected' family of the mother also have an unknown risk.

Category 3   *Asymptomatic test candidates inheriting an intermediate or reduced penetrance allele on an HD haplotype.* A young female requested presymptomatic testing before starting a family (Fig. 7.3, case 3). A maternal grandparent had pathologically confirmed HD, her family was known in the Leiden Roster, and a disease repeat was found in a distant relative. Her mother did not want to discuss HD, because she felt it was a disgrace to the family and refused testing. The daughter described her mother as probably affected. DNA analysis in the daughter showed a normal (17) and an intermediate (34) repeat. The father showed normal alleles. The daughter was given a risk of <1 per cent of developing HD and a risk of about 1 per cent for expansion into a HD allele for her future offspring. She was relieved she had not inherited a disease repeat, but decided to use the option of prenatal diagnosis. She intended to terminate a pregnancy if ≥36 repeats were identified.

Category 4   *Asymptomatic test candidates who are relatives of a newly identified HD patient (no family history).* An adult woman had symptoms of HD and was found to have a disease-causing repeat length (Fig. 7.3, case 4). Her parents were healthy (73 and 78 years) and the father showed an intermediate (33 repeat) allele. The patient's brother and sister, unexpectedly confronted with a possible risk for themselves and their offspring, applied for testing. Both of them showed an intermediate allele of 33 and 34 repeats, respectively, derived from their father. Their personal risk of developing HD was estimated as <1 per cent, and the risk for children of the sister approximately 1 per cent and of the brother 5 per cent. Prenatal testing was discussed with them. We suggested to them that they inform relatives of the result and related consequences.

Category 5   *Asymptomatic partners (no family history) of carriers, tested as a control for prenatal diagnosis.* A couple with one parent carrier of HD (43 repeats) applied for prenatal diagnosis (Fig. 7.3, case 5). DNA analysis was also done on the healthy partner as a control (maternal contamination or homozygosity). The foetus showed a normal and an intermediate (31) repeat, the latter inherited from the healthy partner. The risk of the foetus developing HD is small. In future pregnancies of this couple or of the unborn child, there is a risk of expansion of the repeat in a disease allele. There is also a risk for relatives of the partner with the intermediate allele.

In a Dutch study, intermediate alleles (3.9 per cent) and reduced penetrance alleles (2.5 per cent) were encountered in 71 of 1101 persons, affected and not affected, from 42 different

Huntington families (Maat-Kievit *et al.* 2001). The frequency of intermediate (together with a disease/reduced penetrance allele) and reduced penetrance alleles in the symptomatic population ($n=659$) was 2.6 and 2.4 per cent, respectively, and the frequency of intermediate and reduced penetrance alleles in asymptomatic presymptomatic testing candidates ($n=442$) was 5.8 and 2.7 per cent, respectively. The frequency of intermediate alleles (3.9 per cent) was significantly higher ($p=0.002–0.004$) than previously reported by Kremer *et al.* (1994) and Goldberg *et al.* (1995) in the general population (1.5–1.9 per cent). The intermediate allele range has increased compared with previous reports (currently 27 to 35 repeats as opposed to 30 to 35 (Kremer *et al.* 1994) or 29 to 35 repeats (Goldberg *et al.* 1995)). In addition, the intermediate alleles of relatives of newly identified patients (category 4 above) who became presymptomatic test applicants are included in the Dutch series. Intermediate alleles (mean repeat length 29) in asymptomatic and symptomatic (besides a disease allele) test candidates, inherited from the unaffected family branch, were most frequent (46 per cent). Reduced penetrance alleles in symptomatic test applicants (mean repeat length 39) were also quite frequent (22 per cent). No symptomatic test candidates with an intermediate allele were detected. Categories 4 and 5 were infrequently observed (11 per cent) and only intermediate alleles were found (Table 7.4).

Fourteen out of 43 intermediate test results (33 per cent) were smaller than 30 CAG repeats and analysed before 1998, when the intermediate lower limit was considered to be 30 repeats. These carriers were not informed when the limit was reset at 27 repeats. Obviously, the size of the CAG repeat, through its natural property of variability in transmission, may in a small percentage of asymptomatic individuals be of a class where a straightforward prediction of the phenotype or future disease is not possible. This has consequences for the information that is provided to test candidates.

Identification of the HD status (by family history, pathology, and DNA data) in at least one relative in a family is of paramount importance. Family members who may have had physical or mental complaints that went unnoticed because they were not admitted to hospital, under medical surveillance, or were misdiagnosed should be re-evaluated.

Table 7.4 Frequencies and mean repeat length of intermediate (IA) and reduced penetrance (RP) alleles in symptomatic ($N = 659$) and presymptomatic ($N = 442$) test applicants in Leiden and Rotterdam (1993–98) in the five different categories* of individuals with IA or RP alleles

Test outcome	Frequency (mean repeat length) in category					Total *n*
	1	2	3	4	5	
Symptomatic subject						
IA allele (with disease allele)	—	17 (29)	—	—	—	17
RP allele	16 (39)	0	—	—	—	16
Asymptomatic subject						
IA allele		16 (29)	2 (34)	6 (32)	2 (29)	26
RP allele		3 (36)	9 (39)	0	0	12
Total *n*	16	36	11	6	2	71

*Categories: 1, Symptomatic test applicants inheriting RP allele on HD haplotype; 2, symptomatic and asymptomatic test applicants inheriting IA/RP allele from unaffected parent (no family history); 3, asymptomatic test applicants inheriting IA/RP allele on HD haplotype; 4, asymptomatic test applicants who are relatives of newly identified HD parent (no family history); 5, asymptomatic partners (no family history) of carriers, tested as a control for prenatal testing.

Sometimes it is necessary to perform additional investigations (for example, DNA analysis, neurological/psychiatric examination) in the parent without a family history for interpretation of an intermediate or reduced penetrance allele found in the test candidate. It should be noted that going back to these parents raises issues in itself. Knowing whether there are HD patients or carriers of reduced penetrance or intermediate alleles in the family may have implications for counselling.

It is important to inform test candidates in pre-test sessions about repeat lengths, the possible uncertainties in a few per cent of presymptomatic, diagnostic, or prenatal tests related to the nature of the repeat mechanism, and the chance of intermediate or reduced penetrance alleles. Although it is possible in pre-test sessions to explore the desire to know these uncertain test results, it can be debated whether, in the complex process of decision-making, detailed discussion about risks for expansion and penetrance is appropriate.

The limits of the different categories of the repeat size have changed over time, so normal results might now be classified as intermediate, intermediate as reduced penetrance, and disease as reduced penetrance alleles. Furthermore, the initial analysis included a CCG repeat downstream that was later proven to be polymorphic (De Rooy *et al.* 1993). This may have had consequences for those carrying borderline-sized repeats. In addition, the data currently available do not yet allow provision of exact penetrance risk figures for those who received a disease or an intermediate allele (especially those without a family history), now called reduced penetrance alleles. Nor are we able to give exact risk figures for expansions in the offspring of those (especially those without a family history) who received a normal test result but whom we now call intermediate alleles. In these 'minimal risk' situations, for example, when unaffected parents or partners without a family history are involved, it might be wise to refrain from providing information or re-testing.

The policy with regard to disclosing results is not to communicate the repeat length unless applicants ask for it (Burgess and Hayden 1996). In the case of intermediate or reduced penetrance alleles it is necessary to be specific about the repeat length, because of the possible consequences for test candidates' (future) offspring and relatives.

Carriers of intermediate repeats can inform their adult children about the outcome and the possibility of presymptomatic testing because of the yet unknown risk of expansion. It can be questioned whether it is morally justified and good medical practice to burden other relatives, especially those families without a HD patient, with these uncertain risks for a disorder with which they are not familiar. On the other hand, not informing might prevent individuals from making decisions concerning their life and future. Admittedly, the risk arising from an intermediate allele is markedly less than that of the HD disease allele, but individuals and families may want to reconsider their risks. It remains to be seen whether and how they cope with the new information and situation. Informing relatives of carriers of reduced penetrance alleles (by the carriers) and offering the option of presymptomatic testing is hardly under debate because this risk approximates to the risk of relatives of a disease allele carrier.

It should be borne in mind that a prenatal test always carries a risk for the pregnancy. Prenatal testing for HD has been used by only a minority of at-risk individuals (2 per cent of those under the age of 50) and asymptomatic disease allele carriers (11 per cent) (Maat-Kievit *et al.* 1999). The option of prenatal testing for intermediate allele carriers needs discussion because of the, as yet unquantified, risk of expansion. Prenatal testing for this category resembles prenatal testing for a chromosomal translocation with a small risk of unbalanced offspring or chromosomal abnormalities in women over 36 years. Although no empirical risk figures yet exist, prenatal testing for carriers of reduced penetrance alleles can be an option because of the possibility of full penetrance of the mutation in offspring.

Specific psychological problems may be encountered in individuals who decide to be tested in the hope of relieving their children from the risk of HD and who are unexpectedly told that they have an intermediate repeat. Having received a decreased risk themselves, they must tell their children that they have not yet escaped HD, as there is still a chance of expansion with a consequent risk to them and future generations of developing the disease. The parents and children do not share a common fate, as is usual in dominant disorders, which can result in sustained feelings of guilt in the parents and reproach in the children, as in recessive disorders.

Other concerns may include the difficulty in coping with the uncertainty about the risk of expansion and penetrance, the different implications of an intermediate test result for daughters and sons, and turmoil induced by informing relatives, unaware of a risk, about the uncertain consequences of intermediate and reduced penetrance alleles. It is important to realize that it is difficult for most of these applicants, who are unexpectedly confronted with a risk for themselves and their offspring and relatives, to live with this uncertainty. It is our experience that most applicants, and especially this group, not familiar with HD and testing, wish to know the result as soon as possible in order to restore control over their life. This is an understandable reaction to a far-reaching event, but may lead them to underestimate the ramifications of testing. It is therefore recommended that these individuals, in particular, first become fully aware of what it means to be at-risk, and then to adjust to this awareness. After this, testing could be an option. The international guidelines were published 1 year after identification of the HD gene; they do not take account of the new data on intermediate and reduced penetrance alleles. Suggestions for further adjustment have been provided by Maat-Kievit *et al.* (2001) (Table 7.5).

Table 7.5 Provisional additional guidelines for counselling (possible) carriers of intermediate and reduced penetrance alleles of HD (from Matt-Kievit *et al.* 2001)

Pre-test information
    Family history (neurological/psychiatric examination, DNA-data, pathology)
    Four ranges of repeat sizes
    Chance of unexpected test results
    Uncertainties about risk of expansion of intermediate alleles and penetrance of disease alleles with
      reduced penetrance
    Difference of intermediate test result for sons and daughters
    Chance of additional investigation of the unaffected parent without a family history for
      interpretation of the intermediate or reduced penetrance allele found in the test candidate
    Exploration of the wish to know an intermediate- or reduced penetrance allele test result
Disclosure of repeat size if CAG repeat size is between 27 and 39
Offering the possibility of information and presymptomatic testing to relatives of carriers with repeats
    between 27 and 39 (after adjusting to the awareness of what is means to be at-risk)
Discussing the possibility of prenatal testing with carriers with repeats between 27 and 39 because of
    the yet unknown risk of expansion and penetrance
Psychological support in decision-making, before and after testing for applicant and relatives if
    they wish

Exclusion testing by linkage

'*The purpose of the exclusion test, which was frequently performed before the gene defect itself had been found, is to permit a 50 per cent at-risk person to exclude the possibility of having affected children without changing his or her 50 per cent at-risk status*' (International Guidelines, 7.3).

Individuals at 25 per cent risk and healthy individuals requesting prenatal testing (where the pregnancy is usually at 25 per cent risk) have the option of exclusion testing. As was discussed in the section 'Risk estimation', the actual risk is lower than 25 per cent as the chance that an offspring of an affected parent has inherited the disease-causing mutation decreases with increasing age. Exclusion testing, where linked markers are used in preference to specific mutation testing, is often unfamiliar and confusing to family members and to those involved in genetic counselling. Before 1993, exclusion testing was more widely used, especially in pregnancy. Here, exclusion testing is still carried out using gene tracking by linked markers, which allows information to be derived without providing a result in the at-risk parent (Simpson *et al.* 2001). The concept of exclusion testing is illustrated in Fig. 7.4.

The question to be resolved is whether the individual (or pregnancy) at 25 per cent risk has received from their 50 per cent at-risk parent, the chromosome that originated from the affected or the unaffected grandparent. If the latter is the case, then the risk of HD in the individual or pregnancy at 25 per cent risk is clearly very low, although there is a small chance (1–2 per cent) due to genetic recombination. If it is the affected grandparental chromosome that has been transmitted, then the risk will rise from 25 to 50 per cent, which is the same as that for the parent at risk. There will be nonspecific prediction, since the transmitted grandparental chromosome could equally be the HD or the normal one. Likewise, and most importantly, the 50 per cent risk for the intervening individual is unaltered by the result of the offspring or pregnancy at 25 per cent risk. Exclusion testing could be considered as an important option in two specific situations. The first situation applies when a person at 25 per cent risk wishes to be tested, but his at-risk parent does not want to learn about his genetic status. Exclusion testing offers the possibility of getting a low-risk test result without altering the genetic status of the parent at 50 per cent risk. Second, in case of a pregnancy, an individual at

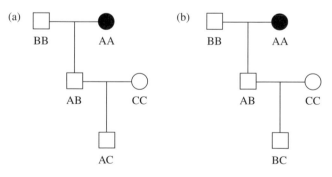

Fig. 7.4 Exclusion testing in HD. In this family the HD gene is associated with marker genotype A. Thus, (a) if the person (or pregnancy) at 25 per cent risk has also inherited genotype A there will be a high risk for developing HD (50 per cent, as for the intervening parent), whereas (b) if genotype B has been inherited (derived from the unaffected grandparent), the risk will be low.

25 per cent risk, not wishing to pass the gene on to future offspring, and not wishing to know their own status, may make use of exclusion testing (see also the section 'Prenatal testing').

A serious limitation of exclusion testing in pregnancy is the implication of an increased (50 per cent) risk. Should the pregnancy be terminated or continued? In the case when the couple decides to terminate the pregnancy, there is a 50 per cent chance that an unaffected pregnancy is terminated. How often can a couple make such a dreadful decision? And what if they find out at a later stage that the at-risk parent is not a carrier of the gene, and the termination has been unnecessary? On the other hand, if a child with 50 per cent risk is carried to term, the parent at risk has to cope with a double burden in the future if they develop symptoms. The couple has the certainty that the child has inherited the HD gene and will develop the disease in the future. This awareness may happen in childhood or adolescence. Therefore, the guidelines recommend that the test should not be performed when the couple at-risk has no intention of terminating a pregnancy with increased risk. In other words, as commented in the guidelines: '*This includes the termination of pregnancies where the foetus is at 50 per cent risk and continuation of pregnancies where the foetus is only at low risk*' (International Guidelines, 7.3, comment).

Neurological and psychological examination

'*Neurologic examinations and psychological appraisal are considered important to establish a baseline evaluation of each individual*' (International Guidelines 6.2).

One of the most cited reasons for wanting presymptomatic testing is to obtain relief from uncertainty. Individuals at risk may have suffered for many years and through several stages of their life from the fear of developing symptoms. They may be continuously preoccupied with mental or physical signs that could be the first announcement of the disease.

I told myself, as I always do, your legs ache because you're not fit (the muscle in your chin jumps because you are tired, carelessness made you drop that glass) and I thought what a fool I was to go out in high heels, in pointed shoes that pinched my toes. It scarcely helped, nothing helps except the ache, the tic, the weakness, going away. [Vine 1989]

Genetic centres involved in presymptomatic testing for HD have adopted different policies with regard to the use of a neurological examination as a part of the testing protocol, to exclude the possibility that the test candidate is showing symptoms of the disease. Some testing centres require a neurological investigation prior to testing with the consequence that early symptoms might be an argument to withhold or refuse testing. Also, in some centres, a psychological or psychiatric assessment is part of the standard evaluation (Meissen *et al.* 1988; Brandt *et al.* 1989). In a study by McCusker *et al.* (2000), 156 test candidates underwent neurological assessment to analyse the association between pre-gene result symptoms and minimal neurological signs. In 61 per cent of the identified carriers minor neurological signs were found (opposed to 8 per cent in non-carriers). In contrast, neurological complaints made by the at-risk group did not distinguish gene status, whereas behavioural and cognitive symptoms were more often reported by the gene-positive group (McCusker *et al.* 2000). The authors concluded that neurological examination remains the most accessible, reliable, and cost-effective means of determining clinical disease onset. However, a Dutch study revealed that there was considerable disagreement between three HD-experienced neurologists with regard to the neurological examinations in the earliest phase of the disease (de Boo *et al.* 1998).

It was only after deliberation that satisfactory levels of interrater agreement were reached but, even then, in 16 per cent of the cases the neurologists came to a false-positive decision and in 9 per cent they could not reach an agreement. Neuropsychological motor assessment proved to be more sensitive to early changes than neurological judgements. Yet, the question that genetic counsellors are most frequently asked is whether an individual will become affected in the future, as will be discussed later.

The aim of the neurological examination is to distinguish the difference between a diagnosis of HD based on clinical symptoms, and the finding that an individual is a gene-carrier. However, test applicants might want to be tested, not because they seek confirmation that they are already showing early signs of the disease, but to find out whether they will develop HD in the future. A person for whom a positive clinical diagnosis has been made may feel that he or she does not need testing. Others, with awareness that their dysfunctions could be associated with HD, may request confirmatory or diagnostic testing. They may feel that they have a slightly increased risk of being a gene-carrier, being relatively close to more overt symptomatology. These people generally expect to get unfavourable test results, and admit after disclosure that the result is not surprising.

Neurological examination can provide information about how closely an individual at risk may need to be followed after learning that he or she is carrier of the disease-causing mutation. The guidelines suggest that the neurological evaluation might also serve as a starting point for long-term follow-up, once carriers have been identified. From a scientific point of view this might be important to gain more insight into the onset and course of HD over time. The clinical relevance for identified gene carriers, however, is small. It remains to be seen whether neurological and neuropsychological follow-up is actually reinforcing a premature medicalization of carriers. On the other hand, identified carriers may feel comfortable and comforted when under surveillance of professionals who are specialized in HD. Moreover, the opportunity to contribute to research projects may be considered as a meaningful experience for gene-carriers. Sometimes, identified carriers ask for surveillance with the provision that the results of examinations are not communicated until they ask for it. To some extent, these carriers need to take control over their personal life and future, and it may be possible to face the reality of their genetic status when the carrier is able to do so. The guidelines comment that individuals with established, unacknowledged symptoms should not automatically be excluded from the test and should receive additional counselling. However, clinical experience has taught us that identified carriers with subtle symptomatology may not need follow-up and additional counselling as this would mean an unwanted confrontation with HD.

If a genetic centre has decided to include a neurological examination as part of the testing protocol, early signs may be observed that are suspiciously like HD, though they may be not sufficient to warrant a diagnosis. In some instances, what are interpreted as early behavioural signs, such as anxiety or depression, may not be related to HD at all. A person with subtle dysfunctions may be at a slightly increased risk of being a gene-carrier or may be relatively close to more overt symptomatology (de Boo *et al.* 1998). The neurological investigation can provide the counsellor with information about how closely an individual may need to be monitored in the time immediately following the test outcome. It should be noted that '*the presymptomatic test indicates whether someone has or has not inherited the gene defect, but it does not make a current clinical diagnosis of HD if the gene is present*' (International Guidelines 5.2.5).

Psychological or psychiatric assessment is carried out because high levels of depression and risk of suicide have been observed in individuals at risk. The probability of adverse emotional reactions can be considered as the test candidate's greatest risk of taking the test. Although it seems important to identify those test candidates who are likely to need more psychosocial support than others, the parameters that should be used, apart from the overt risks for suicide and/or major depression, are not determined. A history of suicidal intentions or depressive moods may reflect a life of prolonged uncertainties and unresolved fears, which can only be relieved by either test result. Moreover, the worldwide study on catastrophic events has shown that serious events were only rarely observed as a reaction to the test results, and occurred mostly in individuals with pre-existing problems (see Chapter 3).

Refusal by professionals to offer a test, on the basis of psychological or psychiatric screening, can be experienced by the test applicant as a personal rejection and lack of trust, instead of cautious medical practice. Unconditional positive regard for the test candidate, one of the cornerstones of the non-directive counselling approach, may be more useful in reaching an appropriate decision taken by the test candidate than a delay of the test based on an authoritative veto. Whilst a proper estimation of the test candidate's mental resources might lead to uncertainties in the counsellor and, consequently, delay of the test, an empathic understanding based on the family history and individual psychological make-up of the test candidate may reassure both the candidate (and companion) and the counsellor. It is obvious that, in the case of a clear psychiatric condition, the test should be discussed with other health-care professionals who are involved. If the counsellor has sincere doubts about the mental condition of a test candidate, it is good medical practice to refer them for a psychological assessment. Counsellors should not violate their professional responsibility by conducting a test against their better judgement. However, refusal to undergo either neurological or psychological examination does not justify withholding the presymptomatic test from an individual at risk who wishes to be tested. Postponement or exclusion from testing have been reported for various reasons: because of manifest symptoms of HD (Bloch *et al.* 1989; Brandt *et al.* 1989), severe depression (Meissen *et al.* 1988; Brandt *et al.* 1989; Codori and Brandt 1994), and evaluation by a psychiatrist (Meissen *et al.* 1988).

Confirmatory presymptomatic testing

Some individuals request presymptomatic testing even though the experienced counsellor clearly observes that characteristic movements betray the beginning onset of the disease.

Example. A man of 44 years of age was married and had a 14-year-old son. His affected mother had died many years ago. He wanted to be tested in order to relieve the uncertainty of his carrier status, to prepare for his own future, and to be able to inform his son. When he and his wife came to the centre he showed intangible features that were suspiciously like HD, but he denied any symptoms, and had no complaints about his functioning as a bus driver. Yet, the memories of his dead mother were still vivid, and he remembered her facial gestures and kicking the table. He had been very nervous during the previous week with the prospect of coming to the centre, and his wife commented with a laugh that he had been presenting those facial gestures and kicking with his legs like his mother did. Cautious references to equivalent features in his mother were dismissed. The couple remained hopeful, but acknowledged that in the case of an unfavourable result they would need extensive professional guidance.

Consequently, the test may in fact be not a presymptomatic but an affirmative one. A non-directive approach does not allow straightforward communication of the counsellor's observations and suspicions. Careful and prudent counselling is needed to find out whether the test candidate is willing to consider the onset of symptoms. Partners often underline the absence of what is noticed by the counsellor. For an inexperienced counsellor this may seem odd, peculiar, and difficult to understand. Yet the psychological meaning of such denial should be acknowledged and appreciated. We must differentiate, however, between those individuals who have a lot of experience of HD in their family, and those who have never seen a HD patient in the various stages of the disease. Besides, the clinical geneticist or genetic counsellor is not always the appropriate professional to communicate the diagnosis which is usually a task for clinicians with experience in the clinical diagnosis of HD.

Denial is a psychological defence strategy often used against the untoward reality of HD. Most people working with HD families develop remarkably sensitive 'antennae' for detecting the individual who is not quite right. This does not necessarily encompass the clear neurological HD abnormality, although equivocal abnormalities may be found and the neurological examination may show changes. It is more a professional intuition that leads one to 'know' that HD seems close to manifestation. The experienced counsellor will have observed—more than incidentally—the inability of individuals from HD families to face up to the presence of prominent characteristic choreic movements. Often, identified carriers suspected of early symptoms are able to acknowledge the onset shortly after disclosure of the test results, while others need a longer time to allow the onset of symptoms to enter their awareness. The best approach is an exploration of whether at-risk carriers have complaints that could relate to onset of disease. If so, referral to a neurologist could follow. Otherwise, DNA testing should be continued with the provision that all conditions for proper testing have been met. It is very important to remain neutral and to ask the person what brings him or her to the centre. In general, people have considered coming for a long time. Once this decision has been made they deserve to be treated with respect and consideration.

There are important quantitative and qualitative differences between the way in which neurologists and geneticists attend to the patient. The neurologist is considering a neurological problem, the side-effects of which may be given some attention but are essentially subsidiary. The geneticist offers more time and pays attention to the meaning of the disease and risks for patients and their families. There is a broader discussion of the impact of the disease on all life issues. This might explain why individuals with initial symptoms may prefer to visit a geneticist instead of a neurologist. A second explanation is that individuals with early signs of the disease may prefer a genetic test instead of a diagnostic test. Being identified as a gene carrier may confirm long-existing fears but allows the admission of being a patient to be delayed.

For once, of course, when experiencing trembling or lack of co-ordination or ordinary failure of manual dexterity, I had no real fear that this was the onset of Huntington's, I knew it was the effect of shock. But I told myself that I must exercise control, I must behave as if nothing had happened. [Vine 1988]

Denial of the awareness of being affected can be supported by the partner who also has understandable reasons to postpone acknowledgement of the feared truth. It remains a point of debate as to whether a clearly affected individual should be allowed to undergo presymptomatic testing or whether they should be referred directly to a neurologist. Rejection of the test and referral to a neurologist would be, however, a coerced choice without showing appreciation of the psychological reasons for coming to a genetic centre.

The request for testing by a person, who shows subtle or obvious signs of the disorder without being willing to consider their current condition, must be appreciated. However, this does not mean that the counsellor should not explore the boundaries of reality. Sometimes the person asks frankly whether the counsellor thinks they are already affected. An honest answer could be postponed until the feelings and thoughts of the applicant are explored. 'I'd like to answer your question, but could you first tell me your personal thoughts, feelings and concerns?'

The most difficult situation occurs perhaps when a person has no idea how HD develops in the early stages, but comes for a presymptomatic test and learns before the test result is disclosed that he or she is probably affected. A careful neurological examination could be important to verify the first clinical impression. The best one can do is to note one's concern, to emphasize that the genetic risks for offspring will be dependent on a person's own status, and to try to maintain contact with the family. It poses a particularly traumatic situation for all concerned, for the individual has come to ask one question: what is the risk of developing HD in the future?—but is faced with an adverse answer to a question that was probably not even raised. The disease is already present. No easy solution can be given as to how to cope best with this situation.

Based on my own experience, communicating the view that the person is affected should be avoided in the initial interview, even if asked directly. It would seem unreasonable to give such important information as a complete stranger and after a single assessment, especially if circumstances have dictated a less than thorough examination. It is best to try to find out from the patient and family whether they have noticed any symptoms. It may become apparent that requesting genetic counselling has been the only way by which medical attention could be sought for symptoms that are recognized but not yet accepted. Again, this information may be obtained only at a second visit. A more detailed neurological assessment could be suggested before disclosing the diagnosis. This may well not show anything that is not already apparent clinically but it will help to exclude other (possibly treatable) disorders and again will give time for adjustment to the situation. It might be preferable not to tell a person that he or she is affected until a later stage. The best policy is to be open and frank about it once it is definite and once there has been adequate time to adjust to the possibility of being affected.

It is my experience that neurologists have offered presymptomatic testing to adult children of an affected parent who has recently been clinically diagnosed, confirmed by mutation analysis. In my opinion, this is unsatisfactory unless the testing meets the international guidelines. In my, and other's experience, however, testing has—more than occasionally—been carried out without sound pre- and post-test counselling. In the Netherlands, the Leiden laboratory would refuse to analyse DNA for presymptomatic reasons when requested by a neurologist or other medical specialist not involved in a presymptomatic testing programme. Laboratories in most other countries have adopted a comparable policy and use the International Guidelines as a framework (IHA/WFN 1994; ACMG/ASHG 1998). The Dutch Association of Neurologists has supported the policy that genetic centres should carry out presymptomatic testing. Indeed, professionals with the most experience of testing, as well as people who have been tested, continue to urge caution. Wherever possible, physicians are strongly advised to refer applicants for testing to the nearest (genetic) centre that has extensive experience with testing for HD. These centres are staffed with the personnel necessary to administer the counselling and other necessary support.

Testing children and adolescents

'The test is available only to individuals who have reached the age of majority (according to the laws of the respective country)' (International Guidelines 2.1).

The general opinion among professionals is that testing in childhood for adult-onset, untreatable disorders holds more potential for harm than benefit (Clarke 1994). Hence, DNA tests for adult-onset diseases on asymptomatic children—at parental request—are generally not performed in most genetic centres. We and others (Ball and Harper 1992; Binedell 1998) have made exceptions to this guideline when testing is sought by an adolescent who is sufficiently mature to make such a profound decision and is able to freely provide fully informed consent. As in adults, it remains difficult to determine competence to consent and strategies for individual assessment have yet to be developed.

Before further discussing testing children and adolescents there is the issue of when to tell children about HD. Parents who receive an unfavourable test result often raise this question. Recommendations have been made that children should be told about the disease between the ages of 14 and 16 years, depending on the maturity of the child (Folstein 1991). However, children may not wait until they are told about the disease, but pose awkward questions with regard to the visible features they have noticed. As the illness progresses in a parent or close relative, symptoms will become more noticeable and may elicit social reactions. In general, truth is better than deceit, and honesty fosters trust and a sense of security (Levebvre 1999). Although doubts have been expressed about whether children can understand the implications of the disease at a younger age, young people in HD families seemed able to discuss the disease and its implications in a rational and thoughtful manner (Korer and Fitzsimmons 1987). Korer and Fitzsimmons found no evidence for the supposition that young people are too emotionally unstable to cope with information about HD. On the other hand, adolescents tend to be present-oriented, attaching too much weight to present as opposed to future concerns and not appreciating that values change over time (Wertz *et al.* 1994). There may not be a need to introduce 'the whole truth'. It is often more humane and effective to share the truth in 'instalments', or easier-to-swallow bites. The child's developmental level and how this affects their reasoning and understanding should be taken into account before launching into a complex explanation about the illness and its causation. Abstract thinking does not develop until adolescence; before then, abstract discussions about genetics will only go over a child's head and confuse them (Fanos 1997; Levebvre 1999).

I was fourteen when they told me. They were right, they had to tell me, but perhaps they could have waited a few more years. What harm would it have done to wait four years? I wasn't likely to have married in those four years, I wasn't likely to have had a baby. . . . It wasn't that my mother's illness was apparent. They weren't even sure she was ill, not physically that is. Mental changes, which is how the books describe her condition, could be attributed to many causes or to none in particular. But they had set fourteen as the age and they stuck to it and told me, not on the birthday itself, which is what happens to the heroes and heroines of romance initiated into family rituals and family secrets on some pre-set coming of age, but two months later, on a wet Sunday afternoon. They must have known it would frighten me and make me unhappy. But did they understand what shock it was? Did they realize they would make me feel as much set apart from the rest of humanity as if I had a hump on my back or was destined to grow seven feet tall? I understood then why I was an only child, though not why I had been born at all. For a while I reproached them for giving me birth, for being irresponsible when even then they knew the facts. And for a while, a long while, I no longer wanted them as parents, I no longer wanted to know them. The rapid progress of my mother's illness made no difference. There is no time in our lives when we are so conspicuously without mercy as in adolescence. I turned from them and their secret, her distorted genes, his watchful eyes and suspenseful waiting for the appearance of signs, to someone who was kind and didn't cause me pain. [Vine 1989]

The most important principle is, no matter how painful it is, for adults in the family, to never deny the possibility that children are aware of the social reactions, and to have a frank discussion about how people tend to fear any 'different behaviour' that they do not understand.

The way in which a family copes with HD is an important factor in the experience of an adolescent and will be of far-reaching influence on their perception and decision-making capacities with regard to presymptomatic testing. Waiting until 18 to find out whether or not a child has inherited HD can be a tremendous stress and constant worry for both parents and children. Even if children are functioning well at school, many of their fears and anxieties, which they are afraid of adding to their parents own fears, may influence their life and friendships deeply. In the absence of evidence or experience of long-term effects of presymptomatic testing of children, the current policy is guided by the ethical principle of 'first do no harm'. In addition to protecting children from the potential harm of test results, there is the motive of safeguarding the child's future right to make an autonomous decision, with confidentiality preserved (Clarke and Flinter 1996). Although withholding minors from presymptomatic testing for HD is based on lack of medical treatment, the psychological costs and benefits are less clear. Surveys on attitudes towards testing children have shown throughout the last three decades that testing of family members under 18 should be made possible (Barette and Marsden 1979; Morris *et al.* 1989; Tibben *et al.* 1993b). More than occasionally, parents ask whether their children can be tested and sometimes children under 18 ask for the test themselves (Morris *et al.* 1989). In my experience, parents do accept the generally adopted policy to not test children for the HD gene if their request is considered seriously, and if they are offered help in coping with the HD issue towards their children. In the discussion about testing for children, less attention has been given to the potential impact of withholding testing of the child on the parents, and the effect on their relationship with the child, than to the potential effects of testing. Unfortunately, there is still no reliable information concerning the most appropriate age to offer testing for HD. The strain of undergoing testing, receiving test results, and adjusting to the new genetic status must be weighed against the stress and uncertainty of living at risk for HD. Moreover, the attack on the child's self-respect by being denied testing and the possible sense of humiliation and helplessness at having one's autonomy undermined could have adverse effects (Bloch *et al.* 1992). Could the child be harmed by the test result? It is assumed that an unfavourable test result might lower the self-esteem of the child. The test might prove self-fulfilling; becoming preoccupied with symptoms may limit use of the childs' emotional, intellectual, and social resources through perceived restricted future prospects. The child may suffer from stigmatization, and could have serious problems in education and career. However, these assumptions are speculative.

There is no doubt that testing prevents the child from having the chance to make a personal decision about testing. Untested children lose their right to be tested, and adults lose their right to have been tested in childhood. Yet, there is no evidence for those assumptions. Children might also benefit from the opportunity to prepare psychologically for the future. Caution in the absence of evidence is second best (Michie 1996). But what if the parents are suffering from uncertainty and the subsequent ambivalent attitude towards their children? Most requests from parents are motivated by a hope that being tested might spare their children the lifelong worry they themselves have experienced, but also from a wish to ensure that their children know themselves to be free of the gene before having their own families in the future. It has been demonstrated that mothers with ambivalent feelings toward their children show disorganized behaviour with the consequence of insecure attachment patterns in the child (Schuengel *et al.* 1999). Some disorders, such as HD, appear to have a major disorganizing effect on families (Wexler 1979). This may lead to adjustment problems in later life (Kessler 1998). Thus, when parents ask for testing of young children, this might benefit the attachment and subsequently the child's personality development. But, again, to allow parents to decide on their children's participation in testing would have broken the primary principles of confidentiality, privacy, and individual justice that are owed to them. It should also be highlighted that allowing a third party to make decisions for an individual at risk could set precedents for others outside the direct family. Adoption agencies, educational institutions, insurance companies, and other third parties could insist on genetic testing for any individuals shown to be at risk.

Another reason for a third party to request the presymptomatic testing of minors might be in an attempt to diagnose an illness in a sick child where HD is a possibility. A case has been described in which clinicians, knowing that a child was at risk of juvenile HD, asked for a test to be performed to assist in diagnosing the child's current illness. This request was denied on the grounds that it would be detrimental to the child at risk. Geneticists were concerned that in obtaining confirmation of the child's status the clinicians may have been deterred from making further investigations that could have identified a treatable cause for the child's illness that was unrelated to HD. The geneticists' concerns were that, if the child recovered from the possibly unrelated illness, a test would have been carried out before the child at risk was capable of giving informed consent. The limited contribution that the test would have on the final diagnosis should be weighed against the psychosocial problems the child at risk would suffer should the illness turn out not to be HD (Craufurd *et al.* 1990).

Support for the view that any HD tests taken should be done with the fully informed and voluntary consent of the individual at risk is given in the international guidelines, which state that a presymptomatic test should be offered only to freely consenting adults. Exceptions could be made to this guideline when a decision to terminate pregnancy in someone under the age of 18 is being considered or where a confirmatory test is required for a symptomatic minor, but the problems mentioned above would have to be taken into consideration.

Binedell (1998) summarized useful information in assessing competence in adolescence:

1. The length of time the adolescent has lived with knowledge of HD in the family and being at risk will be an important factor in the ability to weigh the costs and benefits of learning more precisely about the genetic status.

2. The way in which an adolescent has adjusted to the awareness of HD in the family and being at risk is a predictor of how he or she will cope with a test result.

3. Level of autonomy: is the adolescent able to make an independent decision and what is their reference group with regard to this decision?

4. Does the adolescent have accurate knowledge about the most important aspects of the test procedure, and is he or she able to use the information in the decision process?

5. Is the adolescent able to appreciate the impact of test results for close relatives?

6. Are the decision and the motives for the decision stable and consistent over time?

7. Are there any underlying motives with regard to family dynamics such as resolving family conflicts, undoing beliefs about preselection, etc. that require a different approach and subsequent interventions?

8. Is there any previous evidence of competent decision-making? What is the pattern of shar-
    ing information and making decisions in the family?

For a more general view and a guide to further reading on testing children, see Clarke (1998).

The issues of being at 25 per cent risk (the conflict of interests)

'*Extreme care should be exercised when testing would provide information about another
person who has not requested the test*' (International Guidelines 2.4). One of the important
issues we have encountered in presymptomatic testing, although not frequently, concerns
individuals at 25 per cent risk for diseases such as HD who request genetic testing with full
awareness that the symptom-free parent wishes to remain uninformed about their personal
genetic status. By 25 per cent risk we mean half the risk of the parent at risk. Actually, this
means that the risk should be adjusted for the age of the parent and the decreased computed
risk as the parent's age increases without having symptoms. The probability that an asymptomatic individual at-risk has the HD gene remains 50 per cent during childhood and young
adulthood, but gradually decreases with increasing age (see also the section 'Risk estimation'). The consequence of an unfavourable test result in an individual at 25 per cent risk is
that the genetic status of intervening parent is also 'disclosed'. If there are any untested
siblings, their risk has increased to 50 per cent.

Example. An 18-year-old woman requested DNA testing after referral by the family practitioner; a
schoolteacher accompanied her. She had seen a television programme on HD and was shocked by the
patients presented in the programme. She realized that her parents had not told the whole truth about the
disease in her grandmother. She had discussed this with neither her parents nor her sister who was
6 years older. She had strong intrusive images of HD and was not able to function at school. A visit to
her family doctor led to her to apply for the test.

In counselling our patients, we are guided by the principle of beneficence, which means that
we do not want to impose any evil or harm. We also want to prevent or remove adverse effects,
and we hope that we can promote the favourable. The International Guidelines have emphasized that such cases need extreme care and that every effort should be made by the counsellor and the test candidates to find a solution of this conflict that is satisfactory for all
parties, not only the test candidate. The majority of representatives of patient organizations
acknowledge the right of the adult child to be tested over the right of the parent to remain
ignorant.

   When we consider a request as giving rise to a potential conflict of interest we have a serious counselling problem, whether one approaches the issue from a moral or legal point of
view. The psychological issue, however, is that we do not sufficiently take account of what is
going on in a family and its individual members. We do not know the meaning of the test
request against the background of the entire family system and history. Moreover, when we
deal with such request as a conflict—a conflict that refers to disagreement within the family—
we do not anticipate the consequences a test result might have. The interests of at least one
party are violated. Yet, family members have to go on together after a test result and are chal-
lenged to maintain mutual satisfactory relationships. As far as possible, testing should not
serve as a crowbar. What, then, can be done to serve an individual at 25 per cent risk requiring
a test, and—at the same time—to help reach a satisfactory solution for all parties? For that we

need a family approach and the request for testing ought to be seen in the context of the family history. Every HD family has built its coping strategies, often over two or more generations. Anticipating the test results should be regarded in the light of the near and far future, which may become overshadowed by the disease in one or more relatives. Family members may need each other in the future and a test procedure that is carried out too rashly may jeopardize the mutual relationships irrevocably.

Apart from the obvious reasons for individuals at 25 per cent risk to undergo testing such as relieving anxiety or planning a family, we have observed a variety of underlying reasons. One is the need to resolve the uncertainty in the entire family; the family does not know how to cope with the disease and suffers from the uncertainty without being able to resolve this. Another reason may be that the applicant wishes to reassure his or her parents, to take away the uncertainty about their child. The roles within the family are sometimes reversed: the child takes over the responsibility of the parent to create safety and openness in the family. Older children are sometimes asked to act as chaperones for a parent with HD. Children are sometimes regarded as a source of future support for the non-carrier parent. Guilt feelings towards a partner may be an important reason to request testing. Also, the applicant may wish to break the family's denial of the disease and avoidance of talking about the disease. The presence of such underlying reasons can be considered against the background of developmental tasks in the adolescent and young adult (Fanos 1997).

An important adolescent developmental task is separation or seeking freedom from parental figures. The strong bond with the parent because of HD may delay this separation process or even make it impossible, either on the part of the adolescent or on the part of the parent. A second task is the establishment of a personal identity, which may be hampered by preselection, by stigmatization by peers, or by self-stigmatization. It is generally known that many individuals at risk have adopted an HD identity. Next, coping with sexual feelings and interpersonal intimacy is a task in adolescence. Being at risk for HD may interfere with sexual experimenting, and lead to avoidance of forming relationships; on the other hand, some may express extreme sexual activity for the same reasons (Fanos 1997). Finally, adolescents have to remodel the idealizations of their parents that are created in childhood. The burden of HD in the family may make this process extremely difficult and induce guilt feelings about having a more realistic presentation of the parents and a more realistic representation of early attachments with the parents.

Example continued. The counselling focused on the way the parents and daughters coped with HD, the family experiences, and the threat for all of them. The woman was very anxious about an unfavourable result for herself and the consequences this would have for her father at risk. She intended to keep such a result hidden from her parents. She also missed the support of her parents who were not willing to discuss HD at all. Yet, she realized that her parents might have withheld the genetic information in their daughter's best interests, or that they did not know how to prepare their daughters for HD adequately. She also guessed that her parents would feel guilty knowing that their daughter had gone through testing without them being involved. Actually, she resented her parents avoiding the issue of HD. After three sessions she discussed her application for testing with her parents who joined her in the next session. The parents and their daughter were helped by their mutual communication, which resulted in the father's wish to be the first to have the test. He emphasized that, in the case of an unfavourable test result, his daughter should reconsider what to do and not feel obliged to have a test too.

From a legal point of view the individual at 25 per cent risk is the client. The counsellor can not be responsible for the well-being of the client's parent, as this would adversely interfere in the relationship with the test candidate. Also, the individual at 25 per cent risk cannot be responsible for their parents and siblings as this would reflect a role reversal. However, the individual at 25 per cent risk can be held responsible for the effects his or her behaviour—specifically regarding the test results—has on others.

A family life overshadowed by the risk of HD will obviously influence the way parents perform their parental tasks. An important task with respect to their children is the establishment of a stable and safe environment for the family, which may become difficult if the parents fear the disease. Another task is to explain the facts and circumstances of the grandparent's disease and their personal risks. It requires openness and courage to discuss these issues with ones' children. Parents must be able to understand their childrens' developmental capacities for coping with their risk of a disease and they must be able to express this understanding. They must assist in tolerating and expressing uncertainty and anxiety, and facilitate the change to new relationships and responsibilities.

Having considered the tasks of parents and children, the tasks of the counsellor can be made more explicit. The counsellor can increase the awareness of how HD has specifically affected every member of the family. He or she can help to discuss the traditions, the myths, and the coping strategies in the family with respect to HD. The counsellor can help to explore the underlying motives of the test request and consider this in the light of the developmental and parental tasks. The counsellor can give clarity about the developmental issues and tasks of each member, and facilitate openness and nonreactivity (that is being able to listen, hear the emotions and considerations of the other without counteracting immediately). Such work might increase the cohesion in the family and lead to new, constructive and creative ways to deal with HD. The counsellor serves as a model in discussing HD-related themes.

It takes time, specific training and knowledge, and much experience to be able to recognize and explore the specific themes in the family regarding their development. The themes and issues to be addressed include the individual beliefs, attitudes, and feelings about the disease and its impact in the family. Further, the impact on the current interactional framework of the family needs to be viewed. Subsequently, the way this framework is carried over into social contexts such as work, school, and social life must be considered and, finally, counsellors should investigate what is the common theme that links to family, loyalties and traditions. Counsellors may benefit from the concepts of family system theory, and education in the use of family dynamics could enrich their work.

Test requests should be considered against the background of the specific age- and role-related tasks that each member has in a family with a hereditary disease. The successful achievement of these tasks may have been extremely compromised by the occurrence of HD. The test applicant's motives should be explored to enable him or her to make an informed decision. The decision should be taken in the context of the personal and family history and their future. The decision must be understood as a reflection of the entire family's and the individual's coping mechanisms regarding the risks and the disease. Perhaps the next issue of the guidelines or comments could emphasize more explicitly the need for a family approach.

Prenatal testing

The localization and isolation of the HD mutation have presented new choices regarding reproduction for couples who have an increased risk of HD in a foetus. Although prenatal testing for foetuses at risk for HD is available, it is not a frequently chosen option (Adam *et al.* 1993; Maat-Kievit *et al.* 1999; Simpson *et al.* 2001). A European study, involving seven genetic centres in six countries, has evaluated reproductive decisions as an effect of the outcome of predictive testing. The overall experience, together with the associated legal and ethical issues, has been presented in a recent book (Evers-Kiebooms *et al.* 2002a), as well as in specific papers. A total of 305 prenatal tests were performed between 1993 and 1998. The uptake of prenatal testing was also assessed. Of the prospective parents, 57 per cent were known to have the gene, whereas others had not undergone predictive or diagnostic testing. Sixty-five per cent of the pregnancies were investigated using mutation analysis, the remainder by exclusion testing. In the carrier group prenatal testing occurred in two-thirds of the subsequent pregnancies. Three years after disclosure of the test results, 39 per cent of the identified carriers, who expressed reproductive motives in the pre-test sessions, had subsequent pregnancies (Evers-Kiebooms *et al.* 2002b; Simpson *et al.* 2001). Eight of 131 identified high-risk pregnancies were continued. The uptake of the exclusion test has remained low over the years, and has diminished since the availability of the mutation test. We can distinguish four categories of couples applying for prenatal testing, based on the risk of one of the prospective parents: (1) couples at high risk of developing HD (>95 per cent); (2) the 25 per cent or 50 per cent at-risk parent who does not wish to know his or her precise personal risk; (3) the parent at risk who is a carrier of an intermediate allele; and (4) the prospective parent, coming from a HD family, who is symptomatic. Table 7.6 shows the options that are available for prenatal testing.

It is very important that couples who consider the option of prenatal testing receive preconception counselling because the information about the different choices regarding reproduction, the impact of the possible outcomes of prenatal testing, and the decision-making process is quite complex. The testing protocol is, in general, the same as that for the presymptomatic testing programme (see Table 7.3). It is widely accepted that, in general, prenatal testing for serious genetic disorders in childhood should be available for couples who do not consider termination of a pregnancy. Anticipating the birth of a handicapped child may enable prospective parents to prepare for its birth. However, the couple at risk for HD requesting prenatal testing must be clearly informed that, if they intend to complete the pregnancy if the foetus

Table 7.6 Choices regarding reproduction for couples with an increased risk for HD in the foetus (from Maat-Kievit *et al.* 1999)

Choices regarding reproduction	Parent carrier	Parent 50% at risk
Having children	Yes	Yes
Refrain from having children	Yes	Yes
Adoption/fostering	Yes	Yes
Donor sperm insemination/egg donation + IVF	Yes	Yes
Presymptomatic testing of parent	No	Yes
Prenatal diagnosis	Yes	No
Prenatal exclusion testing	No	Yes
Prenatal exclusion—definitive testing	No	Yes
Prenatal mutation testing of foetus without prior testing of parent	No	Yes
Pre-implantation genetic testing*	Yes	Yes

*Theoretically possible.

proves to be a carrier of the gene defect, then there is no valid reason for performing the test. This safeguards the right of the future child not to know their genetic status.

Also important is the chance that a child, tested mutation-positive, will be harmed by the early knowledge regarding their genetic status. Stigmatization within the family and within their broader social environment might have untoward effects on the child's personality development. Finally, testing a foetus carries with it a small, additional risk of miscarriage. Clinical experience has shown that couples, not considering termination of a mutation-positive pregnancy, usually decide not to pursue prenatal testing when the implications are carefully discussed (Adam *et al.* 1993). Information about the prenatal testing procedures suitable for the family in question and consequences for the foetus, the parent at-risk, and siblings who have not been tested is given and discussed. Much attention should be given to the consequences of a possible change in decisions about prenatal and/or presymptomatic testing in the future.

The couple that decides to have an exclusion test (see Fig. 7.4) must face the possibility that, if they are eventually found not to be a carrier of the gene (by testing or staying asymptomatic at old age), they will have had an unnecessary termination of a foetus at 50 per cent risk. The prenatal exclusion-definitive test is a two-step test. If the foetus is found to be at 50 per cent risk (as a result of exclusion testing), the couple at risk might decide to opt for mutation testing in the foetus. Direct mutation analysis of the foetus, without prior knowledge of the status of the parent at risk, is a better prenatal testing alternative (Maat-Kievit *et al.* 1999). DNA of the future parents and grandparents is not needed and only the mutation in the DNA of the foetus is tested. If the mutation is detected the parent at risk simultaneously receives a result, but the genetic status of the parent at risk is disclosed in 25 per cent, which is only half the risk of an exclusion-definitive test (Table 7.7). According to the International Guidelines it is essential that prenatal testing for the HD mutation should only be performed if the parent has already been tested. Maat-Kievit *et al.* (1999) have proposed an adaptation of the guidelines: couples at risk, opting for specific prenatal diagnosis rather than exclusion testing, should be offered direct mutation testing of the pregnancy because it is quicker and has the smallest risk of disclosure of the genetic status of the parent at risk (Maat-Kievit *et al.* 1999).

Couples with a prospective parent at 50 per cent risk, planning to opt for prenatal testing after they already had children without testing, should be aware that their children have

Table 7.7 Differences between prenatal test options for a parent at 50% risk for HD (from Maat-Kievit *et al.* 1999)

Prenatal test option	Exclusion test	Exclusion—definitive test	Mutation test in foetus only
Grandparent(s)' informed consent and blood needed	Yes	Yes	No
Applicable to every pedigree	No	No	Yes
Time (relative) needed for result	+ +	+ + +	+
Reliability test result (%)	98–99	>99	>99
Risk of 'unnecessary' termination of pregnancy (%)	50	0	0
Risk of disclosure of genetic status of at 50% risk person (%)	0	50	25

different risks (25 per cent in the untested children and 0 per cent in children, tested by exclusion). When the parent becomes ill, the risks of the children at 25 per cent increase to 50 per cent whereas those of the children at 0 per cent remain unchanged. It is extremely important to investigate the motivation for prenatal testing of both parents. It is highly desirable that both parents agree to a prenatal test, and that the eventual decision should be taken according to the personal values and beliefs of both parents. If there is a conflict, every effort should be made by the counsellor and the couple to reach an agreement. The possibility of guilt feelings towards the future child or partner not at risk, unresolved traumas, etc. should be made clear and weighed against the decision to have a test, and subsequent termination of pregnancy after an unfavourable result. A termination of pregnancy cannot be undone, which underlines the need for careful counselling. The issues that may be encountered in the counselling sessions often require much time, and several sessions.

It is obvious that a couple, presenting for prenatal testing when already pregnant, may not have sufficient time to resolve all of the possible conscious and underlying problems of the pregnancy and test outcome. The support a couple receives from family and friends, the meaning of this future child to both parents, and the attitude towards termination of the pregnancy needs full exploration.

If the couple decides to undergo a prenatal test, appointments about disclosure and eventual termination of the pregnancy should be made at the outset of the prenatal test procedure. The genetic status of the foetus can be identified by direct mutation analysis. In the case of exclusion testing, linkage testing is still performed. In prenatal testing, except when only the foetus is tested without testing the at-risk parent, DNA from the prospective parents and from the foetus are needed. In case of an exclusion test, DNA from at least one of the future grandparents should also be taken. In exclusion testing it is possible, unintentionally, to alter the risk of the parent at risk if other family members are genotyped. To avoid this, the results of genotyping from other family members are kept strictly separate from the results of the exclusion test. DNA of the foetus can be extracted from foetal cells obtained by chorionic villus sampling, performed in the 10th to 12th week of the pregnancy, or by amniocentesis in the 15th to 17th week. The risk of miscarriage after amniocentesis is 0.5 to 1 per cent, and 1 to 2 per cent after chorionic villus sampling. DNA obtained from the amniocentesis or chorionic villi can be directly isolated for analysis, although somatic instability of the CAG repeat has been described (Telenius *et al.* 1994) and there is somatic stability in chorionic villi samples and other tissues of affected foetuses (Benitez *et al.* 1994). Availability of the prenatal test results depend on the laboratory that performs the test, but test results are usually available within 10 days to allow termination of the pregnancy by suction-curettage after chorionic villi sampling, or by prostaglandin induction after amniocentesis.

The low uptake of the relatively simple, reliable, and accessible prenatal test is probably related to psychological defences of the couples at risk, the fear of an unfavourable test result, and the risk of a prenatal test to the pregnancy. In addition, ethical reservations about the termination of a pregnancy for a disorder of relatively late onset or the hope that in the future a definitive therapy might become available may explain why couples at risk are reluctant to opt for prenatal testing (Post 1992; Adam *et al.* 1993; Tibben *et al.* 1993c).

Pre-implantation genetic testing is a new option for at-risk couples who wish to avoid the tragedy of (repeated) selective termination of pregnancies. Pre-implantation genetic testing is still experimental and the reliability of the diagnostic tests, as well as the safety of the preparatory biopsy, remain to be proven. The chances of a successful pregnancy using this option, as with all assisted reproductive technologies, should not be overestimated, as the chance of a treatment resulting in a birth is 10–20 per cent per cycle. There are other risks to be taken into account such as ovarian hyperstimulation syndrome, multifetal pregnancies, etc. A European collaborative project on prenatal testing for HD has evaluated in detail the advantages and disadvantages of prenatal testing options, including the ethical aspects (Evers-Kiebooms *et al.* 2002a; Simpson *et al.* 2001).

Insurance

The far-reaching consequences of presymptomatic testing have also made this new technology subject to social, political, and economic forces. Genetic discrimination has been a topic of intense news coverage, and an issue much debated in the professional and lay organizations. The issue of genetic discrimination is one of the most controversial, and it has attracted the attention of legislators and policy-makers all over the world. The fear of genetic discrimination and coercive genetic testing by health insurers and employers is a very sincere one among the IID community. In 2000, the Association of British Insurers (ABI) stated that 'when considering applications for life insurance, insurers should continue to have access to a genetic test for HD previously undergone by the applicant.' This was supported by a government committee, but late in 2001 the insurance industry agreed to a 5-year moratorium on the use or need for disclosure of abnormal test results, including HD, except for very large sums insured. Crosby (2001) has made an international comparison of the current policy and legislation. In the USA, 28 states have passed legislation that prohibits health insurers from accessing genetic information for the purposes of determining eligibility for policies that are provided by the employer or the government. However for those who are self-insured or who live in any of the 22 states without legislation, there is no protection. And there is no existing legislation that covers other forms of insurance such as mortgage or long-term care. The Netherlands has enacted legislation that restricts genetic discrimination in insurance. Australia has attempted to do so. Sweden has signed an agreement with insurers governing their use of genetic information. The German Bundestag has set up a Commission of Inquiry into 'Law and Ethics in Modern Medicine', which will consider, amongst other things, genetic information. Notwithstanding the fact that these countries all agree that some form of regulation of insurers' use of genetic information is required, the type and terms of the protections differ considerably. In Austria neither insurers nor employers may obtain results of genetic test results. In most countries, insurers will not request the results of genetic tests. In some countries, such as France and the Netherlands, the insurers have a moratorium on the use of genetic test results (favourable and unfavourable). There is some variation in legislation, which can be explained by fundamental differences in terms of national provision of health care. For example, the Australian Medicare system provides universal health care to Australians, whereas the overwhelming majority of Americans rely on health insurance to meet their health care needs. The Netherlands and Sweden have both adopted the approach of setting an upper limit, beyond which the. restrictions on insurers' use of genetic information will not apply (Crosby 2001).

The implications of genetic testing are far-reaching, so these issues need to be addressed in the pre-test counselling sessions. Because legislation in the different countries could develop rapidly, the information given here may become outdated very quickly. Therefore, the reader is referred to the websites mentioned at the end of this chapter for up-to-date information.

HD as a family disease

HD affects a family in several ways. An affected parent may have symptoms impeding his or her accessibility for a child or inducing frightening changes in personality (Fanos 1997). The non-affected parent, together with the children, has to take care of the affected parent, and the non-affected parent may seek one of the children as a substitute partner (Hans and Koeppen 1980). A parent may create an emotional distance, feel guilty, or may have fantasies about having transmitted the disease gene (Kessler 1988; Fanos 1997).

Many types of loss must be handled, which may be associated with shame, secretiveness, and social isolation. HD can have a far-reaching impact on families, so it is surprising that the systemic perspective has received little research attention; in particular, there has been no examination of the implications of presymptomatic testing. Implications for the partner have been addressed in some studies. Kessler (1998; Kessler and Bloch 1989) has described the disorganizing effect on the family of keeping HD as a secret from the spouse and the illness of a parent in young family. He discussed the difference between a father or mother becoming affected and the compromises asked of the non-affected spouse, such as the need for autonomy versus care-giving tasks. He pointed out that presymptomatic testing might be especially difficult for the partner as it challenges expectations about the future. A central theme for a counsellor, social worker, or psychologist working with families in which HD occurs is teaching spouses to deal with feelings of guilt and role shifts. Family coping strategies include patient preselection, as the next example clearly illustrates.

Example. A young woman, A, applied for the test. She has an older and a younger sister. Her mother was affected. The older sister had applied for the test a few months earlier; she received good news. Clinical experience has taught us not to expect by definition that A would have learned about her sister's test result, as tested persons sometimes keep these results secret for a variety of reasons. However, on the question 'what makes you wish to have the test for HD?', A replies that she needs to know her genetic status now her sister has had the test. 'You have spoken to your sister?' 'Yes, indeed, she has had an *unfavourable* test result…'. This answer obviously embarrassed the counsellor. A told us that her sister had initially received a favourable test result. The family was not willing to believe and accept this outcome as it was against the family expectations (Kessler referred to this phenomenon as preselection), with the subsequent turmoil (Kessler and Bloch 1989). The sister told her family a week later that the laboratory had made a mistake—for which they were apologetic—but she had indeed inherited the disease. The family could then express their sorrow towards the sister.

This case illustrates dramatically how we need to be informed about the family structure, family coping strategies, etc. to get a profound understanding of the test candidate's motives. Loyalties, encompassing several generations, along with feelings of guilt, debt, and gratitude play an important role in the reactions to a test result. In our work with test candidates the family life cycle framework has become a substantive concept and a useful therapeutic tool for genetic counsellors as well as for family therapists, psychotherapists, and social workers.

The experiences of test candidates with HD can be explored with the stages of the family life cycle in mind: (1) leaving home, single young adults; (2) joining of families through marriage, the new couple; (3) families with young children; (4) families with adolescents; (5) launching children and moving on; and (6) families in later life (Carter and McGoldrick 1998). The flow of anxiety in a family system includes patterns of relating and functioning that are transmitted primarily through the mechanism of emotional triangling. It includes all the family attitudes, taboos, expectations, labels, and loaded issues with which we grow up. In the case of HD families one can think of the family history of dealing with HD, in terms of secrecy, shame, guilt, or openness. Other stressors include the development task of a family, for example, the life cycle transitions and the unpredictable events such as untimely death, chronic illness, accidents, war, etc.

Family stress is often greatest at transition points of the family developmental process, and symptoms are most likely to appear when there is an interruption or dislocation in the unfolding family life cycle. Sometimes a family is not able to cope with the stresses that life offers either because they have not learned how to, or because of the unexpected and uncontrollable nature of events. Families with HD are confronted with chronic neuropsychiatric illness and untimely death through the generations, as HD is hereditary and every child of an affected parent has a 50 per cent risk of inheriting the disease. Nobody knows, however, exactly when and how it will strike an individual member of the family (Rolland 1990).

The test candidate and his or her family are central in the entire testing procedure. Sobel and Cowan (2000) interviewed families of test candidates and found that HD had affected family functioning at the level of individual family membership and in family patterns of communication. Moreover, concerns about future care-giving influenced current relationships (Sobel and Cowan 2000). Awareness of the family context influences the counselling sessions. Medical information and construction of the pedigree illuminate relationships between family members and generations. The pedigree also provides information on the life cycle through time and over more than two generations. It broadens and often provides a change of perspective, new insights, and a corrective experience. There are a number of family system theories that apply to the case of HD.

The model constructed by Rolland (1994), addressing the issue of illness in a family over time, gives a perspective on the psychological demands, family beliefs, and family functioning that result from chronic illness in a family. To be able to respond adequately to illness, a family needs the inclusion of belief systems. His model also considers anticipation of future loss, an experience common to families faced with a genetic disease. In the face of a possible loss, creating meaning for an illness that preserves a sense of competency is a primary task for families. In this regard, a family belief about what and who can influence the course of events is fundamental (Rolland 1990, 1994).

Fifteen years experience

The advent of presymptomatic testing created a revolution, not only in the world of science and health care, but also in politics, insurance, and other social structures. HD was regularly found on the front pages of prominent magazines and at prime time on television and radio. At the level of families with HD, learning about their personal risk for HD was expected to generate profound emotional responses that had to be acknowledged and dealt with. An adverse emotional response was considered the single greatest risk of presymptomatic testing. It is important that the psychological evaluation of emotional stability not be viewed as an obstacle to be jumped in order to get access to testing, but rather as a method of identifying persons likely to need greater emotional support after learning the test results. In some instances, such as overt risk for suicide and/or major depressive symptoms, it is appropriate to delay testing, initiate psychiatric treatment, and establish emotional stability before proceeding with the test.

Indeed, previous studies of the expectations of at-risk individuals had suggested that psychological effects of testing might include severe psychosocial problems such as overalertness for early symptoms, depression, and suicidal behaviour in identified gene-carriers (Kessler *et al.* 1987; Markel *et al.* 1987; Meissen and Berchek 1988). The same studies reported that between 40 and 79 per cent of individuals at risk intended to take the test (see Table 7.8).

There was some relief in the professional community involved in testing that the actual uptake has been much lower. The percentage of individuals at risk who requested testing when approached by registries or testing centres varied from 9 per cent in Wales, 10 per cent in Indiana, 16 per cent in the Manchester area, to 20 per cent in the Vancouver area (Meiser and Dunn 2000). In the Netherlands, of the 1032 individuals at risk who applied for presymptomatic testing in the period 1987–97, 752 decided to be tested: 24 per cent of the at-risk persons registered in the Leiden Roster for HD (Maat-Kievit *et al.* 2000).

An important part of the counselling of test candidates is preparing them for adverse responses and helping them to cope. This requires an estimation of the resources of test candidates. Because there was no experience with presymptomatic testing for late-onset disorders there was a strong urge for follow-up of those individuals who decided to undergo the presymptomatic test. Worldwide, a number of groups started a psychological follow-up programme that accompanied the testing protocol (see Table 7.9).

At the biannual meetings of the Working Group on HD of the WFN, experiences were exchanged and new insights incorporated in the counselling and testing procedures. The most important groups that have published their data include those of Vancouver, Baltimore, Leuven, Stockholm, Leiden–Rotterdam, Rome, Genoa, Cardiff, Manchester, and Aberdeen. Many other centres have since published their quantitative and qualitative data. Nothing illustrates the close cooperation of the various centres more clearly than the worldwide study of catastrophic events. A total of 100 centres in 21 countries have provided follow-up data on the test results and the psychosocial effects (Almqvist *et al.* 1999). In general, the experiences have been unambiguous whilst the studies published have shifted their focus over time. Understandably, the initial concern focused on the newly identified gene-carrier. However, a substantial minority of the non-carriers also proved to experience adjustment problems after the test result. Partners and children initially received little attention but, fortunately, some groups have addressed them in a number of studies.

The studies were initially designed using a variety of standardized psychological instruments and self-developed questionnaires. There was close contact between the groups from the

Table 7.8 Overview of studies on attitudes to genetic testing for HD (from Meiser and Dunn 2000)

Study	Sample	Reporting intention to use test (%)
Schoenfeld *et al.* 1984	21 men/34 women at 50% risk	73
Evers-Kiebooms *et al.* 1987	41 people 50%, 8 at 25% risk	57
Evers-Kiebooms *et al.* 1989	51 men/53 women	66
Kessler *et al.* 1987	27 men/42 women at 50% risk	79
Markel *et al.* 1987	52 men/103 women at 50% risk	63
Mastromauro *et al.* 1987	56 men/75 women at 50% risk	66
Meissen *et al.* 1987	21 men/35 women at 50% risk	65
Jacopini *et al.* 1992	27 men/30 women	40

Table 7.9 Studies on the psychological impact of genetic testing for HD (from Meiser and Dunn 2000)

Study	Type of genetic test*	Sample	Instrument	Carrier versus non-carrier scores[‡] at	
				7–10 days	12 months
Wiggins *et al.* 1992	LA	37 carriers	SCL-90	Higher	NS
		58 non-carriers	GWS	Lower	
		40 no result[§]	BDS	Higher	NS
Tibben *et al.* 1994	LA	20 carriers	IES avoidance	Higher	NS
		44 non-carriers	BHS	Higher	NS
Codori *et al.* 1997	LA/MA	52 carriers	BDI	NA	NS
		108 non-carriers	BHS	NA	Higher
Quaid and Wesson 1995	LA	5 carriers	SCL-90	NA	Higher
		14 non-carriers			
Decruyenaere *et al.* 1996	LA/MA	22 carriers	STAI	NS	NS
		31 non-carriers	BDI	NS	NS
Dudok de Wit *et al.* 1998	MA	9 carriers	IES	NS	NS
		16 non-carriers			

*LA, Linkage analysis; MA, mutation analysis.
[†]BHS, Beck Hopelessness Scale; BDI, Beck Depression Inventory; IES, Impact of Event Scale (higher scores are equivalent to more symptoms); SCL, Symptom CheckList; STAI, Spielberger Anxiety Inventory; GWS, General Wellbeing Scale.
[‡]NS, Not significant; NA, not available.
[§]The 'no result' group includes 23 testing decliners and 17 people who did not receive an informative result.

very beginning with respect to the instruments to be used, to allow cross-cultural comparison. We give just a brief summary of the studies by the groups that have published over the entire period since the test has been available. The studies aimed to describe the experiences with test results, to follow-up the course of adjustment over time, and to find factors that could help to identify those test candidates who might be at risk for extreme adverse reactions and adjustment problems.

The criteria for inclusion in studies on adjustment after test disclosure were age over 18 years and an at-risk status for HD. Exclusion criteria were: having symptoms of HD; severe depression or other major psychiatric illness; or, by personal history, being at risk for suicide (Baltimore Group, USA, Brandt *et al.* 1989; Boston, USA, Meissen *et al.* 1988; Indianapolis, USA, Quaid *et al.* 1989; Leuven Group, Belgium, Evers-Kiebooms *et al.* 1987; Rotterdam/Leiden Group, The Netherlands, Tibben 1993; Vancouver Group, Canada, Fox *et al.* 1989). In the study by Meissen and colleagues secondary exclusion criteria were: a recently experienced stressful event; moderate depression; a suicide attempt more than 10 years before testing, or a family history of suicide (Meissen *et al.* 1988). The Leuven group included risk-carriers with a psychiatric history, provided that social support was available and that the risk-carriers were receiving psychiatric treatment (Decruyenaere 1999, personal communication).

In general, the most important reasons to require testing were to seek relief from uncertainty, and to get some control over the future (particularly with regard to planning a family).

It was expected therefore that a reduction of anxiety and a gain in certainty about one's risk would improve the test candidates' quality of life (Tibben *et al.* 1993c).

Before a test result was given, risk-carriers expressed concern about the future and guilt about the possibility of passing on the gene. During the first period after the test disclosure, half of the identified carriers stated that the results had not influenced their lives; also half of them rarely thought of the result, indicating that denial might play a role. The non-carriers expressed relief in the first weeks after the test result was given, but soon thereafter half of the non-carriers appeared to deny the impact of the test result, as was reflected by absence of relief and emotional numbness. Some of them have expressed survival guilt.

The common experience has been that tested individuals found relief from their prior psychological distress and that they benefited psychologically from testing. Several studies have shown that participants in the testing programmes fell within the normal range of psychological well-being and HD-specific distress, prior to disclosure of the test result (Bloch *et al.* 1989; Brandt *et al.* 1989; Wiggins *et al.* 1992; Codori *et al.* 1997; Tibben *et al.* 1997; Dudok deWit *et al.* 1998). Most test applicants had a normal psychological profile (Decruyenaere *et al.* 1996). A small minority of the applicants were mildly hopeless or mildly depressed. In 20 per cent of the risk-carriers the possible presence of psychiatric morbidity was observed (Bloch *et al.* 1989; Tibben *et al.* 1997). In comparison with the general population, they were more socially extroverted, had higher ego-strength, and reacted more with active coping, palliative coping, social support seeking, and comforting ideas. This could underscore the opinion that the first group of tested people had strong mental resources. In the long term, identified carriers and non-carriers did not differ on general well-being and HD-specific distress.

Although identified gene-carriers showed more depression, hopelessness, and a decrease in general well-being in the first week after disclosure of the results, their mean scores remained in the mild range. A return to baseline levels of anxiety and depression occurred in the first month and remained there several years later. Although not differing from baseline, Wiggins and colleagues (1992) found linear declines for distress and depression in the first year. Only Brandt *et al.* (1989) reported a slight increase in general distress after 1 year. In general, the findings should be interpreted with caution because the drop-out rate in most studies is high.

The non-carriers were more optimistic regarding their future immediately after the test. This optimistic view of the future disappeared thereafter, although anxiety and depression decreased (Wiggins *et al.* 1992; Decruyenaere *et al.* 1996; Tibben *et al.* 1997). Also general distress decreased in the first year after the test result (Brandt *et al.* 1989). The adverse reactions in non-carriers have been referred to as survivor's guilt (Tibben *et al.* 1990; Huggins *et al.* 1992). Williams *et al.* (2000a) found that non-carriers experienced loss of former beliefs about themselves and developed new self-definitions, relationships with family, and roles in society. This coping process evolved from a personal focus to a broader future perspective in the short term. Identifying components of the redefinition process is an important consideration in planning interventions to promote coping with normal gene results in persons within at-risk families (Williams *et al.* 2000a). These reactions in non-carriers are understandable for those who have worked with HD families and the presymptomatic testing programme. However, they must be considered as a maladjustment. Non-carriers have the psychological task and challenge of experiencing relief and developing their lives in accordance with the good test result. Often, traumatic experiences have to be worked through in psychotherapy.

In comparison with a group that did not have a test result, Wiggins *et al.* (1992) found that both carriers and non-carriers scored lower for depression and higher for well-being. However, it cannot be inferred from these findings that testing has benefits, since an uninformative result, in particular, can lead to an increase in distress, the wish for certainty about carrier status having been frustrated. In the Dutch programme it was found that almost all people who were given an uninformative result in the linkage period (before 1993) requested the mutation test, several years later, whereas only 32 per cent of those who could not be tested due to a small family structure took the direct test.

A subgroup of both carriers and non-carriers had difficulties adjusting to their new carrier status. Ten to 20 per cent of carriers and non-carriers showed psychological problems in the post-test period (Huggins *et al.* 1992; Wiggins *et al.* 1992; Tibben *et al.* 1994; Decruyenaere *et al.* 1996; Lawson *et al.* 1996). Interviews with carriers, 3 months after the result, indicated that half of the carriers had periods of severe depression, whereas the other half had suffered a moderate depression (Meissen *et al.* 1988). Therapists identified a minority of carriers and non-carriers as having psychiatric symptoms in the first year after the test. However, very few individuals committed or attempted suicide or needed psychiatric hospitalization after presymptomatic testing (Brandt *et al.* 1989; Almqvist *et al.* 1999).

The observations by Lawson and colleagues (1996) underscore the general impression that both carriers and non-carriers have problems in adapting to the test result, but over different timescales. The number of adverse events was similar for carriers and non-carriers. For the carriers adverse events took place within 10 days after the test result, whereas for non-carriers adverse events occurred 6 months after the result or later. Of these events, 70 per cent were identified by clinical criteria, that is, suicidal ideation, a depression lasting longer than 2 months, substance abuse, and a breakdown of an important relationship, either alone or in conjunction with an elevated score on one or more questionnaires.

HD is a family disease that inevitably will have a profound effect on the life of the partner (Hans and Koeppen 1980). Partners found coping with the mental deterioration and personality changes in the affected spouse or relatives the most difficult things to deal with. The threat that their own children may later develop the same disease is one of the most dramatic aspects they have to deal with (Evers-Kiebooms *et al.* 1990). Partners have reacted to the clinical diagnosis with disbelief and denial but, after full awareness of the threat of transmission to the children, their responses changed to resentment and hostility (Hans and Koeppen 1980). As this was known, it is surprising that partners have received little empirical attention in presymptomatic testing programmes (Evers-Kiebooms *et al.* 1990; Kessler 1993; Tibben *et al.* 1993b; Quaid and Wesson 1995; Williams *et al.* 2000b). The few studies that have addressed this issue found, that spouses were more depressed than their at-risk partners at the first counselling session (Quaid and Wesson 1995), whereas both were equally hopeless, and tended to avoid discussing the test results (Tibben *et al.* 1992). They also reported overwhelming anxious feelings and thoughts about HD and their future. Although Quaid and Wesson found that spouses of prospective carriers were more distressed about their marriage than partners of non-carriers at baseline, there were no differences in the follow-up measures. Williams *et al.* (2000) found that support persons for individuals with a positive gene test were slightly more distressed than those who were support persons for those with negative gene mutation results (Williams *et al.* 2000). In the Dutch study, spouses were more depressed than their at-risk partners were at baseline. Partners of carriers reported the most difficulties in coming to terms with the impending burden (Tibben *et al.* 1993b). Codori and Brandt (1994) reported that the majority of carriers and non-carriers stated that the test result had no impact on their relation-ships. Satisfactory support of partners prior to test disclosure was associated with fewer feelings of hopelessness and avoidance thoughts, which emphasizes the important role of partners (Tibben *et al*. 1993a).

The partners of non-carriers felt relieved and could express this in an uncomplicated manner. Quaid and Wesson found that all partners, independently of the test result, showed comparable distress in the first period after disclosure of the result (Quaid and Wesson 1995).

Whereas distress was similar for carriers and their partners, their attitudes toward the test result differed. Carriers did not report an increase in problems after they received an unfavourable test result. Their partners did mention having problems, but expressed reluctance to seek help or to talk about it with their spouse, due to feelings of guilt and not wanting to hurt them. This was especially the case for those who became aware of the risk for HD at a later stage, for example, after marriage. For the non-carriers, most of them did not experience relief, whereas their partners did (Tibben *et al*. 1992, 1993b).

Having children proved to be an additional stress factor for partners during and after the test procedure. At the first counselling session, partners with children were significantly more hopeless than partners without children. After the test, carrier partners with children reported significantly more hopelessness and distress than those without children (Tibben *et al*. 1997).

Is it possible to find factors that predict problematic adjustment after a test result? Few studies aimed to identify pre-test variables that predict the way subjects adapt to their test result. In general, test outcome did not predict psychological adjustment. Only Codori *et al*. (1997) found carriers to be more likely to be pessimistic about their future than non-carriers.

The level of psychological adaptation after the test (anxiety, depression, hopelessness, intrusion, and avoidance) was predicted by the same measures at baseline (Tibben *et al*. 1993a; Decruyenaere *et al*. 1996; Codori *et al*. 1997; Dudok deWit *et al*. 1998). The more depressive symptoms reported at baseline, the more distress subjects reported at the 1-year follow-up, and the greater the chances that they were rated as having experienced an adverse event, as defined by Lawson *et al*. (1996).

We can conclude that predictive testing has provided relief from anxiety and allowed pru-dent arrangements for the future. However, 15 years experience have taught us the extent of the psychological consequences of an unfavourable test result. Dissemination of knowledge and experience, for the benefit of the HD population and for all other families with late-onset genetic diseases, remains a continuing task.

Internet resources

Huntington's Disease Society of America: www.hdsa.org

Huntington Society of Canada: www.hsc-ca.org

International Huntington Association: www.huntington-assoc.com

The Hereditary Disease Foundation: www.hdfoundation.org

Caring for People with Huntington's Disease: www.kumc.edu/hospital/huntingtons/index.html

Facing Huntington's disease—a handbook for friends and families: neuro-chief-e.mgh.harvard.edu/mcmenemy/facinghd.html

References

ACMG/ASHG (1998). ACMG/ASHG statement. Laboratory guidelines for Huntington disease genetic testing. The American College of Medical Genetics/American Society of Human Genetics Huntington Disease Genetic Testing Working Group. *Am J Hum Genet* **62** (5): 1243–7.

Adam, S., Wiggins, S., *et al.* (1993). Five year study of prenatal testing for Huntington's disease: demand, attitudes, and psychological assessment. *J Med Genet* **30** (7): 549–56.

Almqvist, E.W., Bloch, M., *et al.* (1999). A worldwide assessment of the frequency of suicide, suicide attempts, or psychiatric hospitalization after predictive testing for Huntington disease [see comments]. *Am J Hum Genet* **64** (5): 1293–304.

American Society of Human Genetics, A.H.C. o. G.C. (1975). Genetic counseling. *Am J Hum Genet* **27**: 240–2.

Andrew, S.E., Goldberg, Y.P., *et al.* (1993). The relationship between trinucleotide (CAG) repeat length and clinical features of Huntington's disease. *Nat Genet* **4** (4): 398–403.

—— —— *et al.* (1997). Rethinking genotype and phenotype correlations in polyglutamine expansion disorders. *Hum Mol Genet* **6** (12): 2005–10.

Bachoud-Levi, A.C., Remy, P., *et al.* (2000). Motor and cognitive improvements in patients with Huntington's disease after neural transplantation. *Lancet* **356** (9246): 1975–9.

Baker, D.L., Schuette, J.L., and Uhlmann, W.R. (eds.) (1998). *A guide to genetic counseling.* New York: Wiley-Liss, Inc.

Ball, D.M. and Harper, P.S. (1992). Presymptomatic testing for late-onset genetic disorders: lessons from Huntington's disease. *FASEB J* **6** (10): 2818–19.

Barette, J. and Marsden, C.D. (1979). Attitudes of families to some aspects of Huntington's chorea. *Psychol Med* **9** (2): 327–36.

Bell, J. (1934). Huntington's chorea. In: *The treasury of human inheritance* (ed. R.A. Fisher), Vol. IV, part 1, pp. 1–67. Cambridge: Cambridge University Press.

Benitez, J., Fernandez, E., *et al.* (1994). Trinucleotide (CAG) repeat expansion in chromosomes of Spanish patients with Huntington's disease: somatic stability in chorionic villi samples and other Huntington foetal tissues. *Hum Genet* **94** (5): 563–4.

Benjamin, C.M., Adam, S., *et al.* (1994). Proceed with care: direct predictive testing for Huntington disease. *Am J Hum Genet* **55** (4): 606–17.

Binedell, J. (1998). Adolescent requests for predictive genetic testing. In: *The genetic testing of children* (ed. A.J. Clarke), pp. 123–32. Oxford: BIOS Scientific Publishers Ltd.

Bloch, M., Fahy, M., *et al.* (1989). Predictive testing for Huntington disease: II. Demographic characteristics, life-style patterns, attitudes, and psychosocial assessments of the first fifty-one test candidates. *Am J Med Genet* **32** (2): 217–24.

—— Adam, S., *et al.* (1992). Predictive testing for Huntington disease in Canada: the experience of those receiving an increased risk [see comments]. *Am J Med Genet* **42** (4): 499–507.

Brandt, J., Quaid, K.A., *et al.* (1989). Presymptomatic diagnosis of delayed-onset disease with linked DNA markers. The experience in Huntington's disease [see comments]. *J Am Med Assoc* **261** (21): 3108–14.

Brinkman, R.R., Mezei, M.M., *et al.* (1997). The likelihood of being affected with Huntington disease by a particular age, for a specific CAG size. *Am J Hum Genet* **60** (5): 1202–10.

Burgess, M.M. and Hayden, M.R. (1996). Patients' rights to laboratory data: trinucleotide repeat length in Huntington disease. *Am J Med Genet* **62** (1): 6–9.

Carter, E.A. and McGoldrick, M. (eds.) (1998). *The expanded family life cycle: individual, family, and social perspectives.* Boston: Allyn & Bacon.

Chandler, J.H. (1966). EEG in prediction of Huntington's chorea: an eighteen year follow-up. *Electroencephalogr Clin Neurol* **21**: 79–80.

Chong, S.S., Almqvist, E., *et al.* (1997). Contribution of DNA sequence and CAG size to mutation frequencies of intermediate alleles for Huntington disease: evidence from single sperm analyses. *Hum Mol Genet* **6** (2): 301–9.

Clarke, A. (1994). The genetic testing of children. Working Party of the Clinical Genetics Society (UK). *J Med Genet* **31** (10): 785–97.

—— (ed.) (1998). *The genetic testing of children*. Oxford: BIOS Scientific Publishers Ltd.

—— Flinter, F. (1996). The genetic testing of children: a clinical perspective. In: *The troubled helix: social and psychological implications of the new human genetics* (ed. T. Marteau and M. Richards), pp. 164–76. Cambridge: Cambridge University Press.

Clarke, D.J. and Bundey, S. (1990). Very early onset Huntington's disease: genetic mechanism and risk to siblings. *Clin Genet* **38** (3): 180–6.

Codori, A.M. and Brandt, J. (1994). Psychological costs and benefits of predictive testing for Huntington's disease [see comments]. *Am J Med Genet* **54** (3): 174–84.

—— Slavney, P.R., *et al.* (1997). Predictors of psychological adjustment to genetic testing for Huntington's disease. *Health Psychol* **16** (1): 36–50.

Conneally, P.M. (1984). Huntington disease: genetics and epidemiology. *Am J Hum Genet* **36** (3): 506–26.

Craufurd, D., Donnai, D., *et al.* (1990). Testing of children for adult genetic diseases. *Lancet* **335** (8702): 1406.

Crosby, D. (2001). Protection of genetic information: an international comparison, Human Genetics Commission, London.

de Boo, G., Tibben, A., *et al.* (1998). Subtle involuntary movements are not reliable indicators of incipient Huntington's disease. *Movement Dis* **13** (1): 96–9.

Decruyenaere, M., Evers-Kiebooms, G., *et al.* (1996). Prediction of psychological functioning one year after the predictive test for Huntington's disease and impact of the test result on reproductive decision making. *J Med Genet* **33** (9): 737–43.

De Rooy, K.E., de Koning Gans, P.A.M., *et al.* (1993). Borderline repeat expansions in Huntington's disease. *Lancet* **342**: 1491–92.

Djurdjinovic, L. (1998). Psychosocial counseling. In: *A guide to genetic counseling* (ed. D.L. Baker, J.L. Schuette, and W.R. Uhlmann), pp. 127–70. New York: Wiley-Liss.

Dudok deWit, A.C., Duivenvoorden, H.J., *et al.* (1998). Course of distress experienced by persons at risk for an autosomal dominant inheritable disorder participating in a predictive testing program: an explorative study. Rotterdam/Leiden Genetics Workgroup. *Psychosom Med* **60** (5): 543–9.

Duisterhof, G.M.D. and Tibben, A. (2000). Childhood experiences with a parent with a hereditary late onset disease and the impact on wellbeing: a new direction in research. *J Med Genet* **37** (suppl. II): A9.

Duyao, M., Ambrose, C., *et al.* (1993). Trinucleotide repeat length instability and age of onset in Huntington's disease. *Nat Genet* **4** (4): 387–92.

Evers-Kiebooms, G., Cassiman, J.J., *et al.* (1987). Attitudes towards predictive testing in Huntington's disease: a recent survey in Belgium. *J Med Genet* **24** (5): 275–9.

—— Swerts, A., Cassiman, J.J., and Van den Berghe, H. (1989). The motivation of at-risk individuals and their partners in deciding for or against predictive testing for Huntington's disease. *Clin Genet* **35** (1): 29–40.

—— Swerts, A., *et al.* (1990). Partners of Huntington patients: implications of the disease and opinions about predictive testing and prenatal diagnosis. *Genet Counselling* **1** (2): 151–9.

—— Zoeteweij, M., and Harper, P.S. (eds.) (2002a). Prenatal testing for late onset neurogenetic diseases. Oxford: Bios.

—— Nys, K., *et al.* (2002b). The impact of the predictive test result upon subsequent reproductive decision making in families with Huntington's disease; a European collaborative study. *Eur J Hum Genet* **9** (suppl. 1): 226.

Fanos, J.H. (1997). Developmental tasks of childhood and adolescence: implications for genetic testing. *Am J Med Genet* **71** (1): 22–8.

Farrer, L.A. (1986). Suicide and attempted suicide in Huntington disease: implications for preclinical testing of persons at risk. *Am J Med Genet* **24** (2): 305–11.

Folstein, S.E. (1991). *Huntington's disease. A disorder of families*. Baltimore: The Johns Hopkins University Press.

Fox, S., Bloch, M., *et al.* (1989). Predictive testing for Huntington disease: I. Description of a pilot project in British Columbia. *Am J Med Genet* **32** (2): 211–16.

Gersting, J.M., Conneally, P.M., *et al.* (1984). Huntington's disease research roster data base support with MEGADATS-3M. *J Med Syst* **8** (3): 163–72.

Goldberg, Y.P., Kremer, B., *et al.* (1993). Molecular analysis of new mutations for Huntington's disease: intermediate alleles and sex of origin effects. *Nat Genet* **5** (2): 174–9.

—— McMurray, C.T., *et al.* (1995). Increased instability of intermediate alleles in families with sporadic Huntington disease compared to similar sized intermediate alleles in the general population. *Hum Mol Genet* **4** (10): 1911–18.

Gusella, J.F., Wexler, N.S., *et al.* (1983). A polymorphic DNA marker genetically linked to Huntington's disease. *Nature* **306** (5940): 234–8.

Hans, M.B. and Koeppen, A.H. (1980). Huntington's chorea. Its impact on the spouse. *J Nerv Ment Dis* **168** (4): 209–14.

Harper, P.S. (ed.) (1991). *Huntington's disease*. London: W.B. Saunders Company Ltd.

—— (ed.) (1996). *Huntington's disease*, 2nd edn. London: W.B. Saunders Company Ltd.

—— Newcombe, R.G. (1992). Age at onset and life table risks in genetic counselling for Huntington's disease. *J Med Genet* **29** (4): 239–42.

Hayden, M.R., Soles, J.A., *et al.* (1985). Age of onset in siblings of persons with juvenile Huntington disease. *Clin Genet* **28** (2): 100–5.

Hille, E.T., Siesling, S., *et al.* (1999). Two centuries of mortality in ten large families with Huntington disease: a rising impact of gene carriership. *Epidemiology* **10** (6): 706–10.

Huggins, M., Bloch, M., *et al.* (1992). Predictive testing for Huntington disease in Canada: adverse effects and unexpected results in those receiving a decreased risk. *Am J Med Genet* **42** (4): 508–15.

IHA/WFN (1994). International Huntington Association and the World Federation of Neurology Research Group on Huntington's Chorea. Guidelines for the molecular genetics predictive test in Huntington's disease. *J Med Genet* **31** (7): 555–9.

Imbert, G., Kretz, C., *et al.* (1993). Origin of the expansion mutation in myotonic dystrophy. *Nat Genet* **4** (1): 72–6.

Jacopini, G.A., D'Amico, R., Frontali, M., and Vivona, G. (1992). Attitudes of persons at risk and their partners toward predictive testing. *Birth Defects Orig. Artic. Ser.* **28** (1): 113–17.

Kessler, S. (1988). Invited essay on the psychological aspects of genetic counseling. V. Preselection: a family coping strategy in Huntington disease. *Am J Med Genet* **31** (3): 617–21.

—— (1993). Forgotten person in the Huntington disease family. *Am J Med Genet* **48** (3): 145–50.

—— (1998). Family processes in regard to genetic testing. In: *The genetic testing of children* (ed. A.J. Clarke), pp. 113–22. Oxford: BIOS Scientific Publishers Ltd.

—— M. Bloch (1989). Social system responses to Huntington disease. *Family Process* **28** (1): 59–68.

—— Kessler, H., *et al.* (1984). Psychological aspects of genetic counseling. III. Management of guilt and shame. *Am J Med Genet* **17** (3): 673–97.

—— Field, T., *et al.* (1987). Attitudes of persons at risk for Huntington disease toward predictive testing. *Am J Med Genet* **26** (2): 259–70.

Klawans, H.L., Goetz, C.G., *et al.* (1980). Levodopa and presymptomatic detection of Huntington's disease—eight-year follow-up. *New Engl J Med* **302** (19): 1090.

Korer, J.R. and Fitzsimmons, J.S. (1987). Huntington's chorea and the young people at risk. *Br J Social Work* **17**: 521–34.

Kremer, B., Goldberg, P., *et al.* (1994). A worldwide study of the Huntington's disease mutation. The sensitivity and specificity of measuring CAG repeats. *New Engl J Med* **330** (20): 1401–6.

—— Almqvist, E., *et al.* (1995). Sex-dependent mechanisms for expansions and contractions of the CAG repeat on affected Huntington disease chromosomes. *Am J Hum Genet* **57** (2): 343–50.

Lawson, K., Wiggins, S., *et al.* (1996). Adverse psychological events occurring in the first year after predictive testing for Huntington's disease. The Canadian Collaborative Study of Predictive Testing. *J Med Genet* **33** (10): 856–62.

Leeflang, E.P., Zhang, L., *et al.* (1995). Single sperm analysis of the trinucleotide repeats in the Huntington's disease gene: quantification of the mutation frequency spectrum. *Hum Mol Genet* **4** (9): 1519–26.

Legius, E., Cuppens, H., *et al.* (1994). Limited expansion of the (CAG)*n* repeat of the Huntington gene: a premutation (?). *Eur J Hum Genet* **2** (1): 44–50.

Lefebvre, A. (1999). Talking with children about Huntington disease in the family. Horizon, Huntington Society of Canada. http://www.huntington.assoc.com/children

Losekoot, M., Bakker, B., *et al.* (1999). A European pilot quality assessment scheme for molecular diagnosis of Huntington's disease. *Eur J Hum Genet* **7** (2): 217–22.

Lucotte, G., Turpin, J.C., *et al.* (1995). Confidence intervals for predicted age of onset, given the size of (CAG)*n* repeat, in Huntington's disease. *Hum Genet* **95** (2): 231–2.

Lyle, O.E. and Gottesman, I.I. (1977). Premorbid psychometric indicators of the gene for Huntington's disease. *J Consult Clin Psychol* **45** (6): 1011–22.

Maat-Kievit, A., Vegter-van der Vlis, M., *et al.* (1999). Experience in prenatal testing for Huntington's disease in The Netherlands: procedures, results and guidelines (1987–1997). *Prenatal Diagnos* **19** (5): 450–7.

—— —— *et al.* (2000). Paradox of a better test for Huntington's disease. *J Neurol, Neurosurg Psychiatry* **69** (5): 579–83.

—— Losekoot, M., *et al.* (2001). New problems in testing for Huntington's disease: the issue of intermediate and reduced penetrance alleles. *J Med Genet* **38**: E12.

Maat-Kievit, J. A. (2001). Predictive testing for Huntington disease. PhD thesis, Leiden University, Leiden.

Markel, D.S., Young, A.B., *et al.* (1987). At-risk persons' attitudes toward presymptomatic and prenatal testing of Huntington disease in Michigan. *Am J Med Genet* **26** (2): 295–305.

Martindale, B. (1987). Huntington's chorea: some psychodynamics seen in those at risk and in the responses of the helping professions. *Br J Psychiatry* **150**: 319–23.

Mastromauro, C., Myers, R.H., and Berkman, B. (1987). Attitudes toward presymptomatic testing in Huntington disease. *Am J Med Genet* **26** (2): 271–82.

McCusker, E., Richards, F., *et al.* (2000). Huntington's disease: neurological assessment of potential gene carriers presenting for predictive DNA testing. *J Clin Neurosci* **7** (1): 38–41.

McNeil, S.M., Novelletto, A., *et al.* (1997). Reduced penetrance of the Huntington's disease mutation. *Hum Mol Genet* **6** (5): 775–9.

Meiser, B. and Dunn, S. (2000). Psychological impact of genetic testing for Huntington's disease: an update of the literature. *J Neurol Neurosurg Psychiatry* **69** (5): 574–8.

Meissen, G.J., Berchek, R.L. (1988). Intentions to use predictive testing by those at risk for Huntington's disease: implications for prevention. *Am J Community Psychol* **16** (2): 261–77.

—— Myers, R.H., *et al.* (1988). Predictive testing for Huntington's disease with use of a linked DNA marker. *New Engl J Med* **318** (9): 535–42.

Michie, S. (1996). Predictive genetic testing in children: paternalism or empiricism? In: *The troubled helix: social and psychological implications of the new human genetics* (ed. T. Marteau and M. Richards), pp. 177–83. Cambridge: Cambridge University Press.

Montermini, L., Andermann, E., *et al.* (1997). The Friedreich ataxia GAA triplet repeat: premutation and normal alleles. *Hum Mol Genet* **6** (8): 1261–6.

Morris, M.J., Tyler, A., *et al.* (1989). Problems in genetic prediction for Huntington's disease. *Lancet* **2** (8663): 601–3.

Murray, A., Macpherson, J.N., *et al.* (1997). The role of size, sequence and haplotype in the stability of FRAXA and FRAXE alleles during transmission. *Hum Mol Genet* **6** (2): 173–84.

Myers, R.H., MacDonald, M.E., *et al.* (1993). *De novo* expansion of a (CAG)n repeat in sporadic Huntington's disease. *Nat Genet* **5** (2): 168–73.

Perry, T.L. (1981). Some ethical problems in Huntington's chorea. *Can Med Assoc J* **125** (10): 1098–100.

Platt-Walker, A. (1998). The practice of genetic counseling. In: *A guide to genetic counseling* (ed. D.L. Baker, J.L. Schuette, and W.R. Uhlmann), pp. 1–26. New York: Wiley-Liss.

Post, S.G. (1992). Huntington's disease: prenatal screening for late onset disease. *J Med Ethics* **18** (2): 75–8.

Quaid, K.A. and Wesson, M.K. (1995). Exploration of the effects of predictive testing for Huntington disease on intimate relationships. *Am J Med Genet* **57** (1): 46–51.

—— Brandt, J., *et al.* (1989). Knowledge, attitude, and the decision to be tested for Huntington's disease. *Clin Genet* **36** (6): 431–8.

Quarrell, O.W., Tyler, A., *et al.* (1988). Population studies of Huntington's disease in Wales. *Clin Genet* **33** (3): 189–95.

Rolland, J.S. (1990). Anticipatory loss: a family systems developmental framework. *Family Process* **29** (3): 229–44.

—— (1994). *Families, illness, and disability*. New York: Basic Books.

Rubinsztein, D.C., Leggo, J., *et al.* (1996). Phenotypic characterization of individuals with 30–40 CAG repeats in the Huntington disease (HD) gene reveals HD cases with 36 repeats and apparently normal elderly individuals with 36–39 repeats. *Am J Hum Genet* **59** (1): 16–22.

Schoenfeld, M., Berkman, B., Myers, R.H., and Clark, E. (1984). Attitudes toward marriage and child-bearing of individuals at risk for Huntington's disease. *Soc Work Health Care* **9** (4): 73–81.

Schuengel, C., Bakermans-Kranenburg, M.J., *et al.* (1999). Frightening maternal behavior linking unresolved loss and disorganized infant attachment. *J Consulting Clin Psychol* **67** (1): 54–63.

Simpson, S., Zoeteweij, M., *et al.* (2001). Prenatal testing for Huntington's disease—a description of tests accomplished from 1993–1998; a European collaborative study. *Eur J Hum Genet* **9** (suppl. 1): 226.

Snell, R.G., MacMillan, J.C., *et al.* (1993). Relationship between trinucleotide repeat expansion and phenotypic variation in Huntington's disease. *Nat Genet* **4** (4): 393–7.

Sobel, S.K. and Cowan, D.B. (2000). Impact of genetic testing for Huntington disease on the family system. *Am J Med Genet* **90** (1): 49–59.

Stevanin, G., Giunti, P., *et al.* (1998). *De novo* expansion of intermediate alleles in spinocerebellar ataxia 7. *Hum Mol Genet* **7** (11): 1809–13.

Telenius, H., Kremer, B., *et al.* (1994). Somatic and gonadal mosaicism of the Huntington disease gene CAG repeat in brain and sperm. *Nat Genet* **6** (4): 409–14.

Tibben, A. (1993). *What is knowledge but grieving? On psychological effects of presymptomatic DNA-testing for Huntington's disease*. PhD thesis. Rotterdam: Erasmus University.

—— Vegter-van der Vlis, M., *et al.* (1990). Testing for Huntington's disease with support for all parties. *Lancet* **335** (8688): 553.

—— Vegter-van der Vlis, M., *et al.* (1992). DNA-testing for Huntington's disease in The Netherlands: a retrospective study on psychosocial effects. *Am J Med Genet* **44** (1): 94–9.

—— Duivenvoorden, H.J., *et al.* (1993a). Presymptomatic DNA testing for Huntington disease: identifying the need for psychological intervention. *Am J Med Genet* **48** (3): 137–44.

—— Frets, P.G., *et al.* (1993b). On attitudes and appreciation 6 months after predictive DNA testing for Huntington disease in the Dutch program. *Am J Med Genet* **48** (2): 103–11.

Tibben, A., Frets, P.G., *et al.* (1993c). Presymptomatic DNA-testing for Huntington disease: pretest attitudes and expectations of applicants and their partners in the Dutch program. *Am J Med Genet* **48** (1): 10–16.

—— Duivenvoorden, H.J., *et al.* (1994). Psychological effects of presymptomatic DNA testing for Huntington's disease in the Dutch program. *Psychosom Med* **56** (6): 526–32.

—— Timman, R., *et al.* (1997). Three-year follow-up after presymptomatic testing for Huntington's disease in tested individuals and partners. *Health Psychol* **16** (1): 20–35.

Trottier, Y., Biancalana, V., *et al.* (1994). Instability of CAG repeats in Huntington's disease: relation to parental transmission and age of onset. *J Med Genet* **31** (5): 377–82.

Vine, B. (1989). *The house of stairs*. London: Penguin Books.

Vuillaume, I., Vermersch, P., *et al.* (1998). Genetic polymorphisms adjacent to the CAG repeat influence clinical features at onset in Huntington's disease. *J Neurol Neurosurg Psychiatry* **64** (6): 758–62.

Wertz, D.C., Fanos, J.H., *et al.* (1994). Genetic testing for children and adolescents: who decides? *J Am Med Assoc* **272**: 875–81.

Wexler, N.S. (1979). Genetic Russian roulette: the experience of being 'at risk' for Huntington's disease. In: *Genetic counseling: psychological dimensions* (ed. S. Kessler), pp. 199–200. New York: Academic Press.

Wiggins, S., Whyte, P., *et al.* (1992). The psychological consequences of predictive testing for Huntington's disease. Canadian Collaborative Study of Predictive Testing. *New Engl J Med* **327** (20): 1401–5.

Williams, J.K., Schutte, D.L., *et al.* (2000a). Redefinition: coping with normal results from predictive gene testing for neurodegenerative disorders. *Res Nurs Health* **23** (4): 260–9.

—— —— *et al.* (2000b). Psychosocial impact of predictive testing for Huntington disease on support persons. *Am J Med Genet* **96** (3): 353–9.

Zuhlke, C., Riess, O., *et al.* (1993). Mitotic stability and meiotic variability of the (CAG)n repeat in the Huntington disease gene. *Hum Mol Genet* **2** (12): 2063–7.

Section 3   Neurobiology

8 The neuropathology of Huntington's disease

Claire-Anne Gutekunst, Francine Norflus, and
Steven M. Hersch

This chapter reviews the neuropathology of Huntington's disease (HD) and examines the relationships between the neurodegenerative findings and recent advances in our knowledge of the mutant huntingtin protein. The specific symptoms and progression of HD can be related to its neuropathology, which is characterized by loss of specific neuronal populations in many brain regions. The most striking and best-characterized neuropathology is found in the basal ganglia. Pathology, however, has also been described in other brain regions and new studies continue to provide information about selective cortical and subcortical cell loss. With the relatively recent descriptions of normal huntingtin expression as well as of the progressive formation of nuclear and cytoplasmic huntingtin-containing protein aggregates in HD, further neuropathological features have emerged.

Gross pathology

Macroscopic inspection of the brains of advanced HD patients at autopsy shows the leptomeninges to be thickened and opaque. HD brains weigh less than brains of age-matched controls with the weight being reduced by about 10–20 per cent. Reduction in size occurs in the cerebral hemispheres, the diencephalon, the cerebellum, and also the brainstem and the spinal cord (Forno and Norville 1979). The most striking neuropathological feature is the shrunken appearance of the neostriatum with gross atrophy of the caudate nucleus and putamen with the caudate nucleus reduced to a thin rim of tissue (Fig. 8.1). Reduction in the size of the caudate is accompanied by secondary enlargement of the lateral ventricles. Another notable feature is the reduced amount of white matter under the cortical mantle (Fig. 8.1).

Microscopic pathology

Neostriatum

At the microscopic level, the atrophied neostriatum shows marked neuronal loss and astrogliosis, which has been the topic of many quantitative analyses (Bruyn *et al.* 1979; Vonsattel *et al.* 1985; Myers *et al.* 1988; Roos *et al.* 1985; Heinsen *et al.* 1994). Striatal pathology probably underlies involuntary movements (chorea and dystonia), disordered planning, impulsive behaviours, and diminished emotional control as well as some other symptoms of HD (Reiner *et al.* 1988; DeLong 1990; Crossman 1987; Albin *et al.* 1989). The extent of gross and microscopic striatal pathology provides a basis for dividing the severity of HD pathology into five grades (0 to 4) of increasing pathological severity that correlate with

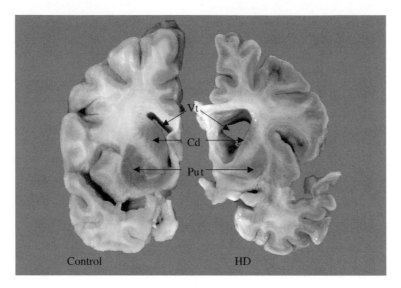

Fig. 8.1 Gross pathology. Photographs of fixed cerebral hemispheres from an HD case (right) and an age-matched normal specimen (left) at a coronal level through the rostral striatum. Note the marked atrophy of the caudate nucleus and putamen, along with cortical atrophy and white matter loss in the HD brain. Vt, Lateral ventricle; Cd, caudate; Put, putamen.

clinical progression (Vonsattel *et al.* 1985; Myers *et al.* 1988). Grade 0 cases have a strong clinical and familial history suggesting HD but no detectable histological neuropathology at autopsy. In grade 1 cases, neuropathological changes can be detected microscopically with as much as 50 per cent depletion of striatal neurones but without visible gross atrophy. In more severe grades (2–4), gross atrophy, neuronal depletion, and gliosis are progressively more pronounced, and pallidal pathology becomes evident. In the most severe grade (4), more than 90 per cent of striatal neurones are lost, and microscopic studies predominantly reveal the remaining astrocytes. There is a dorsal to ventral, anterior to posterior, and medial to lateral progression of neuronal death with the dorsomedial striatum affected earliest and relative sparing of the ventral striatum and nucleus accumbens (Vonsattel *et al.* 1985; Roos *et al.* 1985; Bots and Bruyn 1981).

Neuroanatomy of the basal ganglia

The basal ganglia encompasses the striatum (putamen and caudate), the subthalamic nucleus, globus pallidus (internal and external segments), and the substantia nigra (pars compacta and pars reticulata). The major excitatory inputs to the basal ganglia originate in the cerebral cortex and the thalamus and terminate in the striatum and the subthalamic nucleus. The dopaminergic nigrostriatal projections are an important extrinsic modulating input that act on glutamate release as well as upon the striatal output neurones themselves. The striatum does not receive any direct inputs from peripheral sensory or motor systems. The bulk of the output from the basal ganglia arises from the internal segment of the globus pallidus and the substantia nigra pars reticulata and projects to particular thalamic and brainstem nuclei (Fig. 8.2). There are no direct outputs from the basal ganglia to spinal motor circuits. The output is

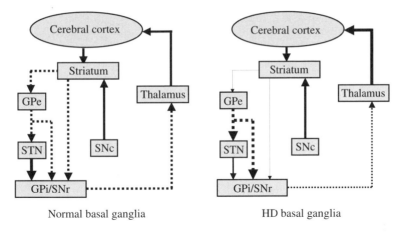

Normal basal ganglia   HD basal ganglia

Fig. 8.2 Basal ganglia pathways. Schematic of some of the interactions in the basal ganglia under normal and HD pathogenesis. The plain and dotted lines indicate excitatory and inhibitory pathways, respectively. The width of each line indicates the relative level of activity of each pathway. GPe, Globus pallidus external segment; GPi, globus pallidus internal segment; STN, subthalamic nucleus; SNr, substantia nigra pars reticulata; SNc, substantia nigra pars compacta.

inhibitory as it results in a decrease in the activity of its targets. In HD it has been postulated that degeneration of the projection neurones in the striatum results in aberrant activation of the basal ganglia output nuclei resulting in uncoordinated (uncontrolled) movements, cognition, and emotional control (Fig. 8.2).

Selective vulnerability

The striatum is composed of a variety of medium to large neurones that differ in their size and dendritic profile as well as neurochemical content and output (see Cicchetti *et al.* 2000 for a thorough review). Quantitative microscopic studies have shown the relative preservation of large striatal neurones and severe loss of medium-sized striatal neurones. Medium spiny neurones are inhibitory projection neurones carrying the output of the striatum to the globus pallidus and the substantia nigra and are the major neuronal type, comprising approximately 95 per cent of the neuronal cells in the striatum. They have large dendritic trees and use γ-aminobutyric acid (GABA) as their neurotransmitter. As these neurones degenerate in HD, the neurochemicals they contain, including glutamic acid decarboxylase (GAD), substance P, enkephalin, calcineurin, calbindin, adenosine receptors, and dopamine receptors, also decrease. The medium spiny neurones are subdivided into two groups according to their connectivity and neurochemical differences. As mentioned earlier, the striatum sends outputs to both the internal (GPi) and external (GPe) segment of the globus pallidus and the substantia nigra pars compacta (SNc) and reticulata (SNr). Medium spiny neurones that express the D1 dopamine receptors and substance P project to GPi and SNc, whereas those expressing D2 and enkephalin project to GPe (Gerfen 1992). Both subpopulations of medium spiny neurones degenerate in HD, but several studies have shown that the two types of projection neurones are differentially affected in the course of the disease. One study of 17 early- and middle-grade HD cases used immunocytochemical techniques to look at the integrity of the axon terminal plexuses arising from the different populations of substance P-containing and enkephalin-containing striatal projection neurones in the striatal target (Reiner *et al.* 1988). They found that enkephalin-containing neurones projecting to GPe were much more affected than substance P-containing neurones projecting to the GPi. Substance P-containing neurones projecting to the SNr were also more affected than those projecting to the SNc. At the most advanced stages of the disease, the study shows that projections to all striatal target areas were depleted, with the exception of some apparent sparing of the striatal projection to the SNc (Reiner *et al.* 1988). In two other studies, also using immunocytochemical techniques, striatal neurones projecting to GPe or the substantia nigra showed evident loss, whereas those projecting to GPi appeared relatively spared at presymptomatic and early stages of symptomatic HD (Albin *et al.* 1990, 1992). Understanding this selective vulnerability of striatal projection neurones has been a major goal in the neuropathological analysis of HD.

In addition to medium spiny neurones, there are a variety of aspiny interneurones in the striatum, expressing other neuroactive substances and sending their axons to contact medium spiny and other striatal neurones. Interneurones of particular interest for HD include the large cholinergic neurones and sparse medium spiny neurones containing somatostatin, neuro-peptide Y, and reduced nicotinamide–adenine dinucleotide phosphate (NADPH) diaphorase, now recognized as a form of nitric oxide synthetase (NOS). These populations of interneurones are relatively resistant to the neurodegenerative process occurring in the projection neurones surrounding them (Ferrante *et al.* 1987a,b; Cicchetti *et al.* 2000). The density of these neur-ones is increased in HD striatum reflecting their survival in a shrinking tissue. Although the intricate mechanism leading to death of subpopulations of these neurones is not fully known, the selective vulnerability of medium spiny neurones and the resistance to degeneration of striatal interneurones could be related to differential susceptibility to disruptions of cellular respiration (for review see Mitchell *et al.* 1999), or perhaps to low levels of expression of endogenous huntingtin (Ferrante *et al.* 1997).

At a higher level of organization, the striatum is also composed of heterogeneous compart-ments that contain distinct neurochemicals and project to distinct target regions. These compartments are termed patches (or striosomes) and matrix (Gerfen 1992; Graybiel 1990). Striosomes consists of discrete zones distributed throughout the striatum in which opiate receptors, substance P, met-enkephalin, and cholecystokinin are concentrated (Fig. 8.3). The intervening matrix is enriched in somatostatin, neuropeptide Y, NADPH-diaphorase, calbindin, choline acetyltransferase, acetylcholinesterase, and cytochrome oxidase.

Several conflicting studies have described what happens to these two compartments as HD progresses. Although the striosome/matrix compartmentation persists in the HD striatum, as determined by acetylcholinesterase or by calbindin, the total area of the matrix is reduced, whereas the total area of the striosomes is unchanged (Seto-Ohshima *et al.* 1988; Ferrante *et al.* 1987b; Hersch and Ferrante 1997). Other studies have suggested that the striosome compartment is affected initially in the disease process (Reiner *et al.* 1988; Morton *et al.* 1993; Hedreen and Folstein 1995). One study showed that early in the disease there is a loss of NADPH diaphorase staining in the neuropil, which is first evident in the striosome com-partment (Morton *et al.* 1993). The authors, however, indicate that in advanced stages of the disease the NADPH diaphorase staining is also greatly reduced in the matrix compartment. In another study (Hedreen and Folstein 1995), immunocytochemical stains for glial fibrillary acidic protein and for markers of the neostriatal striosome–matrix system correlated with astrocytosis and neuronal loss to the striosome compartment in low-grade HD cases. Neuronal loss in the striosomes was present throughout the dorsoventral extent of the caudate

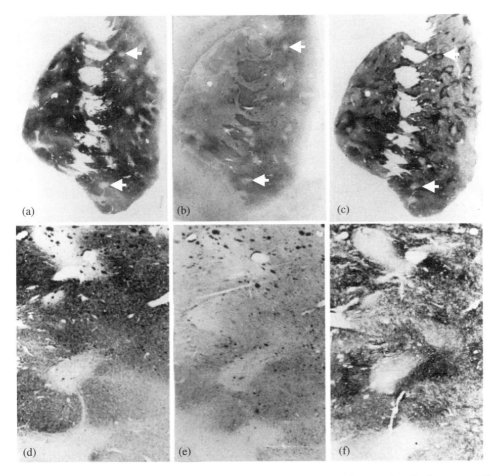

Fig. 8.3 Huntingtin protein expression in the normal striatum. Photomicrographs of adjacent serially cut sections of the rostral striatum demonstrating the patch and matrix compartments using antisera against (a),(d) calbindin D28K, (b),(e) huntingtin, and (c),(f) enkephalin. Areas of low huntingtin immunoreactivity correspond to those of low calbindin D28K immunoreactive areas (patches) in contiguous sections. In patches both neuronal and neuropil huntingtin immunoreactivity were reduced. (Reproduced with permission from Ferrante *et al.* (1997) ©2001 by the Society for Neuroscience.)

nucleus and putamen during the early phase of symptomatic disease, and extended to the most ventral region of the nucleus accumbens in later stages. The authors suggested that early degeneration of neurones in the striosome could produce hyperactivity of the nigrostriatal dopaminergic pathway, causing chorea and other early clinical manifestations of HD (Hedreen and Folstein 1995).

Other basal ganglia regions

Neuronal cell loss is not confined to the neostriatum but is also found in other regions of the basal ganglia. Detailed quantitative studies from the pallidum and substantia nigra certainly established this previously (Dom *et al.* 1976; Lange *et al.* 1976; Oyanagi and Ikuta 1987; Oyanagi *et al.* 1989; Heinsen *et al.* 1994).

Globus pallidus

Pallidal atrophy has long been recognized to occur in HD (Lange *et al.* 1976; Vonsattel *et al.* 1985; Bruyn and von Wolferen 1973). In a quantitative study, it was shown that GPe and GPi can lose more than 50 per cent of their volume and more than 40 per cent of their neurones while glia increase both in concentration and in absolute number (Lange *et al.* 1976). The authors attributed the pallidal loss of neurones to primary degeneration as opposed to a transneuronal consequence of striatal atrophy. As this study also pointed out, pallidal degeneration and loss of pallidal projection neurones have not been sufficiently considered in attempts to explain chorea. More recent studies concerned with pallidal pathology in HD as described above have been more concerned with striatopallidal afferents than with pallidal neurones themselves and their projections (Reiner *et al.* 1988; Albin *et al.* 1990; Storey and Beal 1993).

Ansae peduncularis

One qualitative study was performed in the nucleus ansae peduncularis of 45 cases of HD patients ranging in age and grade (Averback 1981). The ansae peduncularis is a poorly characterized group of large ganglionic cells found amid the substantia innominata near the lateral part of the anterior commissure. In HD, neurones in this region appear massively enlarged and vacuolated and surrounded by glial clusters. No quantitative numbers were given except that 43 of the 45 cases studied contained these degenerating neurones. Little is known about the connectivity, biochemistry, or physiology of this cell group. It is possible that disruption of this nucleus might result in emotional and motivational disturbances.

Subthalamus

Subthalamic lesions in human and non-human primates have been shown to result in ballistic involuntary movements that are similar to those of chorea. The subthalamus may be excessively disinhibited by loss of GABAergic inputs in HD, leading to pallidothalamic excitation and, as previously outlined, this may be the basis for chorea. Furthermore, the subthalamus gives rise to one of the few excitatory pathways in the basal ganglia and thus may be relevant in excitotoxic cell death. Nevertheless, little has been added to our knowledge of subthalamic pathology in HD since the morphometric study by Lange and his colleagues (1976), who found that subthalamic volume and neurone number are reduced by about 25 per cent.

Substantia nigra

There have been reports of loss of striatonigral fibres as well as nigral neurones in HD (Bruyn *et al.* 1979; Forno and Jose 1973; Bugiani *et al.* 1984; Dom *et al.* 1976; Lange *et al.* 1976). Two quantitative studies of nigral pathology in HD were done using distinct methods, which might explain the difference in their results (Oyanagi and Ikuta 1987; Oyanagi *et al.* 1989; Ferrante *et al.* 1989). Both studies found substantial atrophy and gliosis of both the pars compacta (SNc) and pars reticulata (SNr), with a loss in cross-sectional area of as much as 40 per cent. Ferrante and colleagues observed that the SNr, however, had a greater loss of area than the SNc. Both studies also reported that nonpigmented neurones were reduced in both the nigral zones by as much as 45 per cent.

Neuropathology in other brain regions

Many studies have shown that neurodegeneration is not confined to the basal ganglia but also occurs widely in cortical and other subcortical regions. The relative time course of degeneration in these areas is not well understood, as most studies have been performed in advanced cases. In every region analysed in detail at a cellular level, selective vulnerability of particular neuronal populations appears to occur.

Degeneration certainly occurs in the neurones of many brain regions as a direct result of the HD disease process occurring within them. Secondary causes of degeneration may also be significant contributors to the neuropathology of HD. For example, abnormal regulation of glutamatergic corticostriatal afferents could cause excicitotoxic injury to striatal neurones (Chen and Reiner 1996; Cha *et al.* 1998, 1999). On the other hand, deafferentation of target neurones due to loss of the neurones or axons innervating them is also a well-known cause of atrophy or degeneration that could contribute to the neuropathology of HD.

Cerebral cortex
Atrophy of the cerebral cortex has long been recognized as occurring in HD. As mentioned previously, generalized cortical atrophy is usually apparent at autopsy and neuropathological studies have demonstrated thinning of the cerebral cortex and underlying white matter. Many qualitative and quantitative studies of a variety of cortical regions have been performed and show that cortical neuronal degeneration is heterogeneous and ranges from 10 to 55 per cent within the various regions analysed. The neocortex can generally be divided into five or six different layers from pia down to the white matter depending on its regional location. In HD, neuronal loss affects mostly layers III, V, and VI with small and scattered foci of neuronal loss also present in other layers. The alignment of the neurones in layer VI can also appear disturbed. Glial density is greatly increased, more so in the cortex than the adjacent white matter. The subcortical white matter becomes atrophic with loss of both myelin and axons (Tellez-Nagel *et al.* 1973).

Analysis in prefrontal cortices has demonstrated significant reductions in the number of pyramidal neurones (Cudkowicz and Kowall 1990; Sotrel *et al.* 1991) with an average of 30 per cent loss of SMI-32 immunoreactive pyramidal neurones across all grades (Cudkowicz and Kowall 1990). SMI-32 is a non-phosphorylated neurofilament protein that specifically stains the cell body and proximal dendrites of pyramidal neurones (Grotton *et al.* 1995). In the prefrontal area 46, a recent study of eight HD cases revealed increased neuronal (35 per cent) and glial (61 per cent) density as compared to those of normal controls, with substantial cortical thinning suggesting a major reduction of interneuronal neuropil (Selemon *et al.* 1998). Because of its connectivity to the basal ganglia most pathological studies of cortex have focused on the frontal lobes. In a recent study of parietal cortex there was a more dramatic reduction in pyramidal neurones than that predicted from previous studies of cortical pathology (Macdonald *et al.* 1997). This study found up to 55 per cent of pyramidal loss in the angular gyrus, another cortical region projecting to the dorsal part of the caudate. The HD brains had noticeable histological changes including smaller neurones and disruption of the cortical laminar pattern. Neuronal loss in this region approaches the cell loss observed in subcortical regions and may account for the slowing of saccadic eye movements, and deficits in perception and performance of voluntary movements (Macdonald *et al.* 1997). Although the relationship between widespread cortical degeneration and subcortical degeneration is poorly understood, it has been suggested that cortical neurodegeneration might also be involved in personality changes and dementia occurring in HD (Braak and Braak 1992a,b).

Hippocampus

Few studies have addressed changes occurring in the hippocampus. An early study reported a reduction of hippocampal area of about 20 per cent in HD (30 cases) as compared to controls (de la Monte *et al.* 1988). In a later study, cell counts were carried out in nine HD patients. Neuronal densities were quantified using stereological techniques in the granule cell layer of the dentate, and in the CA1, CA3, and CA4 fields of the hippocampus. The neuronal density in the CA1 region was dramatically decreased in the HD brains representing a neuronal loss of about 35 per cent. Changes in the other regions of hippocampus were not significant (Spargo *et al.* 1993). CA1 degeneration also occurs in other diseases and the selective vulnerability of this region of the hippocampus is as yet unclear.

Cerebellum

Reports of cerebellar involvement in HD have been variable with cerebellar atrophy being reported in some cases (Byers *et al.* 1973; Castaigne *et al.* 1976; Rodda 1981; Hattori *et al.* 1984). Purkinje cell loss has been demonstrated, however, and thinning of the granule cell layer has also been observed. One quantitative study examined Purkinje cell loss in 17 HD cases and found a reduction of about 50 per cent of Purkinje cell density in half of the cases (Jeste *et al.* 1984). Although the cerebellum is sometimes considered to be spared in HD, it has not actually been sufficiently studied.

Hypothalamus

Hypothalamic pathology was outlined in several studies and might be related to the cachexia and autonomic disturbance that occur in HD patients. Bruyn and von Wolferen (1973) described significant neuronal loss and gliosis in the supraoptic nucleus and lateral hypothalamic nucleus. A later quantitative study (Kremer *et al.* 1991) revealed up to 90 per cent neuronal loss in the lateral tuberal nucleus, which was worse in patients developing motor symptoms at an early age. The lateral tuberal nucleus is located in the basolateral tuberal hypothalamic region and can be defined by cytoarchitectonic and neurochemical criteria (Kremer 1992). The percentage of astrocytes did not change, whereas oligodendrocytes were reduced by 40 per cent. It was further postulated that the high levels of glutamate receptors normally present in the lateral tuberal nucleus render these neurones selectively susceptible to excitotoxic cell death. Although little is known about the normal function of the lateral tuberal nucleus, the possibility that its degeneration underlies the catabolic state that frequently occurs in HD patients has been proposed. Furthermore, because cell loss is so severe, this nucleus may have value in experimental investigations of cell death and neuroprotection in HD.

Thalamus

Several qualitative studies have focused on pathology occurring in thalamic nuclei. Some have observed diffuse neuronal loss and gliosis in all thalamic nuclei (Byers *et al.* 1973) with global thalamic atrophy (de la Monte *et al.* 1988); others have described more selective atrophy and reduced density of small or 'micro'-neurones in the thalamic ventrolateral nucleus (Dom *et al.* 1976). Two more recent quantitative studies have used stereological methods (Schmitz *et al.* 1999) to compare the number of neurones and glial cells between normal and terminal-stage HD patients (Heinsen *et al.* 1996, 1999) in two thalamic nuclei. The first study (Heinsen *et al.* 1996) found a 55 per cent loss of neurones as well as a slight reduction in glial cells in the thalamic centromedial-parafascicular (TCP) complex in HD. This thalamic nucleus is part of a neuronal loop comprising striatum–globus pallidus–thalamus–striatum and receives its main (collateral) afferents from the internal pallidum via the ansae lenticularis with its principal outputs directed to the sensorimotor territory of the striatum (Parent and Hazrati 1995a, b). The authors have suggested that the neuronal loss observed in HD might contribute to sensorimotor integration deficits. The other study describes a 23.8 per cent reduction in the number of neurones and a 29.7 per cent decrease in glial cell number in the mediodorsal nucleus (MD) of the thalamus (Heinsen *et al.* 1999). In primates, the MD receives and sends inputs to the prefrontal cortex (Barbas *et al.* 1995; Giguere and Glodman-Rakic 1988). Loss of neurones in MD might relate to visuospatial and emotional disturbances frequently seen in HD patients.

Brainstem
Very little has been reported on neuropathological alterations of brainstem nuclei in HD. One study describes neurodegeneration in the olives and the gracile and cuneate nuclei and suggests the involvement of lateral vestibular, dorsal vagal, and hypoglossal nuclei in HD (Roos 1986). Another investigation revealed brainstem atrophy by computerized tomography (CT) in an 11-year-old who had HD since the age of 4 (Hattori *et al.* 1984).

Structural and ultrastructural changes

Neurodegeneration occurring in HD appears to be a gradual process in which neurones undergo stress, express compensatory molecular and structural changes, and gradually decompensate, undergoing both injury and responses to injury, while becoming atrophic, and ultimately perishing and being removed. Though stress and injury and compensatory processes are often conceived as happening to neuronal cell bodies, they may also be evident in axons and dendrites.

Dendritic pathology

Several studies have described structural and ultrastructural changes in HD brain. Alterations observed in the dendritic structure of several types of neurones vulnerable in HD have suggested that both proliferative and degenerative alterations occur for some time before cell death finally ensues. Whether these alterations reflect a primary abnormality in the regulation of dendritic architecture or a secondary compensation and decompensation for altered striatal circuitry is unknown. Early morphological alterations of spiny striatal neurones have been described using Golgi and calbindin immunocytochemical methods (Graveland *et al.* 1985; Ferrante *et al.* 1991). Changes that occur in medium spiny cells prior to degeneration include dendritic remodelling (Ferrante *et al.* 1991), suggesting that these cells undergo a period of stress and injury prior to succumbing. Such changes were found in moderate grades of HD and include prominent recurving of distal dendritic segments, short segments branching along the length of the dendrites, and increased numbers and size of dendritic spines. The early increased numbers of spines may reflect new functional connections and represent a plastic increase in postsynaptic surface to compensate for lost neurones (Ferrante *et al.* 1993). Degenerative atrophic alterations, found mostly in more severe cases, consist of truncated dendritic arbors, focal dendritic swelling, and marked spine loss, indicative of a protracted period of degeneration during which the neurone may be unable to support its processes and their physiological functions.

Axonal pathology

Alterations in the neurofilament network have also been shown in HD medium spiny neurones. One study compared normal and HD striatum using specific antibodies to non-phosphorylated (SMI 32) and phosphorylated (SMI 31) neurofilament and neural cell adhesion molecule (NCAM) (Nihei and Kowall 1992). In normal striatum, SMI 32 identifies medium-sized neuronal perikarya and dendrites. In grade 3–4 HD striatum, SMI 32 neurones were morphologically abnormal and significantly depleted. Dendritic arbors were intensely immunoreactive, tortuous, and fragmented, especially in the subependymal zone. The authors describe the presence of proliferative SMI 32-positive sprout-like structures and axon-like processes. SMI 31 normally stains a fine meshwork of axon-like processes. In HD these processes became intensely immunoreactive, condensed, convoluted, and fragmented. Finally, NCAM staining, which is minimal in normal striatum, stained many dot- and thread-like structures in the HD striatum, especially in the subependymal region. The authors suggest that abnormalities revealed by the various markers reflect an alteration of the neurofilament phosphorylation and that growth-related proteins are again expressed. They also postulated that dephosphorylation and destabilization of the cytoskeleton may contribute to neuronal injury and death in HD. Another more probable explanation in view of the recent evidence of transcriptional dysregulation in HD (Cha 2000) is that neurofilament abormalities might represent a downstream effect of disordered signal transduction. Synaptophysin, a marker of axon terminals, is significantly reduced in HD and suggests depletion of medium spiny neurone local collaterals or degeneration of striatal afferent terminals when they lose their striatal target cells (Goto and Hirano 1990).

The presence of dystrophic neurites (abnormal processes unidentifiable as specifically axonal or dendritic) have also been described in HD (Cammarata *et al.* 1993; Jackson *et al.* 1995). They are mostly found in cortical regions including Brodman areas 7, 8, 10, 18, 24, 28, 33, 38, and 39 (Jackson *et al.* 1995). Within the cortex, dystrophic neurites were mostly seen in layers III, V, and VI. Electron microscopy revealed the presence of a central core of granulofilamentous material (Jackson *et al.* 1995). These morphologically abnormal processes stained positively for ubiquitin and ubiquitin hydrolase, suggestive of degradative processes taking place within them.

Glia in HD

As mentioned earlier, gliosis is seen in HD and has been described in both the neostriatum and the cortex. Specific studies of glial cells are few (Zalneraitis *et al.* 1981). One new study has found activated microglia in the brains of 13 grade 1–4 HD cases using thymosin β-4 as a marker (Sapp *et al.* 2001). Immunoreactive microglia were found in the neostriatum, cortex, and globus pallidus as well as in the subcortical white matter and internal capsule. In the striatum, reactive microglia occurred in all grades of pathology and increased with increasing grade. Interestingly, the cell bodies of the reactive microglia were sometimes found adjacent to neuronal cell bodies containing nuclear aggregates (Fig. 8.4). In the same study, reactive

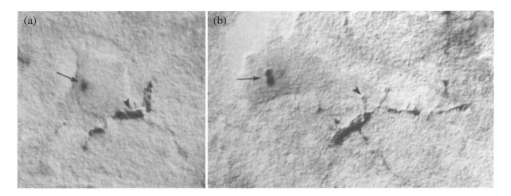

Fig. 8.4 Reactive microglia in HD. (a),(b) Photographs showing perineuronal Tβ4 immunoreactive microglia (arrowheads) in direct contact with pyramidal cell bodies containing nuclear inclusions (small arrows). Photomicrographs were taken using Nomarski interference microscopy. (Reproduced with permission from Sapp *et al.* 2001.)

microglia were also detected using major histocompatibility complex (MHC) class II antibodies. The presence of reactive microglia early in the disease process and in close association with degenerating neurones in the HD brain implies a potential role for activated microglia and inflammatory response in HD pathogenesis.

Huntingtin localization in HD and control brains

To determine the regional and subcellular localization of normal and mutant huntingtin, a variety of antibodies to different regions of the protein have been generated and used in immunocytochemical studies. Although different studies have used different antibodies, the results are generally consistent. This review will primarily describe studies in humans.

Several antibodies have been developed to internal sequences of huntingtin and are able to detect both normal and mutant huntingtin proteins in Western blots and tissue sections. Antibodies made against the *N*-terminal region of huntingtin, the region preceding or encompassing the CAG repeat segment, often predominantly recognize aggregated mutant huntingtin protein when used for immunocytochemistry.

Normal huntingtin

The regional and subcellular localization of huntingtin has been the subject of a number of studies in experimental animals as well as cell lines. Results from these studies are described in Chapters 12 and 13. Only a handful of studies have addressed huntingtin localization in normal and diseased human brain. Immunocytochemistry indicates that huntingtin is widely expressed in neurones throughout the brain (Gutekunst *et al.* 1995; Sharp *et al.* 1995; Persichetti *et al.* 1996; Trottier *et al.* 1995; DiFiglia *et al.* 1995) with high levels evident in cortical pyramidal cells, cerebellar Purkinje cells, and large striatal interneurones (Fig. 8.5).

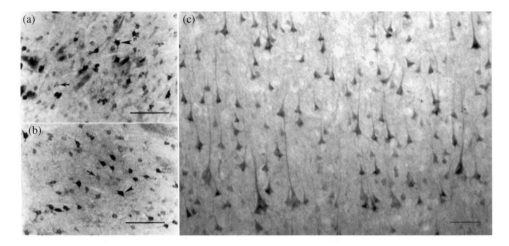

Fig. 8.5 Huntingtin immunoreactivity in normal striatum and cortex. Huntingtin (HDp549: raised against amino acids 549–679) immunoreactivity in the (a) dorsal and (b) ventral striatal matrix of the caudate nucleus and (c) in the frontal cortex. Huntingtin immunoreactivity is present in medium-sized neurones and is confined to the cytoplasm. Marked variability in neuronal immunoreactive intensity is observed. Neurones are immunolabelled either darkly (arrowheads) or lightly (arrows) for huntingtin. Scale bars: (a), (b) 200 μm; (c) 50 μm. ((a) and (b) are reproduced with permission from Ferrante *et al.* (1997) ©2001 by the Society for Neuroscience.)

Its expression, however, is heterogeneous, and we have shown in humans that, in the striatum, the regions and neurones most vulnerable to neurodegeneration normally express the highest levels of huntingtin, while spared interneurones express very little (Ferrante *et al.* 1997). Thus, differences in the endogenous levels of huntingtin expression may in part explain select-ive vulnerability within the striatum. Since, however, there are many neurones in other brain regions with high levels of huntingtin expression that do not readily degenerate, other factors, in addition to huntingtin expression, are likely to contribute to selective vulnerability. At a subcellular level, the protein is found in the cytoplasm in somatodendritic regions (Fig. 8.6) but with some presence in axons as well. Normal huntingtin associates with microtubules, vesicular organelles, and mitochondria and has been proposed as playing a role in organelle transport (Gutekunst *et al.* 1995, 1998; DiFiglia *et al.* 1995).

One study has examined the localization of huntingtin in HD brain with an antibody that recognizes the wild-type and mutant proteins (Sapp *et al.* 1997). Neuronal staining was reduced in areas of the HD striatum depleted of medium-sized neurones; large striatal neur-ones, which are spared in HD, retained normal levels of huntingtin expression. Neuronal labelling was markedly reduced in both segments of the globus pallidus even in HD cases where cell loss in this region was minimal. In some cortical and striatal neurones with normal looking morphology, huntingtin was associated with punctate cytoplasmic granules resembling multivesicular bodies, organelles involved in retrograde transport and protein degradation. Some immunoreactive processes showed blebbing and segmentation similar to that induced experimentally by hypoxic-ischaemic or excitotoxic injury. Huntingtin staining was more concentrated in the perinuclear cytoplasm and reduced or absent in processes of atrophic cortical neurones. Nuclear staining was also evident. Fibres in the subcortical white matter of

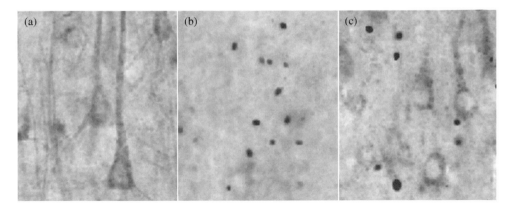

Fig. 8.6 *N*-terminal huntingtin antibodies reveal huntingtin aggregates in HD brain. Neuropil aggregates are not labelled by an antibody to the internal region of huntingtin. Adjacent sections through cerebral cortex from a grade 1 HD case were immunostained with: (a) mHD549 alone (amino acids 549–679); (b) EM48 alone (amino acids 1–256); or (c) EM48 and mHD549 combined. mHD549 staining is found in the perikarya and proximal dendrites of the pyramidal neurones (a,c) but is not found in aggregates. In contrast, EM48 intensively labels the aggregates. (Reproduced with permission from Gutekunst *et al.* (1999) ©2001 by the Society for Neuroscience.)

HD patients had significantly increased huntingtin immunoreactivity compared with those of controls (Sapp *et al.* 1997).

Abnormal huntingtin

In HD, mutant huntingtin cleavage releases *N*-terminal fragments that aggregate and also recruit other proteins. Huntingtin aggregates can be found in any part of a neurone, including the nucleus, perikaryon, dendrites, and axons. These aggregates become ubiquitinated, presumably because they are recognized as containing misfolded proteins that become targeted for degradation. Their persistence suggests that degradation cannot keep pace with aggregate formation. Their ability to recruit other proteins might cause depletion of crucial cellular proteins. *N*-terminal huntingtin aggregates are heterogeneously distributed in different regions of the HD brain (Fig. 8.6). They are primarily observed in grey matter but are also found in white matter. Aggregates are especially frequent in the layers V and VI of cerebral cortex. However, differences between cortical areas within individual HD brains are observed. For example, insular and cingulate cortex may have significantly higher densities of aggregates than prefrontal, temporal association, and premotor cortex (Gutekunst *et al.* 1999). Aggregates have also been observed, but at lower densities, in the caudate, putamen, substantia nigra, hypothalamic nuclei, thalamus, and brainstem nuclei such as nucleus cuneatus, regions in which various degrees of neurodegeneration have been described. In the striatum, aggregates are uncommon but widely scattered without any groupings suggestive of patch or matrix compartmentation. In the substantia nigra, most aggregates are in the pars compacta neuropil and very few in pars reticulata. Aggregates are rarely seen in the globus pallidus, a major target of striatal axons. Aggregates are also rare in the hippocampus and cerebellum although a few are visible in both the molecular and granule cell layers of the cerebellum (Gutekunst *et al.* 1999).

Nuclear aggregates

In HD brain, *N*-terminal fragments of mutant huntingtin accumulate and form inclusions in the nucleus (DiFiglia *et al.* 1997; Becher *et al.* 1998; Gourfinkel-An *et al.* 1998; Maat-Schieman *et al.* 1999; Gutekunst *et al.* 1999). Abnormal nuclear accumulations have also been observed in other triplet-repeat disorders and in a variety of animal and cell models (see Chapters 12–14). Intranuclear aggregates containing *N*-terminal huntingtin fragments have been observed in the striatum and cortex of HD patients (DiFiglia *et al.* 1997; Becher *et al.* 1998; Gourfinkel-An *et al.* 1998; Maat-Schieman *et al.* 1999; Gutekunst *et al.* 1999). Nuclear aggregates are round to fusiform in shape (Fig. 8.7), usually one but occasionally two in number per nucleus, and have long axes ranging from 3 to 5 μm (Becher *et al.* 1998; DiFiglia *et al.* 1997; Gutekunst *et al.* 1999).

Perikaryal aggregates

Neurones containing nuclear aggregates also commonly contain smaller immunolabelled puncta in their perikarya (Fig. 8.7). Labelled perikaryal puncta are round to oval and generally smaller than nuclear or neuropil aggregates, having diameters ranging from 0.3 to 1.5 μm. As described in *in vitro* studies of *N*-terminal huntingtin aggregation (Heiser *et al.* 2000; Huang *et al.* 1998) and animals models of HD (Davies *et al.* 1997), some of the aggregates present in HD striatum and cortex can be stained with Congo red, which is suggestive of amyloid-like structure (McGowan *et al.* 2000).

Neuropil aggregates

Aggregates located in the neuropil (axons, dendrites, and synapses) are by far the most common and range from 60–100 per cent of the total aggregates present in layer III of cortex and 35–98 per cent in layers V/VI (Gutekunst *et al.* 1999). Although most neuropil aggregates are described as being round to oval, more tubular forms that can be hundreds of microns long and appear to fill neuronal processes are also common (Fig. 8.7). In the cerebral cortex, these tubular aggregates frequently have the size and orientation of apical dendrites (Gutekunst *et al.* 1999). These tubular forms are not as intensely immunoreactive as the more punctate forms, suggesting that the protein they contain may not be as condensed. Curved multiform aggregates reminiscent of short dendritic segments and branch points are also seen, some of which appeared to give rise to aggregate-containing dendritic spines. Linear arrays of more intensely stained punctate neuropil aggregates are also observed. In cortex, they are oriented like apical dendrites, whereas in striatum they tend to be curvilinear. These arrays suggest that the tubular and multiform aggregates might condense into a series of separate punctate aggregates. Since larger punctate aggregates are seen in later grade cases, they may continue to grow in size.

As antibodies recognizing *N*-terminal-huntingtin epitopes recognize huntingtin aggregates while internal and *C*-terminal antibodies do not, the aggregates appear to contain primarily *N*-terminal fragments of huntingtin (<549 amino acids) (DiFiglia *et al.* 1997; Gutekunst *et al.* 1999). Aggregates have also been shown to contain α-synuclein (Charles *et al.* 2000) and, more recently, were shown to recruit the transcriptional coactivator cAMP-responsive elements binding protein (CREB)-binding protein, CBP (Nucifora *et al.* 2001). Proteins that are recruited or sequestered within huntingtin aggregates may no longer be available for their normal functions. In the case of CBP, genes under its control were also shown to be dysregulated (Nucifora *et al.* 2001), suggesting a potential cascade of pathological effects (see Chapter 12).

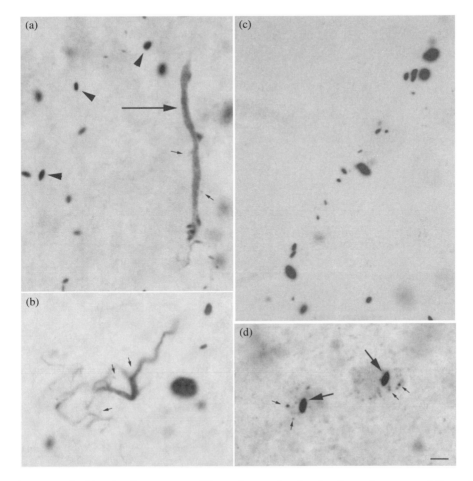

Fig. 8.7 *N*-terminal huntingtin aggregates. Photomicrographs showing the various types of *N*-terminal huntingtin aggregates in HD cortex labelled with EM48 antibodies. Aggregates are present (a)–(c) in the neuropil and (d) in neuronal nuclei long arrows) and perikarya (small arrows). In the neuropil, small spherical or fusiform aggregates are shown either (a) scattered (arrowheads) or (c) arranged in linear arrays reminiscent of neuronal process. EM48 immunoreactivity is also found in (a) long tubular (long arrow) or (b) serpentine elements reminiscent of short dendritic segments and branch points, some of which appeared to give rise to (a),(b) immunoreactive dendritic spines (small arrows). Scale bar for (a)–(d) 10 μm. (Reproduced with permission from Gutekunst *et al.* (1999) ©2001 by the Society for Neuroscience.)

Ultrastructure of nuclear and neuropil aggregates

Huntingtin aggregates have been examined in human brain by electron microscopy (DiFiglia *et al.* 1997; Gutekunst *et al.* 1999), verifying their presence in nuclei, perikarya, dendrites, dendritic spines, and axons. Often, the aggregates completely filled the cross-section of the process being examined (Fig. 8.8). Aggregates are made up of granular and filamentous material and are not membrane-bound. Likewise, no extracellular aggregates have been identified that might have been released from degenerated neurones. In addition, neuropil aggregates do not contain any apparent membrane-bound structures such as vesicles or vacuoles and do not appear to be associated with any particular organelles such as mitochondria or vesicular organelles. The width of the filaments is about 10 nm, and they are often ordered and aligned along the axis of the dendrites. The filamentous material appears to be relatively loose in smaller neuropil aggregates and more compact in larger aggregates. It is conceivable that the aggregates seen in the neuronal processes could disturb intracellular transport. It should be mentioned that nuclear aggregates were originally described as filamentous inclusions in the late 1970s in a descriptive ultrastructural study of neuronal nuclei in HD brains (Roizin *et al.* 1979).

Aggregates in early HD

A few studies have reported on the distribution of huntingtin-containing aggregates in early HD grades (Gutekunst *et al.* 1999; DiFiglia *et al.* 1997; Gomez-Tortosa *et al.* 2001). These studies describe the presence of both nuclear and neuropil aggregates in cortex and striatum and suggest that neuropil aggregates are especially prevalent in the cortical areas in the early stages of HD. In one presymptomatic patient, there was a remarkably high density of neuropil aggregates but almost no nuclear aggregates in the areas of cerebral cortex that were examined (Gutekunst *et al.* 1999). Aggregates were especially frequent in insular, cingulate, and dorsolateral prefrontal cortex but were less common in calcarine and superior parietal cortex and in hippocampus. Most aggregates were located in the neuropil of cortical layers V and VI. The striatum showed degenerative changes dorsally consistent with a grade 1 classification.

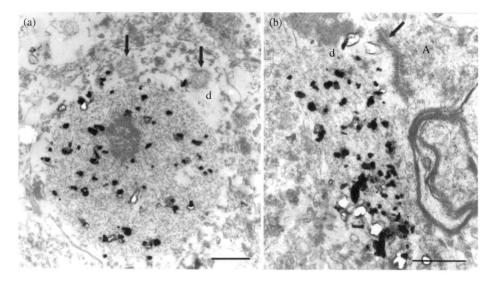

Fig. 8.8 Neuropil aggregates in dendritic profiles. Electron micrographs of EM48 immunogold-labelled aggregates in insular cortex from a grade 1 adult HD brain. Immunogold particles are associated with aggregates made of filamentous material within the dendritic processes. (a) A large-calibre dendrite (d) containing an immunolabelled aggregate. Mitochondria (arrows) are seen in the cytoplasm adjacent to the aggregate. In (b), the filaments consituting the aggregates align with the orientation of the dendrite. Near the aggregate, the dendrite is receiving a synaptic contact (arrow) from an axon terminal (A). Scale bar, 500 nm.

All types of striatal aggregates, however, were very rare, even in the dorsal striatum where degeneration had already started. This unique case indicates that neuropil but not nuclear aggregates may be very common in the brain prior to the development of neurological symptoms. At the same time, nuclear aggregates were exceedingly rare, despite the overall burden of aggregation, at least in cerebral cortex. Most importantly, despite significant neuronal loss in a striatum still containing many normal areas, striatal aggregates seem rarely to correlate with the active degenerative process occurring there, although a more recent study has described the presence of ubiquitinated nuclear aggregates in the tail of the caudate in presymptomatic HD cases (Gomez-Tortosa *et al.* 2001). Although striatal aggregates are uncommon, especially in the early stages of the disease, a connection between the large numbers of cerebral cortical neuropil aggregates and striatal pathology could exist by virtue of the potential importance of glutamatergic corticostriatal projections.

Hypotheses about pathogenesis

Although studies of huntingtin and of transgenic models are producing many leads, a clear pathway from the genetic mutation to neuronal loss has not yet been established. Studies in humans and animal models, however, have led to a number of hypotheses about the final mechanisms of cell death in HD.

Excitotoxicity theory and oxidative stress

The close match of excitotoxin-lesioned animal models and human HD neuropathology strongly suggested excitotoxicity to be the mechanism of cell death (Beal *et al.* 1984, 1989, 1991; Ferrante *et al.* 1993; Bazzett *et al.* 1993; Storey and Beal 1993). Increased glutamate levels, abnormalities in glutamate receptors, or the presence of an endogenous excitotoxin, however, have not been demonstrated in HD brain. It was subsequently suggested that impaired energy metabolism could underlie excitotoxic neuronal death in HD (Beal *et al.* 1993; Beal 1992; Albin and Greenamyre 1992). Many subsequent studies in HD that have supported this idea include positron emission tomography (PET) (Kuhl *et al.* 1985), reductions in several complex activities of the mitochondrial electron transport chain (Brennan *et al.* 1985; Parker *et al.* 1990; Browne *et al.* 1997), and reduced pyruvate dehydrogenase activity in the striatum and hippocampus (Butterworth *et al.* 1985). Cortical biopsies from patients with HD contain abnormal mitochondria (Goebel *et al.* 1978). A marked increase in mitochondrial DNA deletions occurs in the cerebral cortex of HD patients (Polidori *et al.* 1999). Beal and colleagues have identified threefold elevations of lactate in HD cerebral cortex and striatum and the basal ganglia *in vivo* using magnetic resonance (MR) spectroscopy (Jenkins *et al.* 1993; Koroshetz *et al.* 1997), which is further evidence for a defect in oxidative phosphorylation in HD. Increased lactate/pyruvate ratios in cerebrospinal fluid (CSF) of HD patients have also been reported (Koroshetz *et al.* 1997). More recent reports show that molecular epitopes indicative of oxidative damage are greatly increased in the striatum and cortex in HD (Browne *et al.* 1997, 1999). Thus, extensive evidence suggests the involvement of oxidative injury in HD, either as a cause of cell death or as a secondary component of the cell death cascade.

Huntingtin aggregation

It has been proposed that nuclear aggregates are a common cause of neurodegeneration in polyglutamine disorders and that the molecular context of the neurones in which they are expressed accounts for the differences between these diseases (Davies *et al.* 1998; Ross 1997). As mentioned above, the transcriptional coactivator CREB-binding protein (CBP) was found to be depleted from its normal nuclear location and present in polyglutamine aggregates in human HD post-mortem brain as well as in models (Nucifora *et al.* 2001). Such recruitment of CBP into huntingtin aggregates was shown to interfere with CBP-activated gene transcription. The authors suggest that polyglutamine-mediated interference with CBP-regulated gene transcription may constitute a genetic gain of function, underlying the pathogenesis of HD as well as other polyglutamine disorders. In HD, however, it has not yet been shown that huntingtin aggregation or even the presence of nuclear huntingtin is injurious to neurones and not a secondary phenomenon. As mentioned earlier in this chapter, nuclear aggregates in the striatum are not present in the known temporal and spatial patterns of neuronal loss in HD (Gutekunst *et al.* 1999). More importantly, they seem to be rarely found in the neurones most vulnerable in HD (Kuemmerle *et al.* 1999). These facts suggest that nuclear aggregates, as visualized microscopically, are unlikely to play a causative role in HD. Nevertheless, it remains open whether nuclear huntingtin or even whether submicroscopic aggregates of huntingtin in the nucleus might be important (Hodgson *et al.* 1999). An additional possibility is that huntingtin aggregation could be a benign sequestration of a protein fragment resistant to proteolysis (Ordway *et al.* 1999).

Neuronal cell death

Apoptosis is a specific form of programmed cell death characterized morphologically by pyknosis, chromatin condensation and fragmentation, membrane blebbing, and the formation of apoptotic bodies. Necrosis, on the other hand, is characterized by cell and organelle swelling, and lysis and is often associated with significant inflammatory responses. The morphology of neuronal death in human HD remains poorly understood, while in transgenic models of HD cell death does not fit either mechanism well. The molecular events underlying apoptosis and necrosis involve complex signal transduction and protease activations that have also been difficult to identify as occurring in human material. *In situ* hybridization and gel electrophoresis techniques show that neurones of HD patients have increased levels of DNA strand breaks, a possible indicator of apoptosis (Dragunow *et al.* 1997; Butterworth *et al.* 1998; Portera-Cailliau *et al.* 1995). Animal and cellular models are producing more leads as discussed in Chapters 12 and 13 (Ona *et al.* 1999; Turmaine *et al.* 2000; Rigamonti *et al.* 2000, 2001).

Concluding remarks

Neuropathological findings in HD continue to be unveiled and these are essential for the analysis and assessment of the animal models of HD that are being developed in various laboratories. The size of a human brain makes it difficult to evaluate the extent of neurodegeneration that occurs in a disease-specific manner. Novel information from animal models of HD, in turn, will require continued verification from, and will continue to stimulate studies in, human HD brain.

References

Albin, R., Young, A., and Penney, J. (1989). The functional anatomy of basal ganglia disorders. *Trends in Neuroscience* **12**: 366–75.

Albin, R., Young, A., and Penney, J. (1990). Abnormalities of striatal projections neurones and N-methyl-D-aspartate in presymptomatic Huntington's disease. *New England Journal of Medicine* **322**: 1293–8.

Albin, R.L. and Greenamyre, J.T. (1992). Alternative excitotoxic hypotheses. *Neurology* **42**: 733–8.

Albin, R.L., Reiner, A., Anderson, K. D., Dure, L. S., Handelin, B., Balfour, R., Whetsell, W. O., Penney, J. B., and Young, A. B. (1992). Preferential loss of striato-external pallidal projection neurones in presymptomatic Huntington's disease. *Annals of Neurology* **31**: 425–30.

Averback, P. (1981). Lesions of the nucleus ansae peduncularis in neuropsychiatric disease. *Archives of Neurology* **38**: 230–5.

Barbas, H., Henion, T., and Dermon, C. (1995). Diverse thalamic projections to the prefrontal cortex in the rhesus monkey. *Journal of Comparative Neurology* **313**: 65–94.

Bazzett, T.J., Becker, J.B., Kaatz, K.W., and Albin, R.L. (1993). Chronic intrastriatal dialytic administration of quinolinic acid produces selective neural degeneration. *Experimental Neurology* **120**: 177–85.

Beal, M.F. (1992). Does impairment of energy metabolism result in excitotoxic neuronal death in neurodegenerative illnesses? *Annals of Neurology* **31**: 119–30.

—— Bird, E.D., Langlais, P.J., and Martin, J. B. (1984). Somatostatin is increased in the nucleus accumbens in Huntington's disease. *Neurology* **34**: 663–6.

—— Kowall, N.W., Swartz, K.J., Ferrante, R.J., and Martin, J.B. (1989). Differential sparing of somatostatin-neuropeptide Y and cholinergic neurones following striatal excitotoxin lesions. *Synapse* **3**: 38–47.

—— Ferrante, R.J., Swartz, K.J., and Kowall, N.W. (1991). Chronic quinolinic acid lesions in rats closely resemble Huntington's disease. *Journal of Neuroscience* **11**: 1649–59.

—— Brouillet, E., Jenkins, B.G., Ferrante, R.J., Kowall, N.W., Miller, J.M., Storey, E., Srivastava, R., Rosen, B.R., and Hyman, B.T. (1993). Neurochemical and histologic characterization of striatal excitotoxic lesions produced by the mitochondrial toxin 3-nitropropionic acid. *Journal of Neuroscience* **13**: 4181–92.

Becher, M.W., Kotzuk, J.A., Sharp, A.H., Davies, S.W., Bates, G.P., Price, D.L., and Ross, C.A. (1998). Intranuclear neuronal inclusions in Huntington's disease and dentatorubral and pallidoluysian atrophy: correlation between the density of inclusions and IT15 CAG triplet repeat length. *Neurobiology of Diseases* **4**: 387–97.

Bots, G.T. and Bruyn, G.W. (1981). Neuropathological changes of the nucleus accumbens in Huntington's chorea. *Acta Neuropathologica* **55**: 21–2.

Braak, H. and Braak, E. (1992a). Allocortical involvement in Huntington's disease. *Neuropathology and Applied Neurobiology* **18**: 539–47.

—— —— (1992b). The human entorhinal cortex: normal morphology and lamina-specific pathology in various diseases. *Neuroscience Research* **15**: 6–31.

Brennan, W.A. Jr, Bird, E.D., and Aprille, J.R. (1985). Regional mitochondrial respiratory activity in Huntington's disease brain. *Journal of Neurochemistry* **44**: 1948–50.

Browne, S.E., Bowling, A.C., MacGarvey, U., Baik, M.J., Berger, S.C., Muqit, M.M., Bird, E.D., and Beal, M.F. (1997). Oxidative damage and metabolic dysfunction in Huntington's disease: selective vulnerability of the basal ganglia. *Annals of Neurology* **41**: 646–53.

Browne, S.E., Ferrante, R.J., and Beal, M.F. (1999). Oxidative stress in Huntington's disease. *Brain Pathology* **9**: 147–63.

Bruyn, G., Bots, G., and Dom, R. (1979). Huntington's chorea: current neuropathological status. *Advances in Neurology* **1**: 83–93.

Bruyn, G.W. and von Wolferen, W.J. (1973). Pathogenesis of Huntington's chorea. *Lancet* **1**: 1382.

Bugiani, O., Tabaton, M., and Cammarata, S. (1984). Huntington's disease: survival of large striatal neurones in the rigid variant. *Annals of Neurology* **15**: 154–6.

Butterworth, J., Yates, C.M., and Reynolds, G.P. (1985). Distribution of phosphate-activated glutaminase, succinic dehydrogenase, pyruvate dehydrogenase and gamma-glutamyl transpeptidase in post-mortem brain from Huntington's disease and agonal cases. *Journal of Neurological Science* **67**: 161–71.

Butterworth, N.J., Williams, L., Bullock, J.Y., Love, D.R., Faull, R.L., and Dragunow, M. (1998). Trinucleotide (CAG). repeat length is positively correlated with the degree of DNA fragmentation in Huntington's disease striatum. *Neuroscience* **87**: 49–53.

Byers, R.K., Gilles, F.H., and Fung, C. (1973). Huntington's disease in children. Neuropathologic study of four cases. *Neurology* **23**: 561–9.

Cammarata, S., Caponnetto, C., and Tabaton, M. (1993). Ubiquitin-reactive neurites in cerebral cortex of subjects with Huntington's chorea: a pathological correlate of dementia? *Neuroscience Letters* **156**: 96–8.

Castaigne, P., Escourolle, R., and Gray, M. (1976). Huntington's chorea and cerebellar atrophy. A propos of anatomo-clinical case. *Rev Neurol* **132**: 233–40.

Cha, J. (2000). Transcriptional dysregulation in Huntington's disease. *Trends in Neuroscience* **23**: 387–92.

Cha, J.H., Kosinski, C.M., Kerner, J.A., Alsdorf, S.A., Mangiarini, L., Davies, S.W., Penney, J.B., Bates, G.P., and Young, A.B. (1998). Altered brain neurotransmitter receptors in transgenic mice expressing a portion of an abnormal human huntington disease gene. *Proceedings of the National Academy of Sciences, USA* **95**: 6480–5.

Cha, J.H., Frey, A.S., Alsdorf, S.A., Kerner, J.A., Kosinski, C.M., Mangiarini, L., Penney, J.B. Jr, Davies, S.W., Bates, G.P., and Young, A.B. (1999). Altered neurotransmitter receptor expression in transgenic mouse models of Huntington's disease. *Philosophical Transactions of the Royal Society of London, B Biological Science* **354**: 981–9.

Charles, V., Mezey, E., Reddy, P.H., Dehejia, A., Young, T.A., Polymeropoulos, M.H., Brownstein, M.J., and Tagle, D.A. (2000). Alpha-synuclein immunoreactivity of huntingtin polyglutamine aggregates in striatum and cortex of Huntington's disease patients and transgenic mouse models. *Neuroscience Letters* **289**: 29–32.

Chen, Q. and Reiner, A. (1996). Cellular distribution of the NMDA receptor NR2A/2B subunits in the rat striatum. *Brain Research* **743**: 346–52.

Cicchetti, F., Prensa, L., Wu, Y., and Parent, A. (2000). Chemical anatomy of striatal interneurones in normal individuals and in patients with Huntington's Disease. *Brain Research Reviews* **34**: 80–101.

Crossman, A. (1987). Primate model of dyskinesia: The experimental approach to the study of basal ganglia-related involuntary movement disorders. *Neuroscience* **21**: 1–40.

Cudkowicz, M. and Kowall, N.W. (1990). Degeneration of pyramidal projection neurones in Huntington's disease cortex. *Annals of Neurology* **27**: 200–4.

Davies, S.W., Turmaine, M., Cozens, B.A., DiFiglia, M., Sharp, A.H., Ross, C.A., Scherzinger, E., Wanker, E.E., Mangiarini, L., and Bates, G.P. (1997). Formation of neuronal intranuclear inclusions underlies the neurological dysfunction in mice transgenic for the HD mutation. *Cell* **90**: 537–48.

—— Beardsall, K., Turmaine, M., DiFiglia, M., Aronin, N., and Bates, G.P. (1998). Are neuronal intranuclear inclusions the common neuropathology of triplet-repeat disorders with polyglutamine-repeat expansions? *Lancet* **351**: 131–3.

de la Monte, S.M., Vonsattel, J.P., and Richardson, E.P. (1988). Morphometric demonstration of atrophic changes in the cerebral cortex, white matter, and neostriatum in Huntington's disease. *Journal of Neuropathology and Experimental Neurology* **47**: 516–25.

DeLong, M. (1990). Primate models of movement disorders of basal ganglia origin. *Trends in Neuroscience* **13**: 281–285.

DiFiglia, M., Sapp, E., Chase, K., Schwarz, C., Meloni, A., Young, C., Martin, E., Vonsattel, J.-P., Reeves, S., Carraway, R., Boyce, F., and Aronin, N. (1995). Huntingtin is a cytoplasmic protein associated with vesicles in human and rat brain neurones. *Neuron* **14**: 1075–81.

DiFiglia, M., Sapp, E., Chase, K.O., Davies, S.W., Bates, G.P., Vonsattel, J.P., and Aronin, N. (1997). Aggregation of huntingtin in neuronal intranuclear inclusions and dystrophic neurites in brain. *Science* **277**: 1990–3.

Dom, R., Malfroid, M., and Baro, F. (1976). Neuropathology of Huntington's chorea. Studies of the ventrobasal complex of the thalamus. *Neurology* **26**: 64–8.

Dragunow, M., MacGibbon, G.A., Lawlor, P., Butterworth, N., Connor, B., Henderson, C., Walton, M., Woodgate, A., Hughes, P., and Faull, R.L. (1997). Apoptosis, neurotrophic factors and neurodegeneration. *Reviews in the Neurosciences* **8**: 223–65.

Ferrante, R., Kowall, N., and Richardson, E. (1989). Neuronal and neuropil loss in the substantia nigra in Huntington's disease. *Journal of Neuropathology and Experimental Neurology* **48**: 380.

Ferrante, R.J., Beal, M.F., Kowall, N.W., Richardson, E.P., and Martin, J.B. (1987a). Sparing of acetyl-cholinesterase-containing striatal neurones in Huntington's disease. *Brain Research* **411**: 162–6.

Ferrante, R.J., Kowall, N.W., Beal, M.F., Martin, J.B., Bird, E.D., and Richardson, E.P. (1987b). Morphologic and histochemical characteristics of a spared subset of striatal neurones in Huntington's disease. *Journal of Neuropathology and Experimental Neurology* **46**: 12–27.

Ferrante, R.J., Kowall, N.W., and Richardson, E.P. (1991). Proliferative and degenerative changes in striatal spiny neurones in Huntington's disease: a combined study using the section-Golgi method and calbindin D28k immunocytochemistry. *Journal of Neuroscience* **11**: 3877–87.

Ferrante, R.J., Kowall, N.W., Cipolloni, P.B., Storey, E., and Beal, M.F. (1993). Excitotoxin lesions in primates as a model for Huntington's disease: histopathologic and neurochemical characterization. *Experimental Neurology* **119**: 46–71.

Ferrante, R.J., Gutekunst, C.A., Persichetti, F., McNeil, S.M., Kowall, N.W., Gusella, J.F., MacDonald, M.E., Beal, M.F., and Hersch, S.M. (1997). Heterogeneous topographic and cellular distribution of huntingtin expression in the normal human neostriatum. *Journal of Neuroscience* **17**: 3052–63.

Forno, L. and Jose, C. (1973). Huntington's chorea: a pathological study. *Advances in Neurology* **1**: 453–70.

Forno, L. and Norville, R. (1979). Ultrastructure of the neostriatum in Huntington's and Parkinson's disease. *Advances in Neurology* **23**: 123–35.

Gerfen, C. (1992). The neostriatal mosaic: multiple levels of compartmental organization in the basal ganglia. *Annual Reviews in Neuroscience* **15**: 285–320.

Giguere, M. and Glodman-Rakic, P. (1988). Mediodorsal nucleus: areal, laminar, and tangential distribution of afferents and efferents in the frontal lobe of the rhesus monkey. *Journal of Comparative Neurology* **277**: 195–213.

Goebel, H.H., Heipertz, R., Scholz, W., Iqbal, K., and Tellez-Nagel, I. (1978). Juvenile Huntington chorea: clinical, ultrastructural, and biochemical studies. *Neurology* **28**: 23–31.

Gomez-Tortosa, E., MacDonald, M.E., Friend, J.C., Taylor, S.A., Weiler, L.J., Cupples, L.A., Srinidhi, J., Gusella, J.F., Bird, E.D., Vonsattel, J.P., and Myers, R.H. (2001). Quantitative neuropathological changes in presymptomatic Huntington's disease. *Annals of Neurology* **49**: 29–34.

Goto, S. and Hirano, A. (1990). Synaptophysin expression in the striatum in Huntington's disease. *Acta Neuropathologica* **80**: 88–91.

Gourfinkel-An, I., Cancel, G., Duyckaerts, C., Faucheux, B., Hauw, J.J., Trottier, Y., Brice, A., Agid, Y., and Hirsch, E.C. (1998). Neuronal distribution of intranuclear inclusions in Huntington's disease with adult onset. *Neuroreport* **9**: 1823–6.

Graveland, G., Williams, R., and Di Figlia, M. (1985). Evidence for degenerative and regenerative changes in neostriatal spiny neurones in Huntington's disease. *Science* **227**: 770–3.

Graybiel, A. (1990). Neurotransmitters and neuromodulators in the basal ganglia. *Trends in Neuroscience* **13**: 244–54.

Grotton, F., Turetsky, D., and Choi, D. (1995). SMI-32 antibody against non-phosphorylated neurofilaments identifies a subpopulation of cultured cortical neurones hypersensitive to kainate toxicity. *Neuroscience Letters* **194**: 1–4.

Gutekunst, C.-A., Levey, A., Heilman, C., Whaley, W., Yi, H., Nash, N., Rees, H., Madden, J., and Hersch, S. (1995). Identification and localization of huntingtin in brain and lymphoblasts with anti-fusion protein antibodies. *Proceedings of the National Academy of Sciences, USA* **92**: 8710–14.

Gutekunst, C.A., Li, S.H., Yi, H., Ferrante, R.J., Li, X.J., and Hersch, S.M. (1998). The cellular and sub-cellular localization of huntingtin-associated protein 1 (HAP1): comparison with huntingtin in rat and human. *Journal of Neuroscience* **18**: 7674–86.

Gutekunst, C.A., Li, S.H., Yi, H., Mulroy, J.S., Kuemmerle, S., Jones, R., Rye, D., Ferrante, R.J., Hersch, S.M., and Li, X.J. (1999). Nuclear and neuropil aggregates in Huntington's disease: relationship to neuropathology. *Journal of Neuroscience* **19**: 2522–34.

Hattori, H., Takao, T., Ito, M., Nakano, S., Okuno, T., and Mikawa, H. (1984). Cerebellum and brain stem atrophy in a child with Huntington's disease. *Computerized Radiology* **8**: 53–6.

Hedreen, J.C. and Folstein, S.E. (1995). Early loss of neostriatal striosome neurones in Huntington's disease. *Journal of Neuropathology and Experimental Neurology* **54**: 105–20.

Heinsen, H., Strik, M., Bauer, M., Luther, K., Ulmar, G., Gangnus, D., Jungkunz, G., Eisenmenger, W., and Gotz, M. (1994). Cortical and striatal neuron number in Huntington's disease. *Acta Neuropathologica* **88**: 320–33.

Heinsen, H., Rub, U., Gangnus, D., Jungkunz, G., Bauer, M., Ulmar, G., Bethke, B., Schuler, M., Bocker, F., Eisenmenger, W., Gotz, M., and Strik, M. (1996). Nerve cell loss in the thalamic centro-median-parafascicular complex in patients with Huntington's disease. *Acta Neuropathologica* **91**: 161–8.

Heinsen, H., Rub, U., Bauer, M., Ulmar, G., Bethke, B., Schuler, M., Bocker, F., Eisenmenger, W., Gotz, M., Korr, H., and Schmitz, C. (1999). Nerve cell loss in the thalamic mediodorsal nucleus in Huntington's disease. *Acta Neuropathologica* **97**: 613–22.

Heiser, V., Scherzinger, E., Boeddrich, A., Nordhoff, E., Lurz, R., Schugardt, N., Lehrach, H., and Wanker, E.E. (2000). Inhibition of huntingtin fibrillogenesis by specific antibodies and small molecules: implications for Huntington's disease therapy. *Proceedings of the National Academy of Sciences, USA* **97**: 6739–44.

Hersch, S. and Ferrante, R. (1997). In *Movement disorders*: *neurologic principles and practice* (eds. R. Watts and W. Koller). Chapter 36: Neuropathology and Pathophysiology of Huntington's Disease, pp. 503–26. New York: McGraw-Hill.

Hodgson, J., Agopyan, N., Gutekunst, C.-A., Leavitt, B., LePiane, F., Singaraja, R., Smith, D., Bissada, N., McCutcheon, K., Nasir, J., Jamot, L., Li, X., Stevens, M., Rosemond, E., Roder, J., Phillips, A., Rubin, E., Hersch, S., and Hayden, M. (1999). A YAC mouse model for Huntington's disease with full-length mutant huntingtin, cytoplasmic toxicity, and selective striatal neurodegeneration. *Neuron* **23**: 181–92.

Huang, C.C., Faber, P.W., Persichetti, F., Mittal, V., Vonsattel, J.P., MacDonald, M.E., and Gusella, J.F. (1998). Amyloid formation by mutant huntingtin: threshold, progressivity and recruitment of normal polyglutamine proteins. *Somatic Cell Molecular Genetics* **24**: 217–33.

Jackson, M., Gentleman, S., Lennox, G., Ward, L., Gray, T., Randall, K., Morrell, K., and Lowe, J. (1995). The cortical neuritic pathology of Huntington's disease. *Neuropathology and Applied Neurobiology* **21**: 18–26.

Jenkins, B.G., Koroshetz, W.J., Beal, M.F., and Rosen, B.R. (1993). Evidence for impairment of energy metabolism *in vivo* in Huntington's disease using localized 1H NMR spectroscopy. *Neurology* **43**: 2689–95.

Jeste, D., Barban, L., and Parisi, J. (1984). Reduced Purkinje cell density in Huntington's disease. *Experimental Neurology* **85**: 78–86.

Koroshetz, W.J., Jenkins, B.G., Rosen, B.R., and Beal, M.F. (1997). Energy metabolism defects in Huntington's disease and effects of coenzyme Q10. *Annals of Neurology* **41**: 160–5.

Kremer, H.P. (1992). The hypothalamic lateral tuberal nucleus: normal anatomy and changes in neurological diseases. *Progress in Brain Research* **93**: 249–61.

Kremer, H.P., Roos, R.A., Dingjan, G.M., Bots, G.T., Bruyn, G.W., and Hofman, M.A. (1991). The hypothalamic lateral tuberal nucleus and the characteristics of neuronal loss in Huntington's disease. *Neuroscience Letters* **132**: 101–4.

Kuemmerle, S., Gutekunst, C.A., Klein, A.M., Li, X.J., Li, S.H., Beal, M.F., Hersch, S.M., and Ferrante, R.J. (1999). Huntington aggregates may not predict neuronal death in Huntington's disease. *Annals of Neurology* **46**: 842–9.

Kuhl, D.E., Markham, C.H., Metter, E.J., Riege, W.H., Phelps, M.E., and Mazziotta, J.C. (1985). Local cerebral glucose utilization in symptomatic and presymptomatic Huntington's disease. *Research Publications Association for Research in Nervous and Mental Disease* **63**: 199–209.

Lange, H., Thorner, G., Hopf, A., and Schroder, K.F. (1976). Morphometric studies of the neuropathological changes in choreatic diseases. *Journal of Neurological Science* **28**: 401–25.

Maat-Schieman, M.I., Dorsman, J.C., Smoor, M.A., Siesling, S., Van Duinen, S.G., Verschuuren, J.J., den Dunnen, J.T., Van Ommen, G.J., and Roos, R.A. (1999). Distribution of inclusions in neuronal nuclei and dystrophic neurites in Huntington disease brain. *Journal of Neuropathology and Experimental Neurology* **58**: 129–37.

Macdonald, V., Halliday, G.M., Trent, R.J., and McCusker, E.A. (1997). Significant loss of pyramidal neurones in the angular gyrus of patients with Huntington's disease. *Neuropathology and Applied Neurobiology* **23**: 492–5.

McGowan, D.P., van Roon-Mom, W., Holloway, H., Bates, G.P., Mangiarini, L., Cooper, G.J., Faull, R.L., and Snell, R.G. (2000). Amyloid-like inclusions in Huntington's disease. *Neuroscience* **100**: 677–80.

Mitchell, I., Cooper, A., and Griffiths, M. (1999). The selective vulnerability of striatopallidal neurones. *Progress in Neurobiology* **59**: 691–719.

Morton, A.J., Nicholson, L.F., and Faull, R.L. (1993). Compartmental loss of NADPH diaphorase in the neuropil of the human striatum in Huntington's disease. *Neuroscience* **53**: 159–68.

Myers, R., Vonsattel, J., Stevens, T., Cupples, L., Richardson, E., Martin, J., and Bird, E. (1988). Clinical and neuropathologic assessment of severity in Huntington disease. *Neurology* **38**: 341–7.

Nihei, K. and Kowall, N. (1992). Neurofilament and neural cell adhesion molecule immunocytochemistry of Huntington's disease striatum. *Annals of Neurology* **31**: 59–63.

Nucifora, F.C. Jr, Sasaki, M., Peters, M.F., Huang, H., Cooper, J.K., Yamada, M., Takahashi, H., Tsuji, S., Troncoso, J., Dawson, V.L., Dawson, T.M., and Ross, C.A. (2001). Interference by huntingtin and atrophin-1 with cbp-mediated transcription leading to cellular toxicity. *Science* **291**: 2423–8.

Ona, V.O., Li, M., Vonsattel, J.P., Andrews, L.J., Khan, S.Q., Chung, W.M., Frey, A.S., Menon, A.S., Li, X.J., Stieg, P.E., Yuan, J., Penney, J.B., Young, A.B., Cha, J.H., and Friedlander, R.M. (1999). Inhibition of caspase-1 slows disease progression in a mouse model of Huntington's disease [see comments]. *Nature* **399**: 263–7.

Ordway, J.M., Cearley, J.A., and Detloff, P.J. (1999). CAG-polyglutamine-repeat mutations: independence from gene context. *Philosophical Transactions of the Royal Society of London, B Biological Science* **354**: 1083–8.

Oyanagi, K. and Ikuta, F. (1987). A morphometric reevaluation of Huntington's chorea with special reference to the large neurons in the neostriatum. *Clinical Neuropathology* **6**: 71–9.

Oyanagi, K., Takeda, S., Takahashi, H., *et al.* (1989). A quantitative investigation of the substantia nigra in Huntington's disease. *Annals of Neurology* **26**: 13–19.

Parent, A. and Hazrati, L. (1995a). Functional anatomy of the basal ganglia I. The cortico-basal ganglia-thalamo-cortical loop. *Brain Research Review* **20**: 91–127.

Parent, A. and Hazrati, L. (1995b). Functional anatomy of the basal ganglia. 2. The place of subthalamic nucleus and external pallidum in basal ganglia circuitry. *Brain Research Review* **20**: 128–154.

Parker, W. J., Boyson, S., Luder, A., and Parks, J. (1990). Evidence for a defect in NADH: ubiquinone oxidoreductase (complex 1) in Huntington's disease. *Neurology* **40**: 1231–34.

Persichetti, F., Carlee, L., Faber, P.W., McNeil, S.M., Ambrose, C.M., Srinidhi, J., Anderson, M., Barnes, G.T., Gusella, J.F., and MacDonald, M.E. (1996). Differential expression of normal and mutant Huntington's disease gene alleles. *Neurobiology of Diseases* **3**: 183–90.

Polidori, M.C., Mecocci, P., Browne, S.E., Senin, U., and Beal, M.F. (1999). Oxidative damage to mitochondrial DNA in Huntington's disease parietal cortex. *Neuroscience Letters* **272**: 53–6.

Portera-Cailliau, C., Hedreen, J.C., Price, D.L., and Koliatsos, V.E. (1995). Evidence for apoptotic cell death in Huntington disease and excitotoxic animal models. *Journal of Neuroscience* **15**: 3775–87.

Reiner, A., Albin, R.L., Anderson, K.D., D'Amato, C.J., Penney, J.B., and Young, A.B. (1988). Differential loss of striatal projection neurones in Huntington disease. *Proceedings of the National Academy of Sciences, USA* **85**: 5733–7.

Rigamonti, D., Bauer, J. H., De-Fraja, C., Conti, L., Sipione, S., Sciorati, C., Clementi, E., Hackam, A., Hayden, M.R., Li, Y., Cooper, J.K., Ross, C. A., Govoni, S., Vincenz, C., and Cattaneo, E. (2000). Wild-type huntingtin protects from apoptosis upstream of caspase-3. *Journal of Neuroscience* **20**: 3705–13.

—— Sipione, S., Goffredo, D., Zuccato, C., Fossale, E., and Cattaneo, E. (2001). Huntingtin's neuroprotective activity occurs via inhibition of pro caspase-9 processing. *Journal of Biological Chemistry* **5**: 5.

Rodda, R. (1981). Cerebellar atrophy in Huntington's disease. *Journal of Neurological Science* **50**: 147–57.

Roizin, L., Stellar, S., and Liu, J. (1979). Neuronal nuclear–cytoplasmic inclusions in Huntington's disease: electron microscopic investigations. *Advances in Neurology* **23**: 95–122.

Roos, R. (1986). In *Handbook of clinical neurology*, Vol. 49 (ed. P. Vinken, G. Bruyn, and H. Klawan), pp. 315–22. Amsterdam: Elsevier.

—— Pruyt, J., de Vries, J., and Bots, G. (1985). Neuronal distribution in the putamen of in Huntington's disease. *Journal of Neurology, Neurosurgery and Psychiatry* **48**: 422–5.

Ross, C. A. (1997). Intranuclear neuronal inclusions: a common pathogenic mechanism for glutamine-repeat neurodegenerative diseases? *Neuron* **19**: 1147–50.

Sapp, E., Schwarz, C., Chase, K., Bhide, P.G., Young, A.B., Penney, J., Vonsattel, J.P., Aronin, N., and DiFiglia, M. (1997). Huntingtin localization in brains of normal and Huntington's disease patients. *Annals of Neurology* **42**: 604–12.

—— Kegel, K.B., Aronin, N., Hashikawa, T., Uchiyama, Y., Tohyama, K., Bhide, P.G., Vonsattel, J.P., and DiFiglia, M. (2001). Early and progressive accumulation of reactive microglia in the Huntington disease brain. *Journal of Neuropathology and Experimental Neurology* **60**: 161–72.

Schmitz, C., Rub, U., Korr, H., and Heinsen, H. (1999). Nerve cell loss in the thalamic mediodorsal nucleus in Huntington's disease. II. Optimization of a stereological estimation procedure. *Acta Neuropathologica* **97**: 623–8.

Selemon, L.D., Rajkowska, G., and Goldman-Rakic, P.S. (1998). Elevated neuronal density in prefrontal area 46 in brains from schizophrenic patients: application of a three-dimensional, stereologic counting method. *Journal of Comparative Neurology* **392**: 402–12.

Seto-Ohshima, A., Emson, P.C., Lawson, E., Mountjoy, C.Q., and Carrasco, L.H. (1988). Loss of matrix calcium-binding protein-containing neurones in Huntington's disease. *Lancet* **1**: 1252–5.

Sharp, A.H., Loev, S.J., Schilling, G., Li, S.H., Li, X.J., Bao, J., Wagster, M.V., Kotzuk, J.A., Steiner, J.P., Lo, A., *et al.* (1995). Widespread expression of Huntington's disease gene (IT15). protein product. *Neuron* **14**: 1065–74.

Sotrel, A., Paskevich, P.A., Kiely, D.K., Bird, E.D., Williams, R.S., and Myers, R.H. (1991). Morphometric analysis of the prefrontal cortex in Huntington's disease. *Neurology* **41**: 1117–23.

Spargo, E., Everall, I.P., and Lantos, P.L. (1993). Neuronal loss in the hippocampus in Huntington's disease: a comparison with HIV infection. *Journal of Neurology, Neurosurgery and Psychiatry* **56**: 487–91.

Storey, E. and Beal, M. (1993). Neurochemical substrate of rigidity and chorea in Huntington's disease. *Brain* **116**: 1201–22.

Tellez-Nagel, I., Johnson, A., and Terry, R. (1973). Ultrastructural and histochemical study of cerebral cortex biopsies in Huntington's disease. *Advances in Neurology* **1**: 397–8.

Trottier, Y., Devys, D., Imbert, G., Saudou, F., An, I., Lutz, Y., Weber, C., Agid, Y., Hirsch, E.C., and Mandel, J.L. (1995). Cellular localization of the Huntington's disease protein and discrimination of the normal and mutated form. *Nature Genetics* **10**: 104–10.

Turmaine, M., Raza, A., Mahal, A., Mangiarini, L., Bates, G.P., and Davies, S.W. (2000). Nonapoptotic neurodegeneration in a transgenic mouse model of Huntington's disease. *Proceedings of the National Academy of Sciences of the United States of America* **97**: 8093–7.

Vonsattel, J.P., Myers, R.H., Stevens, T.J., Ferrante, R.J., Bird, E.D., and Richardson, E.P. (1985). Neuropathological classification of Huntington's disease. *Journal of Neuropathology and Experimental Neurology* **44**: 559–77.

Zalneraitis, E., Landis, D., Richardson, E., and Selkoe, D. (1981). A comparison of astrocytic structure in cerebral cortex and striatum in Huntington disease. *Neurology* **31**: 151.

9 Neurochemistry of Huntington's disease

George J. Yohrling, IV and Jang-Ho J. Cha

Introduction

Neurochemical alterations in Huntington's disease (HD) have long attracted attention from researchers. Historically, the observations made from analysis of post-mortem human HD brains have given rise to some of the most important modern concepts in human neurodegenerative diseases. The idea that overexcitation of the glutamate neurotransmitter system—*excitoxicity*—could reproduce several neuropathological features of HD was suggested by observations of the effect of injection of analogues of the neurotransmitter glutamate into the striatum of primates or rodents. Additionally, the notion that particular neurochemically defined classes of neurones are selectively vulnerable in HD is now a common theme in many neurological diseases. Indeed, the idea that the neurochemical identity of a neurone could predispose to its demise found its strongest support from observations of post-mortem human HD brain.

And yet, the observations from human post-mortem HD samples have been hampered by the confounding factor of neuronal loss. Simply put, the interpretation of a decrease of a particular neurochemical marker—whether it be neurotransmitter, synthetic enzyme, receptor, or uptake site—is made immensely more complex by the mere fact that neurones have been lost. That is, an apparent decrease in a particular marker may carry no more import beyond confirming that some neurones have disappeared. Conversely, preservation or increase of a marker may in fact be artefactual, caused by the increased cellular density resulting from tissue shrinkage.

Thus, results obtained from human post-mortem samples must be interpreted with caution. Nevertheless, pathological observations strongly suggest that particular neurotransmitter systems are selectively affected or spared in HD (Young and Penney 1984). In addition, the issue of cell loss in post-mortem studies is becoming less problematic, with the advent of positron emission tomography (PET) scanning in living human subjects, as well as animal lesion models and transgenic animal models. Indeed, many of the more recent studies confirm that earlier post-mortem observations were not simply artefactual. It is now clear that some of the earliest pathological changes in HD are indeed neurochemical. It is conceivable that these neurochemical alterations not only produce the characteristic clinical symptoms of HD, but also accelerate the process of cell death, and are thus essential mediators of disease pathogenesis.

The gross pathology of HD is characterized by atrophy of the basal ganglia, specifically the striatum (caudate–putamen) (Vonsattel *et al.* 1985). The basal ganglia are a set of subcortical grey matter structures that are involved in various aspects of motor control, cognition, and sensory pathways (Graybiel 1990). Pathological changes have also been described in the cortex, thalamus, and subthalamic nucleus (Hedreen *et al.* 1991). This characteristic pattern of neuronal damage stands in contrast to the rather ubiquitous distribution of the huntingtin protein (DiFiglia *et al*. 1995; Gutekunst *et al*. 1995; Ferrante *et al*. 1997; Kosinski *et al*. 1997). Neurochemical changes reflect the cell populations affected in the disease, while offering insights into selective neuronal vulnerability. Regional specificity of neuronal damage in HD is not limited to specific nuclei; within the same nuclei certain cell types are more susceptible than others. For example, within the striatum, the structure most affected in HD, projection neurones are preferentially lost while interneurones are relatively spared.

Human studies

The initial studies concerning HD were made using human post-mortem brain samples, investigating levels of neurotransmitters, neurotransmitter synthetic enzymes, receptors, and uptake sites.

GABA

The first neurotransmitter discovered to be decreased in HD brain was γ-aminobutyric acid (GABA). Early evidence suggested decreased levels of GABA and its synthetic enzyme glutamic acid decarboxylase (GAD) in post-mortem HD brain (Perry *et al*. 1973; Bird and Iversen 1974). In the striatum, 90 percent of the neurones are medium spiny neurones, the GABA-containing projection neurones that are preferentially lost in HD (Ferrante *et al*. 1985, 1987a; Vonsattel *et al*. 1985). While it is not yet clear why this population of neurones is especially targeted in HD, this selective cellular vulnerability is a neuropathological hallmark of HD (DiFiglia 1990).

While GABA content was decreased, there was a more complex pattern of alteration in GABA receptors. GABA receptors were decreased in striatum (caudate–putamen) (Lloyd *et al*. 1977; Reisine *et al*. 1979a), unchanged in cortex (Lloyd *et al*. 1977), but increased in the external, or lateral, segment of the globus pallidus (GPe) (Enna *et al*. 1976). The loss of striatal GABA receptors thus most probably represents loss of striatal neurones, whereas the increase in GABA receptors in the GPe, an area that normally receives synaptic input from striatal projections, most probably represents a measure of denervation supersensitivity. Similar findings were made with benzodiazepines, which bind to a modulatory site on the GABA receptor. Benzodiazepine binding sites were decreased in HD striatum, but increased in the substantia nigra pars reticulata (SNr), GP, and the cortex (Reisine *et al*. 1979b, 1980; Walker *et al*. 1984). Penney and Young (1982) found that GABA and benzodiazepine receptors were increased in the internal (medial) and external segments of the globus pallidus (GPi and GPe, respectively), while decreased in the ventrolateral nucleus of the thalamus (VL). These findings suggested that loss of one population of cells, the GABAergic medium spiny striatal neurones, had downstream effects, altering the levels of receptors expressed in synaptic target areas. More specifically, these findings emphasize the importance of taking into account neuronal circuitry: the functioning of specific nuclei can be influenced by changes in their inputs (Albin *et al*. 1989).

Disruptions in the GABA system are not limited to the striatum. Reynolds and Pearson (1987) have shown decreased GABA levels in the hippocampus and cerebral cortex. In addition, levels of the synthetic enzyme glutamic acid decarboxylase (GAD) are reduced throughout the brain, although most markedly in the striatum and GPe (Spokes 1980).

Finally, alterations in the GABA system occur early in the course of the disease. Reynolds and Pearson (1990) report decreased GABA levels in a presymptomatic HD gene carrier, suggesting that alteration in striatal GABA content precedes the appearance of gross clinical symptoms.

Neuropeptides

While most of the striatal neurones are medium spiny GABAergic neurones, they can be further classified by their synaptic target destination, one population projecting to the GPe ('striato-lateral pallidal' neurones), and the other projecting to the GPi and SNr ('striato-medial pallidal' and 'striatonigral' neurones, respectively). The two different populations of medium spiny striatal projection neurones are distinct start points for two separate anatomical pathways, termed the 'direct' and 'indirect' pathways (Albin *et al.* 1989). These two classes of neurones differ in the peptidergic co-neurotransmitter they use in addition to GABA, with striatolateral pallidal neurones also containing enkephalin, and the striatomedial pallidal and striatonigral neurones containing substance P and dynorphin (Reiner and Anderson 1990). Even between the populations of medium spiny neurones, there appears to be a measure of selective vulnerability, with striatolateral pallidal neurones affected to a greater degree than striatonigral neurones (Spokes 1980; Reiner *et al.* 1988; Albin *et al.* 1990a; Pearson *et al.* 1990; Reynolds and Pearson 1990).

Reflecting the preferential impact of striatal medium spiny neurones in HD, decreased concentrations of the co-neurotransmitter peptides have been reported in synaptic target areas. Substance P is decreased in SN and GPi, with lesser reductions having been reported in striatum, SNc, and GPe (Kanazawa *et al.* 1977, 1979, 1985; Gale *et al.* 1978; Emson *et al.* 1980; Buck *et al.* 1981; Kowall *et al.* 1993). Reduction of substance P has also been reported in HD spinal cord (Vacca 1983; Vacca-Galloway 1985). Enkephalin, contained in the GABAergic medium spiny neurones that project to GPe, is decreased in HD patients (Emson *et al.* 1980). Decreases in mRNA for substance P and enkephalin have been detected in early grade HD, indicating that dysfunction of medium spiny neurones is an early event in the pathogenesis of HD, while providing a clue to the mechanism of such transmitter decreases (Augood *et al.* 1996).

By comparing relative levels of substance P and enkephalin, one can assess the relative impact of the disease on the direct and indirect pathways, respectively. Striatal cells projecting to GPe degenerate before striatal cells projecting to GPi, as evidenced by the relative preservation of substance P immunostaining in GPi compared to enkephalin immunostaining in GPe (Reiner *et al.* 1988; Albin *et al.* 1990b; Sapp *et al.* 1995). In one case of a presymptomatic HD person, there was preferential loss of striato-external pallidal projection neurones, suggesting that loss of peptide co-transmitters occurs early, and that the indirect pathway is affected before the direct pathway (Reiner *et al.* 1988; Albin *et al.* 1992; Richfield *et al.* 1995). Another presymptomatic HD patient demonstrated decreased GABA in the striatum and the GPe, but not in the GPi (Reynolds and Pearson 1990). Loss of indirect pathway striato-external pallidal neurones would be predicted to result in a relative excess in involuntary movements, whereas loss of direct pathway striatonigral and striato-internal pallidal neurones would tend to produce bradykinesia (Albin *et al.* 1989). In juvenile-onset HD, characterized instead by a bradykinetic-rigid phenotype and relative absence of chorea, enkephalin and substance P are lost in parallel, suggesting simultaneous degeneration of both the direct and indirect pathways. Similarly, in late-stage HD, also characterized by bradykinesia and absence of chorea, there is massive degeneration of both the direct and indirect pathways (Reiner *et al.* 1988).

In contrast to those neuropeptides that are contained by striatal projection neurones, the levels of peptides contained by striatal interneurones are unchanged or increased in HD, reflecting the relative preservation of interneurone populations (Beal and Martin 1986). Medium aspiny reduced nicotinamide–adenine dinucleotide phosphate (NADPH)-diaphorase-positive, neuronal nitric oxide synthase (nNOS)-positive neurones are relatively spared in HD striatum, as are large aspiny cholinergic interneurones, although to a lesser extent (Ferrante *et al.* 1985, 1987b). Peptides that are increased in concentration in the striatum include somatostatin (Aronin *et al.* 1983; Nemeroff *et al.* 1983; Beal *et al.* 1985, 1986a; Dawbarn *et al.* 1985). As neuropeptide Y and NADPH-diaphorase are co-localized within somatostatin neurones, it is no surprise that these markers are also increased (Dawbarn *et al.* 1985; Ferrante *et al.* 1985). NADPH-diaphorase is the same enzyme as nNOS, an enzyme that generates the gaseous neurotransmitter nitric oxide (NO) upon *N*-methyl-D-aspartate (NMDA) receptor stimulation (Dawson and Dawson 1996). One explanation for the relative preservation of nNOS/NADPH-diaphorase-positive striatal interneurones in HD is that these neurones, upon stimulation by glutamatergic corticostriatal afferents, generate NO, which itself can generate harmful free radicals, thereby killing nearby susceptible projection neurones. Medium aspiny striatal neurones containing calretinin and expressing tachykinin receptors also appear to be relatively spared (Cicchetti *et al.* 1996).

Striatal levels of neurotensin (Nemeroff *et al.* 1983) and thyrotrophin-releasing hormone (Spindel *et al.* 1980; Nemeroff *et al.* 1983) are increased in HD, reflecting their presence on striatal afferents that are largely unaffected in the disease. However, neurotensin receptor levels are not altered (Palacios *et al.* 1991). Cholecystokinin (CCK) receptors have been reported to be decreased in HD brain (Hays *et al.* 1981).

Binding sites for opioid peptides have been found to be decreased in living HD subjects as assessed by PET scanning using [^{11}C]diprenorphine (Weeks *et al.* 1997). Numerous peptides have been found to be unchanged in HD brain, including vasoactive intestinal peptide (VIP) and somatostatin (Arregui *et al.* 1979).

Acetylcholine

Another class of striatal neurones that are relatively spared are the large aspiny neurones that contain acetylcholine (ACh) (Ferrante *et al.* 1987a; Kawaguchi *et al.* 1995). Despite this observation, sparing is relative, as decreases in the acetylcholine synthetic enzyme choline acetyltransferase (ChAT) have been reported in HD striatum, as well as in the nucleus accumbens, the septal nuclei, and hippocampus (Spokes 1980; Ferrante *et al.* 1987a). Muscarinic ACh receptors are decreased in striatum and GPe (Hiley and Bird 1974; Enna *et al.* 1976; Wastek *et al.* 1976), while unchanged in SNr and cortex (Wastek and Yamamura 1978). Among the muscarinic receptors, M2 receptors appear to be decreased to a greater extent than M1 receptors (Joyce *et al.* 1988).

Decreased levels of choline have been found in cerebrospinal fluid samples from HD patients, although, in the same study, the activity of the catabolic enzyme for ACh, acetyl-cholinesterase (AChE), was normal (Manyam *et al.* 1990).

Dopamine

Experiments in the 1970s hinted at dopaminergic abnormalities in HD patients, suggested by altered prolactin or growth hormone responses to dopamine receptor agents (Caraceni *et al.* 1977; Hayden *et al.* 1977; Chalmers *et al.* 1978; Muller *et al.* 1979; Durso *et al.* 1983). Subsequently, a number of investigators have sought to determine dopamine levels in HD brain. Reflecting a preservation of the substantia nigra pars compacta (SNc) combined with tissue atrophy, dopamine levels are unchanged or increased in striatum, nucleus accumbens, and SNc in HD brain (Spokes 1980; Reynolds and Garrett 1986). Kish *et al.* (1987) have reported that there is a regionally specific decrease in dopamine in the caudal subdivision of the caudate nucleus, suggesting pathology within the SNc, the source of dopaminergic afferents to the striatum. While some workers have reported normal levels of the dopamine synthetic enzyme tyrosine hydroxylase (TH) (McGeer and McGeer 1976b; Bird and Iversen 1977), Ferrante and Kowall (1987) have suggested the presence of subtle pathology of the nigrostriatal dopaminergic system. The striatum has been divided into two functional compartments, known as 'striosome' or 'patch' and 'matrix' (Graybiel 1990). In both normal and HD human brain, TH immunoreactivity is enriched in the matrix compartment (Ferrante and Kowall 1987). In HD brain, although there is atrophy of the striatum, there is no change in the density of neuropil fibres that are immunopositive for TH. These authors interpret the result to mean that there has been proportional decrease of TH-positive fibres, in effect 'keeping pace' with the striatal atrophy.

In contrast to measures of dopamine, dopamine receptors are consistently decreased in HD striatum, reflecting their localization on the medium spiny striatal neurones that are preferentially affected (Reisine *et al.* 1977, 1978). Conventional wisdom holds that striatal neurones projecting to the lateral pallidum have D2-type dopamine receptors, whereas striatonigral and striatal neurones projecting to the medial pallidum contain primarily D1-type receptors (Albin *et al.* 1989). Thus, one can assess the health of different populations of medium spiny striatal neurones by separately analysing the D1 and D2 receptor populations. By comparing patterns of striatal loss of D1 or D2 receptors, various authors have concluded: (1) that the D2-containing striato-external pallidal neurones are affected before the striatonigral neurones (Augood *et al.* 1997); (2) that the striatonigral neurones are affected before the striato-external pallidal neurones (Joyce *et al.* 1988; Richfield *et al.* 1991); or (3) that these cell populations are affected in parallel (Cross and Rossor 1983; Weeks *et al.* 1996). One explanation that may resolve these apparently conflicting findings is that the segregation of D1 and D2 dopamine receptors on separate populations of striatal cells is not as strict as had been previously believed (Surmeier *et al.* 1993). One consistent feature found by multiple authors is that the pattern of dopamine receptor loss is patchy in the human striatum, with certain striatal subregions affected and others spared (Richfield *et al.* 1991). These areas of dopamine receptor loss do not correspond to the striatal striosome/patch organization as defined by AChE-defined immunohistochemistry. Again, this heterogeneous pattern of dopamine receptor loss hints at selective neuronal susceptibility to degeneration in HD.

Dopamine receptors are also decreased in target areas of striatal projection neurones. For instance, D1 receptors are decreased in substantia nigra (Filloux *et al.* 1990) as well as the GPe (Reisine *et al.* 1978). Abnormalities of dopaminergic function may not be limited to simple loss of receptor numbers. Seeman *et al.* (1989) have documented a decrease in HD striatum in the normal functional interaction between D1 and D2 receptors.

Dopamine receptors have also been studied in living human subjects with HD (Brandt *et al.* 1990; Brucke *et al.* 1991). For example, [^{123}I]epidepride or [^{123}I]iodobenzamide ([^{123}I]IBZM) single-photon emission tomography has been used to assess D2 dopamine receptors *in vivo* (Leslie *et al.* 1996, 1999; Pirker *et al.* 1997; Staffen *et al.* 1997; see also Chapter 4, this volume). In addition, non-invasive imaging methods have been used to assess dopamine receptors in presymptomatic HD gene positive patients (Ichise *et al.* 1993; Antonini *et al.* 1996; Andrews *et al.* 1999). Even asymptomatic HD mutation carriers were found to have decreased D1 and D2 receptor activities, and these abnormalities correlated with subtle deficits seen in cognitive testing (Backman *et al.* 1997; Lawrence *et al.* 1998). These findings parallel the result of Augood *et al.* (1997) who found decreases of D1 and D2 receptor mRNA in the striatum of human HD patients, even in early-stage HD (Vonsattel grade 0 or grade 1). Thus, decrease in dopamine receptors, both at the mRNA and protein levels, appears to be a reliable and early event in HD pathogenesis. Indeed, serial PET scanning has been proposed as a method to follow onset and progression of disease in human HD patients (Antonini *et al.* 1998; Andrews *et al.* 1999).

Dopamine uptake sites have been reported as unchanged in human HD striatum (Leenders *et al.* 1986; Joyce *et al.* 1988; Mizukawa *et al.* 1993), although studies using the ligand [^{123}I]beta-carbomethoxy-3 beta-(4-iodophenyltropane) ([^{123}I] βCIT) have found decreases in uptake (Ginovart *et al.* 1997; Staffen *et al.* 1997). There is a deficit in the vesicular monoamine transporter type-2 (VMAT2) system, indicative of nigrostriatal pathology in HD subjects (Bohnen *et al.* 2000). Deficits in VMAT2 were most pronounced in the posterior putamen, and more affected in patients with the rigid phenotype of HD compared to those patients with chorea-predominant phenotype.

The overall problem may be a relative excess of dopamine, as therapeutic benefit for chorea has been reported with the dopamine-depleting compound tetrabenazine (Jankovic and Beach 1997). In a similar vein, EMD 23,448, a compound that acts presynaptically to decrease dopamine release, has been reported to have antichoreic effects in a few HD patients (Newman *et al.* 1985). Bromocriptine, a D2 dopamine receptor agonist, has been reported to worsen chorea (Kartzinel *et al.* 1976). Dopamine has also been postulated to play a toxic role in HD, with an excess of dopamine potentially producing neurotoxicity (Jakel and Maragos 2000).

Glutamate

Because the essential amino acid glutamate and some of its analogues are neurotoxic, it has long been proposed that abnormalities of glutamatergic function may play a causal role in neurodegenerative disorders such as HD (DiFiglia 1990). In particular, the pattern of selective neuronal vulnerability seen in HD has implicated NMDA-receptor-mediated toxicity (see the section, 'Animal models'). For example, reminiscent of the pattern seen in human HD, cultured striatal neurones containing NADPH-diaphorase are relatively resistant to NMDA toxicity *in vitro* (Koh and Choi 1988). Blockade of NMDA receptors provides the scientific rationale for a clinical trial in human HD patients (Kieburtz *et al.* 1996).

In 1981, London *et al.* demonstrated reduced [^{3}H]kainic acid binding in HD brain homogenates. Using a quantitative autoradiographic binding technique, [^{3}H]glutamate binding was found to be decreased in HD striatum but relatively preserved in cortex and nucleus basalis of Meynert (Greenamyre *et al.* 1985). One study found no change in NMDA receptors in HD frontal cortex, but did find a decrease in kainate and α-amino-3-hydroxy-5-methyl-4-isoxazolepropionic acid (AMPA) receptors (Wagster *et al.* 1994). Decreased binding to the glycine site associated with the NMDA receptor has also been found (Reynolds *et al.* 1994). Although some studies have suggested the existence of a relatively selective decrease in NMDA receptors (Young *et al.* 1988), other studies have concluded that all subtypes of glutamate receptors are decreased to an equal extent (Dure *et al.* 1991). Altered mRNA expression levels of the NR1 and NR2B subunits of the NMDA receptor have been found in human HD brain, suggesting that the alteration in NMDA receptors in HD brain may not simply be one of abundance, but one of altered subunit stoichiometry (Arzberger *et al.* 1997).

Serotonin

One class of medications that is frequently used in HD patients comprises the antidepressants, which act as inhibitors of serotonin uptake. Alterations in the serotonin system have been documented in HD, including increases in levels of serotonin (5-hydroxytryptamine, 5-HT) and its metabolite 5-hydroxyindoleacetic acid (5-HIAA) in HD cortex and striatum, but not in hippocampus (Reynolds and Pearson 1987). Other authors have reported elevated 5-HT levels in HD striatum (Kish *et al.* 1987). Serotonin receptors have been reported as decreased in HD basal ganglia, including 5-HT_{1B} (Castro *et al.* 1998), 5-HT_{1D} (Waeber and Palacios 1989), 5-HT_3 (Steward *et al.* 1993), and 5-HT_4 binding sites (Wong *et al.* 1996). Interestingly, activated astrocytes found in HD striatum can express increased levels of 5-HT_{2A} receptors, suggestive of a reactive astrocytic response to injury (Wu *et al.* 1999).

Noradrenaline (also called norepinephrine)

Noradrenaline concentrations were found to be increased in HD caudate nucleus, lateral pallidum, and pars reticulata of the substantia nigra, indicating preservation of central noradrenaline pathways (Spokes 1980). Although there was no difference in the density of $\beta 1$ and $\beta 2$ adrenergic receptors in the basal ganglia of grade 2 HD patients, a nearly complete loss of $\beta 1$ binding sites was observed in the basal ganglia of HD patients at later stages of the disease (Waeber *et al.* 1991). The concentration of $\beta 2$ receptors was increased in the posterior putamen of all choreic cases.

Cannabinoids

The distribution of cannabinoid receptors in the human brain holds special relevance for HD; cannibinoid receptors are especially concentrated in the outflow target areas of the basal ganglia (Herkenham *et al.* 1990). Indeed, it is in these outflow areas that cannabinoid receptors are found to be decreased, that is, in the SN, GPe, and GPi (Glass *et al.* 1993; Richfield and Herkenham 1994). The pattern of cannibinoid receptor loss is suggestive of selective neuronal vulnerability in that loss of cannabinoid receptors is more pronounced in the striato-lateral pallidal pathway compared to the striato-medial pallidal pathway (Richfield and Herkenham 1994). The fact that terminal areas (GPe and GPi) are affected to a greater degree than the area in which the cell bodies are located (putamen) suggests that loss of cannabinoid receptors is not simply reflective of cell death, but more probably represents a type of neuronal dysfunction that preferentially affects the distal cellular processes prior to affecting the cell somata (Richfield and Herkenham 1994).

Other neurotransmitter receptors

Decreases in numerous neurotransmitter receptors, including histamine H2 receptors (Martinez-Mir *et al*. 1993), histamine H3 receptors (Goodchild *et al*. 1999), and imidazoline I2 receptors (Reynolds *et al*. 1996), have been reported in human HD brain. There is no change in insulin-like growth factor-1 (IGF-1) in HD frontal cortex and white matter (De Keyser *et al*. 1994).

Second messenger systems

Abnormalities in HD brain have been reported not only for neurotransmitters, but also in associated effector systems. There is evidence of alteration of the inositol phosphate second messenger system (Warsh *et al*. 1991; Tanaka *et al*. 1993). Tanaka *et al*. found decreased binding sites for [^{3}H]inositol triphosphate, as well as for [^{3}H]-4-beta-phorbol 12,13-dibutyrate ([^{3}H]-PDBu), an agent that binds to protein kinase C (PKC). Using immunoquantification methods, they investigated four isoforms of PKC and found a specific decrease in the PKC-βII isoform, an isoform of PKC that is particularly enriched in striatal GABAergic projection neurones (Hashimoto *et al*. 1992).

Other molecules

Several other neurochemical markers have been described as being decreased in post-mortem human HD brain, including the neuronal proteins PEP-19 (Utal *et al*. 1998) and connexin II (Vis *et al*. 1998). Decreases of brain gangliosides (Bernheimer *et al*. 1979) and ornithine aminotransferase activity have been reported (Wong *et al*. 1982). L-type calcium channels have been found to be decreased in HD brains but not in Alzheimer's disease or parkinsonism brains (Sen *et al*. 1993). In addition, adenosine triphosphate (ATP)-sensitive potassium channels have been reported to be mildly decreased in HD brain (Holemans *et al*. 1994). The glucose transporter isoforms GLUT1 and GLUT3 are decreased in late stage (Vonsattel grade 3) HD brain but unchanged in grade 1 brain (Gamberino and Brennan 1994). Angiotensin-converting enzyme (ACE) activity has been found to be decreased in HD SN, GPe, and GPi (Arregui *et al*. 1979).

Animal models

While numerous neurochemical alterations have been described in post-mortem human HD brain (summarized in Table 9.1), there are many difficulties inherent in the interpretation of the data. The significance of neurochemical changes is confounded by the cerebral atrophy that occurs in HD. Furthermore, examination of human post-mortem material has been limited largely to end-stage changes; there are only isolated reports of analyses of early-stage or presymptomatic human HD material. Thus, early changes in neurochemistry have been difficult to capture.

Animal models have provided valuable insights into potential pathogenic mechanisms underlying HD. The first set of relevant HD models were *lesion models* in which excitotoxins were injected into the striatum of primates and rodents, re-creating some of the pathological and neurochemical features of human HD. Lesion models have bolstered arguments for two theories of HD pathogenesis, namely, glutamate excitotoxicity and mitochondrial dysfunction.

Table 9.1 Neurochemical changes in human HD brain*

Component	Str	GPe	GPi	SN	Ctx	Other	References
GABA							
GABA content	↓				↓	↓ hippocampus	Perry et al. 1973; Bird and Iversen 1974; Reynolds and Pearson 1987
GABA receptors	↓	↑	↑		=	↓ thalamus	Enna et al. 1976; Lloyd et al. 1977; Reisine et al. 1979b; Penney and Young 1982; Greenamyre et al. 1985; Young et al. 1988
GAD	↓	↓					Spokes 1980
Peptide							
Enkephalin mRNA	↓	↓					Albin et al. 1991; Augood et al. 1996
Enkephalin peptides	↓	↓	↓	↓, =			Arregui et al. 1979; Emson et al. 1980; Seizinger et al. 1986, Albin et al. 1991, 1992; Weeks et al. 1997
Opiate receptors	↓	↓					Kanazawa et al. 1979; Emson et al. 1980; Buck et al. 1981; Augood et al. 1996
Substance P mRNA	↓	↓	↓	↓			Kowall et al. 1993
Substance P peptide	↓	↓					
Dynorphin	↓	↑	=				Seizinger et al. 1986
IGF-1 receptors	=	=	=				De Keyser et al. 1994
Neurotensin receptors	↓	=			=		Palacios et al. 1991
Somatostatin peptide	↑	=					Arregui et al. 1979
Angiotensin AT1 receptors	↓						Ge and Barnes 1996
Angiotensin AT2 receptors	↑						Ge and Barnes 1996
Cholecytokinin receptors	↓				↓		Hays et al. 1981
Acetylcholine							
Choline acetyltransferase	↓					↓ nucleus accumbens, septum	Spokes 1980
Muscarinic receptors	↓			=			Enna et al. 1976; Wastek et al. 1976; Joyce et al. 1988
Dopamine							
D1 receptor	↓			↓			Reisine et al. 1978; Cross and Rossor 1983; Joyce et al. 1988; Richfield et al. 1991; Backman et al. 1997; Ginovart et al. 1997
D2 receptor	↓	↓					Reisine et al. 1978; Leenders et al. 1986; Hagglund et al. 1987; Seeman et al. 1987; Joyce et al. 1988; Richfield et al. 1991; Brucke et al. 1993; Backman et al. 1997; Ginovart et al. 1997; Staffen et al. 1997

Measure	Change	Other regions	References
Dopamine content	↑, ↓, = ↑	↑ nucleus accumbens	Spokes 1980; Reynolds and Garrett 1986; Kish et al. 1987
Tyrosine hydroxylase	↑, =		McGeer and McGeer 1976; Bird and Iversen 1977; Ferrante and Kowall 1987
Uptake	=, →		Leenders et al. 1986; Joyce et al. 1988; Mizukawa et al. 1993; Ginovart et al. 1997; Staffen et al. 1997
Glutamate			
AMPA	→	=, →	Dure et al. 1991; Wagster et al. 1994
Glutamate receptors	→	=	Greenamyre et al. 1985
Glycine modulatory site	→		Reynolds et al. 1994
Kainate receptors	→	↓ whole brain	Beaumont et al. 1979; London et al. 1981; Wagster et al. 1994
Metabotropic receptors	→	=	Dure et al. 1991
NMDA receptors	→	=	Young et al. 1988; Albin et al. 1990b; Dure et al. 1991; Wagster et al. 1994; Cross et al. 1986
Uptake	→		Reynolds and Pearson 1987
Serotonin			
5-HT content	↑		Reynolds and Pearson 1987
5-HIAA metabolite	↑		Castro et al. 1998
5-HT1B receptors	→		Waeber and Palacios 1989
5-HT1D receptors	→		Steward et al. 1993
5-HT3 receptors	→		Wong et al. 1996
5-HT4 receptors	→		
Noradrenaline (also called norepinephrine)			
Noradrenaline content	↑		Spokes 1980
β1 receptors	↑		Waeber et al. 1991
β2 receptors	↑		Waeber et al. 1991
Cannabinoid			
CB1 receptors	→		Glass et al. 1993; Richfield and Herkenham 1994
Histamine			
H2 receptors	→	↓ nucleus accumbens	Martinez-Mir et al. 1993
H3 receptors	→		Goodchild et al. 1999
Imidazoline			
I2 receptors	→	=	Reynolds et al. 1996

*Str, striatum; GPe, globus pallidus, external segment; GPi, globus pallidus, internal segment; SN, substantia nigra; Ctx, cortex; ↑, increased; =, unchanged; ↓, decreased.

With the discovery of the *HD* gene in 1993, the development of *genetic models* of HD became possible (see Chapter 13). Genetic models, in particular, offer a temporal window into the process of neurochemical alteration in HD. That is, using genetic animal models, one is now able to discern early-stage neurochemical alterations that are unlikely to be confounded by the issue of neuronal loss. Fortuitously, many of the neurochemical alterations that had been previously described in post-mortem human HD brain have been confirmed in transgenic mouse models of HD, lending further credence to the notion that such changes are not merely artefactual, but rather of fundamental importance.

Lesion models

Rodents

A number of analogues of the neurotransmitter amino acid glutamate have been used to create lesions in rodent models. Over the past 25 years, these experiments have supported the viewpoint that the pathological damage that occurs in HD could be the result of overactivity of glutamate neurotransmission, a process termed *excitotoxicity*. Striatal injection of glutamate analogues provided the first approximate replication of neuropathological damage that occurs in HD. Later, mitochondrial toxins, either directly injected into the striatum or systemically administered, were also found to replicate the pattern of neuronal damage found in the HD striatum.

The first animal models for HD were reported in 1976 (Coyle and Schwarcz 1976; McGeer and McGeer 1976a). Independently, Coyle and Schwarcz and the McGeers found that stereotaxic kainic acid (KA) injections into the striatum of rats caused a selective neuronal degeneration reminiscent of HD in that projection neurones were destroyed to a greater degree than interneurones. KA is a potent neuroexcitant that is present in some species of seaweed and is structurally related to glutamic acid. Injection of KA resulted in decreased GAD and ChAT activities 48 hours post-injection (Coyle and Schwarcz 1976; McGeer and McGeer 1976a). TH activity was increased in KA-lesioned rats. TH is the rate-limiting enzyme in the biosynthesis of the catecholamines dopamine, adrenaline, and noradrenaline. KA injection caused immediate diarrhoea and cessation of all grooming behaviour in these rats and, within 3 days, severe bleeding in the nose and urinary tract was observed (McGeer and McGeer 1976a). These abnormal physiological responses may have contributed to the significant increase in TH activity, since stress is a known positive regulator of TH activity. However, a more likely explanation is that destruction of striatal projection neurones, which normally serve to inhibit the activity of the substantia nigra, results in disinhibition of substantia nigra neurones, thereby increasing TH activity (Albin *et al.* 1989). These lesions replicated the earlier post-mortem HD findings of selective degradation of the GABAergic and cholinergic systems of the striatum, with relative sparing of the afferent dopaminergic system. Finally, the KA-lesioned rat first suggested that abnormal glutamate neurotransmission may play a role in the aetiology of HD and other neurodegenerative disorders.

Similarly, striatal injection of another glutamate analogue, ibotenic acid (IA), into the striatum resulted in a significant reduction in GAD and ChAT activity (Isacson *et al.* 1985). IA injections also produced a slow decline in dopamine content, different from that seen in KA-lesioned rats. IA is an agonist at both NMDA-type glutamate receptors as well as metabotropic glutamate receptors (Monaghan *et al.* 1989). Recent evidence suggests that striatal toxicity depends on simultaneous stimulation of NMDA and metabotropic glutamate receptors (Beal *et al.* 1993b; Orlando *et al.* 1995; Calabresi *et al.* 1999). Thus, IA may produce a different type of lesion by virtue of its agonist activity at both NMDA and metabotropic receptors.

A more faithful replication of HD pathology was produced by Schwarcz and colleagues (1983), who demonstrated that striatal injections of the selective NMDA receptor agonist quinolinic acid (QA) produced an HD-like phenotype in rats. QA is a metabolite of the amino acid tryptophan and is a known convulsant and cortical neurone excitant. Thus, in contrast to exogenously administered KA or IA, QA is an endogenous molecule with neurotoxic potential. QA-induced lesions resulted in a depletion of the neurotransmitters contained within striatal spiny neurones (GABA), while dopamine levels were unaffected. QA recreates the neuropathology of HD better than other glutamate analogues, in that QA causes marked depletion of GABA and substance P, while NADPH-diaphorase/nNOS/somatostatin/neuropeptide-Y-positive neurones are relatively spared (Beal and Martin 1986). Lesions caused by KA, IA, or NMDA lesions affect all striatal cell types without selective sparing of the NADPH-diaphorase/nNOS/somatostatin/neuropeptide-Y-positive neurones (Beal *et al.* 1986b). Although there does appear to be some selectivity of QA lesions, this selectivity is only relative: in the centre of the lesion area, all neurones degenerate. Other researchers have not been able to replicate the cellular specificity of the QA striatal lesion (Davies and Roberts 1987). Of interest is the disparity between the profile of QA and NMDA. QA is an agonist at NMDA receptors, and thus would be expected to have the same effect as NMDA. However, recent evidence suggests the presence of multiple types of NMDA receptors with differing affinities for agonists and antagonists (Monaghan *et al.* 1988). One possibility is that QA activates a specific subset of NMDA receptor that is especially present on susceptible projection neurones. Indeed, recent work suggests that striatal cell populations have distinct types of NMDA receptors (Calabresi *et al.* 1998; Standaert *et al.* 1999).

Homocysteic acid (L-HCA), is a sulfated amino acid that is also present in mammalian striatum and, similarly to QA, is able to produce HD-like striatal lesions (Beal *et al.* 1990). L-HCA, when injected into rat striatum, decreased levels of substance P, enkephalin, and GABA, while relatively sparing NOS/somatostatin/neuropeptide-Y-positive neurones. Similarly to what is seen with QA, L-HCA lesions are blocked by MK-801, an antagonist of NMDA receptors, indicating that L-HCA is acting at NMDA receptors.

In addition, receptor antagonists have recently been used and found to be efficacious in the treatment of some HD symptoms in the QA-lesioned rats. Blockade of presynaptic inhibitory α2-adrenergic autoreceptors facilitates noradrenaline release. The α2-adrenoceptor antagonists, (+)-efaroxan and (+/−)-idazoxan, were evaluated in QA-lesioned rats (Martel *et al.* 1998). Both antagonists reduced the circling response to apomorphine and reduced the ChAT deficit in the lesioned striatum. These results suggest that α2-adrenoceptor antagonists may be beneficial in neurodegenerative disorders where excitotoxicity has been implicated.

In addition to glutamate receptor agonists, mitochondrial inhibitors can also replicate certain features of HD. A number of these toxins, such as aminooxyacetic acid (AOAA), 3-nitropropionic acid (3-NP), malonate, and azide have been administered to rats to investigate neurochemical changes in HD. Local or systemic injections of these compounds cause secondary excitotoxic lesions by selectively inhibiting the mitochondrial respiratory chain. All of these compounds generate an increase in striatal lactate levels (Beal *et al.* 1991b; Jenkins *et al.* 1996). The toxicity mediated by these compounds is due, at least in part, to glutamatergic transmission. Blockade of glutamate receptors with the selective antagonist MK-801 reduced lesion size as well as lactate levels. However, lesion size and lactate levels were also diminished by energy repletion with ubiquinone and nicotinamide, indicating that mitochondrial (energy) involvement and dysfunction are important in HD and other neurodegenerative diseases (Jenkins *et al.* 1996). Overall, glutamate receptor antagonists and other agents that improve energy metabolism can prevent striatal degeneration (Albin and Greenamyre 1992; Ikonomidou and Turski 1996).

Damage induced by the reversible inhibitor of succinate dehydrogenase (complex II of the mitochondrial electron transport chain), malonate, and the irreversible inhibitor, 3-NP, closely resembles the histological, neurochemical, and clinical features of HD in both rats and non-human primates. These compounds disrupt oxidative phosphorylation resulting in decreased levels of ATP. Low intracellular ATP levels cause a cellular depolarization and a secondary activation of the voltage-dependent NMDA receptors. Activation of the NMDA receptors causes a cycle of deleterious events including increasing calcium entry. Increased intracellular calcium levels cause an activation of calcium-dependent enzymes, such as nNOS. nNOS produces NO, which can react to form dangerous free-radicals and the nitrating agent, peroxynitrite, both of which could exacerbate the damage already caused by inhibiting the electron transport chain (Schulz *et al.* 1997; see also Chapter 10).

The idea of energy metabolism as a possible pathological mechanism in HD was further supported when it was shown that mutant huntingtin can bind to the glycolytic enzyme glyceraldehyde-3-phosphate dehydrogenase (GAPDH) (Burke *et al.* 1996). This interaction appears to inhibit GAPDH activity in HD (Mazzola and Sirover 2001). Intrastriatal administration of the GAPDH inhibitor, iodoacetate, produces striatal lesions in rats and suggests that the inhibition of GAPDH could contribute to neuronal degeneration in HD (Matthews *et al.* 1997).

Systemic administration of the mitochondrial toxin 3-NP to rats also results in selective striatal lesions and serves as an additional experimental model of HD (Beal *et al.* 1993a; Vis *et al.* 1999). 3-NP lesion experiments add credence to the idea that the striatal lesion in HD results from a systemic excitotoxic insult. Whereas other agents such as KA or QA need to be directly injected into the striatum in order to produce pathology, 3-NP produces lesions that are most notable within the striatum, even following systemic administration, thus providing proof of the principle that a diffuse metabolic insult could produce strikingly focal pathological damage. However, 3-NP affects markers for both the spiny and aspiny striatal population. It was recently determined that administration of 3-NP, followed by acute methamphetamine exposure, increased the frequency of striatal lesions in rats (Reynolds *et al.* 1998). This effect was blocked by the administration of dopamine receptor antagonists, suggesting that dopamine may play an important role in the formation of striatal lesions in HD. Therefore, the modulation of dopamine neurotransmission may also aid in the treatment of HD.

Analyses of the numerous rat lesion models of HD suggest that the chronic QA lesions most closely resemble the neurochemical features of HD. These findings imply that an NMDA receptor-mediated excitotoxic process is playing a role in the pathogenesis of HD (Beal *et al.* 1991a). Further adaptation of the rodent models of HD to the non-human primate has also allowed investigators to examine lesion-induced motor dysfunction more comparable to that in human HD (DiFiglia 1990).

Primates

It has been well documented that excess glutamate in the corticostriatal afferents (inputs) results in neuronal cell death (Choi and Rothman 1990; DiFiglia 1990; Bittigau and Ikonomidou 1997). Both unilateral and bilateral injections of excitatory amino acids produce neuropathology and a phenotype in primates similar to that of humans with HD. Expansion of the HD models to include primates is critical from an obvious evolutionary standpoint. In addition, primate models permit a better glimpse into the early pathogenic events in HD, a major limitation of human post-mortem studies.

The monkey striatum is anatomically more similar to the human striatum, thus providing one advantage over rodent models. Lesion models, in which monkeys receive intrastriatal excitotoxin injection, have been used to study chorea. Kanazawa *et al.* (1986, 1993) reproduced choreic movements in the monkey by creating a striatal kainic acid lesion followed by the administration of L-dihydroxyphenylalanine (L-dopa). These authors observed increased TH activity in the unlesioned striatum and increased 2-deoxyglucose (2DG) uptake at the presynaptic dopaminergic nerve terminals in and around the lesioned area. The authors propose that the mechanism of choreic movements is the presynaptic activation of the nigrostriatal dopaminergic pathways in the putamen, rather than postsynaptic receptor activation.

IA, a glutamate receptor agonist, has also been injected unilaterally into the baboon caudate–putamen to achieve a neural degeneration model in the primate (Isacson *et al.* 1989). Such treatment has also succeeded in producing neuropathology similar to that found in HD. This model replicates the findings found in the rat and has been used to test neural transplantation as a means of treating the striatal degeneration of HD. This model was used to determine if positive effects could be achieved in these baboons following rat striatal cell replacement. Neurochemical markers for AChE and the opiate Leu-enkephalin, which are normally found in the caudate–putamen, were distributed in an appropriate patchy manner in the striatal implants, although there was no phenotypic improvement.

The functional status of the dopaminergic system of this baboon model of HD was investigated with PET using 6-[^{18}F]fluoro-L-dopa as specific tracer for the presynaptic dopaminergic terminals and [^{76}Br]bromolisuride as selective dopamine D2 receptor marker. *In vivo* PET studies performed 3 to 6 months after the IA injections revealed a dose-dependent reduction in D2 binding sites in the lesioned striatum of all IA-injected animals. Re-uptake into the presynaptic terminal of the HD baboons was also decreased, suggesting a possible loss of nigral dopamine cell function in HD (Hantraye *et al.* 1992).

Another primate model of HD was generated with unilateral injections of QA into the caudate nucleus and putamen of rhesus monkeys. It has been demonstrated that 3-hydroxyanthranilic acid oxidase, the synthetic enzyme for QA, is increased in HD brain (Schwarcz *et al.* 1988). As seen in human studies, the medium-sized spiny neurones containing calbindin D28k, enkephalin, and substance P were lost, while aspiny neuronal subpopulations containing NADPH diaphorase (NADPH-d) and ChAT activity were spared. QA-lesioned monkeys exhibited losses of GABA and substance P-like immunoreactivity, while no significant decreases in somatostatin-like immunoreactivity or neuropeptide Y-like immunoreactivity were seen. MK-801, a noncompetitive NMDA antagonist, blocked striatal QA neurotoxicity in these animals. Overall, these QA lesion monkeys display overall neuropathology similar to that of human HD and strengthen the possibility that the pathogenesis of HD involves an NMDA-receptor-mediated excitotoxic process (Ferrante *et al.* 1993).

Mitochondrial dysfunction has also been postulated to play a role in the pathogenesis of HD (see Chapter 10). Malonate, the reversible inhibitor of succinate dehydrogenase (complex II of the electron transport chain), and the irreversible inhibitor, 3-NP, produce dyskinesia and pathology in baboons similar to that in HD (Palfi *et al.* 1996). Both agents closely parallel the histological, neurochemical, and clinical features of HD in both rats and non-human primates

(Schulz *et al.* 1997). 3-NP caused selective caudate–putamen lesions, cognitive decline, and spontaneous abnormal movements. These results add to the growing notion of dysfunctional energy metabolism in HD. In an independent study, malonate and 3-NP produced striatal lesions in primates (Brouillet *et al.* 1999). The inhibition of the electron transport chain leads to decreases in ATP formation and activation of the voltage-dependent NMDA receptors. The latter results in an increase in intracellular calcium concentration, which may trigger excitotoxicity and thus actually exacerbate the clinical manifestations of HD. Extensive neuropathological evaluations of rodents and non-human primates following chronic blockade of succinate oxidation with systemic administration of 3-NP showed that a partial, yet prolonged energy impairment resulting from 3-NP is sufficient to replicate most of the clinical and pathophysiological hallmarks of HD. 3-NP preferentially affected the medium-sized spiny GABAergic neurones while sparing the interneurones and afferents, as was observed in HD striatum. It has been argued that any impairment of neuronal energy metabolism would render susceptible neurones vulnerable to glutamate-mediated excitoxicity, the so-called 'weak excitotoxic hypothesis' (Albin and Greenamyre 1992).

Pharmacological administration of several other compounds has also been found to generate an HD-like phenotype. The effects of these compounds further emphasize the importance of basal ganglia connectional circuitry. For example, injection of the GABA antagonist, bicuculline, into the GPe produces an HD-like phenotype (Crossman *et al.* 1988). Injection of this type of agent does not generate a lesion, unlike the glutamate analogues. The mode of action of bicuculline is suggested to be interruption of GABAergic transmission from the striatum to GPe. Since this alteration occurs in HD, the authors propose that the experimental chorea induced with bicuculline in the monkey is a useful model of the dyskinesia seen in human HD.

Use of the selective dopamine receptor antagonists, SCH 39166 (D1-selective) and raclopride (D2-selective), produced dose-dependent slowing of reaction time performance in rhesus monkeys (Weed and Gold 1998). The authors suggested that the effect of blockade, of either D1-like or D2-like dopamine receptors, on reaction time performance in rhesus monkeys may serve as a useful paradigm to study movement dysfunction in non-human primates. It has been hypothesized that error in feedback control may be one of the earliest detectable signs of HD in humans (Smith *et al.* 2000). Additional neurochemical analysis of the pharmacological primate models remains to be accomplished, yet is pivotal to confirm the appropriateness of these models for studying HD.

While the use of injections of receptor agonist or antagonist agents may provide some insight into the genesis of phenotypic symptoms of HD, these experiments are unlikely to yield further insight into the pathogenesis of how HD actually arises. That is, we may derive a better understanding of why a person with HD has chorea or altered reaction time by understanding the neurotransmitter systems involved. However, in order to understand *why* these neurotransmitter systems are altered in HD in the first place, genetic models hold more promise.

Genetic models of HD

Mice

Following the identification of the aberrant gene in HD in 1993 (Huntington's Disease Collaborative Research Group 1993), the field of HD research has seen rapid progress. At the forefront has been the development of a number of genetic mouse models, including transgenic mice and so-called 'knock-in' mice (Mangiarini *et al.* 1996; Reddy *et al.* 1998; Hodgson *et al.* 1999; Levine *et al.* 1999; Sathasivam *et al.* 1999; Shelbourne *et al.* 1999). The most widely reported transgenic HD mice are the R6 lines (Mangiarini *et al.* 1996; Bogdanov *et al.* 1998; Cha *et al.* 1998, 1999; Dunnett *et al.* 1998; Carter *et al.* 1999; Hansson *et al.* 1999; Hurlbert *et al.* 1999; Kosinski *et al.* 1999; Chen *et al.* 2000; Ferrante *et al.* 2000; Luthi-Carter *et al.* 2000; Murphy *et al.* 2000; van Dellen *et al.* 2000). R6 lines express exon 1 of the human HD gene, which contains a large CAG expansion (141–157 CAG), and 262 bp of intron 1, with expression driven by 1 kb of the human HD gene promoter. The CAG mutation is hypothesized to initiate a dominant gain of function; however, the exact mechanism by which CAG expansion leads to neuronal dysfunction and cell death remains unknown. These mice exhibit a progressive neurological phenotype that includes motor disturbances, as well as neuronal and cognitive deficits similar to those observed in human HD. The transgenic mouse models of HD are discussed in detail in Chapter 13. Development of these transgenic mouse models of HD creates a promise of uncovering the molecular basis of this disease, as well as a hope of developing efficacious therapies.

It was in these mice that formation of protein aggregates and nuclear inclusion bodies was observed (Davies *et al.* 1997). Loss of neurotransmitter receptors, especially glutamate and dopamine receptors, is one of the pathological hallmarks of HD. Cha *et al.* (1998) were the first to characterize the changes in these important receptor systems for the R6/2 mice using [^{3}H]glutamate receptor binding, protein immunoblotting, and *in situ* hybridization. When compared with age-matched littermate controls, symptomatic 12-week-old R6/2 mice showed decreases in certain metabotropic glutamate receptors—mGluR1, mGluR2, and mGluR3— but not in the mGluR5 subtype of G protein-linked mGluR. Ionotropic AMPA and kainate receptors were also decreased, while NMDA receptors were unchanged in the R6/2 line. It was also shown that dopamine and muscarinic cholinergic, but not GABA, receptors were significantly decreased. Interestingly, decreases in D1 binding and expression could be observed after just 4 weeks, well before the onset of behavioural and motor symptoms in these mice. These findings indicated that mouse models of HD replicated the pattern of receptor alterations that has been observed in human HD. In addition, receptor alterations were specific, in that certain receptors were altered while others were not. Finally, these receptor alterations were detectable at a timepoint when there was little neuronal death, indicating that receptor decreases were not simply a measure of cell loss.

Similar studies were performed to characterize the neurotransmitter changes in a number of different HD mouse models (Cha *et al.* 1999). Decreases in adenosine A2a, dopamine D1, and dopamine D2 receptor binding were observed in the R6/1, R6/2, and R6/5 HD mouse lines. All of these lines develop an abnormal phenotype, albeit at different time points (Mangiarini *et al.* 1996). Transgenic mice expressing exon 1 of the human HD gene with 18 CAG repeats did not show any significant changes in neurotransmitters, indicating that receptor alterations were caused by the presence of the abnormally expanded CAG repeats present in the R6 lines. Receptor binding decreases were preceded by selective decreases in the corresponding mRNA species. Significant decreases in D1 mRNA were observed in 4-week-old R6/2 mice, without a corresponding decrease in D1 binding. This early-stage decrease in dopamine receptor mRNA is reminiscent of that which has been reported for human HD cases (Augood *et al.* 1997). This suggests that the altered transcription of specific genes might contribute to the development of clinical symptoms in HD, and that transcriptional dysregulation may be a key pathological mechanism in HD (Cha 2000; see also Chapter 12).

Recently, evidence for alterations in dopamine signalling of presymptomatic R6/2 mice has been described (Bibb *et al.* 2000). Once again, at 4 weeks of age, the R6/2 mice displayed severe deficiencies in dopamine signalling in the striatum. The neurochemical changes included selective reductions in striatal dopamine- and cyclic adenosine monophosphate (cAMP)-regulated phosphoprotein, DARPP-32, as well as other dopamine-regulated phosphoprotein markers of medium spiny neurones. At 6 weeks of age, the R6/2 mice resembled DARPP32 knock-out mice, which also have abnormal dopamine signalling (Greengard *et al.* 1999). Dopamine signalling is known to regulate gene transcription. These observations provide more credence to the idea of a dysregulation of the transcriptional machinery in HD.

Recently, glutamate receptor sensitivity and striatal electrophysiology were investigated in two different HD mouse models, the R6/2 line and a CAG repeat knock-in line with 71 or 94 CAG repeats (Levine *et al.* 1999). Unlike the R6/2 line, the CAG71 and CAG94 knock-in lines do not exhibit neuropathological or behavioural abnormalities. However, CAG94 and R6/2 mice displayed a significant increase in striatal cell swelling when brain slices were subjected to glutamate receptor activation with NMDA. This effect was specific to NMDA receptors in that AMPA or kainate exposure failed to induce cellular swelling. The R6/2 and CAG94 lines also exhibited significant changes in their membrane depolarization states when compared to the CAG71 and control mice. This suggests that an increased sensitivity to NMDA occurs early in the disease process, before the onset of symptoms and, therefore, that NMDA antagonists may be useful in the treatment of HD.

The expression of several neurotransmitters, neuropeptides, and GAD has also been examined in the R6/2 and CAG71 and CAG94 HD mice (Menalled *et al.* 2000). Both types of mice showed significant decreases in enkephalin mRNA in the striatum with quantitative *in situ* hybridization. Surprisingly, immunohistochemistry did not reveal any significant protein changes for enkephalin, substance P, GAD_{65}, GAD_{67}, somatostatin, or ChAT. This report and other studies suggest that decreased expression of particular mRNA species precedes detectable decreases in protein abundance (Cha *et al.* 1998).

Reynolds and colleagues (1999) first characterized the levels of many neurotransmitters in the R6/2 mice. High-performance liquid chromatography (HPLC) was used to determine the concentrations of GABA, glutamate, and the monoamine neurotransmitters in four brain regions, at times before and after the emergence of an HD-like phenotype. When compared to the human post-mortem findings, several noteworthy disparities were observed. Striatal GABA in the R6/2 mice was normal. This finding suggests that loss of GABA-containing neurones is not an important early pathogenetic event in the transgenic mice, and that the GABA decreases described in human HD most probably simply reflect cell loss. In the striatum of 12-week-old R6/2 mice, significant decreases in the levels of dopamine and serotonin were recorded. A significant drop in striatal 5-HIAA levels, the major metabolite of serotonin, was seen in 4-, 8-, and 12-week-old animals. Similar decreases were observed at 8 and 12 weeks of age only in the hippocampus and brainstem of the R6/2 mice. Noradrenaline levels were only decreased in the hippocampus and brainstem. These data appear to indicate that the R6/2 model of HD has severely disrupted serotonergic and dopaminergic systems.

One early gene change observed in post-mortem HD patients was a decrease in the cannabinoid receptor (CB1) binding (Glass *et al.* 1993). This observation was in a grade 1 (minimal neuropathology) patient. Cannabinoids are important modulators of the dopaminergic system, which is also disrupted in HD. Northern blots and *in situ* hybridization were performed on 4- to 10-week-old R6/2 mice to investigate CB1 receptors (Denovan-Wright and

Robertson 2000). Significant decreases in CB1 mRNA were observed in the lateral striatum by 6 weeks of age, also before the onset of HD-like motor symptoms. R6/2 mice also showed a loss of CB1 mRNA within a subset of neurones in the cortex and hippocampus. These data suggest that the early dysregulation of the cannabinoid system (receptor loss) may affect the progression of HD, especially the cognitive and motor decline seen in these patients. For this reason, CB1 receptor agonists, such as anandamide, may be ultimately prove useful in the treatment of these symptoms.

A specific and progressive loss of complexin II in the R6/2 line has been observed (Morton and Edwardson 2001). Complexin II is known to bind to the SNARE complex of proteins, which are critical in vesicular release. Complexin II was also found to co-aggregate with huntingtin to form intranuclear inclusions. This observation suggests that mutant huntingtin may disrupt neurotransmitter release by sequestering complexin II into aggregates and rendering the presynaptic vesicles unable to release neurotransmitter.

Neurotransmitter release has also been investigated in the R6/1 line. Investigators have found that basal striatal dialysate glutamate levels were reduced by 42 per cent in 16-week-old, asymptomatic R6/1 mice compared to control mice after induction with NMDA (Nicniocaill *et al.* 2001). Release of aspartate and GABA release was normal. This observation provides further evidence that striatal neurotransmitter release becomes dysfunctional before the onset of an HD phenotype. Interestingly, both CB1 and mGluR2 receptors decreased in transgenic mouse brain are postulated to be involved with neurotransmitter release (Kim and Thayer 2000).

Among non-transmitter neurochemical alterations that have been described in transgenic HD mice, a decrease in *N*-acetyl aspartate (NAA), considered to be a marker of neuronal viability, has been observed with magnetic resonance spectroscopy (Jenkins *et al.* 2000). These authors also noted an increase in concentrations of glutamine, a finding that these authors interpreted as an indication of an underlying metabolic defect.

Numerous researchers have begun using gene expression profiling (microarray technologies) to elucidate the changes in transcription of mRNA in the numerous mouse models of HD. From the recent data, it is clear that alterations in gene expression for a number of neurochemical gene markers may play significant roles in the aetiology of the disease. Recently, oligonucleotide microarrays have been used to investigate mRNA expression changes in R6/2 mice at 6 and 12 weeks of age (Luthi-Carter *et al.* 2000). The ages of these mice represent both early- and late-stage HD phenotypes. In addition, gene changes in the N171–18Q and N171–82Q transgenic mice models of HD were investigated. The N171 mice have a transgene encoding the first 171 amino acids of the human HD gene with either 18 or 82 polyglutamine repeats (Schilling *et al.* 1999). N171–82Q mice display a delayed phenotype, when compared to the R6/2 mice. Four-month-old (late symptomatic) N171–82Q mice were used for gene expression analysis. The mRNAs that were decreased in both the R6/2 and N171–82Q mice are critical neurotransmitter, calcium, and retinoid signalling pathway genes. In addition, gene expression analysis confirmed previously described mRNA alterations such as decreases of the dopamine D1 and D2 receptors. Such microarray experiments confirm the involvement of many neurotransmitter systems, but also demonstrate that expression changes are not confined to neurotransmitter-related molecules. DNA hybridization technologies have been used to investigate gene changes in other mouse models of HD, such as the R6/1 line (Iannicola *et al.* 2000) . Further use of this type of technology will help researchers identify a reliable gene expression 'signature' for HD, or any other disease, that will facilitate the development of targeted therapies.

Cellular models

Despite the surge of data coming from the new mouse models of HD, *in vitro* systems to analyse huntingtin function are necessary to bypass some of the limitations of whole animal research (see also Chapter 12). Cell models allow researchers to accelerate their search for promising therapeutics for HD by enabling high-throughput screening of potentially useful compounds.

In 1981, cultured fibroblasts from HD patients were analysed for GAD activity and GABA concentration changes compared to control patient fibroblasts, as well as other well-described cell lines (Hamel *et al.* 1981). However, in contrast to what has been reported for HD brain, these studies failed to report significant changes in GAD activity or GABA in the HD fibroblasts. Immortalized fibroblasts have been used to study CAG repeat instability, but these cells are unable to replicate the characteristic neurochemical changes of HD *in vitro* (Manley *et al.* 1999). Lymphoblasts from HD patients have also been used to investigate calcium homeostasis (Panov *et al.* 1999; Sawa *et al.* 1999). Thus, non-neuronal cells may be useful for exploring certain abnormal physiological processes, but they are unlikely to shed light on the neurochemical alterations that occur in HD.

Slice cultures of striatal tissue from newborn rats have also been prepared in an attempt to generate another *in vitro* HD model (Ostergaard *et al.* 1995). However, these cells do not contain the mutant huntingtin protein and do not display the cell pathology observed in HD. In addition, little neurochemistry on this cell system has been performed. However, it is possible that primary striatal cells could be exposed to certain excitotoxic or mitochondrial stressors that are hypothesized to play a role in HD to generate a cellular phenotype similar to that observed in HD. In particular, several groups are now experimenting with slice cultures prepared from transgenic HD mouse models.

Transiently transfected cultured cells have been used to investigate the cellular effects of huntingtin (Saudou *et al.* 1998; Li and Li 1998; Peters *et al.* 1999; Chen *et al.* 1999). To assess the function of particular NMDA receptors in the presence of huntingtin, cells were co-transfected with huntingtin containing either 138 (pathogenic) or 15 (non-pathogenic) glutamines, and NMDA receptors (Chen *et al.* 1999). Patch-clamp electrophysiology demonstrated that the receptors composed of the NR1 and NR2B subunits have a larger current in the presence of pathogenic huntingtin. This effect was specific for NR2B. The NR1/NR2A receptors showed no change in current in response to co-expression with either the mutant or normal huntingtin. Western analysis showed no difference in cell surface protein levels for NR1/NR2B. Therefore, it is proposed that mutant huntingtin may alter function of NR1/NR2B receptors. Interestingly, this variety of NMDA receptor is predominantly localized in the medium spiny neurones of the striatum, which undergo extensive degeneration in HD.

Cellular studies reinforce the relevance of dopamine. Dopamine treatment of clonal striatal cells alters the subcellular localization of huntingtin (Kim *et al.* 1999). In the presence of dopamine, huntingtin increases its localization to clathrin-enriched membrane fractions. This dopaminergic response was eliminated in a cell line lacking D1 receptors. This suggests that proper cellular localization of the huntingtin protein depends upon activation of adenylyl cyclase and stimulation of dopamine D1 receptors. It is conceivable that the decrease in D1 mRNA commonly observed in HD may result in a heretofore undescribed loss of huntingtin function.

Numerous stable cellular models of HD have been developed using PC12 cells, neuroblastoma cell lines, or immortalized striatal neurones (Lunkes and Mandel 1998; Li *et al.* 1999;

Lunkes *et al.* 1999; Rigamonti *et al.* 2000; Varani *et al.* 2001; Wyttenbach *et al.* 2001). In certain cell lines, the expression of full-length or truncated forms of wild-type and mutant huntingtin is inducible upon the addition of specific drugs to the media. These cell lines typically generate cytoplasmic and nuclear inclusions containing huntingtin but, like their predecessors, the neurochemical changes in these cells remain to be elucidated.

Other HD models

Insight into the function and pathogenesis of mutant huntingtin is now coming from the development of innovative model systems (see also Chapter 14). For example, a *Drosophila* model for HD has recently been described. Expression of the expanded polyglutamine huntingtin causes neuronal degeneration and, as in all models of HD, nuclear inclusions are identified before the visible degeneration (Jackson *et al.* 1998). The toxic formation of the huntingtin protein is the expanded polyglutamine repeat. It has been found that expression of polyglutamine chains alone in *Drosophila* is toxic depending on cell type. Paradoxically, the toxic effect of polyglutamines can be neutralized by the protein context in which they reside (Marsh *et al.* 2000).

Caenorhabditis elegans (*C. elegans*) is another model organism of choice for a growing number of HD researchers. The simplicity and availability of a complete genome sequence for *C. elegans* makes this organism ideal for gaining insight into gene function (Aboobaker and Blaxter 2000). With this said, a *C. elegans* model for HD now exists (Faber *et al.* 1999). The expression of human huntingtin with a pathogenic number of CAG repeats (150) results in the degeneration of the ASH sensory neurones. This cell death was dependent upon the function of a particular caspase. Like the other cell models for HD, no neurochemical information is available.

Summary

HD has been well characterized with respect to the neurochemical changes occurring in the human brain. The alterations offer insight into the pathogenesis of HD and, more specifically, the nature of susceptibility of vulnerable neuronal populations. Widespread alterations of neurotransmitter synthetic enzymes, neurotransmitter concentrations, and neurotransmitter receptors most probably account for the clinical symptoms of HD. Symptomatic therapies directed at correcting altered neurotransmitter systems may therefore be useful in the treatment of HD. Recently developed cellular and animal models confirm the importance and relevance of neurochemical alterations that occur in HD. The use of such model systems will certainly reveal the underlying mechanisms causing such characteristic alterations.

References

Aboobaker, A. A. and Blaxter, M. L. (2000). Medical significance of *Caenorhabditis elegans*. *Annals of Medicine* **32**, 23–30.

Albin, R. L. and Greenamyre, J. T. (1992). Alternative excitotoxic hypotheses. *Neurology* **42**, 733–738.

—— Young, A. B., and Penney, J. B. (1989). The functional anatomy of basal ganglia disorders. *Trends in Neurosciences* **12**, 366–375.

Albin, R. L., Reiner, A., Anderson, K. D., Penney, J. B., and Young, A. B. (1990a). Striatal and nigral neuron subpopulations in rigid Huntington's disease: implications for the functional anatomy of chorea and rigidity-akinesia. *Annals of Neurology* **27**, 357–365.

—— Young, A. B., Penney, J. B., Handelin, B., Balfour, R., Anderson, K. D., Markel, D. S., Tourtellotte, W. W., and Reiner, A. (1990b). Abnormalities of striatal projection neurons and N-methyl-D-aspartate receptors in presymptomatic Huntington's disease. *New England Journal of Medicine* **322**, 1293–1298.

—— Qin, Y., Young, A. B., Penney, J. B., and Chesselet, M. F. (1991). Preproenkephalin messenger mRNA-containing neurons in striatum of patients with symptomatic and presymptomatic Huntington's disease: an *in situ* hybridization study. *Annals of Neurology* **30**, 542–549.

—— Reiner, A., Anderson, K. D., Dure, L. S., Handelin, B., Balfour, R., Whetsell, W. O., Jr., Penney, J. B., and Young, A. B. (1992). Preferential loss of striato-external pallidal projection neurons in presymptomatic Huntington's disease. *Annals of Neurology* **31**, 425–430.

Andrews, T. C., Weeks, R. A., Turjanski, N., Gunn, R. N., Watkins, L. H., Sahakian, B., Hodges, J. R., Rosser, A. E., Wood, N. W., and Brooks, D. J. (1999). Huntington's disease progression. PET and clinical observations. *Brain* **122**, 2353–2363.

Antonini, A., Leenders, K. L., Spiegel, R., Meier, D., Vontobel, P., Weigell-Weber, M., Sanchez-Pernaute, R., De Yebenez, J. G., Boesiger, P., Weindl, A., and Maguire, R. P. (1996). Striatal glucose metabolism and dopamine D2 receptor binding in asymptomatic gene carriers and patients with Huntington's disease. *Brain* **119**, 2085–2095.

—— —— Eidelberg, D. (1998). [11C]raclopride-PET studies of the Huntington's disease rate of progression: relevance of the trinucleotide repeat length. *Annals of Neurology* **43**, 253–255.

Aronin, N., Cooper, P. E., Lorenz, L. J., Bird, E. D., Sagar, S. M., Leeman, S. E., and Martin, J. B. (1983). Somatostatin is increased in the basal ganglia in Huntington disease. *Annals of Neurology* **13**, 519–526.

Arregui, A., Iversen, L. L., Spokes, E. G. S., and Emson, P. C. (1979). Alteration in postmortem brain angiotensin-converting enzyme activity and some neuropeptides in Huntington's disease. In *Advances in neurology*, Vol. 23 (ed. T. N. Chase, N. S. Wexler, and A. Barbeau), pp. 517–525. Raven Press, New York.

Arzberger, T., Krampfl, K., Leimgruber, S., and Weindl, A. (1997). Changes of NMDA receptor subunit (NR1, NR2B) and glutamate transporter (GLT1) mRNA expression in Huntington's disease—an *in situ* hybridization study. *Journal of Neuropathology and Experimental Neurology* **56**, 440–454.

Augood, S. J., Faull, R. L. M., Love, D. R., and Emson, P. C. (1996). Reduction in enkephalin and substance P messenger RNA in the striatum of early grade Huntington's disease: a detailed cellular *in situ* hybridization study. *Neuroscience* **72**, 1023–1036.

—— —— Emson, P. C. (1997). Dopamine D1 and D2 receptor gene expression in the striatum in Huntington's disease. *Annals of Neurology* **42**, 215–221.

Backman, L., Robins-Wahlin, T. B., Lundin, A., Ginovart, N., and Farde, L. (1997). Cognitive deficits in Huntington's disease are predicted by dopaminergic PET markers and brain volumes. *Brain* **120**, 2207–2217.

Beal, M. F. and Martin, J. B. (1986). Neuropeptides in neurological disease. *Annals of Neurology* **20**, 547–565.

—— Benoit, R., Bird, E. D., and Martin, J. B. (1985). Immunoreactive somatostatin-28(1–12) is increased in Huntington's disease. *Neuroscience Letters* **56**, 377–380.

—— —— Mazurek, M. F., Bird, E. D., and Martin, J. B. (1986a). Somatostatin-28(1–12)-like immunoreactivity is reduced in Alzheimer's disease cerebral cortex. *Brain Research* **368**, 380–383.

—— Kowall, N. W., Ellison, D. W., Mazurek, M. F., Swartz, K. J., and Martin, J. B. (1986b). Replication of the neurochemical characteristics of Huntington's disease by quinolinic acid. *Nature* **321**, 168–171.

—— —— Swartz, K. J., and Ferrante, R. J. (1990). Homocysteic acid lesions in rat striatum spare somatostatin–neuropeptide Y (NADPH-diaphorase) neurons. *Neuroscience Letters* **108**, 36–42.

—— Ferrante, R. J., Swartz, K. J., and Kowall, N. W. (1991a). Chronic quinolinic acid lesions in rats closely resemble Huntington's disease. *Journal of Neuroscience* **11**, 1649–1659.

—— Swartz, K. J., Hyman, B. T., Storey, E., Finn, S. F., and Koroshetz, W. (1991b). Aminooxyacetic acid results in excitotoxin lesions by a novel indirect mechanism. *Journal of Neurochemistry* **57**, 1068–1073.

—— Brouillet, E., Jenkins, B. G., Ferrante, R. J., Kowall, N. W., Miller, J. M., Storey, E., Srivastava, R., Rosen, B. R., and Hyman, B. T. (1993a). Neurochemical and histologic characterization of striatal excitotoxic lesions produced by the mitochondrial toxin 3-nitropropionic acid. *Journal of Neuroscience* **13**, 4181–4192.

—— Finn, S. F., and Brouillet, E. (1993b). Evidence for the involvement of metabotropic glutamate receptors in striatal excitotoxin lesions *in vivo*. *Neurodegeneration* **2**, 81–91.

Beaumont, K., Maurin, Y., Reisine, T. D., Fields, J. Z., Spoles, E., Bird, E. D., and Yamamura, H. I. (1979). Huntington's disease and its animal model: alterations in kainic acid binding. *Life Sciences* **24**, 809–816.

Bernheimer, H., Sperk, G., Price, K. S., and Hornykiewicz, O. (1979). Brain gangliosides in Huntington's disease. In *Advances in neurology*, Vol. 23 (ed. T. N. Chase, N. S. Wexler, and A. Barbeau), pp. 463–471. Raven Press, New York.

Bibb, J. A., Yan, Z., Svenningsson, P., Snyder, G. L., Pieribone, V. A., Horiuchi, A., Nairn, A. C., Messer, A., and Greengard, P. (2000). Severe deficiencies in dopamine signaling in presymptomatic Huntington's disease mice. *Proceedings of the National Academy of Sciences, USA* **97**, 6809–6814.

Bird, E. D. and Iversen, L. L. (1974). Huntington's chorea. Post mortem measurement of glutamic acid decarboxylase, choline acetyltransferase and dopamine in basal ganglia. *Brain* **97**, 457–472.

—— —— (1977). Neurochemical findings in Huntington's chorea. *Essays in Neurochemistry and Neuropharmacology* **1**, 177–195.

Bittigau, P. and Ikonomidou, C. (1997). Glutamate in neurologic diseases. *J Child Neurology* **12**, 471–485.

Bogdanov, M. B., Ferrante, R. J., Kuemmerle, S., Klivenyi, P., and Beal, M. F. (1998). Increased vulnerability to 3-nitropropionic acid in an animal model of Huntington's disease. *Journal of Neurochemistry* **71**, 2642–2644.

Bohnen, N. I., Koeppe, R. A., Meyer, P., Ficaro, E., Wernette, K., Kilbourn, M. R., Kuhl, D. E., Frey, K. A., and Albin, R. L. (2000). Decreased striatal monoaminergic terminals in Huntington disease. *Neurology* **54**, 1753–1759.

Brandt, J., Folstein, S. E., Wong, D. F., Links, J., Dannals, R. F., McDonnell-Sill, A., Starkstein, S., Anders, P., Strauss, M. E., Tune, L. E., *et al.* (1990). D2 receptors in Huntington's disease: positron emission tomography findings and clinical correlates. *Journal of Neuropsychiatry and Clinical Neuroscience* **2**, 20–27.

Brouillet, E., Conde, F., Beal, M. F., and Hantraye, P. (1999). Replicating Huntington's disease phenotype in experimental animals. *Progress in Neurobiology* **59**, 427–468.

Brucke, T., Podreka, I., Angelberger, P., Wenger, S., Topitz, A., Kufferle, B., Muller, C., and Deecke, L. (1991). Dopamine D2 receptor imaging with SPECT: studies in different neuropsychiatric disorders. *Journal of Cerebral Blood Flow Metabolism* **11**, 220–228.

—— Wenger, S., Asenbaum, S., Fertl, E., Pfafflmeyer, N., Muller, C., Podreka, I., and Angelberger, P. (1993). Dopamine D2 receptor imaging and measurement with SPECT. *Advances in Neurology* **60**, 494–500.

Buck, S. H., Burks, T. F., Brown, M. R., and Yamamura, H. I. (1981). Reduction in basal ganglia and substantia nigra substance P levels in Huntington's disease. *Brain Research* **209**, 464–469.

Burke, J. R., Enghild, J. J., Martin, M. E., Jou, Y. S., Myers, R. M., Roses, A. D., Vance, J. M., and Strittmatter, W. J. (1996). Huntingtin and DRPLA proteins selectively interact with the enzyme GAPDH. *Nature Medicine* **2**, 347–350.

Calabresi, P., Centonze, D., Pisani, A., Sancesario, G., Gubellini, P., Marfia, G. A., and Bernardi, G. (1998). Striatal spiny neurons and cholinergic interneurons express differential ionotropic glutamatergic responses and vulnerability: implications for ischemia and Huntington's disease. *Annals of Neurology* **43**, 586–597.

Calabresi, P., Centonze, D., Pisani, A., and Bernardi, G. (1999). Metabotropic glutamate receptors and cell-type-specific vulnerability in the striatum: implication for ischemia and Huntington's disease. *Experimental Neurology* **158**, 97–108.

Caraceni, T., Panerai, A. E., Paratl, E. A., Cocchi, D., and Muller, E. E. (1977). Altered growth hormone and prolactin responses to dopaminergic stimulation in Huntington's chorea. *Journal of Clinical Endocrinology and Metabolism* **44**, 870–875.

Carter, R. J., Lione, L. A., Humby, T., Mangiarini, L., Mahal, A., Bates, G. P., Dunnett, S. B., and Morton, A. J. (1999). Characterization of progressive motor deficits in mice transgenic for the human Huntington's disease mutation. *Journal of Neuroscience* **19**, 3248–3257.

Castro, M. E., Pascual, J., Romon, T., Berciano, J., Figols, J., and Pazos, A. (1998). 5-HT1B receptor binding in degenerative movement disorders. *Brain Research* **790**, 323–328.

Cha, J.-H. J. (2000). Transcriptional dysregulation in Huntington's disease. *Trends in Neurosciences* **23**, 387–392.

—— Kosinski, C. M., Kerner, J. A., Alsdorf, S. A., Mangiarini, L., Davies, S. W., Penney, J. B., Bates, G. P., and Young, A. B. (1998). Altered brain neurotransmitter receptors in transgenic mice expressing a portion of an abnormal human Huntington disease gene. *Proceedings of the National Academy of Sciences, USA* **95**, 6480–6485.

—— Frey, A. S., Alsdorf, S. A., Kerner, J. A., Kosinski, C. M., Mangiarini, L., Penney, J. B. Jr, Davies, S. W., Bates, G. P., and Young, A. B. (1999). Altered neurotransmitter receptor expression in transgenic mouse models of Huntington's disease. *Philosophical Transactions of the Royal Society of London B Biological Sciences* **354**, 981–989.

Chalmers, R. J., Johnson, R. H., Keogh, H. J., and Nanda, R. N. (1978). Growth hormone and prolactin response to bromocriptine in patients with Huntington's chorea. *Journal of Neurology, Neurosurgery and Psychiatry* **41**, 135–139.

Chen, M., Ona, V. O., Li, M., Ferrante, R. J., Fink, K. B., Zhu, S., Bian, J., Guo, L., Farrell, L. A., Hersch, S. M., Hobbs, W., Vonsattel, J. P., Cha, J. H., and Friedlander, R. M. (2000). Minocycline inhibits caspase-1 and caspase-3 expression and delays mortality in a transgenic mouse model of Huntington disease. *Nature Medicine* **6**, 797–801.

Chen, N., Luo, T., Wellington, C., Metzler, M., McCutcheon, K., Hayden, M. R., and Raymond, L. A. (1999). Subtype-specific enhancement of NMDA receptor currents by mutant huntingtin. *Journal of Neurochemistry* **72**, 1890–1898.

Choi, D. W. and Rothman, S. M. (1990). The role of glutamate neurotoxicity in hypoxic-ischemic neuronal death. *Annual Review of Neuroscience* **13**, 171–182.

Cicchetti, F., Gould, P. V., and Parent, A. (1996). Sparing of striatal neurons coexpressing calretinin and substance P (NK1) receptor in Huntington's disease. *Brain Research* **730**, 232–237.

Coyle, J. T. and Schwarcz, R. (1976). Lesion of striatal neurones with kainic acid provides a model for Huntington's chorea. *Nature* **263**, 244–246.

Cross, A. and Rossor, M. (1983). Dopamine D-1 and D-2 receptors in Huntington's disease. *European Journal of Pharmacology* **88**, 223–229.

Cross, A. J., Slater, P., and Reynolds, G. P. (1986). Reduced high-affinity glutamate uptake sites in the brains of patients with Huntington's disease. *Neuroscience Letters* **67**, 198–202.

Crossman, A. R., Mitchell, I. J., Sambrook, M. A., and Jackson, A. (1988). Chorea and myoclonus in the monkey induced by gamma-aminobutyric acid antagonism in the lentiform complex. The site of drug action and a hypothesis for the neural mechanisms of chorea. *Brain* **111**, 1211–1233.

Davies, S. W. and Roberts, P. J. (1987). No evidence for preservation of somatostatin-containing neurons after intrastriatal injections of quinoloinic acid. *Nature* **327**, 326–329.

—— Turmaine, M., Cozens, B. A., DiFiglia, M., Sharp, A. H., Ross, C. A., Scherzinger, E., Wanker, E. E., Mangiarini, L., and Bates, G. P. (1997). Formation of neuronal intranuclear inclusions underlies the neurological dysfunction in mice transgenic for the HD mutation. *Cell* **90**, 537–548.

Dawbarn, D., Dequidt, M. E., and Emson, P. C. (1985). Survival of basal ganglia neuropeptide Y-somatostatin neurones in Huntington's disease. *Brain Research* **340**, 251–260.

Dawson, V. L. and Dawson, T. M. (1996). Nitric oxide neurotoxicity. *Journal of Chemical Neuroanatomy* **10**, 179–190.

De Keyser, J., Wilczak, N., and Goossens, A. (1994). Insulin-like growth factor-I receptor densities in human frontal cortex and white matter during aging, in Alzheimer's disease, and in Huntington's disease. *Neuroscience Letters* **172**, 93–96.

Denovan-Wright, E. M. and Robertson, H. A. (2000). Cannabinoid receptor messenger RNA levels decrease in a subset of neurons of the lateral striatum, cortex and hippocampus of transgenic Huntington's disease mice. *Neuroscience* **98**, 705–713.

DiFiglia, M. (1990). Excitotoxic injury of the neostriatum: a model for Huntington's disease. *Trends in Neurosciences* **13**, 286–289.

—— Sapp, E., Chase, K., Schwarz, C., Meloni, A., Young, C., Martin, E., Vonsattel, J. P., Carraway, R., Reeves, S. A., Boyce, F. M., and Aronin, N. (1995). Huntingtin is a cytoplasmic protein associated with vesicles in human and rat brain neurons. *Neuron* **14**, 1075–1081.

Dunnett, S. B., Carter, R. J., Watts, C., Torres, E. M., Mahal, A., Mangiarini, L., Bates, G., and Morton, A. J. (1998). Striatal transplantation in a transgenic mouse model of Huntington's disease. *Experimental Neurology* **154**, 31–40.

Dure, L. S., IV, Young, A. B., and Penney, J. B. (1991). Excitatory amino acid binding sites in the caudate nucleus and frontal cortex of Huntington's disease. *Annals of Neurology* **30**, 785–793.

Durso, R., Tamminga, C. A., Denaro, A., Ruggeri, S., and Chase, T. N. (1983). Plasma growth hormone and prolactin response to dopaminergic GABAmimetic and cholinergic stimulation in Huntington's disease. *Neurology* **33**, 1229–1232.

Emson, P. C., Arregui, A., Clement-Jones, V., Sandberg, B. E., and Rossor, M. (1980). Regional distribution of methionine-enkephalin and substance P-like immunoreactivity in normal human brain and in Huntington's disease. *Brain Research* **199**, 147–160.

Enna, S. J., Bennett, J. P., Jr., Bylund, D. B., Snyder, S. H., Bird, E. D., and Iversen, L. L. (1976). Alterations of brain neurotransmitter receptor binding in Huntington's chorea. *Brain Research* **116**, 531–537.

Faber, P. W., Alter, J. R., MacDonald, M. E., and Hart, A. C. (1999). Polyglutamine-mediated dysfunction and apoptotic death of a Caenorhabditis elegans sensory neuron. *Proceedings of the National Academy of Sciences, USA* **96**, 179–184.

Ferrante, R. J. and Kowall, N. W. (1987). Tyrosine hydroxylase-like immunoreactivity is distributed in the matrix compartment of normal human and Huntington's disease striatum. *Brain Research* **416**, 141–146.

—— —— Beal, M. F., Richardson, E. P. Jr, Bird, E. D., and Martin, J. B. (1985). Selective sparing of a class of striatal neurons in Huntington's disease. *Science* **230**, 561–564.

—— Beal, M. F., Kowall, N. W., Richardson, E. P., and Martin, J. B. (1987a). Sparing of acetylcholinesterase-containing striatal neurons in Huntington's disease. *Brain Research* **411**, 162–166.

—— Kowall, N. W., Beal, M. F., Martin, J. B., Bird, E. D., and Richardson, E. P. (1987b). Morphologic and histochemical characteristics of a spared subset of striatal neurons in Huntington's disease. *Journal of Neuropathology and Experimental Neurology* **46** (1), 12–27.

—— —— Cipolloni, P. B., Storey, E., and Flint Beal, M. (1993). Excitotoxin lesions in primates as a model for Huntington's disease: histopathologic and neurochemical characterization. *Experimental Neurology* **119**, 46–71.

—— Gutekunst, C. A., Persichetti, F., McNeil, S. M., Kowall, N. W., Gusella, J. F., MacDonald, M. E., Beal, M. F., and Hersch, S. M. (1997). Heterogeneous topographic and cellular distribution of huntingtin expression in the normal human neostriatum. *Journal of Neuroscience* **17**, 3052–3063.

—— Andreassen, O. A., Jenkins, B. G., Dedeoglu, A., Kuemmerle, S., Kubilus, J. K., Kaddurah-Daouk, R., Hersch, S. M., and Beal, M. F. (2000). Neuroprotective effects of creatine in a transgenic mouse model of Huntington's disease. *Journal of Neuroscience* **20**, 4389–4397.

Filloux, F., Wagster, M. V., Folstein, S., Price, D. L., Hedreen, J. C., Dawson, T. M., and Wamsley, J. K. (1990). Nigral dopamine type-1 receptors are reduced in Huntington's disease: A postmortem autoradiographic study using [3H]SCH 23390 and correlation with [3H]forskolin binding. *Experimental Neurology* **110**, 219–227.

Gale, J. S., Bird, E. D., Spoke, E. G., Ivejsen, L. L., and Jessel, T. (1978). Human brain substance P: distribution in controls and Huntington's chorea. *Journal of Neurochemistry* **30**, 633–634.

Gamberino, W. C. and Brennan, W. A. Jr (1994). Glucose transporter isoform expression in Huntington's disease brain. *Journal of Neurochemistry* **63**, 1392–1397.

Ge, J. and Barnes, N. M. (1996). Alterations in angiotensin AT1 and AT2 receptor subtype levels in brain regions from patients with neurodegenerative disorders. *European Journal of Pharmacology* **297**, 299–306.

Ginovart, N., Lundin, A., Farde, L., Halldin, C., Backman, L., Swahn, C. G., Pauli, S., and Sedvall, G. (1997). PET study of the pre- and post-synaptic dopaminergic markers for the neurodegenerative process in Huntington's disease. *Brain* **120**, 503–514.

Glass, M., Faull, R. L. M., and Dragunow, M. (1993). Loss of cannabinoid receptors in the substantia nigra in Huntington's disease. *Neuroscience* **56**, 523–527.

Goodchild, R. E., Court, J. A., Hobson, I., Piggott, M. A., Perry, R. H., Ince, P., Jaros, E., and Perry, E. K. (1999). Distribution of histamine H3-receptor binding in the normal human basal ganglia: comparison with Huntington's and Parkinson's disease cases. *European Journal of Neuroscience* **11**, 449–456.

Graybiel, A. M. (1990). Neurotransmitters and neuromodulators in the basal ganglia. *Trends in Neurosciences* **13**, 244–254.

Greenamyre, J. T., Penney, J. B., and Young, A. B. (1985). Alterations in L-glutamate binding in Alzheimer's and Huntington's diseases. *Science* **227**, 1496–1499.

Greengard, P., Allen, P. B., and Nairn, A. C. (1999). Beyond the dopamine receptor: the DARPP-32/ protein phosphatase-1 cascade. *Neuron* **23**, 435–447.

Gutekunst, C. A., Levey, A. I., Heilman, C. J., Whaley, W. L., Yi, H., Nash, N. R., Rees, H. D., Madden, J. J., and Hersch, S. M. (1995). Identification and localization of huntingtin in brain and human lymphoblastoid cell lines with anti-fusion protein antibodies. *Proceedings of the National Academy of Sciences, USA* **92**, 8710–8714.

Hagglund, J., Aquilonius, S. M., Eckernas, S. A., Hartrig, P., Lundquist, H., Gullberg, P., and Langstrom, B. (1987). Dopamine receptor properties in Parkinson's disease and Huntington's chorea evaluated by positron emission tomography using ^{11}C-N-methyl-spiperone. *Acta Neurologica Scandinavica* **75**, 87–94.

Hamel, E., Goetz, I. E., and Roberts, E. (1981). Glutamic acid decarboxylase and gamma-aminobutyric acid in Huntington's disease fibroblasts and other cultured cells, determined by a [3H]muscimol radioreceptor assay. *Journal of Neurochemistry* **37**, 1032–1038.

Hansson, O. A. P. N., Leist, M., Nicotera, P., Castilho, R. F., and Brundin, P. (1999). Transgenic mice expressing a Huntington's disease mutation are resistant to quinolinic acid-induced striatal excitotoxicity. *Proceedings of the National Academy of Sciences, USA* **96**, 8727–8732.

Hantraye, P., Loc, H. C., Maziere, B., Khalili-Varasteh, M., Crouzel, C., Fournier, D., Yorke, J. C., Stulzaft, O., Riche, D., Isacson, O., *et al.* (1992). 6-[18F]fluoro-L-dopa uptake and [76Br]bromolisuride binding in the excitotoxically lesioned caudate–putamen of nonhuman primates studied using positron emission tomography. *Experimental Neurology* **115**, 218–227.

Hashimoto, T., Kitamura, N., Saito, N., Komure, O., Nishino, N., and Tanaka, C. (1992). The loss of BetaII-protein kinase C in the striatum from patients with Huntington's disease. *Brain Research* **585**, 303–306.

Hayden, M. R., Vinik, A. I., Paul, M., and Beighton, P. (1977). Impaired prolactin release in Huntington's chorea. Evidence for dopaminergic excess. *Lancet* **2**, 423–426.

Hays, S. E., Goodwin, F. K., and Paul, S. M. (1981). Cholecystokinin receptors are decreased in basal ganglia and cerebral cortex of Huntington's disease. *Brain Research* **225**, 452–456.

Hedreen, J. C., Peyser, C. E., Folstein, S. E., and Ross, C. A. (1991). Neuronal loss in layers V and VI of cerebral cortex in Huntington's disease. *Neuroscience Letters* **133**, 257–261.

Herkenham, M., Lynn, A. B., Little, M. D., Johnson, M. R., Melvin, L. S., de Costa, B. R., and Rice, K. C. (1990). Cannabinoid receptor localization in brain. *Proceedings of the National Academy of Sciences, USA* **87**, 1932–1936.

Hiley, C. R. and Bird, E. D. (1974). Decreased muscarinic receptor concentration in post-mortem brain in Huntington's chorea. *Brain Research* **80**, 355–358.

Hodgson, J. G., Agopyan, N., Gutekunst, C. A., Leavitt, B. R., LePiane, F., Singaraja, R., Smith, D. J., Bissada, N., McCutcheon, K., Nasir, J., Jamot, L., Li, X. J., Stevens, M. E., Rosemond, E., Roder, J. C., Phillips, A. G., Rubin, E. M., Hersch, S. M., and Hayden, M. R. (1999). A YAC mouse model for Huntington's disease with full-length mutant huntingtin, cytoplasmic toxicity, and selective striatal neurodegeneration. *Neuron* **23**, 181–192.

Holemans, S., Javoy-Agid, F., Agid, Y., De Paermentier, F., Laterre, E. C., and Maloteaux, J. M. (1994). Sulfonylurea binding sites in normal human brain and in Parkinson's disease, progressive supranuclear palsy and Huntington's disease. *Brain Research* **642**, 327–333.

Huntington's Disease Collaborative Research Group. (1993). A novel gene containing a trinucleotide repeat that is unstable in Huntington's disease chromosomes. *Cell* **72**, 971–983.

Hurlbert, M. S., Zhou, W., Wasmeier, C., Kaddis, F. G., Hutton, J. C., and Freed, C. R. (1999). Mice transgenic for an expanded CAG repeat in the Huntington's disese gene develop diabetes mellitus. *Diabetes* **48**, 649–651.

Iannicola, C., Moreno, S., Oliverio, S., Nardacci, R., Ciofi-Luzzatto, A., and Piacentini, M. (2000). Early alterations in gene expression and cell morphology in a mouse model of Huntington's disease. *Journal of Neurochemistry* **75**, 830–839.

Ichise, M., Toyama, H., Fornazzari, L., Ballinger, J. R., and Kirsh, J. C. (1993). Iodine-123-IBZM dopamine D2 receptor and Technetium-99m-HMPAO brain perfusion SPECT in the evaluation of patients with and subjects at risk for Huntington's disease. *Journal of Nuclear Medicine* **34**, 1274–1281.

Ikonomidou, C. and Turski, L. (1996). Neurodegenerative disorders: clues from glutamate and energy metabolism. *Critical Reviews of Neurobiology* **10**, 239–263.

Isacson, O., Brundin, P., Gage, F. H., and Bjorklund, A. (1985). Neural grafting in a rat model of Huntington's disease: progressive neurochemical changes after neostriatal ibotenate lesions and striatal tissue grafting. *Neuroscience* **16**, 799–817.

—— Riche, D., Hantraye, P., Sofroniew, M. V., and Maziere, M. (1989). A primate model of Huntington's disease: cross-species implantation of striatal precursor cells to the excitotoxically lesioned baboon caudate-putamen. *Experimental Brain Research* **75**, 213–220.

Jackson, G. R., Salecker, I., Dong, X., Yao, X., Arnheim, N., Faber, P. W., MacDonald, M. E., and Zipursky, S. L. (1998). Polyglutamine-expanded human huntingtin transgenes induce degeneration of *Drosophila* photoreceptor neurons. *Neuron* **21**, 633–642.

Jakel, R. J. and Maragos, W. F. (2000). Neuronal cell death in Huntington's disease: a potential role for dopamine. *Trends in Neurosciences* **23**, 239–245.

Jankovic, J. and Beach, J. (1997). Long-term effects of tetrabenazine in hyperkinetic movement disorders. *Neurology* **48**, 358–362.

Jenkins, B. G., Brouillet, E., Chen, Y. C., Storey, E., Schulz, J. B., Kirschner, P., Beal, M. F., and Rosen, B. R. (1996). Non-invasive neurochemical analysis of focal excitotoxic lesions in models of neurodegenerative illness using spectroscopic imaging. *Journal of Cerebral Blood Flow Metabolism* **16**, 450–461.

—— Klivenyi, P., Kustermann, E., Andreassen, O. A., Ferrante, R. J., Rosen, B. R., and Beal, M. F. (2000). Nonlinear decrease over time in N-acetyl aspartate levels in the absence of neuronal loss and increases in glutamine and glucose in transgenic Huntington's disease mice. *Journal of Neurochemistry* **74**, 2108–2119.

Joyce, J. N., Lexow, N., Bird, E., and Winokur, A. (1988). Organization of dopamine D1 and D2 receptors in human striatum: receptor autoradiographic studies in Huntington's disease and schizophrenia. *Synapse* **2**, 546–557.

Kanazawa, I., Bird, E., O'Connell, R., and Powell, D. (1977). Evidence for a decrease in substance P content of substantia nigra in Huntington's chorea. *Brain Research* **120**, 387–392.

Kanazawa, I., Bird, E., Gale, J. S., Iversen, L. L., Jessell, T. M., Muramoto, O., Spokes, E. G., and Sutoo, D. (1979). Substance P: decrease in substantia nigra and globus pallidus in Huntington's disease. In *Advances in neurology*, Vol. 23 (ed. T. N. Chase, N. S. Wexler, and A. Barbeau), pp. 495–505. Raven Press, New York.

—— Sasaki, H., Muramoto, O., Matsushita, M., Mizutani, T., Iwabuchi, K., Ikeda, T., and Takahata, N. (1985). Studies on neurotransmitter markers and striatal neuronal cell density in Huntington's disease and dentatorubropallidoluysian atrophy. *Journal of the Neurological Sciences* **70**, 151–165.

—— Tanaka, Y., and Cho, F. (1986). 'Choreic' movement induced by unilateral kainate lesion of the striatum and L-DOPA administration in monkey. *Neuroscience Letters* **71**, 241–246.

—— Murata, M., and Kimura, M. (1993). Roles of dopamine and its receptors in generation of choreic movements. *Advances in Neurology* **60**, 107–112.

Kartzinel, R., Hunt, R. D., and Calne, D. B. (1976). Bromocriptine in Huntington chorea. *Archives of Neurology* **33**, 517–518.

Kawaguchi, Y., Wilson, C. J., Augood, S. J., and Emson, P. C. (1995). Striatal interneurones: chemical, physiological and morphological characterization. *Trends in Neurosciences* **18**, 527–535.

Kieburtz, K., Feigin, A., McDermott, M., Como, P., Abwender, D., Zimmerman, C., Hickey, C., Orme, C., Claude, K., Sotack, J., Greenamyre, J. T., Dunn, C., and Shoulson, I. (1996). A controlled trial of remacemide hydrochloride in Huntington's disease. *Movement Disorders* **11**, 273–277.

Kim, D. J. and Thayer, S. A. (2000). Activation of CB1 cannabinoid receptors inhibits neurotransmitter release from identified synaptic sites in rat hippocampal cultures. *Brain Research* **852**, 398–405.

Kim, M., Velier, J., Chase, K., Laforet, G., Kalchman, M. A., Hayden, M. R., Won, L., Heller, A., Aronin, N., and Difiglia, M. (1999). Forskolin and dopamine D1 receptor activation increase huntingtin's association with endosomes in immortalized neuronal cells of striatal origin. *Neuroscience* **89**, 1159–1167.

Kish, S. J., Shannak, K., and Hornykiewicz, O. (1987). Elevated serotonin and reduced dopamine in subregionally divided Huntingtons disease striatum. *Annals of Neurology* **22**, 386–389.

Koh, J.-Y. and Choi, D. W. (1988). Cultured striatal neurons containing NADPH-diaphorase or acetylcholinesterase are selectively resistant to injury by NMDA receptor agonists. *Brain Research* **446**, 374–378.

Kosinski, C. M., Cha, J. H., Young, A. B., Persichetti, F., MacDonald, M., Gusella, J. F., Penney, J. B., and Standaert, D. G. (1997). Huntingtin immunoreactivity in the rat neostriatum: differential accumulation in projection and interneurons. *Experimental Neurology* **144**, 239–247.

—— —— —— Mangiarini, L., Bates, G., Schiefer, J., and Schwarz, M. (1999). Intranuclear inclusions in subtypes of striatal neurons in Huntington's disease transgenic mice. *NeuroReport* **10**, 3891–3896.

Kowall, N. W., Quigley, B. J., Jr., Krause, J. E., Lu, F., Kosofsky, B. E., and Ferrante, R. J. (1993). Substance P and substance P receptor histochemistry in human neurodegenerative diseases. *Regulatory Peptides* **46**, 174–185.

Lawrence, A. D., Weeks, R. A., Brooks, D. J., Andrews, T. C., Watkins, L. H., Harding, A. E., Robbins, T. W., and Sahakian, B. J. (1998). The relationship between striatal dopamine receptor binding and cognitive performance in Huntington's disease. *Brain* **121**, 1343–1355.

Leenders, K. L., Frackowiak, R. S., Quinn, N., and Marsden, C. D. (1986). Brain energy metabolism and dopaminergic function in Huntington's disease measured *in vivo* using positron emission tomography. *Movement Disorders* **1**, 69–77.

Leslie, W. D., Abrams, D. N., Greenberg, C. R., and Hobson, D. (1996). Comparison of iodine-123-epidepride and iodine-123-IBZM for dopamine D2 receptor imaging [see comments]. *Journal of Nuclear Medicine* **37**, 1589–1591.

—— Greenberg, C. R., Abrams, D. N., and Hobson, D. (1999). Clinical deficits in Huntington disease correlate with reduced striatal uptake on iodine-123 epidepride single-photon emission tomography. *European Journal of Nuclear Medicine* **26**, 1458–1464.

Levine, M. S., Klapstein, G. J., Koppel, A., Gruen, E., Cepeda, C., Vargas, M. E., Jokel, E. S., Carpenter, E. M., Zanjani, H., Hurst, R. S., Efstratiadis, A., Zeitlin, S., and Chesselet, M. F. (1999). Enhanced sensitivity to N-methyl-D-aspartate receptor activation in transgenic and knockin mouse models of Huntington's disease. *Journal of Neuroscience Research* **58**, 515–532.

Li, S. H. and Li, X. J. (1998). Aggregation of N-terminal huntingtin is dependent on the length of its glutamine repeats. *Human Molecular Genetics* **7**, 777–782.

—— Cheng, A. L., Li, H., and Li, X. J. (1999). Cellular defects and altered gene expression in PC12 cells stably expressing mutant huntingtin. *Journal of Neuroscience* **19**, 5159–5172.

Lloyd, K. G., Dreksler, S., and Bird, E. D. (1977). Alterations in 3H-GABA binding in Huntington's chorea. *Life Sciences* **21**, 747–753.

London, E. D., Yamamura, H. I., Bird, E. D., and Coyle, J. T. (1981). Decreased receptor-binding sites for kainic acid in brains of patients with Huntington's disease. *Biological Psychiatry* **16**, 155–162.

Lunkes, A. and Mandel, J. L. (1998). A cellular model that recapitulates major pathogenic steps of Huntington's disease. *Human Molecular Genetics* **7**, 1355–1361.

—— Trottier, Y., Fagart, J., Schultz, P., Zeder-Lutz, G., Moras, D., and Mandel, J. L. (1999). Properties of polyglutamine expansion in vitro and in a cellular model for Huntington's disease. *Philosophical Transactions of the Royal Society of London B Biological Sciences* **354**, 1013–1019.

Luthi-Carter, R., Strand, A., Peters, N. L., Solano, S. M., Hollingsworth, Z. R., Menon, A. S., Frey, A. S., Spektor, B. S., Penney, E. B., Schilling, G., Ross, C. A., Borchelt, D. R., Tapscott, S. J., Young, A. B., Cha, J.-H. J., and Olson, J. M. (2000). Decreased expression of striatal signaling genes in a mouse model of Huntington's disease. *Human Molecular Genetics* **9**, 1259–1271.

Mangiarini, L., Sathasivam, K., Seller, M., Cozens, B., Harper, A., Hetherington, C., Lawton, M., Trottier, Y., Lehrach, H., Davies, S. W., and Bates, G. P. (1996). Exon 1 of the *HD* gene with an expanded CAG repeat is sufficient to cause a progressive neurological phenotype in transgenic mice. *Cell* **87**, 493–506.

Manley, K., Pugh, J., and Messer, A. (1999). Instability of the CAG repeat in immortalized fibroblast cell cultures from Huntington's disease transgenic mice. *Brain Research* **835**, 74–79.

Manyam, B. V., Giacobini, E., and Colliver, J. A. (1990). Cerebrospinal fluid acetylcholinesterase and choline measurements in Huntington's disease. *Journal of Neurology* **237**, 281–284.

Marsh, J. L., Walker, H., Theisen, H., Zhu, Y. Z., Fielder, T., Purcell, J., and Thompson, L. M. (2000). Expanded polyglutamine peptides alone are intrinsically cytotoxic and cause neurodegeneration in *Drosophila*. *Human Molecular Genetics* **9**, 13–25.

Martel, J. C., Chopin, P., Colpaert, F., and Marien, M. (1998). Neuroprotective effects of the α2-adrenoceptor antagonists, (+)-efaroxan and (+/−)-idazoxan, against quinolinic acid-induced lesions in the rat striatum. *Experimental Neurology* **154**, 595–601.

Martinez-Mir, M. I., Pollard, H., Moreau, J., Traiffort, E., Ruat, M., Schwartz, J. C., and Palacios, J. M. (1993). Loss of striatal histamine H2 receptors in Huntington's chorea but not in Parkinson's disease: comparison with animal models. *Synapse* **15**, 209–220.

Matthews, R. T., Ferrante, R. J., Jenkins, B. G., Browne, S. E., Goetz, K., Berger, S., Chen, I. Y.-C., and Beal, M. F. (1997). Iodoacetate produces striatal excitotoxic lesions. *Journal of Neurochemistry* **69**, 285–289.

Mazzola, J. L. and Sirover, M. A. (2001). Reduction of glyceraldehyde-3-phosphate dehydrogenase activity in Alzheimer's disease and in Huntington's disease fibroblasts. *Journal of Neurochemistry* **76**, 442–449.

McGeer, E. G. and McGeer, P. L. (1976a). Duplication of biochemical changes of Huntington's chorea by intrastriatal injections of glutamic acid and kainic acids. *Nature* **263**, 517–519.

McGeer, P. L. and McGeer, E. G. (1976b). Enzymes associated with the metabolism of catecholamines, acetylcholine and gaba in human controls and patients with Parkinson's disease and Huntington's chorea. *Journal of Neurochemistry* **26**, 65–76.

Menalled, L., Zanjani, H., MacKenzie, L., Koppel, A., Carpenter, E., Zeitlin, S., and Chesselet, M. F. (2000). Decrease in striatal enkephalin mRNA in mouse models of Huntington's disease. *Experimental Neurology* **162**, 328–342.

Mizukawa, K., McGeer, E. G., and McGeer, P. L. (1993). Autoradiographic study on dopamine uptake sites and their correlation with dopamine levels and their striata from patients with Parkinson disease, Alzheimer disease, and neurologically normal controls. *Molecular Chemistry and Neuropathology* **18**, 133–144.

Monaghan, D., Bridges, R., and Cotman, C. (1989). The excitatory amino acid receptors: their classes, pharmacology, and distinct properties in the function of the central nervous system. *Annual Review of Pharmacology and Toxicology* **29**, 365–402.

Monaghan, D. T., Olverman, H. J., Nguyen, L., Watkins, J. C., and Cotman, C. W. (1988). Two classes of N-methyl-D-aspartate recognition sites: differential distribution and differential regulation by glycine. *Proceedings of the National Academy of Sciences, USA* **85**, 9836–9840.

Morton, A. J. and Edwardson, J. M. (2001). Progressive depletion of complexin II in a transgenic mouse model of Huntington's disease. *Journal of Neurochemistry* **76**, 166–172.

Muller, E. E., Parati, E. A., Panerai, A. E., Cocchi, D., and Caraceni, T. (1979). Growth hormone hyper-responsiveness to dopaminergic stimulation in Huntington's chorea. *Neuroendocrinology* **28**, 313–319.

Murphy, K. P. S. J., Carter, R. J., Lione, L. A., Mangiarini, L., Mahal, A., Bates, G. P., Dunnett, S. P., and Morton, A. J. (2000). Abnormal synaptic plasticity and impaired spatial cognition in mice transgenic for exon 1 of the human Huntington's disease mutation. *Journal of Neuroscience* **20**, 5115–5123.

Nemeroff, C. B., Youngblood, W. W., Manberg, P. J., Prange, A. J., and Kizer, J. S. (1983). Regional brain concentrations of neuropeptides in Huntington's chorea and schizophrenia. *Science* **221**, 972–975.

Newman, R. P., Tamminga, C. A., Chase, T. N., and LeWitt, P. A. (1985). EMD 23,448: effects of a putative dopamine autoreceptor agonist in chorea. *Journal of Neural Transmission* **61**, 125–129.

Nicniocaill, B., Haraldsson, B., Hansson, O., O'Connor, W. T., and Brundin, P. (2001). Altered striatal amino acid neurotransmitter release monitored using microdialysis in R6/1 Huntington transgenic mice. *European Journal of Neuroscience* **13**, 206–210.

Orlando, L. R., Standaert, D. G., Penney Jr, J. B., and Young, A. B. (1995). Metabotropic glutamate receptors in excitotoxicity: (S)-4-carboxy-3-hydroxyphenylglycine ((S)-4C3HPG) protects against striatal quinolinic acid lesions. *Neuroscience Letters* **202**, 109–112.

Ostergaard, K., Finsen, B., and Zimmer, J. (1995). Organotypic slice cultures of the rat striatum: an immunocytochemical, histochemical and *in situ* hybridization study of somatostatin, neuropeptide Y, nicotinamide adenine dinucleotide phosphate-diaphorase, and enkephalin. *Experimental Brain Research* **103**, 70–84.

Palacios, J. M., Chinaglia, G., Rigo, M., Ulrich, J., and Probst, A. (1991). Neurotensin receptor binding levels in basal ganglia are not altered in Huntington's chorea or schizophrenia. *Synapse* **7**, 114–122.

Palfi, S. P., Ferrante, R. J., Brouillet, E., Beal, M. F., Dolan, R., Guyot, M. C., Peschanski, M., and Hantraye, P. (1996). Chronic 3-nitropropionic acid treatment in baboons replicates the cognitive and motor deficits of Huntington's disease. *Journal of Neuroscience* **16**, 3019–3025.

Panov, A., Obertone, T., Bennett-Desmelik, J., and Greenamyre, J. T. (1999). Ca(2+)-dependent permeability transition and complex I activity in lymphoblast mitochondria from normal individuals and patients with Huntington's or Alzheimer's disease. *Annals of the New York Academy of Science* **893**, 365–368.

Pearson, S. J., Heathfield, K. W., and Reynolds, G. P. (1990). Pallidal GABA and chorea in Huntington's disease. *Journal of Neural Transmission, Genetics Section* **81**, 241–246.

Penney, J. B. Jr and Young, A. B. (1982). Quantitative autoradiography of neurotransmitter receptors in Huntington's disease. *Neurology* **32**, 1391–1395.

Perry, T. L., Hansen, S., and Kloster, M. (1973). Huntington's chorea: deficiency of gamma-aminobutyric acid in brain. *New England Journal of Medicine* **288**, 337–342.

Peters, M. F., Nucifora, F. C., Jr., Kushi, J., Seaman, H. C., Cooper, J. K., Herring, W. J., Dawson, V. L., Dawson, T. M., and Ross, C. A. (1999). Nuclear targeting of mutant huntingtin increases toxicity. *Molecular Cellular Neuroscience* **14**, 121–128.

Pirker, W., Asenbaum, S., Wenger, S., Kornhuber, J., Angelberger, P., Deecke, L., Podreka, I., and Brucke, T. (1997). Iodine-123-epidepride-SPECT: studies in Parkinson's disease, multiple system atrophy and Huntington's disease. *Journal of Nuclear Medicine* **38**, 1711–1717.

Reddy, P. H., Williams, M., Charles, V., Garrett, L., Pike-Buchanan, L., Whetsell, W. O. Jr, Miller, G., and Tagle, D. A. (1998). Behavioural abnormalities and selective neuronal loss in HD transgenic mice expressing mutated full-length HD cDNA. *Nature Genetics* **20**, 198–202.

Reiner, A. and Anderson, K. D. (1990). The patterns of neurotransmitter and neuropeptide co-occurrence among striatal projection neurons: conclusions based on recent findings. *Brain Research Reviews* **15**, 251–265.

—— Albin, R. L., Anderson, K. D., D'Amato, C. J., Penney, J. B., and Young, A. B. (1988). Differential loss of striatal projection neurons in Huntington disease. *Proceedings of the National Academy of Sciences, USA* **85**, 5733–5737.

Reisine, T. D., Fields, J. Z., Stern, L. Z., Johnson, P. C., Bird, E. D., and Yamamura, H. I. (1977). Alterations in dopaminergic receptors in Huntington's disease. *Life Sciences* **21**, 1123–1128.

—— —— Bird, E. D., Spokes, E., and Yamamura, H. I. (1978). Characterization of brain dopaminergic receptors in Huntington's disease. *Communications in Psychopharmacology* **2**, 79–84.

—— Beaumont, K., Bird, E. D., Spokes, E., and Yamamura, H. I. (1979a). Huntington's disease: alterations in neurotransmitter receptor binding in the human brain. *Advances in Neurology* **23**, 717–726.

—— Wastek, G. J., Speth, R. C., Bird, E. D., and Yamamura, H. I. (1979b). Alterations in the benzodiazepine receptor of Huntington's diseased human brain. *Brain Research* **165**, 183–187.

—— Overstreet, D., Gale, K., Rossor, M., Iversen, L., and Yamamura, H. I. (1980). Benzodiazepine receptors: the effect of GABA on their characteristics in human brain and their alteration in Huntington's disease. *Brain Research* **199**, 79–88.

Reynolds, D. S., Carter, R. J., and Morton, A. J. (1998). Dopamine modulates the susceptibility of striatal neurons to 3- nitropropionic acid in the rat model of Huntington's disease. *Journal of Neuroscience* **18**, 10116–10127.

Reynolds, G. P. and Garrett, N. J. (1986). Striatal dopamine and homovanillic acid in Huntington's disease. *Journal of Neural Transmission* **65**, 151–155.

—— Pearson, S. J. (1987). Decreased glutamic acid and increased 5-hydroxytryptamine in Huntington's disease brain. *Neuroscience Letters* **78**, 233–238.

—— —— (1990). Brain GABA levels in asymptomatic Huntington's disease. *New England Journal of Medicine* **323**, 682.

—— —— Hutson, P. H. (1994). Deficit of [3H]L-689,560 binding to the glycine site of the glutamate/ NMDA receptor in the brain in Huntington's disease. *Journal of Neurologic Sciences* **125**, 46–49.

—— Boulton, R. M., Pearson, S. J., Hudson, A. L., and Nutt, D. J. (1996). Imidazoline binding sites in Huntington's and Parkinson's disease putamen. *European Journal of Pharmacology* **301**, R19–R21.

—— Dalton, C. F., Tillery, C. L., Mangiarini, L., Davies, S. W., and Bates, G. P. (1999). Brain neurotransmitter deficits in mice transgenic for the Huntington's disease mutation. *Journal of Neurochemistry* **72**, 1773–1776.

Richfield, E. K. and Herkenham, M. (1994). Selective vulnerability in Huntington's disease: preferential loss of cannabinoid receptors in lateral globus pallidus. *Annals of Neurology* **36**, 577–584.

—— O'Brien, C. F., Eskin, T., and Shoulson, I. (1991). Heterogeneous dopamine receptor changes in early and late Huntington's disease. *Neuroscience Letters* **132**, 121–126.

—— Maguire-Zeiss, K. A., Vonkeman, H. E., and Voorn, P. (1995). Preferential loss of preproenkephalin versus preprotachykinin neurons from the striatum of Huntington's disease patients. *Annals of Neurology* **38**, 852–861.

Rigamonti, D., Bauer, J. H., De-Fraja, C., Conti, L., Sipione, S., Sciorati, C., Clementi, E., Hackam, A., Hayden, M. R., Li, Y., Cooper, J. K., Ross, C. A., Govoni, S., Vincenz, C., and Cattaneo, E. (2000). Wild-type huntingtin protects from apoptosis upstream of caspase-3. *Journal of Neuroscience* **20**, 3705–3713.

Sapp, E., Ge, P., Aizawa, H., Bird, E., Penney, J., Young, A. B., Vonsattel, J. P., and DiFiglia, M. (1995). Evidence for a preferential loss of enkephalin immunoreactivity in the external globus pallidus in low grade Huntington's disease using high resolution image analysis. *Neuroscience* **64**, 397–404.

Sathasivam, K., Hobbs, C., Mangiarini, L., Mahal, A., Turmaine, M., Doherty, P., Davies, S. W., and Bates, G. P. (1999). Transgenic models of Huntington's disease. *Philosophical Transaction of the Royal Society of London B Biological Sciences* **354**, 963–969.

Saudou, F., Finkbeiner, S., Devys, D., and Greenberg, M. E. (1998). Huntingtin acts in the nucleus to induce apoptosis but death does not correlate with the formation of intranuclear inclusions. *Cell* **95**, 55–66.

Sawa, A., Wiegand, G. W., Cooper, J., Margolis, R. L., Sharp, A. H., Lawler, J. F. Jr, Greenamyre, J. T., Snyder, S. H., and Ross, C. A. (1999). Increased apoptosis of Huntington disease lymphoblasts associated with repeat length-dependent mitochondrial depolarization. *Nature Medicine* **5**, 1194–1198.

Schilling, G., Becher, M. W., Sharp, A. H., Jinnah, H. A., Duan, K., Kotzuk, J. A., Slunt, H. H., Ratovitski, T., Cooper, J. K., Jenkins, N. A., Copeland, N. G., Price, D. L., Ross, C. A., and Borchelt, D. R. (1999). Intranuclear inclusions and neuritic aggregates in transgenic mice expressing a mutant N-terminal fragment of huntingtin. *Human Molecular Genetics* **8**, 397–407.

Schulz, J. B., Matthews, R. T., Klockgether, T., Dichgans, J., and Beal, M. F. (1997). The role of mitochondrial dysfunction and neuronal nitric oxide in animal models of neurodegenerative diseases. *Molecular Cellular Biochemistry* **174**, 193–197.

Schwarcz, R., Whetsell W. O. Jr, and Mangano, R. M. (1983). Quinolinic acid: an endogenous metabolite that produces axon-sparing lesions in rat brain. *Science* **219**, 316–318.

Schwarcz, R., Tamminga, C. A., Kurlan, R., and Shoulson, I. (1988). Cerebrospinal fluid levels of quinolinic acid in Huntington's disease and schizophrenia. *Annals of Neurology* **24**, 580–582.

Seeman, P., Bzowej, N. H., Guan, H. C., Bergeron, C., Reynolds, G. P., Bird, E. D., Riederer, P., Jellinger, K., and Tourtellotte, W. (1987). Human brain D1 and D2 dopamine receptors in schizophrenia, Alzheimer's, Parkinson's, and Huntington's diseases. *Neuropsychopharmacology* **1**, 5–15.

—— Niznik, H. B., Guan, H.-C., Booth, G., and Ulpian, C. (1989). Link between D1 and D2 dopamine receptors is reduced in schizophrenia and Huntington diseased brain. *Proceedings of the National Academy of Sciences, USA* **86**, 10156–10160.

Sen, A. P., Boksa, P., and Quirion, R. (1993). Brain calcium channel related dihydropyridine and phenylalkylamine binding sites in Alzheimer's, Parkinson's and Huntington's diseases. *Brain Research* **611**, 216–221.

Seizinger, B. R., Lidbisch, D. C., Kish, S. J., Arendt, R. M., Hornykiewicz, O., and Herz, A. (1986). Opioid peptides in Huntington's disease: alterations in prodynorphin and proenkephalin system. *Brain Research* **378**, 405–408.

Shelbourne, P. F., Killeen, N., Hevner, R. F., Johnston, H. M., Tecott, L., Lewandoski, M., Ennis, M., Ramirez, L., Li, Z., Iannicola, C., Littman, D. R., and Myers, R. M. (1999). A Huntington's disease CAG expansion at the murine Hdh locus is unstable and associated with behavioural abnormalities in mice. *Human Molecular Genetics* **8**, 763–774.

Smith, M. A., Brandt, J., and Shadmehr, R. (2000). Motor disorder in Huntington's disease begins as a dysfunction in error feedback control [see comments]. *Nature* **403**, 544–549.

Spindel, E. R., Wurtman, R. J., and Bird, E. D. (1980). Increased TRH content of the basal ganglia in Huntington's disease [letter]. *New England Journal of Medicine* **303**, 1235–1236.

Spokes, E. G. (1980). Neurochemical alterations in Huntington's chorea: a study of post-mortem brain tissue. *Brain* **103**, 179–210.

Staffen, W., Hondl, N., Trinka, E., Zenzmaier, R., and Ladurner, G. (1997). SPET investigations in extrapyramidal diseases using specific ligands. *Nuclear Medicine Communications* **18**, 159–163.

Standaert, D. G., Friberg, I. K., Landwehrmeyer, G. B., Young, A. B., and Penney, J. B. Jr (1999). Expression of NMDA glutamate receptor subunit mRNAs in neurochemically identified projection and interneurons in the striatum of the rat. *Brain Research Molecular Brain Research* **64**, 11–23.

Steward, L. J., Bufton, K. E., Hopkins, P. C., Davies, W. E., and Barnes, N. M. (1993). Reduced levels of 5-HT3 receptor recognition sites in the putamen of patients with Huntington's disease. *European Journal of Pharmacology* **242**, 137–143.

Surmeier, D. J., Reiner, A., Levine, M. S., and Ariano, M. A. (1993). Are neostriatal dopamine receptors co-localized? *Trends in Neurosciences* **16**, 299–305.

Tanaka, C., Nishino, N., Hashimoto, T., Kitamura, N., Yoshihara, C., and Saito, N. (1993). Second messenger systems in brains of patients with Parkinson's or Huntington's disease. *Advances in Neurology* **60**, 175–180.

Utal, A. K., Stopka, A. L., Roy, M., and Coleman, P. D. (1998). PEP-19 immunohistochemistry defines the basal ganglia and associated structures in the adult human brain, and is dramatically reduced in Huntington's disease. *Neuroscience* **86**, 1055–1063.

Vacca, L. L. (1983). Substance P appears reduced in Huntington's disease: immunocytochemical findings in substantia nigra and substantia gelatinosa. *Journal of Submicroscopical Cytology* **15**, 569–582.

Vacca-Galloway, L. L. (1985). Differential immunostaining for substance P in Huntington's diseased and normal spinal cord: significance of serial (optimal, supra-optimal and end-point) dilutions of primary anti-serum in comparing biological specimens. *Histochemistry* **83**, 561–569.

van Dellen, A., Blakemore, C., Deacon, R., York, D., and Hannan, A. J. (2000). Environmental enrichment delays disease onset in a mouse model of Huntington's disease. *Nature* **404**, 721–722.

Varani, K., Rigamonti, D., Sipione, S., Camurri, A., Borea, P. A., Cattabeni, F., Abbracchio, M. P., and Cattaneo, E. (2001). Aberrant amplification of A2A receptor signaling in striatal cells expressing mutant huntingtin. *FASEB J* **5**, 5.

Vis, J. C., Nicholson, L. F. B., Faull, R. L. M., Evans, W. H., Severs, N. J., and Green, C. R. (1998). Connexin expression in Huntington's diseased human brain. *Cell Biology International* **22**, 837–847.

—— Verbeek, M. M., De Waal, R. M., Ten Donkelaar, H. J., and Kremer, H. P. (1999). 3-Nitropropionic acid induces a spectrum of Huntington's disease-like neuropathology in rat striatum. *Neuropathology and Applied Neurobiology* **25**, 513–521.

Vonsattel, J. P., Myers, R. H., Stevens, T. J., Ferrante, R. J., Bird, E. D., and Richardson, E. P. (1985). Neuropathological classification of Huntington's disease. *Journal of Neuropathology and Experimental Neurology* **44**, 559–577.

Waeber, C. and Palacios, J. M. (1989). Serotonin-1 receptor binding sites in the human basal ganglia are decreased in Huntington's chorea but not in Parkinson's disease: a quantitative *in vitro* autoradiography study. *Neuroscience* **32**, 337–347.

—— Rigo, M., Chinaglia, G., Probst, A., and Palacios, J. M. (1991). Beta-adrenergic receptor subtypes in the basal ganglia of patients with Huntington's chorea and Parkinson's disease. *Synapse* **8**, 270–280.

Wagster, M. V., Hedreen, J. C., Peyser, C. E., Folstein, S. E., and Ross, C. A. (1994). Selective loss of [3H]kainic acid and [3H]AMPA binding in layer VI of frontal cortex in Huntington's disease. *Experimental Neurology* **127**, 70–75.

Walker, F. O., Young, A. B., Penney, J. B., Dorovini-Zis, K., and Shoulson, I. (1984). Benzodiazepine receptors in early Huntington's disease. *Neurology* **34**, 1237–1240.

Warsh, J. J., Politsky, J. M., Li, P. P., Kish, S. J., and Hornykiewicz, O. (1991). Reduced striatal [3H]inositol 1,4,5-trisphosphate binding in Huntington's disease. *Journal of Neurochemistry* **56**, 1417–1422.

Wastek, G. J. and Yamamura, H. I. (1978). Biochemical characterization of the muscarinic cholinergic receptor in human brain: alterations in Huntington's disease. *Molecular Pharmacology* **14**, 768–780.

—— Johnson, P. C., Stern, L. Z., and Yamamura, H. I. (1976). Alterations in brain muscarinic cholinergic receptor binding and choline acetyltransferase activity in Huntington's disease. *Proceedings of the Western Pharmacology Society* **19**, 170–171.

Weed, M. R. and Gold, L. H. (1998). The effects of dopaminergic agents on reaction time in rhesus monkeys. *Psychopharmacology (Berlin)* **137**, 33–42.

Weeks, R. A., Piccini, P., Harding, A. E., and Brooks, D. J. (1996). Striatal D1 and D2 dopamine receptor loss in asymptomatic mutation carriers of Huntington's disease. *Annals of Neurology* **40**, 49–54.

—— Cunningham, V. J., Piccini, P., Waters, S., Harding, A. E., and Brooks, D. J. (1997). 11C-diprenorphine binding in Huntington's disease: a comparison of region of interest analysis with statistical parametric mapping. *Journal of Cerebral Blood Flow Metabolism* **17**, 943–949.

Wong, E. H., Reynolds, G. P., Bonhaus, D. W., Hsu, S., and Eglen, R. M. (1996). Characterization of [3H]GR 113808 binding to 5-HT4 receptors in brain tissues from patients with neurodegenerative disorders. *Behavioural Brain Research* **73**, 249–252.

Wong, P. T., McGeer, P. L., Rossor, M., and McGeer, E. G. (1982). Ornithine aminotransferase in Huntington's disease. *Brain Research* **231**, 466–471.

Wu, C., Singh, S. K., Dias, P., Kumar, S., and Mann, D. M. (1999). Activated astrocytes display increased 5-HT2a receptor expression in pathological states. *Experimental Neurology* **158**, 529–533.

Wyttenbach, A., Swartz, J., Kita, H., Thykjaer, T., Carmichael, J., Bradley, J., Brown, R., Maxwell, M., Schapira, A., Orntoft, T. F., Kato, K., and Rubinsztein, D. C. (2001). Polyglutamine expansions cause decreased CRE-mediated transcription and early gene expression changes prior to cell death in an inducible cell model of Huntington's disease. *Human Molecular Genetics* **10**, 1829–1845.

Young, A. B. and Penney, J. B. (1984). Neurochemical anatomy of movement disorders. *Neurological Clinics* **2**, 417–433.

—— Greenamyre, J. T., Hollingsworth, Z., Albin, R., D'Amato, C., Shoulson, I., and Penney, J. B. (1988). NMDA receptor losses in putamen from patients with Huntington's disease. *Science* **241**, 981–983.

10   Energy metabolism and Huntington's disease

C. Turner and A.H.V. Schapira

Introduction

Huntington's disease (HD) is clinically characterized by a movement disorder and dementia. It is an autosomal dominant condition caused by a CAG repeat expansion within the IT15 gene on chromosome 4, which encodes a 349 kDa protein, huntingtin, of unknown function (Huntington's Disease Collaborative Research Group 1993). There is widespread neuropathology in the HD brain, but it is especially severe in the caudate nucleus where the medium γ-aminobutyric acid (GABA)ergic spiny neurones are mostly affected. The putamen and cortex are less affected and the cerebellum is relatively spared (Vonsattel *et al.* 1985). The cause of such specific neuronal loss is uncertain. There has been increasing evidence over the past 20 years that there is a defect in energy metabolism in HD. An energy defect may lead or contribute to free radical generation, slow excitotoxicity, mitochondrial dysfunction, decreased mitochondrial membrane potential, a lower threshold for apoptosis, and alterations in the haemodynamic responsivity of the cerebral vessels. Some or all of these processes could lead to neurodegeneration. In this chapter, we will review the evidence for defects in energy metabolism in HD and discuss their putative role in the pathogenesis of neurodegeneration in this disorder.

The role of imaging in detecting metabolic defects

Positron emission tomography

During the 1980s positron emission tomography (PET) in conjunction with [18F]deoxyglucose was used extensively to investigate regional utilization of glucose in HD brains. Most studies demonstrated a decrease in striatal regional cerebral metabolic rates for glucose and oxygen (rCMRGlc and rCMRO$_2$, respectively) in symptomatic HD patients (Kuhl *et al.* 1982; Leenders *et al.* 1986). More recent studies have demonstrated a defect in the cerebral cortex and striatum but not in the thalamus and cerebellum (Kuwert *et al.* 1990; Martin *et al.* 1992). The degree of dementia and the duration of chorea correlated with the severity of the defects in most cortical regions and the caudate nucleus. The severity of the chorea correlated more specifically with the defect in the lentiform nucleus, whereas the degree of disability correlated with defects in most cortical regions except the occipital and superior frontal cortex. These initial studies provided evidence that there are widespread changes in HD brains, which involve cortical as well as subcortical structures.

Further studies examined individuals at risk of HD. Before genetic testing became available in the late 1990s, it was suggested that striatal hypometabolism could be used as a method of presymptomatic diagnosis. Striatal defects have been described in presymptomatic/chorea-free/at-risk patients (Mazziotta *et al.* 1987; Grafton *et al.* 1990, 1992; Kuwert *et al.* 1993). In one study (Mazziotta *et al.* 1987), 31 per cent of individuals at risk for HD had reduced caudate glucose metabolism bilaterally compared to an expected gene frequency in this group of 34 per cent. As these studies were performed before genetic testing was available, precise correlation between genotype and PET data could not be made. The similarity between the predicted frequency of HD in the at-risk populations and the frequency of hypometabolism in the striatum suggested that there was an association between presymptomatic HD and a striatal energy defect. All the presymptomatic patients with striatal hypometabolism had a normal computerized tomography (CT) brain scan, which suggested that the metabolic defect preceded gross tissue loss and dysfunction.

In conclusion, PET studies are suggestive of a defect in energy utilization in HD striatum and cortex and imply that the dementia seen in HD is not purely subcortical. The PET studies do not distinguish between failure of energy utilization secondary to atrophy, which cannot be detected on a CT scan, and a primary defect in energy metabolism within the neurones. There is the potential for using PET to monitor progression of disease and putative treatments in the future, although the advent of nuclear magnetic resonance spectroscopy (MRS) has made it possible to study metabolic defects more accurately and in greater detail. Further details of imaging studies are discussed in Chapter 4.

Nuclear magnetic resonance spectroscopy

An initial study using ^{1}H MRS in HD demonstrated elevated lactate levels in the occipital cortex and variable rises in the basal ganglia of symptomatic patients (Jenkins *et al.* 1993). The level of occipital lactate also correlated with the duration of illness. Unfortunately, there was wide variability in the data from the striatum possibly because of spectroscopic artefacts but also due to relatively fewer living neurones in the striatum. The striatal levels of *N*-acetyl aspartate (NAA), a putative neuronal marker, were reduced and those of choline (Ch), a putative glial marker, were elevated. This suggested that there was striatal neurodegeneration and gliosis. Further studies confirmed these findings (Davie *et al.* 1994; Martin *et al.* 1996).

Subsequently, ^{1}H MRS demonstrated increased lactate in the frontal cortex of approximately 50 per cent of symptomatic HD patients and four presymptomatic individuals (Harms *et al.* 1997). A reduced NAA/Ch ratio in the symptomatic patients was also found and this was related to disease severity. There has been much interest in the role of NAA as a marker of neuronal health in NMR and choline as a marker of gliosis. The reduced ratio in HD suggested that there was selective neuronal degeneration. In the same study, there was no reduction in the NAA/Ch ratio in the presymptomatic HD individuals, suggesting that defects in energy metabolism occur before gross neuronal loss and before phenotypic expression.

A further study using ^{31}P MRS demonstrated that there was a significant decrease in the phosphocreatine to inorganic phosphate ratio in symptomatic HD patients' muscle. This suggested a widespread defect in energy metabolism in HD that was not confined to the nervous system. In the same study it was demonstrated that the oral administration of coenzyme Q_{10}, an essential component of the mitochondrial respiratory chain, significantly reduced occipital cortex lactate levels as measured by ^{1}H MRS in symptomatic HD patients. The levels of lactate returned to pretreatment values when the coenzyme Q_{10} was stopped, supporting a treatment-related effect (Koroshetz *et al.* 1997). A recent randomized placebo-controlled trial of coenzyme Q_{10} and remacemide (a noncompetitive *N*-methyl-D-aspartate (NMDA) receptor antagonist) demonstrated no significant benefit in early HD. There was a trend towards slower disease progression with coenzyme Q_{10}, but remacemide had no clinical benefit. Unfortunately, the trial was designed to identify an approximate 35–40 per cent reduction in functional decline and so smaller benefits would have been missed (Huntington Study Group 2001).

A larger cohort of symptomatic HD patients have been studied using ^{1}H MRS and an elevated lactate level in the occipital cortex was confirmed as well as variable increases in the frontal and parietal cortices. They also demonstrated, using extremely small voxels (2–4 µl), highly elevated lactate levels in the striata of HD patients that showed a marked asymmetry towards higher levels in the left striatum. This has been related to asymmetric activation of the striata, as all patients were right-handed. The lactate levels were independent of NAA and choline levels suggesting a metabolic effect as opposed to differences in neuronal and glial populations. They also demonstrated that CAG repeat length, especially when over 45, correlated with levels of striatal lactate. Three of the eight asymptomatic patients they studied demonstrated elevated striatal lactate suggesting that energy-related defects occur before clinical diagnosis is possible (Jenkins *et al.* 1998).

A recent study examined *in vivo* muscle energy metabolism in HD and dentatorubropallidoluyusian atrophy (DRPLA) using ^{31}P MRS. At rest, there was a reduced phosphocreatine (PCr)/inorganic phosphate ratio in the symptomatic patients only. Muscle adenosine triphosphate (ATP)/(PCr+inorganic phosphate) was significantly reduced in both symptomatic and presymptomatic patients. During recovery from exercise the maximum rate of ATP production (V_{max}) in muscle was also reduced. The V_{max} deficit over age also correlated with CAG repeat length (Fig. 10.1). These findings support a role for mitochondrial dysfunction in the pathogenesis of HD. They also suggest that ^{31}P MRS may act as a surrogate marker by which to study disease progression and response to therapy (Lodi *et al.* 2000).

Defects in creatine and NAA levels have been found in presymptomatic (30 per cent) and symptomatic (60 per cent) HD caudate on ^{1}H MRS. The levels of creatine also correlated with CAG repeat length and performance in cognitive timed tests (Sanchez-Pernaute *et al.* 1999).

^{1}H MRS has been performed on the cerebrospinal fluid (CSF) of patients with HD. A slight but significant reduction in lactate and citrate was found in HD patients but not Parkinson's disease (PD) patients. The significance of these observations is uncertain but may relate to impaired glycolysis and Kreb's cycle function or to gross neuronal loss (Garseth *et al.* 2000).

Several studies have found an elevated lactate to pyruvate ratio in symptomatic HD CSF samples, which directly supports the data obtained from NMR of the brain but not that of the CSF (Koroshetz *et al.* 1997).

A more recent study using ^{1}H and ^{31}P MRS failed to demonstrate a significant increase in putaminal or occipital cortical lactate levels or a decrease in the phosphocreatine or ATP levels. The authors suggested that contamination from surrounding CSF might explain apparent increases in HD brain lactate (Hoang *et al.* 1998).

There are alternative explanations for the elevated lactate levels observed in HD patients. Enhanced neuronal stimulation leads to elevated lactate levels due to increased anaerobic glycolysis. This explanation appears unlikely as one would then expect elevated glucose utilization in the cortex and striatum but PET studies suggest that there is a reduction (Kuhl *et al.* 1982; Leenders *et al.* 1986). Mismatching of blood flow and neural activity might also cause elevated lactate levels but the little data available on regional blood flow suggest that it is normal in HD (Weinberger *et al.* 1998).

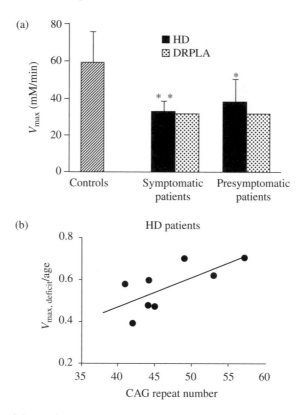

Fig. 10.1 (a) Deficit of the maximum rate of mitochondrial adenosine triphosphate production (V_{max}) in the skeletal muscle of symptomatic (8 HD and 1 dentatorubropallidoluysian atrophy (DRPLA)) and presymptomatic (4 HD and 1 DRPLA) patients compared with that in 12 controls (**$p = 0.0007$, *$p = 0.04$). (b) Correlation between skeletal muscle V_{max} deficit over age and the number of CAG repeats in the 8 symptomatic HD patients ($r = 0.71$, $p = 0.04$). (Reproduced with permission, from Lodi *et al.* (2000, © John Wiley & Sons, Inc.)

Imaging in animal models of HD

The development of the 'MicroPET' has enabled functional *in vivo* studies in rodents. Rats with unilateral quinolinic acid-induced striatal lesions demonstrated decreased 2-deoxy-2-[^{18}F]fluoro-D-glucose (FDG) uptake in the lesioned side 1 week after injection, consistent with a defect in energy metabolism secondary to excitotoxic damage to the striatum (Araujo *et al.* 2000).

The R6/2 mouse was the first transgenic mouse model of HD. The transgene contains the first exon of huntingtin with an expanded CAG repeat length between 141 and 157 (Mangiarini *et al.* 1996; further details are available in Chapter 13, this volume). NMR analysis of R6/2 mice brains has demonstrated a large nonlinear drop in NAA levels, commencing at 6 weeks of age, coincident with the onset of symptoms and the presence of intranuclear inclusions but in the absence of neuronal death (Jenkins *et al.* 2000). *In vitro* NMR analysis also revealed significant increases in glutamine taurine, cholines, and inositol and decreases in glutamate and succinate. It is speculated that the elevation in glutamine represents a profound metabolic defect associated with a decrease in activity of glutaminase. This is a mitochondrial enzyme in neurones, responsible for the conversion of glutamine to glutamate, and is probably involved in the glutamate/glutamine neuronal/glial cycling system.

Further studies using the R6/2 mouse have demonstrated that dietary supplementation with creatine enhances brain creatine levels and reduces the drop in NAA with time. This suggests that enriching metabolic pathways with creatine may slow neuronal dysfunction (Ferrante *et al.* 2000).

Chronic systemic administration of 3-nitropropionic acid (3-NP), which is an inhibitor of succinate dehydrogenase (SDH) or complex II, reproduces most of the motor, cognitive, and histopathological features of HD in primates, rodents, and humans. The temporal and spatial evolution of lesions induced by 3-NP in rats has been studied using magnetic resonance imaging (MRI), where diffusion-weighted images were more sensitive at detecting lesions than T2-weighted images (3 hours versus 4.5 hours post-dose) and lesions were observed in the striatum, hippocampus, and corpus callosum but not the cerebral cortex (Chyi and Chang 1999).

Serial ^{1}H MRS has been used to assess the striatal and occipital cortical concentrations of NAA, phosphocreatine/creatine, choline, and lactate every 2 weeks in 3-NP-treated baboons (Dautry *et al.* 1999). A region-selective increase in lactate was detected in the striatum in association with the formation of a lesion in the dorsolateral putamen on T2-weighted MRI. There was also a region-specific and progressive decrease in NAA, creatine, and choline occurring 3 weeks before the first reduction in lactate. This suggested that NMR might be used to detect the early stages of brain metabolic impairment. The inhibition of SDH by 3-NP occurs throughout the brain but there are selective decreases in NAA and creatine in the striatum, which suggests that there is preferential vulnerability of the striatum to impairment of mitochondrial function by 3-NP.

The mitochondrial respiratory chain in HD

Recently, there has been much interest in the role of mitochondria in neurodegenerative diseases. This is based on the finding of several primary mitochondrial mutations associated with various neurological phenotypes, for example, Leber's hereditary optic neuropathy, as well as *in vitro* and *in vivo* evidence for mitochondrial respiratory chain dysfunction in several neurodegenerative conditions such as PD, Friedreich's ataxia, and HD (Schapira 1999). It is postulated that a defect in mitochondrial function could lead to a defect in energy metabolism that in turn produces depleted intracellular levels of ATP and an increased susceptibility to excitotoxic damage, increased free-radical production, and apoptosis.

Mitochondrial cell biology

The bacterial hypothesis of the origin of mitochondria suggests that alpha-purple bacteria were incorporated into eukaryotic cells and, during evolution, these bacteria transferred many of their essential genes to the nuclear chromosomes (Gray 1992). The mitochondria still have remnants of their bacterial origin such as the use of *N*-formylmethionyl-tRNA as the initiator of protein synthesis (Galper and Darnell 1969; Epler *et al.* 1970).

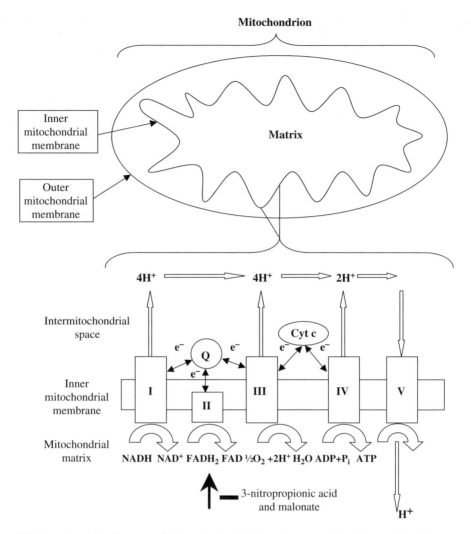

Fig. 10.2 A schematic diagram of the mitochondrial respiratory chain. Cyt c, Cytochrome c; Q, ubiquinone.

The mitochondrial respiratory chain consists of five multisubunit protein complexes, which are located in the inner mitochondrial membrane, and two mobile electron carriers, cytochrome c and ubiquinone (Fig. 10.2). The respiratory chain produces ATP by the production of a proton gradient across the inner mitochondrial membrane, which drives ATP production by ATP synthase or complex V. The proton gradient is produced by the release of protons from complexes I, III, and IV into the intermembranous space. The energy for this process is yielded from the transfer of electrons from NADH/FADH$_2$ through the protein complexes to the final electron acceptor, oxygen. Complex V couples the re-entry of protons to the mitochondrial matrix with the production of ATP. Complex III and, to a lesser extent, complex I are major sites of generation of potentially toxic reactive oxygen species (ROS) (Beal *et al.* 1997).

Each mitochondrion contains 2–10 molecules of circular double-stranded mitochondrial DNA (mtDNA), which encode 22 transfer RNAs, two ribosomal RNAs, and 13 proteins: seven subunits of complex I; cytochrome b of complex III; cytochrome oxidase (COX)I; COXII and COXIII of complex IV; and subunits 6 and 8 of complex V (ATPase) (Anderson et al. 1981; Taanman 1999). mtDNA is inherited through the maternal line. More than 80 mtDNA mutations have been associated with a wide spectrum of human disease (Chinnery et al. 1999). Heteroplasmy is usual, that is, the mutations coexist with normal wild-type molecules (Lightowlers et al. 1997). The proportion of the mutant form varies between tissues depending on segregation during mitosis. A high level of the mutant form is required to produce respiratory chain dysfunction, although this is partly determined by the level of dependence of the tissue on oxidative metabolism. Thus, tissues with a high level of dependence on oxidative respiration, such as neurones, require a high level of ATP production to restore ionic homeostasis following the controlled flux of ions across the cell membrane during electrical signalling. Most of the ATP utilized by Na^+/K^+ ATPase and Ca^{2+} ATPase in maintaining ionic homeostasis is generated in mitochondria.

The mitochondrial hypothesis in neurodegeneration

The mitochondrial hypothesis in neurodegeneration suggests that defects in mitochondrial metabolism lead to a chronic depletion in cellular ATP and a lowered threshold for apoptosis. This may trigger the neurone to enter apoptosis leading to neurodegeneration. Mitochondrial dysfunction may be precipitated by exogenous and endogenous oxidative phosphorylation (OXPHOS) inhibitors or by mutations in nuclear or mitochondrial DNA-encoded OXPHOS subunits or proteins involved in other aspects of mitochondrial function (Leonard and Schapira 2000a, b). This hypothesis is supported by evidence that disorders of mitochondrial function caused by mutations in mtDNA or mitochondrial inhibitors have a role in a variety of neurodegenerative diseases. Indeed, normal ageing may be associated with a gradual reduction in mitochondrial function secondary to mtDNA mutations or other mitochondrial inhibitory processes.

Mitochondrial respiratory chain (MRC) function in HD tissues

Many defects in oxidative phosphorylation in HD post-mortem tissue have been described over the past 30 years. The respiratory chain is illustrated in Fig. 10.2. The early studies demonstrated a complex II defect (Stahl and Swanson 1974; Butterworth et al. 1985). One of the first studies to examine regional mitochondrial respiratory activity in HD isolated mitochondrial membranes from caudate and cerebral cortex and found a reduction in caudate COX activity, and in cytochrome aa3 (complex IV subunit), whereas cytochromes c_1 and b were normal There were no abnormalities in cortical tissue. However, this study did not account for activities relative to a marker of mitochondrial number such as citrate synthase (CS) (Brennan et al. 1985). It was demonstrated subsequently that there was a 77 per cent decrease in caudate complex II/III activity, corrected for CS activities. Activities of complexes I and IV were similar to those of control values (Mann et al. 1990). At the same time, a complex I defect was found in symptomatic HD patients' platelet mitochondria. Complexes II/III and IV were not statistically different from those in controls and at-risk individuals. Again, these results were corrected for protein content only and not for a mitochondrial protein such as CS (Parker et al. 1990). This abnormality of complex I has not subsequently been reproduced (Turner and Schapira, personal communication).

The direct measurement of respiratory chain activity in post-mortem HD caudate nucleus homogenate subsequently demonstrated a severe deficiency of complexes II/III (56 per cent) and IV (33 per cent) activity (Gu *et al.* 1996). Platelet mitochondrial function was not found to be different from that in controls in contrast to an earlier study (Parker *et al.* 1990).

One of the largest post-mortem studies (18 HD patients and 29 controls) examined MRC function in mitochondrial fractions from the frontal and parietal cortex, caudate, putamen, and cerebellum (Browne *et al.* 1997). They found a significant reduction in complex II/III activity in caudate and putamen but not in cortex or cerebellum. A defect in complex IV was also observed in putamen but not elsewhere. This pattern of mitochondrial defect parallels the neuronal cell loss in HD brain. Similar defects have not been described in PD or multiple system atrophy (MSA) suggesting that it is not secondary to nonspecific cell loss. There were also increased levels of 8-hydroxy deoxyguanosine (OH^{8}dG), a marker of free radical generation, in caudate but not putaminal nuclear DNA. There was no effect on caudate or putaminal superoxide dismutase (SOD) or glyceraldehyde-3-phosphate dehydrogenase (GAPDH) activity (Browne *et al.* 1997). A similar but less severe pattern was observed in HD putamen but not cortex, cerebellum, or cultured HD fibroblasts (Tabrizi *et al.* 1999). In agreement with Browne *et al.* (1997), no defect in GADPH activity was found.

Aconitase deficiency was found in HD caudate (92 per cent), putamen (73 per cent), and cortex (48 per cent) but not cerebellum and this deficiency closely follows the pathology in HD (Tabrizi *et al.* 1999). Aconitase is an iron–sulphur (FeS)-containing enzyme that is involved in the Kreb cycle and iron homeostasis. Its activity is especially susceptible to inhibition by $O_2^{\bullet-}$ and by the reaction product of $O_2^{\bullet-}$ with NO$^{\bullet}$, ONOO$^-$, or peroxynitrate (Hausladen and Fridovich 1994; Gardner *et al.* 1994; Patel *et al.* 1996). Complexes II and III are also FeS–containing compounds and they are also susceptible to inhibition by these free radicals. Thus the pattern of enzyme loss in HD suggests that free radicals and excitotoxity have a role in the pathogenesis of the disease.

In contrast to brain, skeletal muscle offers a tissue that can be relatively easily biopsied and has many characteristics in common with neurones, for instance they are post-mitotic cells with a high dependence on oxidative metabolism. ^{31}P MRS has demonstrated a defect of ATP synthesis in skeletal muscle in symptomatic and presymptomatic HD patients that correlates with the length of the CAG repeat. A complex I deficiency has also been described in 3 of 4 muscle biopsies from symptomatic HD patients (Arenas *et al.* 1998). This supports a direct role for a mitochondrial defect secondary to an expanded CAG repeat in HD outside of the central nervous system (CNS) and independent of excitotoxicity. We are currently studying respiratory chain activity in muscle from presymptomatic and symptomatic HD patients. If a mitochondrial defect is found presymptomatically, this will add further weight to the direct role of mitochondrial dysfunction in HD (Shapira 1997, 1999). HD lymphoblasts demonstrated an increased mitochondrial depolarization in response to cyanide, a complex IV inhibitor, but not in response to complex I, II, or III inhibitors. The degree of depolarization was correlated with the CAG repeat length (Sawa *et al.* 1999). Thus a widespread peripheral as well as CNS defect in the MRC seems to occur in HD.

3-Nitropropionic acid: mitochondrial inhibitor and model of HD

The toxin 3-nitropropionic acid (3-NP) irreversibly inhibits succinate dehydrogenase or complex II. It is a widely distributed plant and fungal neurotoxin that causes damage to the basal ganglia, hippocampus, spinal tracts, and peripheral nerves in animals (Alexi *et al.* 1998a). Reports from northern China have suggested that 3-NP can cause putaminal necrosis and delayed dystonia in children who have eaten mildewed sugar cane (Ludolph *et al.* 1991). Accidental ingestion of 3-NP in humans leads to nausea, vomiting, encephalopathy, coma, and, when the subject survives, chorea and dystonia and basal ganglia degeneration (Ludolph *et al.* 1991).

In rats, intrastriatal administration of 3-NP causes dose-dependent ATP depletion, increased lactate concentration, and neuronal loss in the striatum (Beal *et al.* 1993a). The neuronal loss is ameliorated by decortication of the rats. This suggests that the glutaminergic input from the corticostriatal pathway may be required to cause excitotoxic damage in 3-NP-mediated cell death. NMDA receptor antagonists also block the toxic effects of 3-NP, indicating that mitochondrial respiratory chain dysfunction and impaired energy metabolism may predispose to excitotoxic damage (Beal *et al.* 1993b). A reversible SDH inhibitor, malonate, has also been injected intrastriatally into rats to produce lesions similar to but milder than those seen with 3-NP. These lesions are also reduced by glutamate antagonists suggestive of an excitotoxic mechanism (Greene and Greenamyre 1995). The chronic systemic administration of 3-NP in rats produces an animal model displaying lesions that closely resemble the neuropathological features of HD with selective loss of striatal medium spiny neurones. This suggests that the cell population that is most vulnerable in HD is sensitive to energy impairment. Younger animals display more resistance to the neurotoxic effects of 3-NP, suggesting that cellular handling of 3-NP is increasingly impaired with age (Beal *et al.* 1993a).

Three to six weeks of systemic 3-NP administration in primates is sufficient to cause choreiform movements, foot and limb dystonia, and dyskinesia induced by apomorphine. More prolonged exposure results in spontaneous dystonia and dyskinesia accompanied by lesions in the caudate and putamen on MRI. The histopathology is similar to that of HD with depletion of calbindin neurones, gliosis, sparing of NADPH-diaphorase neurones, and growth-related proliferative changes in dendrites of spiny neurones. There is also preservation of the striosomal organization of the striatum and nucleus accumbens, which are features seen in HD (Brouillet *et al.* 1995).

The mechanism linking 3-NP-induced mitochondrial inhibition and cell death is uncertain. In the 3-NP rat model the isolation of striatal and cortical synaptosomes revealed increased levels of protein carbonyls prior to the appearance of morphological changes. Brain synaptosomal proteins also demonstrated a decrease in the W/S ratio, the relevant electron paramagnetic resonance (EPR) parameter used to determine levels of protein oxidation. These results suggest that 3-NP causes widespread and early oxidation of protein and would be consistent with oxidative stress as a link between mitochondrial dysfunction and cell death (La Fontaine *et al.* 2000).

Further insight into possible mechanisms has come from studying the effects of 3-NP in different rodents. The Sprague–Dawley rat appears more susceptible to 3-NP than BALB/c ByJ mice. The rats also demonstrate striatal apoptosis as demonstrated by TUNEL staining, whereas this is not observed in the mice (Alexi *et al.* 1998b). This suggests that there are different mediating factors, such as genetic background, that confer susceptibility to 3-NP. Dissecting out these factors may help further the understanding of the molecular sequence of events that leads to cell death induced by mitochondrial inhibition.

Mitochondrial dysfunction and the R6/2 mouse

Over the past 5 years there have been many different transgenic mouse models produced (Chapter 13). The R6/2 transgenic mouse exhibits progressive neurological disease from

2 months of age, and both the light microscopic and ultrastructural pathology are very similar to those seen in HD brain. These neuropathological features occur approximately 4 weeks prior to a progressive movement disorder and muscle wasting and 10 weeks before neuronal cell death in selected brain regions. This suggests that, in this model, neuronal dysfunction is responsible for the initial phenotype rather than cell death.

Several defects in the respiratory chain have recently been characterized in the R6/2 mouse. These include a reduction in complex IV in the striatum and cerebral cortex and a reduction in aconitase in the striatum (Tabrizi *et al.* 2000; see Fig. 10.3). They were associated with increased immunostaining for inducible nitric oxide synthase (iNOS) and nitrotyrosine (a marker of increased peroxynitrate generation) in the mouse brains. An increase in the lesion size produced by 3-NP in the R6/2 mice and increased striatal 3,4-dihydroxybenzoic acid (a marker of ROS) also support a role for mitochondrial dysfunction and free radical damage (Bogdanov *et al.* 1998).

Recently, creatine has been found to have a protective effect in the R6/2 mouse. Dietary creatine improved survival, slowed the development of brain atrophy, and delayed degeneration of striatal neurones and the formation of intranuclear inclusions. The onset of diabetes was also delayed. NMR in these mice demonstrated delayed decreases in NAA and elevated concentrations of brain creatine (Ferrante *et al.* 2000).

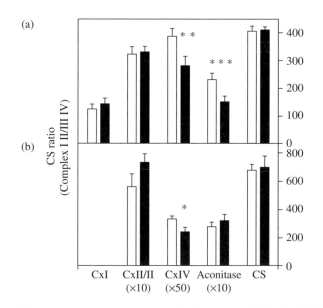

Fig. 10.3 Mitochondrial respiratory chain complex I (Cx I), complex II/III (Cx II/III), and complex IV (Cx IV) citrate synthase (CS) ratios and aconitase activities in (a) striatum and (b) cerebral cortex. Activity data are mean ± SEM values for control (open column) and R6/2 mice for 15 striatum and six cortical samples. Statistical significance by Mann–Whitney U test: $*p < 0.05$; $**p < 0.01$; $***p < 0.005$. (Reproduced with permission from Tabrizi *et al.* (2000), © John Wiley & Sons, Inc.)

Weight loss and HD

It is a well recorded but unexplained observation that HD patients suffer extreme weight loss in spite of an adequate calorific intake. Further studies have found that a higher body mass index (BMI; the ratio of the patient's weight in kilograms to the square of his/her height in metres) at presentation is associated with slower disease progression (Myers *et al.* 1991). These features have also been observed in the R6/2 transgenic mouse. Initially, weight loss was not found to be related to the severity of chorea, but a recent study did find a relationship between the severity of chorea and energy expenditure (Pratley *et al.* 2000). Patient's sedentary energy expenditure is proportionately related to the severity of the movement disorder, but total energy expenditure was the same as that of controls because HD patients tended to not take part in as much voluntary physical activity. Further studies will elucidate whether there is a widespread metabolic defect that can explain this weight loss often observed in HD.

Glyceraldehyde-3-phosphate dehydrogenase (GAPDH)

GAPDH has an essential role in glycolysis. It binds to normal and mutant huntingtin *in vitro* and both GAPDH and huntingtin are present in the cytoplasm and nucleus. The intrastriatal administration of the GAPDH inhibitor iodoacetate produces striatal lesions that are attenuated by decortication, suggesting an excitotoxic mechanism (Matthews *et al.* 1997). Striatal murine cultures are more sensitive than cortical cultures to the GAPDH inhibitor, alpha-monochlorohydrin, with selective sparing of nicotinamide–adenine dinucleotide phosphate (NADPH) diaphorase-positive neurones (Sheline and Choi 1998). Cell death can be attenuated in these experiments by the addition of supraphysiological levels of pyruvate.

Several studies have found normal GAPDH activity in HD post-mortem brain tissue (Browne *et al.* 1997; Tabrizi *et al.* 1999) or unstressed HD fibroblasts (Cooper *et al.* 1998). However, a recent study examined the activity of GAPDH in skin fibroblasts from patients with symptomatic HD and Alzheimer's disease (AD). They found impairment of GAPDH glycolytic function in subcellular fractions in spite of unchanged gene expression in the AD and HD patients. In HD this was most prominent in the nuclear fraction and suggested that the inhibition was a posttranslational event. This suggests that preparation of whole cell or brain tissue destroys subcellular GAPDH interactions that inhibit its glycolytic activity (Mazzola and Sirover 2001). GADPH activity has also been found to be decreased in metabolically stressed HD fibroblasts (Cooper *et al.* 1997). Tissue transglutaminase may cross-link GAPDH with proteins produced from mutant huntingtin processing resulting in reduced GAPDH activity (Gentile *et al.* 1998). The nuclear translocation of GAPDH has been linked to the induction of apoptosis and the finding of markedly reduced activity in the nuclear fraction may indicate a change in catalytic function and an involvement in apoptosis. The changes in function may be induced by the nuclear localization of truncated mutant huntingtin.

Impaired energy metabolism and cell death

Impaired energy metabolism reduces the threshold for glutamate toxicity and can lead to activation of excitotoxic mechanisms and increased production of reactive oxygen species.

Energy depletion can result in partial depolarization of the outer membrane and releases the voltage-dependent Mg^{2+} ion block of the Ca^{2+} channel in the NMDA receptor. Na^+ can also enter via the NMDA receptor and, under conditions of reduced ATP, the Na^+/K^+ ATPase will less effectively extrude Na^+ and intracellular Na^+ levels will rise. This will in turn reduce the efficacy of the Na^+/Ca^{2+} antiport system and also cause an accumulation of Ca^{2+}. Mitochondria, as well as the endoplasmic reticulum and Golgi apparatus, are involved in Ca^{2+} homeostasis in neurones. Calcium entry into mitochondria is linked with opening of the mitochondrial permeability transition pore and cell death (Rizzuto 2001). This function is impaired if the inner mitochondrial membrane potential is more positive than normal because of impaired energy metabolism and a reduced ability to extrude protons (Petersen *et al.* 1999).

Conclusions

The presence of defects in respiratory chain activity associated with excitotoxicity and increased free radical production is now well established in HD. The interaction between these factors and their contribution to the pathogenesis of HD are less well established. The transgenic mouse models of HD enable the dissection of the sequence of molecular events from CAG expansion through to defects in energy metabolism, to neuronal cell dysfunction, and death. The mechanism by which a non-mitochondrial protein, huntingtin, exerts its effect on energy metabolism and mitochondrial function remains elusive and will be the subject of much further research. Future therapeutic strategies will aim to target the primary causes and the defects in energy metabolism with the hope of slowing the neuro-degenerative process.

Acknowledgements

The authors' work described in this review was supported by the Medical Research Council and Wellcome Trust.

References

Alexi T, Hughes PE, Faull RL, Williams CE (1998a). 3-nitropropionic acid's lethal triplet: cooperative pathways of neurodegeneration. *Neuroreport* **9**: R57–64.

——— ——— Knusel B, Tobin AJ (1998b). Metabolic compromise with systemic 3-nitropropionic acid produces striatal apoptosis in Sprague–Dawley rats but not in BALB/c ByJ mice. *Exp Neurol* **153**: 74–93.

Anderson S, Bankier AT, Barrell BG, *et al.* (1981). Sequence and organisation of the human mitochondrial genome. *Nature* **290**: 457–65.

Araujo DM, Cherry SR, Tatsukawa KJ, Toyokuni T, Kornblum HI (2000). Deficits in striatal dopamine D_2 receptors and energy metabolism detected by *in vivo* MicroPET imaging in a rat model of Huntington's disease. *Exp Neurol* **166**: 287–97.

Arenas J, Campos Y, Ribacoba R, *et al.* (1998). Complex I defect in muscle from patients with Huntington's disease. *Ann Neurol* **43**: 397–400.

Beal MF, Brouillet E, Jenkins BG, *et al.* (1993a). Neurochemical and histological characterisation of striatal excitotoxic lesions produced by the mitochondrial toxin 3-nitropropionic acid. *J Neurosci* **13**: 4181–92.

—— —— —— Henshaw R, Rosen BR, Hyman BT (1993b). Age-dependent striatal excitotoxic lesions produced by the endogenous mitochondrial inhibitor malonate. *J Neurochem* **61**: 1147–50.

—— Howell N, Bodis-Wollner I .(1997). *Mitochondria and free radicals in neurodegenerative diseases*. New York: Wiley-Liss.

Bogdanov M, Ferrante RJ, Kuemmerle S, Klivenyi P, Beal MF (1998). Increased vulnerability to 3-nitropropionic acid in an animal model of Huntington's disease. *J Neurochem* **71**: 2642–4.

Brennan WA, Bird ED, Aprille JR (1985). Regional mitochondrial respiratory activity in Huntington's disease brain. *J Neurochem* **44**: 1948–50.

Brouillet E, Hantraye P, Ferrante RJ, *et al.* (1995).Chronic mitochondrial energy impairment produces selective striatal degeneration and abnormal choreiform movements in primates. *Proc Natl Acad Sci USA* **92**: 7105–9.

Browne SE, Bowling AC, MacGarvey U, *et al.* (1997). Oxidative damage and metabolic dysfunction in Huntington's disease: selective vulnerability of the basal ganglia. *Ann Neurol* **41**: 646–53.

Butterworth J, Yates CM, Reynolds GP (1985). Distribution of phosphate-activated glutaminase, succinic dehydrogenase, pyruvate dehydrogenase, and α-glutamyl transpeptidase in post-mortem brain from Huntington's disease and agonal cases. *J Neurol Sci* **67**: 161–71.

Chinnery PF, Howell N, Andrews RA (1999). Clinical mitochondrial genetics. *J Med Genet* **36**: 425–36.

Chyi T, Chang C (1999). Temporal evolution of 3-nitropropionic acid-induced neurodegeneration in the rat brain by T2-weighted, diffusion-weighted, and perfusion resonance imaging. *Neuroscience* **92**: 1035–41.

Cooper AJL, Sheu KFR, Burke JR, *et al.* (1997). Transglutaminase-catalysed inactivation of glyceraldehyde 3-phosphate dehydrogenase and α-ketoglutarate dehydrogenase complexes by polyglutamine domains of pathological length. *Proc Natl Acad Sci USA* **94**: 12604–9.

—— —— —— Srittmatter WJ, Blass JP (1998). Glyceraldehyde 3-phosphate dehydrogenase abnormality in metabolically stressed Huntington disease fibroblasts. *Dev Neurosci* **20**: 462–8.

Dautry C, Conde F, Brouillet E, *et al.* (1999). Serial 1H-NMR spectroscopy study of metabolic impairment in primates chronically treated with the succinate dehydrogenase inhibitor 3-nitropropionic acid. *Neurobiol Dis* **6**:259–68.

Davie CA, Barker GC, Quinn N, Tofts PS, Miller DH (1994). Proton MRS in Huntington's disease. *Lancet* **343**: 1580.

Epler JL, Shugart LR, Barnett WE (1970). N-formylmethionyl transfer ribonucleic acid in mitochondria from *Neurospora*. *Biochemistry* **9**: 3575–9.

Ferrante RJ, Andreassen OA, Jenkins BG, *et al.* (2000). Neuroprotective effects of creatine in a transgenic mouse model of Huntington's disease. *J Neurosci* **20**: 4389–97.

Galper JB, Darnell JE (1969). The presence of N-formyl-methionyl-tRNA in HeLa cell mitochondria. *Biochem Biophys Res Commun* **34**: 205–14.

Gardner PR, Nguyen DH, White CW (1994). Aconitase is a sensitive and critical target of oxygen poisoning in cultured mammalian cells and in rat lungs. *Proc Natl Acad Sci USA* **91**: 12248–52.

Garseth M, Sonnewald U, White LR, *et al.* (2000). Proton magnetic resonance spectroscopy of cerebrospinal fluid in neurodegenerative disease: indication of glial energy impairment in Huntington's chorea, but not Parkinson's disease. *J Neurosci Res* **60**: 779–82.

Gentile V, Sepe C, Calvani M, *et al.* (1998). Tissue transglutaminase-catalyzed formation of high-molecular-weight aggregates *in vitro* is favored with long polyglutamine domains: a possible mechanism contributing to CAG-triplet diseases. *Arch Biochem Biophys* **352**: 314–21.

Grafton ST, Mazziotta JC, Pahl JJ, *et al.* (1990). A comparison of neurological, metabolic, structural and genetic evaluations in persons at risk for Huntington's disease. *Ann Neurol* **5**: 614–21.

—— Mazziotta JC, Pahl JJ, *et al.* (1992). Serial changes of cerebral glucose metabolism and caudate size in persons at risk for Huntington's disease. *Arch Neurol* **11**: 1161–7.

Gray MW (1992). The endosymbiont hypothesis revisited. *Int Rev Cytol* **141**: 233–357.

Greene JG, Greenamyre JT (1995). Characterization of the excitotoxic potential of the reversible succinate dehydrogenase inhibitor malonate. *J Neurochem* **64**: 430–6.

Gu M, Gash MT, Mann VM, Javoy-Agid F, Cooper JM, Schapira AHV (1996). Mitochondrial defect in Huntington's disease caudate nucleus. *Ann Neurol* **39**: 385–9.

Harms L, Meierkord H, Timm G, Pfeiffer L, Ludolph AC (1997). Decreased N-acetyl-aspartate/choline ratio and increased lactate in the frontal lobes of patients with Huntington's disease: a proton magnetic resonance spectroscopy study. *J Neurol Neurosurg Psychiatry* **62**: 27–30.

Hausladen A, Fridovich I (1994). Superoxide and peroxynitrite inactivate aconitases, but nitric oxide does not. *J Biol Chem* **269**: 29405–8.

Hoang TQ, Bluml S, Dubowitz DJ, *et al.* (1998). Quantitative proton-decoupled ^{31}P MRS and ^{1}H MRS in the evaluation of Huntington's and Parkinson's diseases. *Neurology* **50**: 1033–40.

Huntington's Disease Collaborative Research Group (HDCRG) (1993). A novel gene containing a trinucleotide repeat that is expanded and unstable on Huntington's disease chromosomes. *Cell* **172**: 971–83.

Huntington Study Group (2001). A randomised, placebo-controlled trial of the coenzyme Q_{10} and remacemide in Huntington's disease. *Neurology* **57**: 397–404.

Jenkins BG, Koroshetz WJ, Beal MF, Rosen BR (1993). Evidence for impairment of energy metabolism *in vivo* in Huntington's disease using localised ^{1}H NMR spectroscopy. *Neurology* **43**: 2689–95.

—— Rosas HD, Chen YCI, *et al.* (1998). ^{1}H NMR spectroscopy studies of Huntington's disease. Correlations with CAG repeat numbers. *Neurology* **50**: 1357–65.

Jenkins BG, Klivenyi P, Kustermann E, *et al.* (2000). Nonlinear decrease over time in N-acetyl aspartate levels in the absence of neuronal loss and increases in glutamine and glucose in transgenic Huntington's disease mice. *J Neurochem* **74**: 2108–19.

Koroshetz WJ, Jenkins BG, Rosen BR, Beal MF (1997). Energy metabolism defects in Huntington's disease and effects of coenzyme Q_{10}. *Ann Neurol* **41**: 160–5.

Kuhl DE, Phelps ME, Markham CH, Metter EJ, Riege WH, Winter J (1982). Cerebral metabolism and atrophy in Huntington's disease determined by 18FDG and computed tomographic scan. *Ann Neurol* **12**: 425–34.

Kuwert T, Lange HW, Langen K-J, Herzog H, Albrecht A, Feinendegen LE (1990). Cortical and subcortical glucose consumption measured by PET in patients with Huntington's disease. *Brain* **113**: 1405–23.

—— Boecker H, *et al.* (1993). Striatal glucose consumption in chorea-free subjects at risk of Huntington's disease. *J Neurol* **241**: 31–6.

La Fontaine MA, Geddes JW, Banks A, Butterfield DA (2000). 3-nitropropionic acid induced *in vivo* protein oxidation in striatal and cortical synaptosomes: insights into Huntington's disease. *Brain Res* **858**: 356–62.

Leenders KL, Frackowiak RSJ, Quinn N, Marsden CD (1986). Brain energy metabolism and dopaminergic function in Huntington's disease measured *in vivo* using positron emission tomography. *Mov Disord* **1**: 69–77.

Leonard JV, Schapira AHV (2000a). Mitochondrial respiratory chain disorders I: mitochondrial DNA defects. *Lancet* **355**: 299–304.

—— —— (2000b). Mitochondrial respiratory chain disorders II: neurodegenerative disorders and nuclear gene defects. *Lancet* **355**: 389–94.

Lightowlers RN, Chinnery PF, Turnbull DM, Howell N (1997). Mammalian mitochondrial genetics: heredity, heteroplasmy and disease. *Trends Genet* **13**: 450–5.

Lodi R, Schapira AH, Manners D, *et al.* (2000). Abnormal *in vivo* skeletal muscle energy metabolism in Huntington's disease and dentatorubropallidoluysian atrophy. *Ann Neurol* **48**: 72–6.

Ludolph AC, He F, Spencer PS, Hammerstad J, Sabri M (1991). 3-nitropropionic acid-exogenous animal neurotoxin and possible human striatal toxin. *Can J Neurol Sci* **18**: 492–8.

Mangiarini L, Sathasivam K, Seller M, *et al.* (1996). Exon 1 of the HD gene with an expanded CAG repeat is sufficient to cause a progressive neurological phenotype in transgenic mice. *Cell* **87**: 493–506.

Mann V, Cooper JM, Javoy-Agid F, Agid Y, Jenner P, Schapira AHV (1990). Mitochondrial function and parental sex effect in Huntington's disease. *Lancet* **336**: 749.

Martin WRW, Clark C, Ammann W, Stoessl AJ, Shtybel W, Hayden MR (1992). Cortical glucose metabolism in Huntington's disease. *Neurology* **42**: 223–9.

—— Hanstock C, Hodder J, Allen JS (1996). Brain energy metabolism in Huntington's disease measured with *in vivo* proton magnetic resonance spectroscopy. *Ann Neurol* **40**: 538.

Matthews RT, Ferrante RJ, Jenkins BG, *et al.* (1997). Iodoacetate produces striatal excitotoxic lesions. *J Neurochem* **69**: 285–9.

Mazziotta JC, Phelps ME, Pahl JJ, *et al.* (1987). Reduced cerebral glucose metabolism in asymptomatic subjects at risk for Huntington's disease. *New Engl J Med* **316**: 357–62.

Mazzola JL, Sirover MA (2001). Reduction of glyceraldehyde-3-phosphate dehydrogenase activity in Alzheimer's disease and Huntington's disease fibroblasts. *J Neurochem* **76**: 442–9.

Myers RH, Sax DS, Koroshetz WJ, *et al.* (1991). Factors associated with slow progression in Huntington's disease. *Arch Neurol* **48**: 800–4.

Parker WD, Boyson SJ, Luder AS, Parks JK (1990). Evidence for a defect in NADH:ubiquinone oxidoreductase (complex I) in Huntington's disease. *Neurology* **40**: 1231–4.

Patel M, Day BJ, Crapo JD, Fridowich I, McNamara JO (1996). Requirement for superoxide in excitotoxic cell death. *Neuron* **16**: 345–55.

Petersen A, Mani K, Brundin P (1999). Recent advances on the pathogenesis of Huntington's disease. *Exp Neurol* **157**:1–18.

Pratley RE, Salbe AD, Ravussin E, Caviness JN (2000). Higher sedentary energy expenditure in patients with Huntington's disease. *Ann Neurol* **47**:64–70.

Rizzuto R (2001) Intracellular Ca^{2+} pools in neuronal signalling. *Curr Opin Neurobiol* **11**: 306–311.

Sanchez-Pernaute R, Garcia-Segura, JM, del Barrio Alba A, Viano J, de Yebenes JG (1999). Clinical correlation of ^1H MRS changes in Huntington's disease. *Neurology* **53**: 806.

Sawa A, Wiegand GW, Cooper J, *et al.* (1999). Increased apoptosis of Huntington disease lymphoblasts associated with repeat-length dependent mitochondrial depolarisation. *Nature Med* **5**: 1194–8.

Schapira AHV (1997). Mitochondrial function in Huntington's disease: clues for the pathogenesis and prospects for treatment. *Ann Neurol* **41**: 141–2.

—— (1999). Mitochondrial involvement in Parkinson's disease, Huntington's disease, hereditary spastic paraplegia, and Friedreich's ataxia. *Biochim Biophys Acta* **1210**: 159–70.

Sheline CT, Choi DW (1998). Neuronal death in cultured murine cortical cells is induced by inhibition of GAPDH and triosephosphate isomerase. *Neurobiol Dis* **5**: 47–54.

Stahl Wl, Swanson PD (1974). Biochemical abnormalities in Huntington's chorea brains. *Neurology* **24**: 813–19.

Taanman JW (1999). The human mitochondrial genome: structure, transcription, translation and replication. *Biochim Biophys Acta* **1410**: 103–23.

Tabrizi, SJ, Cleeter MWJ, Xuereb J, Taanman JW, Cooper JM, Schapira AHV (1999). Biochemical abnormalities and excitotoxicity in Huntington's disease brain. *Ann Neurol* **45**: 25–32.

—— Workman J, Hart P, *et al.* (2000). Mitochondrial dysfunction and free radical damage in the huntington R6/2 transgenic mouse. *Ann Neurol* **47**: 80–6.

Vonsattel JP, Myers RH, Stevens TJ, Ferrante RJ, Bird ED, Richardson EP (1985). Neuropathological classification of Huntington's disease. *J Neuropathol Exp Neurol* **44**: 559–77.

Weinberger DR, Berman KF, Iadarola M, Driesen N, Zec RF (1998). Prefrontal cortical blood flow and cognitive function in Huntington's disease. *J Neurol Neurosurg Psychiatry* **51**: 94–104.

Section 4 Molecular biology of Huntington's disease

11 Structural biology of Huntington's disease

Erich E. Wanker and Anja Dröge

Introduction

Huntington's disease (HD) is an autosomal dominant progressive neurodegenerative disorder (Harper 1991) characterized by neuronal loss in the cortex and striatum. HD patients suffer from personality changes, motor impairment, and subcortical dementia. The genetic defect underlying HD has been localized to the first exon of the *IT15* gene, which encodes a 348 kDa protein, termed huntingtin (Huntington's Disease Collaborative Research Group 1993). The disease-causing mutation is the expansion of a polymorphic CAG repeat that is completely penetrant once it has reached 40 triplets (Rubinsztein *et al.* 1996; Sathasivam *et al.* 1997). The CAG repeat is translated into a polyglutamine stretch situated 17 amino acids from the *N*-terminus of huntingtin. The length of the abnormal CAG/polyglutamine (polyQ) stretch correlates with the age of onset and severity of the disease, with higher repeat numbers leading to earlier onset.

Huntingtin is a predominantly cytosolic protein, which is widely expressed, with the highest level found in brain (Sharp *et al.* 1995). As suggested by its phylogenetic conservation, huntingtin is an essential protein. It plays an important role during embryonic development including neurogenesis (White *et al.* 1997), gastrulation (Dragatsis *et al.* 1998; Duyao *et al.* 1995; Nasir *et al.* 1995; Zeitlin *et al.* 1995), and formation of extraneuronal tissue (Dragatsis *et al.* 1998). The precise role of huntingtin remains to be elucidated. However, there is growing evidence that the protein is involved in RNA biogenesis (Boutell *et al.* 1999; Faber *et al.* 1998; Passani *et al.* 2000; Takagaki and Manley 2000), vesicle trafficking (Kalchman *et al.* 1997; Li *et al.* 1995; Wanker *et al.* 1997), and iron homeostasis (Hilditch-Maguire *et al.* 2000). Even though the loss of normal huntingtin function may be a factor that contributes to HD pathogenesis (Cattaneo *et al.* 2001), it is generally accepted that a toxic 'gain of function' of mutant huntingtin is the major cause of the disease. Toxicity is clearly associated with the polyQ extension as is demonstrated by the fact that elongated polyQ stretches alone (Ikeda *et al.* 1996) or as part of the huntingtin exon 1 fragment (Mangiarini *et al.* 1996) or even in the context of a completely unrelated protein (Ordway *et al.* 1997) cause neurological symptoms in mice.

The most striking feature of mutant huntingtin is its tendency to form insoluble protein aggregates with a fibrillar morphology *in vivo* and *in vitro* (Davies *et al.* 1997; Scherzinger *et al.* 1997). Formation of huntingtin protein aggregates in neuronal inclusions of affected individuals is a hallmark of HD (DiFiglia *et al.* 1997; Gutekunst *et al.* 1999; Sieradzan *et al.* 1999). Insoluble polyQ-containing aggregates were also observed in yeast (Krobitsch and Lindquist 2000; Muchowski *et al.* 2000), flies (Jackson *et al.* 1998; Kazemi-Esfarjani and Benzer 2000; Marsh *et al.* 2000; Warrick *et al.* 1998), *Caenorhabditis elegans* (Faber *et al.* 1999; Satyal *et al.* 2000), transgenic mice (Davies *et al.* 1997; Li *et al.* 2000; Reddy *et al.*

1998; Schilling *et al.* 1999), and various cell culture model systems (Kazantsev *et al.* 1999; Lunkes and Mandel 1998; Martindale *et al.* 1998; Waelter *et al.* 2001). These observations have led to the proposal that HD and several related polyQ repeat disorders, including spinal bulbar muscular atrophy (SBMA or Kennedy's disease), dentatorubral pallidoluysian atrophy (DRPLA), and spinocerebellar ataxias (SCA) types 1, 2, 3, 6, and 7 (reviewed, for example, by Klockgether and Evert 1998 and Zhuchenko *et al.* 1997), could be the result of the accumulation of insoluble protein aggregates, as has been proposed for Alzheimer's disease (AD), parkinsonism (PD), amyotrophic lateral sclerosis (ALS), and the prion diseases (Harper and Lansbury 1997; Koo *et al.* 1999). However, experimental evidence against this hypothesis has also been presented. Saudou *et al.* (1998), for example, found that nuclear localization of mutant huntingtin, but not the formation of insoluble polyQ-containing protein aggregates, is required to induce neurotoxicity in a cell culture model of HD.

Although the detailed mechanisms by which the elongated polyQ sequence in huntingtin causes selective neurodegeneration are still unclear, it seems likely that abnormal protein folding and aggregation play a key role in the pathogenesis of HD. Therefore, determination of the structure of long polyQ stretches and their aggregates as well as the elucidation of the molecular pathways of protein aggregation and its effect on disease progression and neurodegeneration could open up new avenues for therapeutic intervention.

Aggregation of mutant huntingtin via enzymatic cross-linking

Green (1993) proposed that increasing the number of glutamines in the huntingtin protein beyond a certain threshold may result in the protein becoming a transglutaminase substrate. Transglutaminases are a family of calcium-dependent enzymes that catalyse the formation of covalent ε-(γ-glutamyl)-lysine isopeptide bonds between substrate proteins, resulting in the formation of insoluble cross-linked protein complexes (Greenberg *et al.* 1991). Thus, aggregation in HD could be caused by the cross-linking of mutant huntingtin to itself or to other proteins acting as lysyl donors. Transglutaminase activity has been found within neurones of the brain (Appelt *et al.* 1996; Lesort *et al.* 1999) and is increased in areas specifically affected in HD (Karpuj *et al.* 1999; Lesort *et al.* 1999).

In vitro evidence in support of the transglutaminase hypothesis has been presented (Kahlem *et al.* 1996). Using a number of short peptides containing variable lengths of polyQ, Kahlem and co-workers have shown that these peptides can be cross-linked to radiolabelled glycine-ethyl ester by purified type II transglutaminase. Lengthening of the polyQ reiteration increased the reactivity of the glutamine residues (Kahlem *et al.* 1996). In the presence of transglutaminase, polyQ-containing peptides formed insoluble aggregates with certain proteins of brain extracts. These aggregates contained glutamyl-lysine cross-links, which were detected by high-pressure liquid chromatography (HPLC).

In a separate study Kahlem *et al.* (1998) showed that huntingtin is a substrate for tissue and brain transglutaminase. When protein extracts from lymphoblastoid cell lines derived from HD patients, containing mutant and wild-type huntingtin, were incubated with transglutaminase *in vitro*, insoluble protein aggregates were formed preferentially from mutant huntingtin. The rate of the reaction significantly increased with increasing polyQ sequences. The conversion of huntingtin with expanded polyQ sequences into the polymeric form was prevented by inhibitors of transglutaminases, suggesting that transglutaminase-mediated cross-linking of mutant huntingtin is involved in the formation of the nuclear inclusions found in HD brains.

In support of this hypothesis, Karpuj *et al.* (1999) showed that transglutaminase activity in HD brains is significantly increased compared to that in controls. Furthermore, in HD brains, but not in the control brains, transglutaminase activity was detected in neuronal nuclei, suggesting that formation of nuclear inclusions, a characteristic feature of HD and related glutamine repeat disorders, could be caused by transglutaminase action. However, experimental evidence confirming the role of transglutaminases as mediators for protein aggregation *in vivo* is still lacking. Recently, evidence has been presented that tissue transglutaminases do not directly contribute to the formation of mutant huntingtin aggregates (Chun *et al.* 2001). In human neuroblastoma SH-SY5Y cells expressing a truncated huntingtin fragment with a glutamine repeat in the pathological range (82 glutamines), numerous sodium dodecyl sulfate (SDS)-resistant protein aggregates were detected both in the cytoplasm and the nucleus. Interestingly, the transglutaminase protein itself was not present in these aggregates and neither increasing nor decreasing the level of transglutaminase had any effect on the number of aggregates and their intracellular localization (Chun *et al.* 2001). These findings clearly demonstrate that transglutaminase activity is not involved in the aggregation process, at least in the cell culture model of HD examined. To prove that transglutaminases have any effect on huntingtin aggregation in HD brains it will be necessary to demonstrate the presence of Nε-(γ-glutamyl)-lysine cross-links in the insoluble huntingtin protein aggregates.

Structure of glutamine repeats

After the discovery that HD will always develop in individuals expressing a mutant huntingtin protein with more than 41 glutamines (39 CAG repeats) (Rubinsztein *et al.* 1996), Perutz *et al.* (1994) and colleagues computer-generated an atomic model of poly-L-glutamine (Fig. 11.1). In this model, also termed the 'polar zipper' model, antiparallel β-strands of polyQ are linked together by hydrogen bonds between the main-chain and side-chain amides. Perutz *et al.* (1994) proposed that elongated polyQ chains form stable hairpins when the number of glutamines exceeds 41. Hairpins associate with each other causing the huntingtin protein to aggregate and precipitate in neurones. He proposed that neurological symptoms start when the precipitates in the cell have reached a critical size.

To test this hypothesis *in vitro*, Perutz and co-workers synthesized the polypeptide Asp_2–Glu_{15}–Lys_2. This peptide is soluble at acidic pH, but precipitates to high-molecular weight aggregates at neutral pH. Analysis of the polyQ-containing aggregates by circular dichroism and electron- and X-ray diffraction showed that they consist of β-pleated sheets, consistent with the polar zipper model (Perutz *et al.* 1994). In a separate study, a 10-glutamine repeat was inserted into the external loop of a small protein of known structure, the chymotrypsin inhibitor 2 from barley seed (CI2) (Stott *et al.* 1995). The recombinant protein was expressed in *Escherichia coli* and fast performance liquid chromatography (FPLC) fractionation of crude protein extracts showed that they contained a mixture of monomers, dimers, and trimers of CI2. This observation initially suggested that the recombinant CI2 protein associates via its polyQ sequence. However, attempts to determine the dissociation constants of the oligomers failed, because they could not be separated without completely denaturing the protein. It was concluded that the oligomers were not held together by hydrogen bonds between their polyQ sequences, but were generated by the exchange of domains during protein folding (Stott *et al.* 1995).

The structure of polyQ was also examined by Altschuler *et al.* (1997) using various polyQ-containing peptides. Circular dichroism (CD) measurements showed that the percentage of

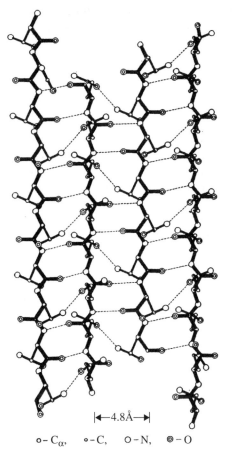

|←—4.8Å—→|

o – C_α,   o – C,   O – N,   ◎ – O

Fig. 11.1 Computer-generated structure of paired antiparallel β-strands of polyglutamine linked together by hydrogen bonds between the main-chain and side-chain amides. (Reprinted from Perutz (1996) with permission from Excerpta Medica Inc.)

random coil structure in these peptides increased with increasing polyQ-length, indicating that polyQ in soluble form has a random coil conformation. However, more recently, Sharma *et al.*, (1999) found that polyQ peptides with or without interruptions adopt a β-sheet, and not a random coil structure. Molecular modelling of homopolymeric polyQ sequences using various modelling packages such as AMBER or CHARMM was also performed. Lathrop *et al.* (1998) presented four polyQ structural motifs: two β-sheet motifs (parallel and anti-parallel) both very similar to the polar zipper model (Perutz *et al.* 1994), and two novel helix motifs. In comparison, a detailed molecular-mechanical investigation of a polypeptide chain with 40 glutamine residues revealed a β-hairpin as well as a highly compact random coil structure (Starikov *et al.* 1999). Clearly, future molecular studies using nuclear magnetic resonance (NMR) or X-ray crystallography will be necessary to determine the exact structure of polyQ in the soluble huntingtin disease protein.

Self-assembly of mutant huntingtin fragments into aggregates

In order to assess the polar zipper hypothesis of Max Perutz, Scherzinger *et al.* (1997) produced glutathione S-transferase (GST)–HD exon 1 fusion proteins with 20, 30, 51, 83, and

122 glutamines in *E. coli*. The recombinant proteins were purified in soluble form by affinity chromatography on glutathione-sepharose. Site-specific proteolysis of the GST–HD exon 1 fusion proteins revealed that the huntingtin fragments with polyQ tracts in the pathological range (51–122 glutamines), but not with polyQ tracts in the normal range (20 and 30 gluta-mines) readily form high-molecular-weight protein aggregates with a fibrillar or ribbon-like morphology (Fig. 11.2). Using a comparable experimental approach, Huang *et al.* (1998) obtained similar results. Monitoring the initial stage of huntingtin fibrillogenesis by dynamic light scattering confirmed these electronmicroscopic observations (Georgalis *et al.* 1998). The structure of the huntingtin fibrils formed *in vitro* is reminiscent of scrapie prion rods (Prusiner *et al.* 1998), α-synuclein fibres in parkinsonism (Conway *et al.* 1998), and β-amyloid fibrils in Alzheimer's disease (Caputo *et al.* 1992). As revealed by electron microscopy, the aggreg-ated huntingtin fibrils obtained after digestion of GST fusion proteins with factor Xa have a diameter of 10–12 nm and a variable length, ranging from 100 nm up to several micrometres. Moreover, the fibrils formed *in vitro* stained with Congo red and showed green birefringence when examined under polarized light. This tinctorial property is characteristic of amyloids (Glenner 1980) and indicates that the huntingtin fibrils formed *in vitro*, similarly to the Asp_2–Glu_{15}–Lys_2 aggregates analysed by Perutz *et al.* (1994), consist of β-pleated sheets held together by hydrogen bonds. Interestingly, huntingtin aggregates prepared from HD brains also exhibit green birefringence after staining with Congo red (Huang *et al.* 1998), indicating that ordered fibrils are not only formed *in vitro* but also *in vivo* in neuronal cells.

A more detailed study of the aggregation behaviour of HD exon 1 proteins with polyQ repeats in the normal and pathological range revealed that the threshold for huntingtin aggre-gation *in vitro* and in a cell culture system is between 32 and 37 glutamines (Scherzinger *et al.*

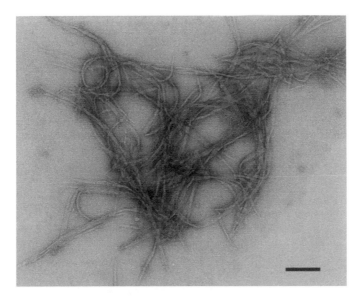

Fig. 11.2 Electron micrograph of HD exon 1 fibrils *in vitro*. Fibril formation was induced by trypsin digestion of GST-HD45Q fusion protein. Cleavage products were negatively stained with 1 per cent uranyl acetate. The bar represents 200 nm.

1999). The pathological threshold in HD is 38–41 glutamines. No case of HD has been reported with fewer than 38 glutamines (36 CAG repeats), nor has any individual with more than 41 glutamines (39 CAG repeats) been found to remain free from HD (Rubinsztein *et al.* 1996). This remarkable correlation is unlikely to have arisen through chance and supports the hypothesis that the pathology of HD and related glutamine-repeat diseases is due to an intrinsic tendency of polyQ sequences of more than 40 residues to self-assemble into aggregates.

Proposed mechanism for the self-assembly of mutant huntingtin into aggregates

In vitro studies using purified GST–HD exon 1 fusion proteins demonstrated that formation of SDS-insoluble huntingtin aggregates, similarly to β-amyloid (Harper and Lansbury 1997) and α-synuclein aggregates (Wood *et al.* 1999), occurs by a nucleation-dependent polymerization mechanism (Scherzinger *et al.* 1999). This means that the formation of a nucleus is the rate-limiting step in the aggregation process. Huntingtin aggregates are only formed when a critical protein concentration is exceeded. Furthermore, polymerization of mutant huntingtin protein does not start immediately, but after a lag time during which dimers, trimers, and longer oligomers are formed. Accordingly, lowering the huntingtin concentration in patient brains should delay the onset and progression of HD. *In vivo* evidence in support of this hypothesis has been presented. Yamamoto *et al.* (2000) showed that switching off the expression of a mutant huntingtin fragment with a polyQ repeat in the pathological range (94 glutamines) in a transgenic mouse model results in the disappearance of insoluble huntingtin protein aggregates and the accompanying motor dysfunction.

A model for the formation of insoluble polyQ-containing protein aggregates is shown in Fig. 11.3. A polyQ sequence in the pathological range is a prerequisite for the self-assembly of huntingtin fibrils. As proposed by Perutz *et al.* (1994), the first step in the aggregation process is a phase change from a potential random coil structure into a hydrogen-bonded hairpin (toxic fold). When the number of glutamines exceeds a certain critical length (for example, 41 glutamines), the formation of the hairpin may become strongly favoured by a gain of entropy due to the liberation of water molecules. Once the hairpin has formed and the protein concentration exceeds a critical value, ordered intermediate structures (nuclei) are formed very slowly and then rapidly grow up to high-molecular-weight ordered fibrillar structures

Soluble protein   Toxic fold   Nucleus   Amyloid fibrils

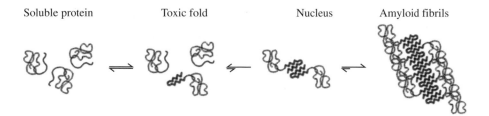

Fig. 11.3 Proposed model of huntingtin aggregation. The elongated polyQ stretch present in mutant huntingtin eventually undergoes a structural transition from a potential random coil into a β-sheet structure (toxic fold, hairpin). Once a hairpin has formed, association with other polyQ-containing hairpins leads to the formation of an unstable nucleus, followed by the generation of insoluble, ordered fibrils.

(amyloid-like fibrils). In neuronal cells, cleavage of the mutant huntingtin protein by specific proteases and/or binding of other cellular proteins to huntingtin (for example, stress-related factors (Welch and Gambetti 1998) or the interacting protein SH3GL3 (Sittler *et al.* 1998)) may accelerate the process of aggregate formation. On the other hand, the association of chaperones and/or components of the proteasome with mutant huntingtin may slow down or prevent its assembly into aggregates *in vivo* (Carmichael *et al.* 2000; Muchowski *et al.* 2000). A detailed understanding of the mechanisms by which these or other cellular factors modulate huntingtin aggregation in HD neurones will be informative with regard to the disease development and, in addition, open up novel approaches to therapy.

Huntingtin protein aggregation *in vivo*

Initially, huntingtin protein aggregates with a fibrillar morphology were discovered in a transgenic mouse model of HD expressing huntingtin exon 1 fragment with a glutamine repeat in the pathological range (115–156 glutamines) (Davies *et al.* 1997). In these mice, formation of insoluble aggregates in neuronal intranuclear inclusions (NIIs) was observed prior to the development of a progressive neurological phenotype displaying symptoms reminiscent of HD (Davies *et al.* 1997). These results suggested that the process of aggregate formation *in vivo* is a prerequisite for the development of neuronal dysfunction and neurodegeneration in HD. Ultrastructural and immunocytochemical studies revealed that the NIIs can be stained with anti-ubiquitin antibodies, indicating that the huntingtin protein in the inclusion bodies is ubiquitinated and marked for, but resists, degradation by the ubiquitin–proteasome system. Aside from NIIs, aggregated huntingtin protein was also discovered in axons and axon terminals of the transgenic mice (Li *et al.* 1999, 2000). These structures were termed neuropil aggregates and it is likely that they affect specific neuronal functions such as axonal transport and neurotransmitter release. Several other laboratories using a variety of transgenic mouse models have confirmed this finding (Hodgson *et al.* 1999; Reddy *et al.* 1998; Schilling *et al.* 1999; Wheeler *et al.* 2000).

Following the initial discovery of insoluble huntingtin protein aggregates in transgenic animals, they were also detected in patient brains (DiFiglia *et al.* 1997; Gutekunst et al. 1999; Sieradzan *et al.* 1999). As was the case for the transgenic mice, ubiquitinated nuclear and cytoplasmic huntingtin aggregates with an amorphous or fibrillar morphology were observed. In addition, dystrophic neurites containing aggregated huntingtin protein were detected (DiFiglia *et al.* 1997). Dystrophic neurites are known to result from dysfunction of neuronal retrograde transport. Interestingly, NIIs in patient brains were only detected by antibodies directed against the *N*-terminus of huntingtin. They were not recognized by antibodies against the *C*-terminus of the protein, indicating that truncated *N*-terminal huntingtin fragments, rather than the full-length protein, are accumulating in neuronal cells (DiFiglia *et al.* 1997).

The formation of insoluble huntingtin protein aggregates was subsequently reproduced in ycast (Krobitsch and Lindquist 2000; Muchowski *et al.* 2000), *C. elegans* (Faber *et al.* 1999; Satyal *et al.* 2000), flies (Jackson *et al.* 1998), and various cell culture model systems (Cooper *et al.* 1998; Li and Li 1998; Lunkes and Mandel 1998; Waelter *et al.* 2001). As shown in Fig. 11.4(a), overexpression of a mutant HD exon 1 protein with 83 glutamines in a 293 Tet-Off cell line mainly results in the accumulation of perinuclear inclusion bodies (Waelter *et al.* 2001). Analysis at the ultrastructural level revealed that these inclusions are large, membrane-free

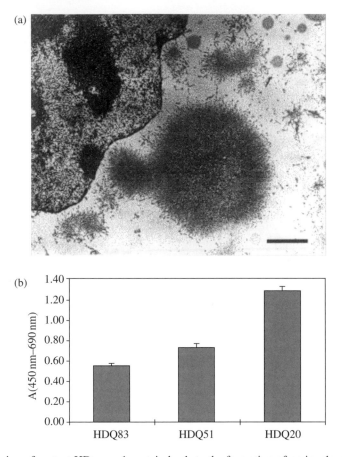

Fig. 11.4 Expression of mutant HD exon 1 protein leads to the formation of perinuclear aggregates and toxicity in induced 293 Tet-Off cells. (a) Electron micrograph of a 293 Tet-Off cell containing a perinuclear inclusion body with aggregated HDQ83 protein. The bar represents 2 μm. (b) Cell viability upon expression of HD exon 1 proteins with 20 (HDQ20), 51 (HDQ51), and 83 (HDQ83) glutamines as determined by the XTT assay. ((b) is reprinted from Waelter *et al.* 2001 with permission of the American Society for Cell Biology.)

structures composed of electron-dense filamentous material. At higher magnification it was possible to determine that the fibrous region consists of individual filaments with a diameter of ~10 nm. These fibrillar structures closely resemble the HD exon 1 fibrils that have been produced from GST-HD exon 1 proteins *in vitro* (Scherzinger *et al.* 1997) as well as in the HD transgenic mouse model (Davies *et al.* 1997). Thus, the current body of evidence from both *in vitro* and *in vivo* studies supports the hypothesis that the accumulation of insoluble huntingtin aggregates in neuronal cells is caused by a conformational change of the elongated glutamine repeat that leads to self-assembly of the disease protein into amyloid-like fibrillar structures, most probably by a nucleation-dependent polymerization.

Aggregation of polyQ-containing proteins and toxicity

The question of whether the formation of huntingtin aggregates is toxic for neuronal cells is controversial. First, Ikeda *et al.* (1996) showed that overexpression of a truncated fragment of the Machado–Joseph disease protein with a polyQ repeat in the pathological range induces cell death in cultured COS cells. These results were confirmed by several other laboratories using truncated fragments of the huntingtin protein in various cell culture model systems (Carmichael *et al.* 2000; Hackam *et al.* 1999; Lunkes and Mandel 1998; Martindale *et al.* 1998). Waelter *et al.* (2001), for example, produced huntingtin exon 1 fragments with 20 (HDQ20), 51 (HDQ51), and 83 (HDQ83) glutamines in inducible 293 Tet-Off cells. They found that overexpression of HD exon 1 protein fragments with a polyQ repeat in the pathological range (51 and 83 glutamines), but not with a polyQ repeat in the normal range (20 glutamines), results in the formation of massive cytoplasmic inclusions containing aggregated huntingtin protein and that these inclusions are toxic for 293 Tet-Off cells (Fig. 11.4(b)). However, evidence that aggregation of a mutant huntingtin fragment in cultured striatal cells is not required to induce cell death has also been presented. Saudou *et al.* (1998) have shown that translocation of mutant huntingtin into neuronal nuclei, but not the formation of microscopic aggregates, is required for the induction of cell death. Similar results were obtained by Klement *et al.* (1998) who found that nuclear localization of mutant ataxin-1 is crucial for the induction of cell death in SCA-1 transgenic mice. However, the neurodegeneration in the SCA-1 transgenic mice was not progressive, indicating that the pathogenic mechanism in this mouse model is different from that in SCA-1 and HD patients, who clearly show a late-onset, progressive neurological phenotype.

There are several possibilities as to the mechanism by which the formation of insoluble huntingtin protein aggregates in patient brains could be toxic for neuronal cells. First, it is possible that polyQ-containing aggregates *per se* are toxic for neuronal cells. Second, toxicity in cells could be induced because proteins that are crucial for cell viability are recruited into the aggregates. Within the last couple of years evidence has been presented that transcription factors (Kazantsev *et al.* 1999; McCampbell *et al.* 2000; Perez *et al.* 1998; Steffan *et al.* 2000), caspases (Sanchez *et al.* 1999), protein kinases (Meriin *et al.* 2001), and components of the proteasome (Cummings *et al.* 1998; Waelter *et al.* 2001) are recruited into huntingtin aggregates. Recently, for example, Suhr *et al.* (2001) found that ubiquitin, the cell cycle-regulating proteins p53 and mdm-2, Hsp70, the transcription factor TFIID, the cytoskeleton protein actin, and proteins of the nuclear pore complex are sequestered at relatively high levels into polyQ-containing protein aggregates. In addition, Nucifora *et al.* (2001) demonstrated that accumulation of CBP, the transcriptional coactivator CREB-binding protein, in insoluble huntingtin and atrophin-1 aggregates alters gene expression at the mRNA level and leads to toxicity in cell culture model systems. CBP is a major mediator of survival signals in mature neurones and has been previously identified as constituent of polyQ aggregates *in vitro* and *in vivo* (McCampbell *et al.* 2000; Steffan *et al.* 2000). Thus, polyQ-mediated interference with CBP-regulated transcription may constitute a gain of function underlying the pathogenesis of HD.

Finally, toxicity in neuronal cells could also be induced because the aggregated huntingtin in nuclear and cytoplasmic inclusions is resistant to proteolytic digestion by the ubiquitin–proteasome system. In fact, immunohistochemical and ultrastructural studies have shown that aggregated huntingtin in inclusions of HD transgenic mice (Davies *et al.* 1997),

HD patients (DiFiglia 1997), and cell culture model systems (Waelter *et al.* 2001) is ubiquitinated. Furthermore, ubiquitin-positive nuclear and cytoplasmic inclusions stain positively for the 20S proteasome. Together, these findings suggest that the redistribution of the proteasomal machinery and molecular chaperones to polyQ-containing protein aggregates is a natural response of cells to remove misfolded aggregation-prone proteins. The accumulating huntingtin fibrils, however, may inhibit the proteasomal activity and thereby obstruct the cellular stress response pathway for misfolded proteins. Experimental evidence in support of this hypothesis has been presented recently (Bence *et al.* 2001). Since it has been shown that the primary function of the proteasome is the rapid degradation of proteins with abnormal folding (Voges *et al.* 1999), the formation of huntingtin aggregates in patient brains may indirectly lead to the accumulation of vital regulatory proteins such as oncogene products, tumour suppressors, and rate-limiting enzymes and this might be highly toxic for mammalian cells.

Inhibition of huntingtin aggregation by small molecules, peptides, antibodies, and oligonucleotides

Abnormal folding of the disease proteins into β-sheets and the accumulation of insoluble protein aggregates with an amorphous or fibrillar morphology in neuronal cells is a common feature of HD and the related glutamine repeat disorders. If the process of aggregate formation is critical for the development of neuronal dysfunction and degeneration, inhibition of aggregate formation in patients may postpone the disease onset and progression. Therefore, efforts are underway to develop screens for chemical compounds, peptides, and antibodies that potentially inhibit aggregation of the expanded polyQ sequence. Additionally, antisense-mediated strategies are being developed to downregulate the expression of mutant huntingtin.

For the detection and quantification of SDS-insoluble HD exon 1 aggregates a sensitive filter retardation assay has been developed, which has proven useful for high-throughput screenings of small molecules that prevent aggregate formation (Wanker *et al.* 1999). This assay is based on the finding that polyQ-containing aggregates are resistant to boiling in SDS and, after filtration, are retained on a cellulose acetate membrane (Fig. 11.5(a)), while the monomeric form of the protein does not bind to this filter membrane. The captured aggregates then can be detected by simple immunoblotting using specific anti-huntingtin antibodies (Scherzinger *et al.* 1997; Wanker *et al.* 1999). Using this filtration assay, Heiser *et al.* (2000) have recently identified several small molecules that prevent huntingtin aggregation *in vitro*. They found that the chemical compounds Congo red (Fig. 11.5(b)), thioflavine S, chrysamine G, and Direct fast yellow inhibit HD exon 1 aggregation in a dose-dependent manner, whereas other potential inhibitors of β-amyloid formation such as thioflavine T, gossypol, melatonin, and rifampicin (Tomiyama *et al.* 1994) had little or no effect on huntingtin aggregation. The results obtained by the filter retardation assay were confirmed by electron microscopy, sodium dodecyl sulfate polyacrylamide gel electrophoresis (SDS-PAGE), and mass spectrometry. Furthermore, Congo red at micromolar concentrations suppressed HD exon 1 aggregation in a cell culture model system (Heiser *et al.* 2000). Similar results were obtained after incubation of organotypic slices prepared from brains of HD transgenic mice expressing mutant HD exon 1 protein (Smith *et al.* 2001). Moreover, feeding of transgenic flies expressing a polyQ tract in the pathological range with Congo red markedly suppressed degeneration of photoreceptors and cell toxicity (L. Thompson, personal communication). These results

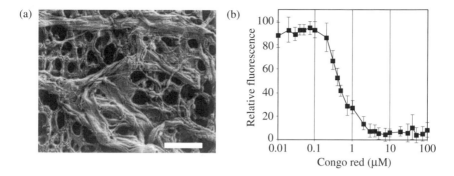

Fig. 11.5 Filter retention of huntingtin aggregates and inhibition of aggregate formation by Congo red. (a) Scanning electron migrograph of aggregated GST–HDQ51 trypsin cleavage products on a cellulose acetate membrane (Heinrich Lündsdorf, GBF, Braunschweig, Germany). The bar represents 5 μm. (b) Inhibition of HD exon 1 aggregation by Congo red. Fibril formation *in vitro* was performed in presence of different concentrations of the inhibitor. Aggregates were detected by the filter retardation assay. (Data and figures were taken from Heiser *et al.* (2000), copyright (2000) National Academy of Science, USA.)

strongly support the notion that the development of huntingtin aggregation inhibitors may be effective in treating HD.

In order to find new chemical compounds that prevent huntingtin aggregation *in vitro* a high-throughput screening assay based on automated cellulose acetate membrane filtration has been developed. Using this assay, approximately 180 000 different chemical compounds have been screened, 700 of which turned out to be potential aggregation inhibitors. These compounds are currently tested in cell culture model systems for their ability to prevent HD exon 1 aggregation *in vivo* (E. Wanker and V. Heiser, unpublished results).

Efforts to find peptides and antibodies that prevent huntingtin aggregation have also been undertaken. Heiser *et al.* (2000) showed that the monoclonal antibody 1C2, which specifically recognizes the elongated polyQ tract in huntingtin (Trottier *et al.* 1995), is able to prevent the formation of SDS-resistant HD exon 1 fibrils *in vitro*. After addition of this antibody to the aggregation reactions, instead of the characteristic fibrillar structures, amorphous aggregates consisting of HD exon 1 protein and antibody were observed by electron microscopy. These structures were soluble in SDS and were no longer resistant to protease treatment. These results suggest that the antibody has a chaperone-like activity and blocks aggregation by stabilizing the native conformation of the elongated polyQ tract, whereas Congo red and its derivatives, which are known to selectively bind to β-sheets (Klunk *et al.* 1998), may inhibit huntingtin aggregation by interfering with nucleus formation (Heiser *et al.* 2000). Using a phage display screening assay, Nagai *et al.* (2000) selected several tryptophan-rich peptides that preferentially bind to elongated polyQ tracts and inhibit polyQ aggregation both *in vitro* and in transfected COS-7 cells. Similarly, Lecerf *et al.* (2001) selected a human single-chain Fv antibody from a phage display library that specifically recognizes the 17 *N*-terminal amino acids of huntingtin. This antibody was tested in a cell culture model of HD expressing a mutant huntingtin exon 1 protein fused to the green fluorescent protein (GFP). Co-expression of the anti-huntingtin Fv antibody with the abnormal huntingtin–GFP fusion protein dramatically reduced the number of aggregates compared to controls. Thus, the development of 'intrabodies' that counteract huntingtin aggregation *in vivo* may also contribute to the treatment of HD and related glutamine repeat diseases.

As the concentration of mutant huntingtin is very critical for the formation of insoluble protein aggregates (Scherzinger *et al.* 1999), selective inhibition of huntingtin synthesis in neurones is another potential strategy to slow down disease progression. Nellemann *et al.* (2000) have demonstrated that huntingtin synthesis can be efficiently inhibited in embryonic teratocarcinoma cells (NT2) and postmitotic neurones (NT2N) using antisense oligodeoxynucleotides. Antisense-mediated downregulation of human huntingtin expression was also observed in PC-12 cells, suggesting that this, in principle, is a suitable approach for the development of a new therapy for HD (Boado *et al.* 2000). However, the delivery of antisense-based therapeutics to the brain is compromised by the poor stability of the oligodeoxynucleotides *in vivo* and by the presence of the blood–brain barrier. Therefore, further research will be necessary to develop antisense molecules that can be applied with success to patients.

Inhibition of huntingtin aggregation by chaperones

Chaperones are known to assist in the folding, refolding, and elimination of proteins under both normal and stress conditions (Hartl 1996). Thus, the recruitment of chaperones and other stress proteins to aggregation-prone huntingtin could be a defence mechanism to protect neuronal cells from the toxicity of the misfolded disease protein. Cummings *et al.* (1998) were the first to show that the molecular chaperone DnaJ (Hsp40) associates with ataxin-1 aggregates in SCA1 patient tissues. Subsequently, co-localization of heat shock proteins, Hsp40 and Hsp70, with polyQ-containing protein aggregates of ataxin-1, ataxin-3, huntingtin, and the androgen receptor protein has been observed in various cell culture and fly model systems (Chai *et al.* 1999; Stenoien *et al.* 1999; Waelter *et al.* 2001). These data support the hypothesis that redistribution of molecular chaperones to insoluble protein aggregates belongs to the natural response of cells to remove misfolded aggregation-prone proteins. Interestingly, overexpression of molecular chaperones significantly suppresses polyQ-aggregation in cell culture, yeast, *C. elegans*, and *Drosophila* model systems (Cummings *et al.* 1998; Chai *et al.* 1999; Kobayashi *et al.* 2000; Muchowski *et al.* 2000; Satyal *et al.* 2000; Chan *et al.* 2000), suggesting that the activation of a heat shock response or the direct overexpression of chaperones in patients may have the potential to diminish polyQ toxicity and neurodegeneration. In support of this hypothesis, Warrick *et al.* (1998) showed that expression of the molecular chaperone Hsp70 suppressed polyQ-mediated neurodegeneration in a *Drosophila* model of SCA3. Surprisingly, suppression of neurodegeneration by Hsp70 occurred without a visible effect on NII formation, suggesting that polyglutamine-toxicity can be dissociated from the formation of large aggregates. On the other hand, Muchowski *et al.* (2000), using mutant HD exon 1 proteins, have found that Hsp70 together with its co-chaperone Hsp40 suppresses the self-assembly of amyloid-like huntingtin fibrils, causing the formation of detergent-soluble amorphous aggregates instead (Fig. 11.6). Thus, the reduction of neurotoxicity seen in the SCA3 *Drosophila* model (Warrick *et al.* 1998) could be due to the ability of the chaperones to shift the self-association pathway of the polyQ-containing proteins from insoluble fibrillar to

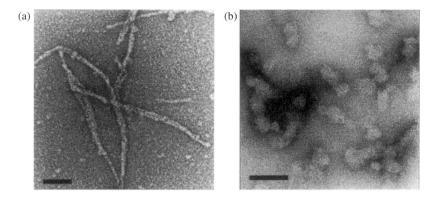

Fig. 11.6 Suppression of HD exon 1 fibril formation by the molecular chaperones. Fibril formation *in vitro* was performed in (a) the absence or (b) the presence of the chaperones Hsc70 and Hdj-1. Samples were negatively stained and analysed by electron microsopy scale bar, 100 nm. (Taken from Muchowski *et al.* 2000, copyright (2000) National Academy of Science, USA.)

more soluble amorphous aggregates that are less toxic. In support of this hypothesis, Chan *et al.* (2000) presented evidence that the chaperone-mediated suppression of polyQ neurotoxicity in *Drosophila* is associated with altered solubility properties of the disease protein.

The current body of evidence suggests that searching for ways to increase the levels of Hsp70/Hsp40 in neurones of patients may open up promising avenues for a therapy of HD and perhaps also other neurodegenerative disorders caused by amyloidogenic proteins. Recently, Sittler *et al.* (2001) have shown that treatment of mammalian cells with the antitumour drug geldanamycin induces the expression of the molecular chaperones Hsp70, Hsp40, and Hsp90 and thereby inhibits HD exon 1 protein aggregation. Similar results were also obtained by overexpression of Hsp40 and Hsp70 in a separate cell culture model of HD. These findings may provide the basis for the development of a novel pharmacotherapy for HD, because activation of a heat shock response by chemical compounds in patient brains may prevent neurodegeneration and disease progression. However, additional drug screens to find chemical compounds that like geldanamycin activate a heat shock response but are less toxic and capable of crossing the blood–brain barrier will be necessary.

Conclusions

Although to date it has not been formally proven whether the process of huntingtin aggregation is the cause or merely a consequence of disease, several lines of experimental evidence support the hypothesis that the accumulation of high-molecular-weight aggregates in neuronal cells is crucial for the development and progression of the disease. First, SDS-insoluble huntingtin aggregates with a fibrillar morphology will only form *in vitro* when the polyQ tract exceeds a critical length of 37 glutamines. Thus, the threshold for protein aggregation is very similar to the pathological threshold found in HD patients. Second, for the formation of ordered fibrils by a nucleation-dependent mechanism long periods of time and a critical protein concentration are required. HD is a late-onset neurodegenerative disorder. The lag time observed *in vitro* and in cell culture model systems could explain the late onset of the disease in patients given that an intracellular concentration of huntingtin in the submicromolar range is required. It could take years in patient brains until enough toxic material is accumulated to initiate a cell death programme. Third, in most animal model systems the process of huntingtin aggregation is linked to disease progression. Consistent with this, the rate of aggregate formation *in vitro* directly correlates with the polyQ repeat length in huntingtin. The longer the poly Q tract, the faster the aggregation rate and the faster also the development of neurological symptoms in HD.

Several lines of evidence support the hypothesis that the pathogenesis of HD is linked to abnormal protein folding and aggregation in neuronal cells. It is very likely that the first step in the disease mechanism is the abnormal folding of the polyQ repeat into a pathological conformation that is rich in β-sheets. Once this conformation is arrived at, the mutant huntingtin protein self-assembles into insoluble protein aggregates by a nucleation dependent polymerization that eventually leads to neuronal dysfunction and toxicity (Perutz and Windle 2001). Currently, it is unknown whether the altered conformation of mutant huntingtin *per se*, transient microaggregates, or high-molecular-weight huntingtin aggregates induce neurotoxicity. However, it is clear from *in vitro* and *in vivo* studies that the process of aggregate formation always correlates with disease progression. Thus, suppression of polyQ aggregation by small molecules that directly interfere with the aggregation process or induce a heat shock response are very promising therapeutic strategies. In addition, drugs that stimulate the degradation of mutant huntingtin are also expected to delay of the onset and progression of HD. The future challenge will be to find small molecules that are nontoxic, cross the blood–brain barrier, and can be administered to patients over relatively long periods of time.

Acknowledgements

We thank E. Scherzinger and S. Schnögl for critical reading of the manuscript. This work was supported by the Max-Planck-Gesellschaft and grants from the Huntington's Disease Society of America, HFSP, Deutsche Forschungsgemeinschaft (SFB 577) and the BMBF (BioFuture project: 0311853).

References

Altschuler, E. L., Hud, N. V., Mazrimas, J. A., and Rupp, B. (1997). Random coil conformation for extended polyglutamine stretches in aqueous soluble monomeric peptides. *Journal of Peptide Research* **50** (1), 73–75.

Appelt, D. M., Kopen, G. C., Boyne, L. J., and Balin, B. J. (1996). Localization of transglutaminase in hippocampal neurons: implications for Alzheimer's disease. *Journal of Histochemistry and Cytochemistry* **44** (12), 1421–1427.

Bence, N., Sampat, R., and Kopito, R. (2001). Impairment of the ubiquitin–proteasome system by protein aggregation. *Science* **292** (5521), 1552–1555.

Boado, R. J., Kazantsev, A., Apostol, B. L., Thompson, L. M., and Pardridge, W. M. (2000). Antisense-mediated down-regulation of the human huntingtin gene. *Journal of Pharmacology and Experimental Therapeutics* **295** (1), 239–243.

Boutell, J. M., Thomas, P., Neal, J. W., Weston, V. J., Duce, J., Harper, P. S., and Jones, A. L. (1999). Aberrant interactions of transcriptional repressor proteins with the Huntington's disease gene product, huntingtin. *Human Molecular Genetics* **8** (9), 1647–1655.

Caputo, C. B., Fraser, P. E., Sobel, I. E., and Kirschner, D. A. (1992). Amyloid-like properties of a synthetic peptide corresponding to the carboxy terminus of beta-amyloid protein precursor. *Archives of Biochemistry and Biophysics* **292** (1), 199–205.

Carmichael, J., Chatellier, J., Woolfson, A., Milstein, C., Fersht, A. R., and Rubinsztein, D. C. (2000). Bacterial and yeast chaperones reduce both aggregate formation and cell death in mammalian cell models of Huntington's disease. *Proceedings of the National Academy of Sciences of the United States of America* **97**, 9701–9705.

Cattaneo, E., Rigamonti, D., Goffredo, D., Zuccato, C., Squitieri, F., and Sipione, S. (2001). Loss of normal huntingtin function: new developments in Huntington's disease research. *Trends inNeurosciences* **24** (3), 182–188.

Chai, Y., Koppenhafer, S. L., Bonini, N. M., and Paulson, H. L. (1999). Analysis of the role of heat shock protein (Hsp) molecular chaperones in polyglutamine disease. *Journal of Neuroscience* **19**, 10338–10347.

Chan, H. Y., Warrick, J. M., Gray-Board, G. L., Paulson, H. L., and Bonini, N. M. (2000). Mechanisms of chaperone suppression of polyglutamine disease: selectivity, synergy and modulation of protein solubility in drosophila. *Human Molecular Genetics* **9** (19), 2811–20.

Chun, W., Lesort, M., Tucholski, J., Ross, C. A., and Johnson, G. V. W. (2001). Tissue transglutaminase does not contribute to the formation of mutant huntingtin aggregates. *Journal of Cell Biology* **153** (1), 25–34.

Conway, K. A., Harper, J. D., and Lansbury, P. T. (1998). Accelerated *in vitro* fibril formation by a mutant α-synuclein linked to early-onset Parkinson disease. *Nature Medicine* **4**, 1318–1320.

Cooper, J. K., Schilling, G., Peters, M. F., Herring, W. J., Sharp, A. H., Kaminsky, Z., Masone, J., Khan, F. A., Delanoy, M., Borchelt, D. R., Dawson, V. L., Dawson, T. M., and Ross, C. A. (1998). Truncated N-terminal fragments of huntingtin with expanded glutamine repeats form nuclear and cytoplasmic aggregates in cell culture. *Human Molecular Genetics* **7** (5), 783–790.

Cummings, C. J., Mancini, M. A., Antalffy, B., DeFranco, D. B., Orr, H. T., and Zoghbi, H. Y. (1998). Chaperone suppression of aggregation and altered subcellular proteasome localization imply protein misfolding in SCA1. *Nature Genetics* **19** (2), 148–154.

Davies, S. W., Turmaine, M., Cozens, B. A., DiFiglia, M., Sharp, A. H., Ross, C. A., Scherzinger, E., Wanker, E. E., Mangiarini, L., and Bates, G. P. (1997). Formation of neuronal intranuclear inclusions underlies the neurological dysfunction in mice transgenic for the HD mutation. *Cell* **90** (3), 537–548.

DiFiglia, M., Sapp, E., Chase, K. O., Davies, S. W., Bates, G. P., Vonsattel, J. P., and Aronin, N. (1997). Aggregation of huntingtin in neuronal intranuclear inclusions and dystrophic neurites in brain. *Science* **277** (5334), 1990–1993.

Dragatsis, I., Efstratiadis, A., and Zeitlin, A. (1998). Mouse mutant embryos lacking huntingtin are rescued from lethality by wild-type extraembryonic tissues. *Development* **125** (8), 1529–1539.

Duyao, M. P., Auerbach, A. B., Ryan, A., Persichetti, F., Barnes, G. T., McNeil, S. M., Ge, P., Vonsattel, J. P., Gusella, J. F., Joyner, A. L., *et al.* (1995). Inactivation of the mouse Huntington's disease gene homolog Hdh. *Science* **269** (5222), 407–410.

Faber, P. W., Barnes, G. T., Srinidhi, J., Chen, J., Gusella, J. F., and MacDonald, M. E. (1998). Huntingtin interacts with a family of WW domain proteins. *Human Molecular Genetics* **7** (9), 1463–1474.

—— Alter, J. R., MacDonald, M. E., and Hart, A. C. (1999). Polyglutamine-mediated dysfunction and apoptotic death of a *Caenorhabditis elegans* sensory neuron. *Proceedings of the National Academy of Sciences of the United States of America* **96** (1), 179–184.

Georgalis, Y., Starikov, E. B., Hollenbach, B., Lurz, R., Scherzinger, E., Saenger, W., Lehrach, H., and Wanker, E. E. (1998). Huntingtin aggregation monitored by dynamic light scattering. *Proceedings of the National Academy of Sciences of the United States of America* **95** (11), 6118–6121.

Glenner, G. G. (1980). Amyloid deposits and amyloidosis—the beta-fibrilloses. 1. *New England Journal of Medicine* **302** (23), 1283–1292.

Green, H. (1993). Human genetic diseases due to codon reiteration: relationship to an evolutionary mechanism. *Cell* **74**, 955–956.

Greenberg, C. S., Birckbichler, P. J., and Rice, R. H. (1991). Transglutaminases—multifunctional cross-linking enzymes that stabilize tissues. *FASEB Journal* **5** (15), 3071–3077.

Gutekunst, C.-A., Li, S.-H., Yi, H., Mulroy, J. S., Kuemmerle, S., Jones, R., Rye, D., Ferrante, R. J., Hersch, S. M., and Li, X.-J. (1999). Nuclear and neuropil aggregates in Huntington's disease: relationship to neuropathology. *Journal of Neuroscience* **19**, 2522–2534.

Hackam, A. S., Singaraja, R., Zhang, T., Gan, L., and Hayden, M. R. (1999). *In vitro* evidence for both the nucleus and cytoplasmas subcellular sites of pathogenesis in Huntington's disease. *Human Molecular Genetics* **8** (1), 25–33.

Harper, J. D. and Lansbury, P. T., Jr. (1997). Models of amyloid seeding in Alzheimer's disease and scrapie: mechanistic truths and physiological consequences of the time-dependent solubility of amyloid proteins. *Annual Review of Biochemistry* **66**, 385–407.

Harper, P. S. (ed.) (1991). *Huntington's disease*, 1st edn. W.B. Saunders, London.

Hartl, F. U. (1996). Molecular chaperones in cellular protein folding. *Nature* **381** (6583), 571–580.

Heiser, V., Scherzinger, E., Boeddrich, A., Nordhoff, E., Lurz, R., Schugardt, N., Lehrach, H., and Wanker, E. E. (2000). Inhibition of huntingtin fibrillogenesis by specific antibodies and small molecules: implications for Huntington's disease therapy. *Proceedings of the National Academy of Sciences of the United States of America* **97** (12), 6739–44.

Hilditch-Maguire, P., Trettel, F., Passani, L. A., Auerbach, A., Persichetti, F., and MacDonald, M. E. (2000). Huntingtin: an iron-regulated protein essential for normal nuclear and perinuclear organelles. *Human Molecular Genetics* **9** (19), 2789–2797.

Hodgson, J. G., Agopyan, N., Gutekunst, C. A., Leavitt, B. R., LePiane, F., Singaraja, R., Smith, D. J., Bissada, N., McCutcheon, K., Nasir, J., Jamot, L., Li, X. J., Stevens, M. E., Rosemond, E., Roder, J. C., Phillips, A. G., Rubin, E. M., Hersch, S. M., and Hayden, M. R. (1999). A YAC mouse model for Huntington's disease with full-length mutant huntingtin, cytoplasmic toxicity, and selective striatal neurodegeneration. *Neuron* **23** (1), 181–92.

Huang, C. C., Faber, P. W., Persichetti, F., Mittal, V., Vonsattel, J.-P., MacDonald, M. E., and Gusella, J. F. (1998). Amyloid formation by mutant huntingtin: threshold, progressivity and recruitment of normal polyglutamine proteins. *Somatic Cell and Molecular Genetics* **24**, 217–233.

Huntington's Disease Collaborative Research Group (1993). A novel gene containing a trinucleotide repeat that is expanded and unstable on Huntington's disease chromosomes. *Cell* **172**, 971–973.

Ikeda, H., Yamaguchi, M., Sugai, S., Aze, Y., Narumiya, S., and Kakizuka, A. (1996). Expanded polyglutamine in the Machado–Joseph disease protein induces cell death *in vitro* and *in vivo*. *Nature Genetics* **13**, 196–202.

Jackson, G. R., Salecker, I., Dong, X., Yao, X., Arnheim, N., Faber, P. W., MacDonald, M. E., and Zipursky, S. L. (1998). Polyglutamine-expanded human huntingtin transgenes induce degeneration of *Drosophila* photoreceptor neurons. *Neuron* **21** (3), 633–42.

Kahlem, P., Terre, C., Green, H., and Djian, P. (1996). Peptides containing glutamine repeats as substrates for transglutaminase-catalyzed cross-linking: relevance to diseases of the nervous system [see comments]. *Proceedings of the National Academy of Sciences of the United States of America* **93** (25), 14580–14585.

—— Green, H., and Djian, P. (1998). Transglutaminase action imitates Huntington's disease: selective polymerization of huntingtin containing expanded polyglutamine. *Molecular Cell* **1** (4), 595–601.

Kalchman, M. A., Koide, H. B., McCutcheon, K., Graham, R. K., Nichol, K., Nishiyama, K., Kazemi-Esfarjani, P., Lynn, F. C., Wellington, C., Metzler, M., Goldberg, Y. P., Kanazawa, I., Gietz, R. D., and Hayden, M. R. (1997). HIP1, a human homologue of *S. cerevisiae* Sla2p, interacts with membrane-associated huntingtin in the brain. *Nature Genetics* **16** (1), 44–53.

Karpuj, M. V., Garren, H., Slunt, H., Price, D. L., Gusella, J., Becher, M. W., and Steinman, L. (1999a). Transglutaminase aggregates huntingtin into nonamyloidogenic polymers, and its enzymatic activity increases in Huntington's disease brain nuclei. *Proceedings of the National Academy of Sciences of the United States of America* **96**, 7388–7393.

Kazantsev, A., Preisinger, E., Dranovsky, A., Goldgaber, D., and Housman, D. (1999). Insoluble detergent-resistant aggregates form between pathological and nonpathological lengths of polyglutamine in mammalian cells. *Proceedings of the National Academy of Sciences of the United States of America* **96** (20), 11404–11409.

Kazemi-Esfarjani, P. and Benzer, S. (2000). Genetic suppression of polyglutamine toxicity in *Drosophila. Science* **287** (5459), 1837–1840.

Klement, I. A., Skinner, P. J., Kaytor, M. D., Yi, H., Hersch, S. M., Clark, H. B., Zoghbi, H. Y., and Orr, H. T. (1998). Ataxin-1 nuclear localization and aggregation: role in polyglutamine-induced disease in SCA1 transgenic mice [see comments]. *Cell* **95** (1), 41–53.

Klockgether, T. and Evert, B. (1998). Genes involved in hereditary ataxias. *Trends in Neuroscience* **21** (9), 413–418.

Klunk, W. E., Debnath, M. L., Koros, A. M., and Pettegrew, J. W. (1998). Chrysamine-G, a lipophilic analogue of Congo red, inhibits A beta-induced toxicity in PC12 cells. *Life Sciences* **63** (20), 1807–1814.

Kobayashi, Y., Kume, A., Li, M., Doyu, M., Hata, M., Ohtsuka, K., and Sobue, G. (2000). Chaperones Hsp70 and Hsp40 suppress aggregate formation and apoptosis in cultured neuronal cells expressing truncated androgen receptor protein with expanded polyglutamine tract. *Journal of Biological Chemistry* **275** (12), 8772–8778.

Koo, E. H., Lansbury, P. T., and Kelly, J. W. (1999). Amyloid diseases: abnormal protein aggregation in neurodegeneration. *Proceedings of the National Academy of Sciences of the United States of America* **96** (18), 9989–9990.

Krobitsch, S. and Lindquist, S. (2000). Aggregation of huntingtin in yeast varies with the length of the polyglutamine expansion and the expression of chaperone proteins. *Proceedings of the National Academy of Sciences of the United States of America* **97** (4), 1589–1594.

Lathrop, R. H., Casale, M., Tobias, D. J., Marsh, J. L., and Thompson, L. M. (1998). Modeling protein homopolymeric repeats: possible polyglutamine structural motifs for Huntington's disease. *Proceedings International Conference on Intelligent Systems for Molecular Biology ISMB. International Conference on Intelligent Systems for Molecular Biology,* **6**, 105–114.

Lecerf, J. M., Shirley, T. L., Zhu, Q., Kazantsev, A., Amersdorfer, P., Housman, D. E., Messer, A., and Huston, J. S. (2001). Human single-chain Fv intrabodies counteract *in situ* huntingtin aggregation in cellular models of Huntington's disease. *Proceedings of the National Academy of Sciences of the United States of America* **98** (8), 4764–4769.

Lesort, M., Chun, W. J., Johnson, G. V. W., and Ferrante, R. J. (1999). Tissue transglutaminase is increased in Huntington's disease brain. *Journal of Neurochemistry* **73** (5), 2018–2027.

Li, H., Li, S. H., Johnston, H., Shelbourne, P. F., and Li, X. J. (2000). Amino-terminal fragments of mutant huntingtin show selective accumulation in striatal neurons and synaptic toxicity. *Nature Genetics* **25**, 385–389.

Li, S. H. and Li, X. J. (1998). Aggregation of N-terminal huntingtin is dependent on the length of its glutamine repeats. *Human Molecular Genetics* **7** (5), 777–82.

Li, X. J., Li, S. H., Sharp, A. H., Nucifora, F. C. Jr, Schilling, G., Lanahan, A., Worley, P., Snyder, S. H., and Ross, C. A. (1995). A huntingtin-associated protein enriched in brain with implications for pathology. *Nature* **378** (6555), 398–402.

Li, Z., Karlovich, C. A., Fish, M. P., Scott, M. P., and Myers, R. M. (1999). A putative *Drosophila* homolog of the Huntington's disease gene. *Human Molecular Genetics* **8** (9), 1807–15.

Lunkes, A. and Mandel, J. L. (1998). A cellular model that recapitulates major pathogenic steps of Huntington's disease. *Human Molecular Genetics* **7** (9), 1355–61.

Mangiarini, L., Sathasivam, K., Seller, M., Cozens, B., Harper, A., Hetherington, C., Lawton, M., Trottier, Y., Lehrach, H., Davies, S. W., and Bates, G. P. (1996). Exon 1 of the Huntington's disease gene containing a highly expanded CAG repeat is sufficient to cause a progressive neurological phenotype in transgenic mice. *Cell* **87** (3), 493–506.

Marsh, J. L., Walker, H., Theisen, H., Zhu, Y. Z., Fielder, T., Purcell, J., and Thompson, L. M. (2000). Expanded polyglutamine peptides alone are intrinsically cytotoxic and cause neurodegeneration in *Drosophila*. *Human Molecular Genetics* **9** (1), 13–25.

Martindale, D., Hackam, A., Wieczorek, A., Ellerby, L., Wellington, C., McCutcheon, K., Singaraja, R., Kazemi-Esfarjani, P., Devon, R., Kim, S. U., Bredesen, D. E., Tufaro, F., and Hayden, M. R. (1998). Length of huntingtin and its polyglutamine tract influences localization and frequency of intracellular aggregates. *Nature Genetics* **18** (2), 150–154.

McCampbell, A., Taylor, J. P., Taye, A. A., Robitschek, J., Li, M., Walcott, J., Merry, D., Chai, Y. H., Paulson, H., Sobue, G., and Fischbeck, K. H. (2000). CREB-binding protein sequestration by expanded polyglutamine. *Human Molecular Genetics* **9** (14), 2197–2202.

Meriin, A., Mabuchi, K., Gabai, V., Yaglom, J., Kazantsev, A., and Sherman, M. (2001). Intracellular aggregation of polypeptides with expanded polyglutamine domain is stimulated by stress-activated kinase MEKK1. *Journal of Cell Biology* **153** (4), 851–864.

Muchowski, P. J., Schaffar, G., Sittler, A., Wanker, E. E., Hayer-Hartl, M. K., and Hartl, F. U. (2000). Hsp70 and hsp40 chaperones can inhibit self-assembly of polyglutamine proteins into amyloid-like fibrils. *Proceedings of the National Academy of Sciences of the United States of America* **97** (14), 7841–7846.

Nagai, Y., Tucker, T., Ren, H. Z., Kenan, D. J., Henderson, B. S., Keene, J. D., Strittmatter, W. J., and Burke, J. R. (2000). Inhibition of polyglutamine protein aggregation and cell death by novel peptides identified by phage display screening. *Journal of Biological Chemistry* **275** (14), 10437–10442.

Nasir, J., Floresco, S. B., O'Kusky, J. R., Diewert, V. M., Richman, J. M., Zeisler, J., Borowski, A., Marth, J. D., Phillips, A. G., and Hayden, M. R. (1995). Targeted disruption of the Huntington's disease gene results in embryonic lethality and behavioral and morphological changes in heterozygotes. *Cell* **81** (5), 811–823.

Nellemann, C., Abell, K., Norremolle, A., Lokkegaard, T., Naver, B., Ropke, C., Rygaard, J., Sorensen, S. A., and Hasholt, L. (2000). Inhibition of huntingtin synthesis by antisense oligodeoxynucleotides. *Molecular and Cellular Neuroscience* **16** (4), 313–323.

Nucifora, F. C., Sasaki, M., Peters, M. F., Huang, H., Cooper, J. K., Yamada, M., Takahashi, H., Tsuji, S., Troncoso, J., Dawson, V. L., Dawson, T. M., and Ross, C. A. (2001). Interference by huntingtin and atrophin-1 with CBP-mediated transcription leading to cellular toxicity. *Science* **291** (5512), 2423–2428.

Ordway, J. M., Tallaksen-Greene, S., Gutekunst, C. A., Bernstein, E. M., Cearly, J. A., Wiener, H. W., Dure, L. S., Lindsey, R., Hersch, S. M., Jope, R. S., Albin, R. L., and Detloff, P. J. (1997). Ectopically expressed CAG repeat cause intranuclear inclusions and a progressive late onset neurological phenotype in the mouse. *Cell* **91**, 753–763.

Passani, L. A., Bedford, M. T., Faber, P. W., McGinnis, K. M., Sharp, A. H., Gusella, J. F., Vonsattel, J. P., and MacDonald, M. E. (2000). Huntingtin's WW domain partners in Huntington's disease post-mortem brain fulfill genetic criteria for direct involvement in Huntington's disease pathogenesis. *Human Molecular Genetics* **9** (14), 2175–2182.

Perez, M. K., Paulson, H. L., Pendse, S. J., Saionz, S. J., Bonini, N. M., and Pittman, R. N. (1998). Recruitment and the role of nuclear localization in polyglutamine-mediated aggregation. *Journal of Cell Biology* **143** (6), 1457–70.

Perutz, M. F. (1996). Glutamine repeats and inherited neurodegenerative diseases: molecular aspects. *Current Opinion in Structural Biology* **6**, 848–858.

—— and Windle A. H. (2001). Cause of neural death in neurodegenerative diseases attributable to expansion of glutamine repeats. *Nature* **412**, 143–144.

—— Johnson, T., Suzuki, M., and Finch, J. T. (1994). Glutamine repeats as polar zippers: their possible role in inherited neurodegenerative diseases. *Proceedings of the National Academy of Sciences of the United States of America* **91** (12), 5355–8.

Prusiner, S. B., Scott, M. R., DeArmond, S. J., and Cohen, F. E. (1998). Prion protein biology. *Cell* **93** (3), 337–348.

Reddy, P. H., Williams, M., Charles, V., Garrett, L., Pike-Buchanan, L., Whetsell, W. O. Jr, Miller, G., and Tagle, D. A. (1998). Behavioural abnormalities and selective neuronal loss in HD transgenic mice expressing mutated full-length HD cDNA. *Nature Genetics* **20** (2), 198–202.

Rubinsztein, D. C., Leggo, J., Coles, R., Almqvist, E., Biancalana, V., Cassiman, J.-J., Chotai, K., Connarty, M., Crauford, D., Curtis, A., Curtis, D., Davidson, M. J., Differ, A.-M., Dode, C., Dodge, A., Frontali, M., Ranen, N. G., Stine, O. C., Sherr, M., Abbott, M. H., Franz, M. L., Graham, C. A., Harper, P. S., Hedreen, J. C., Jackson, A., Kaplan, J.-C., Losekoot, M., MacMillan, J. C., Morrison, P., Trottier, Y., Novelletto, A., Simpson, S. A., Theilmann, J., Whittaker, J. L., Folstein, S. E., Ross, C. A., and Hayden, M. R. (1996b). Phenotypic characterisation of individuals with 30–40 CAG repeats in the Huntington's disease (HD) gene reveals HD cases with 36 repeats and apparently normal elderly individuals with 36–39 repeats. *American Journal of Human Genetics* **59**, 16–22.

Sanchez, I., Xu, C. J., Juo, P., Kakizaka, A., Blenis, J., and Yuan, J. (1999). Caspase-8 is required for cell death induced by expanded polyglutamine repeats. *Neuron* **22** (3), 623–633.

Sathasivam, K., Amaechi, I., Mangiarini, L., and Bates, G. (1997). Identification of an HD patient with a (CAG)180 repeat expansion and the propagation of highly expanded CAG repeats in lambda phage. *Human Genetics* **99** (5), 692–695.

Satyal, S. H., Schmidt, E., Kitagawa, K., Sondheimer, N., Lindquist, S., Kramer, J. M., and Morimoto, R. I. (2000). Polyglutamine aggregates alter protein folding homeostasis in *Caenorhabditis elegans*. *Proceedings of the National Academy of Sciences of the United States of America* **97** (11), 5750–5755.

Saudou, F., Finkbeiner, S., Devys, D., and Greenberg, M. E. (1998). Huntingtin acts in the nucleus to induce apoptosis but death does not correlate with the formation of intranuclear inclusions. *Cell* **95** (1), 55–66.

Scherzinger, E., Lurz, R., Turmaine, M., Mangiarini, L., Hollenbach, B., Hasenbank, R., Bates, G. P., Davies, S. W., Lehrach, H., and Wanker, E. E. (1997). Huntingtin-encoded polyglutamine expansions form amyloid-like protein aggregates *in vitro* and *in vivo*. *Cell* **90** (3), 549–558.

—— Sittler, A., Schweiger, K., Heiser, V., Lurz, R., Hasenbank, R., Bates, G. P., Lehrach, H., and Wanker, E. E. (1999). Self-assembly of polyglutamine-containing huntingtin fragments into amyloid-like fibrils: implications for Huntington's disease pathology. *Proceedings of the National Academy of Sciences of the United States of America* **96** (8), 4604–4609.

Schilling, G., Becher, M. W., Sharp, A. H., Jinnah, H. A., Duan, K., Kotzuk, J. A., Slunt, H. H., Ratovitski, T., Cooper, J. K., Jenkins, N. A., Copeland, N. G., Price, D. L., Ross, C. A., and Borchelt, D. R. (1999). Intranuclear inclusions and neuritic aggregates in transgenic mice expressing a mutant N-terminal fragment of huntingtin [published erratum appears in *Human Molecular Genetics* 1999 May; **8** (5), 943]. *Human Molecular Genetics* **8** (3), 397–407.

Sharma, D., Sharma, S., Pasha, S., and Brahmachari, S. K. (1999). Peptide models for inherited neurodegenerative disorders: conformation and aggregation properties of long polyglutamine peptides with and without interruptions. *FEBS Letters* **456** (1), 181–185.

Sharp, A. H., Loev, S. J., Schilling, G., Li, S.-H., Li, X.-J., Bao, J., Wagster, M. V., Kotzuk, J. A., Steiner, J. P., Lo, A., Hedreen, J., Sisodia, S., Snyder, S. H., Dawson, T. M., Ryugo, D. K., and Ross, C. A. (1995). Widespread expression of Huntington's disease gene (IT15) protein product. *Neuron* **14**, 1065–1074.

Sieradzan, K. A., Mechan, A. O., Jones, L., Wanker, E. E., Nukina, N., and Mann, D. M. (1999). Huntington's disease intranuclear inclusions contain truncated, ubiquitinated huntingtin protein. *Experimental Neurology* **156** (1), 92–99.

Sittler, A., Walter, S., Wedemeyer, N., Hasenbank, R., Scherzinger, E., Eickhoff, H., Bates, G. P., Lehrach, H., and Wanker, E. E. (1998). SH3GL3 associates with the Huntingtin exon 1 protein and promotes the formation of polygln-containing protein aggregates. *Molecular Cell* **2** (4), 427–36.

Sittler, A., Lurz, R., Lueder, G., Priller, J., Lehrach, H., Hayer-Hartl, M., Hartl, F. U., and Wanker, E. E. (2001). Geldanamycin activates a heat schock response and inhibits huntingtin aggregation in a cell culture model of Huntington's disease. *Human Molecular Genetics* **10**, 1307–1315.

Smith, D.L., Portier, R., Woodman, B., Hockly, E., Mahal, A., Klunk, W.E., Li, X.-J., Wanker, E.E., Murray, K.D., and Bates, G.P. (2001) Inhibition of polyglutamine aggregation in R6/2 HD brain slices—complex dose response profiles. *Neurobiology of Disease* **8** (6), 1017–1026.

Starikov, E. B., Lehrach, H., and Wanker, E. E. (1999). Folding of oligoglutamines: a theoretical approach based upon thermodynamics and molecular mechanics. *Journal of Biomolecular Structure and Dynamics* **17** (3), 409–427.

Steffan, J. S., Kazantsev, A., Spasic-Boskovic, O., Greenwald, M., Zhu, Y. Z., Gohler, H., Wanker, E. E., Bates, G. P., Housman, D. E., and Thompson, L. M. (2000). The Huntington's disease protein interacts with p53 and CREB-binding protein and represses transcription. *Proceedings of the National Academy of Sciences of the United States of America* **97** (12), 6763–6768.

Stenoien, D. L., Cummings, C. J., Adams, H. P., Mancini, M. G., Patel, K., DeMartino, G. N., Marcelli, M., Weigel, N. L., and Mancini, M. A. (1999). Polyglutamine-expanded androgen receptors form aggregates that sequester heat shock proteins, proteasome components and SRC-1, and are suppressed by the HDJ-2 chaperone. *Human Molecular Genetics* **8** (5), 731–741.

Stott, K., Blackburn, J. M., Butler, P. J. G., and Perutz, M. (1995). Incorporation of glutamine repeats makes protein oligomerize: implications for neurodegenerative diseases. *Proceedings of the National Academy of Sciences of the United States of America* **92**, 6509–6513.

Suhr, S. T., Senut, M. C., Whitelegge, J. P., Faull, K. E., Cuizon, D. B., and Gage, F. H. (2001). Identities of sequestered proteins in aggregates from cells with induced polyglutamine expression. *Journal of Cell Biology* **153** (2), 283–294.

Takagaki, Y. and Manley, J. L. (2000). Complex protein interactions within the human polyadenylation machinery identify a novel component. *Molecular and Cellular Biology* **20** (5), 1515–1525.

Tomiyama, T., Asano, S., Suwa, Y., Morita, T., Kataoka, K., Mori, H., and Endo, N. (1994). Rifampicin prevents the aggregation and neurotoxicity of amyloid beta protein *in vitro*. *Biochemical and Biophysical Research Communications* **204** (1), 76–83.

Trottier, Y., Devys, D., Imbert, G., Sandou, F., An, I., Lutz, Y., Weber, C., Agid, Y., Hirsch, E. C., and Mandel, J.-L. (1995). Cellular localisation of the Huntington's disease protein and discrimination of the normal and mutated forms. *Nature Genetics* **10**, 104–110.

Voges, D., Zwickl, P., and Baumeister, W. (1999). The 26S proteasome: a molecular machine designed for controlled proteolysis. *Annual Review of Biochemistry* **68**, 1015–1068.

Waelter, S., Boeddrich, A., Lurz, R., Scherzinger, E., Lueder, G., Lehrach, H., and Wanker, E. (2001). Accummulation of mutant huntingtin fragments in aggresome-like inclusion bodies as a result of insufficient protein degradation. *Molecular Biology of the Cell* **12**, 1393–1407.

Wanker, E. E., Rovira, C., Scherzinger, E., Hasenbank, R., Walter, S., Tait, D., Colicelli, J., and Lehrach, H. (1997). HIP-I: a huntingtin interacting protein isolated by the yeast two-hybrid system. *Human Molecular Genetics* **6** (3), 487–95.

—— Scherzinger, E., Heiser, V., Sittler, A., Eickhoff, H., and Lehrach, H. (1999). Membrane filter assay for detection of amyloid-like polyglutamine-containing protein aggregates. *Methods in Enzymology* **309**, 375–86.

Warrick, J. M., Paulson, H. L., Gray-Board, G. L., Bui, Q. T., Fischbeck, K. H., Pittman, R. N., and Bonini, N. M. (1998). Expanded polyglutamine protein forms nuclear inclusions and causes neural degeneration in *Drosophila*. *Cell* **93** (6), 939–49.

Welch, W. J. and Gambetti, P. (1998). Neurodegeneration—chaperoning brain diseases. *Nature* **392** (6671), 23–24.

Wheeler, V. C., White, J. K., Gutekunst, C. A., Vrbanac, V., Weaver, M., Li, X. J., Li, S. H., Yi, H., Vonsattel, J. P., Gusella, J. F., Hersch, S., Auerbach, W., Joyner, A. L., and MacDonald, M. E. (2000).

Long glutamine tracts cause nuclear localization of a novel form of huntingtin in medium spiny striatal neurons in HdhQ92 and HdhQ111 knock-in mice. *Human Molecular Genetics* **9** (4), 503–513.

White, J. K., Auerbach, W., Duyao, M. P., Vonsattel, J. P., Gusella, J. F., Joyner, A. L., and MacDonald, M. E. (1997). Huntingtin is required for neurogenesis and is not impaired by the Huntington's disease CAG expansion. *Nature Genetics* **17** (4), 404–410.

Wood, S. J., Wypych, J., Steavenson, S., Louis, J.-C., Citron, M., and Biere, A. L. (1999). α-Synuclein fibrillogenesis is nucleation-dependent. *Journal of Biological Chemistry* **274**, 19509–19515.

Yamamoto, A., Lucas, J. J., and Hen, R. (2000). Reversal of neuropathology and motor dysfunction in a conditional model of Huntington's disease. *Cell* **101**, 57–66.

Zeitlin, S., Liu, J. P., Chapman, D. L., Papaioannou, V. E., and Efstratiadis, A. (1995). Increased apoptosis and early embryonic lethality in mice nullizygous for the Huntington's disease gene homologue. *Nature Genetics* **11** (2), 155–163.

Zhuchenko, O., Bailey, J., Bonnen, P., Ashizawa, T., Stockton, D. W., Amos, C., Dobyns, W. B., Subramony, S. H., Zoghbi, H. Y., and Lee, C. C. (1997). Autosomal dominant cerebellar ataxia (SCA6) associated with small polyglutamine expansions in the alpha(1A)-voltage-dependent calcium channel. *Nature Genetics* **15** (1), 62–69.

12 The cell biology of Huntington's disease

Lesley Jones

Introduction

Huntington's disease (HD) remains a biological conundrum, despite the discovery of the gene and mutation leading to the disease in 1993, as described in Chapter 5 (Huntington's Disease Collaborative Research Group 1993). The protein, huntingtin, expressed from the HD gene has over 3000 amino acids, giving a molecular mass of around 350 kDa—this is a large protein, represented diagrammatically in Fig. 12.1. Close to the beginning of huntingtin lies a glutamine tract, encoded by the expanded CAG codon stretch in exon 1 of the HD gene (see Chapter 5). An expansion of this glutamine tract in huntingtin is the primary cause of the symptoms of HD described in detail in Chapters 2 and 15.

Huntingtin and its gene

The glutamine tract in huntingtin is polymorphic with 8 to 37 glutamines in the normal population and 41 or more glutamines in those with HD. There is an intermediate area from 38 to 41 glutamines as explained in Chapter 5; people can manifest HD with 38 or more glutamines, but occasional cases of people with up to 41 glutamines living into old age with no discernible symptoms have been reported (Rubinsztein *et al*. 1996). The discrepancy in numbering glutamines as against CAG codons arises from the presence of a CAACAG sequence following the CAG tract—both CAA and CAG encode glutamine so the number of glutamines is always two greater than the number of CAGs except in rare instances where no CAA is present (Gellera *et al*. 1996).

    The protein had no homologues identifiable in the databases when it was cloned (Huntington's Disease Collaborative Research Group 1993) and still does not, although several motifs can be identified including the polyglutamine and polyproline tracts close to the *N*-terminus and the several HEAT repeats found just downstream of the proline-rich regions *C*-terminal to the glutamine tract (Andrade and Bork 1995). The function of the HEAT repeats is unknown although they appear to be found in proteins that have a role in cytoplasmic transport processes, a suggested role for huntingtin (Block-Galarza *et al*. 1997; Cha *et al*. 1998;

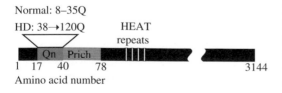

Normal: 8–35Q

HD: 38→120Q   HEAT repeats

Qn Prich

1 17   40   78   3144

Amino acid number

Fig. 12.1 Structure of huntingtin, with the known features marked on to the linear molecule. There is no information about the structure of native huntingtin; thus the position of the polyglutamine region and its effect on the protein's structure remain unknown.

Velier *et al.* 1998) that is discussed further in the section 'Huntingtin's role in cellular processes'. Notably, polyglutamine and polyproline tracts are most commonly found in transcriptionally active proteins (Gerber *et al.* 1994) and the evidence for the possible roles of huntingtin in transcriptional processes is also addressed further in the section 'Huntingtin's role in cellular processes'. These motifs account for a very small proportion of the full protein; thus we cannot assign a function to huntingtin by extrapolation from homologous or orthologous proteins. The rat and mouse *Hdh* orthologues are over 90 per cent homologous to human huntingtin, but have notably smaller polyglutamine repeats, at 8 and 7 glutamines, respectively (Barnes *et al.* 1994; Schmitt *et al.* 1995), and recognizable orthologues with 4 glutamines occur in both *Fugu rubripes* (Baxendale *et al.* 1995) and zebrafish (*Danio rerio*; http://www.ncbi.nlm.nih.gov/UniGene/clust.cgi?ORG=DR&CID=586)(85 and 71 per cent homologous, respectively). There is also a much less well-conserved *Drosophila* homologue (Li *et al.* 1999a).

But how does the expanded glutamine tract in mutant huntingtin exert its pathological effect? HD is a dominantly inherited disease and thus the three possible molecular explanations that can be considered are: (1) haploinsufficiency—a single copy of a gene produces insufficient protein product and this leads to the observed symptoms; (2) a dominant negative effect: the mutant protein ablates the function of the normal protein, for instance, by acting in a multimeric complex—each complex with one or more mutant subunits is inactive, thus only 25 per cent of homodimers, 6.25 per cent of homotetramers, and so on, would be active; or (3) the mutant protein is cytotoxic. Haploinsufficiency itself cannot explain the disease as there is at least one reported case of a translocation of the relevant part of chromosome 4p, leaving only one copy of the functional HD gene, in a person who did not develop HD (Ambrose *et al.* 1994). Most current molecular evidence points to a true dominant effect—that mutant huntingtin is cytotoxic—but there is also some evidence that the normal function of huntingtin is ablated by the mutant isoform, a dominant negative effect, and that this occurs through the binding properties of the polyglutamine region itself. The existence of rare homozygotes for the mutant allele who have a disease no different from that which would be seen in a heterozygote (Durr *et al.* 1999; Myers *et al.* 1989; Wexler *et al.* 1987) might point to a true genetic dominance, but variation seen in parameters measured, such as age of disease onset, is so wide, and the numbers of homozygotes so few, that this evidence is at best only suggestive. Molecular studies of the mutation and its behaviour in cells have also suggested a true dominant effect (Narain *et al.* 1999; Trettel *et al.* 2000).

Mutant huntingtin and cellular inclusions

Whatever the other downstream effects of the expanded glutamine tract, no discussion of the cell biology of HD can avoid an examination of the characteristic pathological hallmark of the disease, huntingtin-containing intranuclear and extranuclear inclusions (Davies *et al.* 1997; DiFiglia *et al.* 1997; Sieradzan *et al.* 1999). At a minimum, the presence of these huntingtin aggregates demonstrates that huntingtin with an expanded glutamine tract is processed differently from the normal protein to form these insoluble inclusions. The possible structures and dynamics of aggregate formation are discussed in detail in Chapter 11. The relationship of the inclusions to the death of neurones and development of the disease remains unclear, but of abiding interest, because of the inescapable fact that such inclusions are not found in normal brains. Indeed, the facts that most neurodegenerative diseases involve insoluble protein deposits of various types in the brain (Trojanowski and Lee 2000) and that ectopic expression of polyglutamine in the hypoxanthine ribosyl transferase gene gives a neurological phenotype with inclusions (Ordway *et al.* 1997) are surely telling us something important about the processes underlying HD and other neurodegenerations.

There has been intense research over the past decade devoted to finding out how the expanded polyglutamine tracts of huntingtin and the other polyglutamine proteins cause neurodegeneration. Work has proceeded at every level, from *in vitro* biochemical studies through to cellular systems, in models developed in a number of different organisms from yeast through to mammals and in further detailed study of patient cohorts. Research at each level has informed research at the other levels and thus a large body of knowledge has accrued, but the detailed pathway by which expanded polyglutamine leads to HD is still unknown and, although we have clues to some of the processes that may be important in the disease, nevertheless it remains difficult to pick out which process leads to pathogenesis. To summarize some of the main experimental work that will be discussed below Table 12.1 gives the proteins detected as interacting directly with huntingtin and Table 12.2 a selection of the most relevant cellular models mentioned here, with a brief description of their main characteristics and major experimental findings. Further details of the transgenic mouse models will be found in Chapter 13, the neurochemistry and neuropathology of HD in Chapters 8 and 9, respectively, huntingtin structural biology in Chapter 11, and the other polyglutamine diseases in Chapter 14.

The downstream effects of the huntingtin mutation must account for the dysfunction and death of neuronal cells in particular areas of the brain. Other proteins containing expanded polyglutamine that cause similar neurodegenerations (Chapter 14) cause a cell dysfunction and death that is assumed to occur through a pathway similar to that operating in HD, but in different neuronal populations, so any satisfactory explanation must account for the specificity of degeneration. There are a number of possible pathways downstream of the production of huntingtin with an expanded glutamine tract, which could explain this specificity. What follows is a description, as far as it is known, of how huntingtin is hatched, matched, and despatched—synthesized, interacted with, and degraded—along with what it may do in between. It is patchy and probably contains both grains of truth and red herrings—misleading clues—and the challenge is sorting one from the other. The many model systems now available, and further genetics, should produce more insights into the role of huntingtin in cellular processes, but it is a little like doing a jigsaw puzzle without knowing what the eventual picture should look like—many of the pieces have not yet been put into place, and neither do we know how many pieces are missing. The proteasome dysfunction hypothesis is promising (Bence *et al.* 2001; Jana *et al.* 2001) and there is a growing body of evidence in support of huntingtin causing transcriptional changes leading to altered gene expression (Boutell *et al.* 1999; Cha *et al.* 1999; Nucifora, Jr. *et al.* 2001; Steffan *et al.* 2000). Both of these hypotheses could account for the observed cellular dysfunction and eventual death of neurones in HD. However, much work remains to elucidate either the normal or pathological function of huntingtin and the outline presented here is both partial, of necessity, and also partisan, as any view must be.

The basic biology of huntingtin: synthesis, processing, and degradation

Despite the fact that only neurones, and specific groups of neurones at that, die in HD, huntingtin is ubiquitously expressed. The most vulnerable cells are the medium spiny neurones of

Table 12.1 Huntingtin-interacting proteins

Interactor	Alternative names	Homologies	Possible cellular role	References	Repeat-length dependence
CBP strong			Transcriptional regulation	Kazantsev et al. 1999	Yes, very strong
CBS			Formation of cystathionine from homocysteine	Boutell et al. 1998	No
HAP 1	None		Involved in intracellular trafficking?	Li et al. 1995	Yes
HIP 1	HIP1R, Sla2p, talin, ZK370.3 (C. elegans)		Vesicle–cytoskeletal attachment, endocytosis	Kalchman et al. 1997; Wanker et al. 1997	Yes—inverse
HIP 2	Ubiquitin-conjugating enzyme	E2–25K (bovine)	Ubiquitinates proteins marking for degradation by 26S proteasome	Kalchman et al. 1996	No
HIP 3		Akr1 (yeast)	Akr1 essential for endocytosis in yeast	Sittler et al. 1998	Yes—inverse
HYP A		FBP11 (mouse) WW domains	Spliceosome function	Faber et al. 1998; Gusella & MacDonald 1998	Yes
HYP B	DNA binding factor	WW domains	Unknown	Faber et al. 1998; Gusella & MacDonald 1998	Yes
HYP C		WW domains	Unknown	Faber et al. 1998; Gusella & MacDonald 1998	Yes
HYP F	P31 subunit of 26S proteasome		Degradation of ubiquitinated proteins	Gusella & MacDonald 1998	
HYP I	Symplekin		Unknown, but found in tight junctions and nuclei	Gusella & MacDonald 1998	
HYP J	α-adaptin C	None	Endocytosis and membrane recycling	Gusella & MacDonald 1998	
HYPs E, H,K,L,M			Unknown	Gusella & MacDonald 1998	
N-CoR, SMRT			Transcriptional regulation	Boutell et al. 1998; Jones, unpublished	No
SH3GL3	Endophilin III, SH3p13, EENB2	Endophilins I and II	Endocytosis, synaptic vesicle recycling	Sittler et al. 1998	Yes

CBP, CREB-binding protein; CBS, cystathionine β-synthase; FBP, formin binding protein; HAP1, huntingtin associated protein 1; HIP, huntingtin interacting protein; HYP, huntingtin yeast partner; N-CoR, nuclear receptor co-repressor; SMRT, silencing mediator of retinoic acid and thyroid hormone receptors.

Table 12.2 Cellular models of HD*

Cell line(s)	Size polyQ tract	Section of huntingtin	Promoter	Expression	Reference	Major findings
NG108-15	15/73/116	FL, 502, 80	Tet	Stable inducible	Lunkes and Mandel 1998	Nuclear and cytoplasmic inclusions, formation faster with truncation of huntingtin. Increased apoptosis correlated to inclusion load
HEK293, N2a	23, 82	FL, 171, 63	CMV	Transient	Cooper et al. 1998	FL constructs gave diffuse staining, nuclear and cytoplasmic aggregates with 82Q truncated proteins and increased susceptibility to apoptosis
Primarystriatal/ hippocampal rat neurones	17/68	480, 171	CMV	Transient	Saudou et al. 1998	Nuclear localization but not aggregation important in huntingtin-induced cell death
Primary cortical rat neurones, 2–2 HEK293 cells	15, 44, 128	651, 145	CMV	Viral transient?	Martindale et al. 1998, Hackam et al. 1998	Truncation of huntingtin and increasing glutamine length increase cytotoxicity
PC12	20, 150	Exon1	CMV	Stable	Li et al. 1999c	150Q diffuse in nucleus, 20Q in cytoplasm. 150Q poor neurite development and susceptible to stress
Mouse primary striatal cells	18, 46, 100	FL,1073	CMV	Transient	Kim et al. 1999	Mutant huntingtin formed inclusions in time- and polyQ-dependent manner. Apoptosis induced in cells expressing mutant huntingtin
N2a	19, 56	PolyQ only	Tet	Inducible	Miyashita et al. 1999	56Q gave nuclear localization and apoptotic changes including activation of caspase 3
N2a	23, 75	63	CMV	Transient	Peters et al., 1999	Nuclear localization of mutant huntingtin important to toxicity
Rat embryonic primary neurones	79Q only	None	CMV	Transient	Sanchez et al.1999	Q79 recruits and activates caspase 8
HEK293, HN33	15, 138	FL	CMV	Transient	Wellington et al. 2000	Caspase inhibitors reduce toxicity of mutant huntingtin
SK-N-SH, Cos7	21, 72	Exon1	CMV	Transient	Ho et al. 2001	WT huntingtin protective against effects of mutant huntingtin
N2a	16, 60, 150	Exon 1	pIND	Stable inducible	Jana et al. 2001	Increased polyQ expression, decreased proteasomal processing, disrupted mitochondrial membrane, PMF, released cyt c and activated caspases
HEK293	15, 138	FL, 548 and NMDA subunits	CMV	Transient	Zeron et al. 2001	NR2B co-expression with 138Q makes cells more susceptible to apoptosis

FL, full length; WT, wild type; Q, glutamine; CMV, cytomegalovirus intermediate early promoter; Tet, tetracycline inducible promoter; pIND, ecdysone inducible promoter system.
*This is not an exhaustive table of all cellular models of HD, but reflects those that have contributed to our knowledge of the behaviour of huntingtin and its mutation, and that are cited in this chapter.

the striatum, which die first, although other neuronal populations in the cortex and basal ganglia also atrophy at later stages of the disease; a detailed discussion can be found in Chapter 8. Huntingtin is expressed in all cells so far investigated, with highest levels of expression in the brain and testes (Sapp *et al.* 1997; Sharp *et al.* 1995; Strong *et al.* 1993). There are two expressed mRNAs, which differ in size at 10 and 13 kb. More of the larger form appears to be expressed in brain, although it is unclear whether this form is responsible for the higher levels of expression in brain (Strong *et al.* 1993). Although expressed at low but significant levels in glial cells, huntingtin is expressed at much higher levels in neurones (Dure *et al.* 1994). Even very detailed studies have not managed to reveal whether the most vulnerable cells express more huntingtin or actually contain higher concentrations of the mutant protein in humans, although it is true that intense immunoreactivity for huntingtin in some abnormal neurones implies that they have high concentrations of the protein (Sapp *et al.* 1997): this is discussed in more detail below. One study of endogenous huntingtin immunoreactivity in rat brain detected the highest concentrations of huntingtin in those cells of the striatum that would be the most vulnerable in humans (Kosinski *et al.* 1997).

In HD both normal and mutant alleles are expressed from early in development and the presence of the mutation appears not to affect expression (Ambrose *et al.* 1994; Bhide *et al.* 1996; Persichetti *et al.* 1996; Schmitt *et al.* 1995a), although generally expression in non-neuronal tissues is downregulated during development (Schmitt *et al.* 1995b). That huntingtin is essential in development is demonstrated by the deaths of three different lines of huntingtin null mice at embryonic days 6–10 (Duyao *et al.* 1995; Nasir *et al.* 1995; Zeitlin *et al.* 1995), although, despite the observed lethality in animals, lack of huntingtin does not kill cells in culture (Metzler *et al.* 1999). HD$^{-/-}$ embryonic stem (ES) cells grow in culture and differentiate into a neuronal phenotype that raises the issue of the exact processes in gastrulation for which huntingtin is essential (Metzler *et al.* 1999). *Hdh* null mice can be rescued from lethality by wild-type extraembryonic tissues and the underlying defect seems to be in the support of embryonic nutrition by these tissues (Dragatsis *et al.* 2000), so the defect may be in transport functions. This is consistent with the putative role proposed for huntingtin in cellular transport (Sapp *et al.* 1999). It has also been observed that reducing the total amount of normal protein leads to abnormalities in brain development and functioning in transgenic mice, although these changes do not directly recapitulate HD (O'Kusky *et al.* 1999; White *et al.* 1997). However, expression of the normal protein also appears to ameliorate some of the toxic effects of mutated huntingtin (Dragatsis *et al.* 2000; Ho *et al.* 2001; Leavitt *et al.* 2001) and these two findings might imply a role for haploinsufficiency or a dominant negative effect in HD, as the mutated protein is known to sequester the normal protein into inclusions (Hackam *et al.* 1998).

Part of the protective effect of wild-type huntingtin may be explained by the observations of Zuccato *et al.* (2001) who observed upregulation of brain-derived neurotrophic factor (BDNF) in cortical neurones, mediated by wild-type huntingtin. Indeed, expressing full-length mutant huntingtin in their conditionally immortalized central nervous system (CNS) cell lines reduced BDNF expression to around half the normal levels, implying a dominant negative effect of mutant huntingtin on this activity of wild-type huntingtin. Mice carrying a transgene consisting of full-length mutant huntingtin with 72 CAG also demonstrated a 50 per cent reduction in cortically derived BDNF and similar results were obtained in human HD brain (Zuccato *et al.* 2001). It is therefore possible that the mutation causes a dominant negative effect by ablating wild-type huntingtin's beneficial effects, as BDNF is an important neuronal survival factor generated in cortical neurones and released and effective in the striatum (Canals *et al.* 2001).

It should also be noted that other ubiquitously expressed proteins can cause localized lesions and that systemic administration of chemical compounds, such as malonate, that inhibit complex II of the mitochondrial respiratory chain can give rise to lesions that are localized in a very similar way to the HD lesions (Beal *et al.* 1993; see also Chapter 10). This implies that the cells affected in the disease are particularly vulnerable to deficits in energy metabolism and that this in turn may disrupt maintenance of the cellular polarization through less efficient operation of the $Na^+K^+ATPase$. This is the basis of the dysfunctional energy metabolism theory of degeneration in HD, discussed in detail in Chapter 10.

Promoter structure and huntingtin expression

Examination of the HD gene promoter reveals that transcriptional activity resides between -221 and $+4$ base pairs relative to the translational start site (Coles *et al.* 1998; Holzmann *et al.* 2001), and this region contains a number of specific upstream sites for transcriptional regulatory proteins but no TATA or CCAAT boxes (Lin *et al.* 1995). Genes constitutively expressed in most tissues and cell types tend to lack these elements and huntingtin is ubiquitously expressed. There is some indication that the promoter may be more active in neuronal than in non-neuronal cell types (Coles *et al.* 1998), which is reflected in *in vivo* expression studies (Dure *et al.* 1994; Lin *et al.* 1993; Persichetti *et al.* 1996; Sharp *et al.* 1995; Strong *et al.* 1993). Promoter activity *in vitro* is largely controlled by two Sp1 (specificity protein 1) sites that act synergistically. Sp1 sites are GC boxes and binding of Sp1 to these sites can have positive (enhancer sequence) or negative (silencer sequence) regulatory effects depending on their exact context and the cell type (Philipsen and Suske 1999). The Sp1 sites are contained in a tandem 20 bp repeat region but, although this is polymorphic with around 1 per cent of the population having only one copy and thus only one Sp1-binding site, giving reduced transcriptional efficacy *in vitro* (Coles *et al.* 1998), this did not appear to influence age of onset of HD (Coles *et al.* 1998). Other putative regulatory sequences are present in the 5' flanking region of the HD gene, but their functionality remains unknown (Holzmann *et al.* 2001). The detailed expression analysis of Landwehrmeyer *et al.* (1995) demonstrated that huntingtin was expressed at higher levels in neurones than glia, but that the cell types that died did not have significantly different expression levels compared with other neurones that do survive in HD. Differential expression therefore, appears unable to explain the specific pattern of neuronal vulnerability in HD. To examine the regionally specific nature of the degeneration, the interacting partners of huntingtin and their roles in different cell types have been examined extensively and some of this evidence is presented below, starting with the intracellular localization of huntingtin.

Tissue mosaicism

One striking observation that could account for the vulnerability of striatal neurones is the dramatic somatic instability of the CAG repeat region in the DNA of these neurones seen by Kennedy and Shelbourne (2000) in their knock-in mice carrying 70–80 CAGs. A confirmation of this finding in human HD would transform the search for factors relating to the specificity of cell death. If translated then these very expanded polyglutamine tracts would undoubtedly have a very deleterious effect on cells as experimental systems using very long repeats demonstrate (Kazantsev *et al.* 1999; Marsh *et al.* 2000; Moulder *et al.* 1999). If this is not the case, for instance, if these repeats are not transcribed or translated, then cells with shorter repeats that are transcribed and translated must be responsible for the neurodegeneration. The issue of somatic mosaicism in HD is discussed in more detail in Chapter 5.

The cellular localization of huntingtin

The localization of huntingtin within cells has been the subject of much debate since the first antibodies were generated subsequent to the gene being cloned (Strong *et al.* 1993). The pathological observation of intranuclear inclusions, immunoreactive for the polyglutamine tract and the areas of the huntingtin protein surrounding the repeat region, was revolutionary, partly because most previous observations had placed huntingtin in the cytoplasm (DiFiglia *et al.* 1995; Gutekunst *et al.* 1995). There were a few reports of huntingtin in the nucleus in particular cell types (De Rooij *et al.* 1996; Sapp *et al.* 1997), although examination of the literature after the observation of inclusions in the transgenic mouse models of HD revealed that structures that were almost certainly intranuclear inclusions had been observed in HD brain previously, but that their significance had gone unrecognized (Roizin *et al.* 1979). Of course, at that time there was no indication of their molecular composition. In neurones, huntingtin is observed throughout the neuropil, in axons, dendrites, and pre- and post-synaptic regions (Gutekunst *et al.* 1999; Sharp *et al.* 1995). Diffuse huntingtin immunoreactivity in the neuronal nucleus of transgenic mice has now also been observed, where it appears before the appearance of nuclear inclusions (Wheeler *et al.* 2000). This can also be seen, rarely, in human Vonsattel grade 0 and 1 HD brain (Jones L., unpublished data), in cells of a type that are known to develop inclusions. The most parsimonious explanation of these observations is that huntingtin is transported into the nucleus and subsequently aggregates into an inclusion. Presumably this diffuse pattern of huntingtin immunoreactivity is observed infrequently in human brain as, by the end stage of the disease, most of the vulnerable neurones either have frank inclusions or have died. This is a very slow process in human HD; the disease can progress for 10 to 20 years and changes are almost certainly occurring before frank symptoms are seen (Gomez-Tortosa *et al.* 2001; Kirkwood *et al.* 2000a,b). However, the knock-in mouse models of HD (Lin *et al.* 2001; Shelbourne *et al.* 1999; Wheeler *et al.* 1999), in particular, give us an opportunity to study this process in detail and determine its relevance to the aetiology of the disease.

It is also interesting that, although it is clear that medium spiny projection neurones in the striatum are most vulnerable in HD, inclusions are more common in the cortex (Gutekunst *et al.* 1999; Sieradzan and Mann 1998) and inclusion load in the cortex correlates better with CAG expansion size than inclusion load in the striatum (Sieradzan and Mann 1998). Brain inclusion load in adult-onset HD is notably low with generally <5 per cent of neurones in any area found to contain inclusions. This may reflect the loss of inclusion-containing neurones in the striatum, or may result from anteriograde or retrograde degeneration from projection of inclusion-containing neurones on to the striatal neurones. Accumulation of *N*-terminal huntingtin altering transport in axons and leading to degeneration of the corticostriatal pathway was suggested by Sapp *et al.* (1999). The finding that mutant huntingtin can lower BDNF expression in cortical neurones projecting to the striatum may indicate a possible anteriograde mechanism of degeneration operating in HD brain (Zuccato *et al.* 2001).

The intranuclear inclusions are not the only huntingtin aggregates detected in HD brain; neuropil aggregates are also found, especially in cortical layers V and VI (Gutekunst *et al.* 1999;

Sapp *et al.* 1997, 1999) and these can be extensive in axons, dendrites, and dendritic spines. Several different HD transgenic mice also demonstrate similar aggregates (Li *et al.* 1999b, 2000; Lin *et al.* 2001; Reddy *et al.* 1998; Schilling *et al.* 1999; Wheeler *et al.* 2000). The cytoplasmic aggregates are more variable than the nuclear ones, with a greater range of morphologies (Gutekunst *et al.* 1998; Sapp *et al.* 1997) and contain longer *N*-terminal fragments of huntingtin than the nuclear inclusions (Aronin *et al.* 1999). However, all of these aggregated forms of huntingtin have been truncated, so how does this occur and is it specific to mutant HD and thus part of the HD pathological process?

The toxicity of mutated huntingtin is affected by its localization. Several sets of experiments have used nuclear import and export signals to investigate the relevance of cellular location to cell dysfunction and death after expression of full-length or fragments of the mutant protein. Full-length huntingtin is unable to enter the nucleus through nuclear pores, as it is too large, although truncated fragments may enter the nucleus by this route. The possible mechanisms of huntingtin truncation are discussed below. A variety of cell culture experiments have shown that successive truncations of the mutant protein, increased polyglutamine length, and nuclear localization increase cytotoxicity (Cooper *et al.* 1998; Hackam *et al.* 1998; Kazantsev *et al.* 1999; Lunkes and Mandel 1998; Martindale *et al.* 1998; Peters *et al.* 1999). Proteolysis of the full-length protein is discussed below. A similar result is found in the other polyglutamine diseases (Chapter 14). In contrast, Saudou *et al.* (1998) found a subtly different result: nuclear localization indeed increased mutated huntingtin toxicity, but prevention of inclusion formation actually increased toxicity of mutant huntingtin to clonal striatal cells. However, the mechanism used to prevent aggregation of huntingtin involved interference with ubiquitination and may have had other deleterious side-effects on cellular viability. It is also true that some aggregation may have taken place, into protofibrils, soluble structures that appear diffuse but are in effect submicroscopic aggregates. Recent evidence in Alzheimer's disease indicates that these small protofibrillar structures may be the toxic moiety, rather than the large and visible amyloid plaques (Nilsberth *et al.* 2001). Further evidence for the importance of huntingtin aggregation to cytotoxicity comes from studies of various transgenic mouse models where intra- or extranuclear aggregate formation correlates with phenotype progression (Davies *et al.* 1997; Morton *et al.* 2000) and altering the rate of inclusion formation by delaying it using inhibitors (Ona *et al.* 1999) or by switching off the transgene in an inducible animal model (Yamamoto *et al.* 2000) correspondingly alters the phenotype.

Huntingtin processing

There are no reports of huntingtin undergoing any covalent posttranslational processing, although there is also a dearth of published work on any processing other than truncation. It appears a relatively stable protein, in both the normal and mutated forms: pulse-chase labelling experiments in lymphoblasts from HD patients showed a half-life of at least 24 hours (Persichetti *et al.* 1996). However, one of the clearest differences between the normal and mutated protein is their relative susceptibility to proteolysis. Mutated huntingtin, which aggregates, is truncated and only the *N*-terminal fragment is deposited in any of the observed cellular inclusions (DiFiglia *et al.* 1997; Gutekunst *et al.* 1999; Sapp *et al.* 1999) and, the more truncated the fragment and the longer the glutamine repeat, the faster aggregation occurs (Cooper *et al.* 1998; Hackam *et al.* 1998; Kazantsev *et al.* 1999; Kim *et al.* 1999;

Lunkes and Mandel 1998; Marsh *et al.* 2000; Martindale *et al.* 1998; Peters *et al.* 1999). Non-mutated full-length huntingtin does not appear to undergo any cleavage process (Kim *et al.* 1999; Lunkes and Mandel 1998). Aggregation only occurs if the glutamine tract is expanded beyond 37 residues. The exact molecular size of huntingtin that is present in aggregates is not clear, but epitopes from the *N*-terminus and polyglutamine tract are detected, whereas more *C*-terminal epitopes are not. The identity of the proteases involved in the *N*-terminal truncation is not known, although caspases have been suggested to be involved (Wellington *et al.* 1998). Their role and that of apoptosis in mediating HD neuronal death is explored further below.

Although we know that truncation of huntingtin renders it more toxic to cells (Marsh *et al.* 2000; Martindale *et al.* 1998) and makes it aggregate faster (Hackam *et al.* 1998), the relationship between these two facts is unclear. The ability of the proteasome to degrade the mutant protein also seems to be important to the speed of aggregation (Jana *et al.* 2001). Aggregation is related to the physical nature of the polyglutamine region as demonstrated by its aggregation *in vitro* (Scherzinger *et al.* 1997) and its occurrence in almost every cell type or animal species forced to express long polyglutamine tracts, from yeast upwards (Faber *et al.* 1999; Krobitsch and Lindquist 2000; Marsh *et al.* 2000; Ordway *et al.* 1997). It is, however, impossible to discuss huntingtin truncation further without considering the involvement of apoptosis.

Cell death in HD
Cells demonstrably die in HD. What is not clear is, first, how this occurs and, second, whether the dying cells have been dysfunctional for a considerable time before cell death. Evidence for the classical apoptotic pathway operating in HD is unclear, although much evidence for the involvement of various players in the pathway is reported (see Fig. 12.2). In some of the

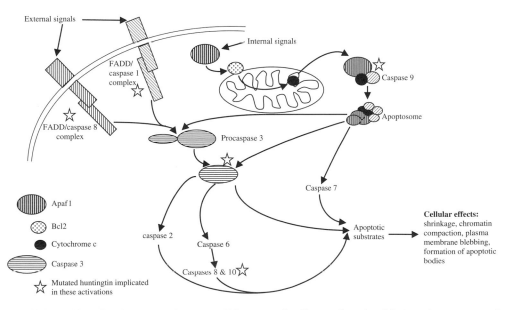

Fig. 12.2 Outline of major apoptotic events. This composite diagram is a simplified version of some of the major cascades showing the relationship of various caspases to each other and to other important molecules in the pathway to apoptosis. Points at which huntingtin has been suggested to have an involvement are indicated by a star and these are referred to in the subsection 'Cell death in HD'.

transgenic animal models there is no evidence for any cell death, apoptotic or otherwise, previous to clear behavioural phenotypes (Davies *et al.* 1997), which suggests that neuronal dysfunction is important in HD. Animal models, however, are not just small versions of humans with HD, although they may recapitulate many aspects of the disease. In particular, their relatively short life span means that either overexpression of the HD gene or fragments of it, or very long polyglutamine lengths, are necessary to produce a phenotype within the life span of the animal (Lin *et al.* 2001; Mangiarini *et al.* 1996; Shelbourne *et al.* 1999; Wheeler *et al.* 1999, 2000; see also Chapter 13). There is, however, considerable evidence for the involvement of apoptosis-related genes as a downstream effect of the expanded glutamine tract in cells (Hackam *et al.* 1998; Jana *et al.* 2001; Kim *et al.* 1999; Li *et al.* 1999c; Liu 1998; Martindale *et al.* 1998; Miyashita *et al.* 1999; Sanchez *et al.* 1999; Wang *et al.* 1999a; Wellington *et al.* 2000).

Apoptosis is programmed cell death operating, for instance, in the wave of neuronal deaths that occurs postnatally in the brains of many animals. It is an active and directed process requiring energy and mediated through the operation of a cascade of signal and effector proteins (Shearwin-Whyatt and Kumar 1999). This is outlined in Fig. 12.2 with an indication of the points at which huntingtin activity has been suggested to play a role, including mitochondrial involvement (see Chapter 10). One class of proteins that contains molecules that may be either apoptotic signals or effectors is the caspases, which activate other proteins though a proteolytic cascade leading to apoptotic cell death.

Caspases can themselves cleave huntingtin and some of the other polyglutamine proteins (Goldberg *et al.* 1996; Wellington *et al.* 1998, 2000), but the relationship of this observation to the *in vivo* cleavage of huntingtin is unclear. In particular, the relative affinity of the caspases for huntingtin compared with their usual substrates in the cell death pathways has not been reported. Wild-type full-length huntingtin protein does not appear to be routinely truncated, but the mutated protein is (Kim *et al.* 1999; Lunkes and Mandel 1998; Wellington *et al.* 2000). What remains unclear is whether it is truncated because its intrinsic structural properties render it more susceptible to proteolysis or because it initiates a process that then causes that truncation.

Caspase 3 is an apoptotic effector molecule, which has a number of consensus proteolytic sites in huntingtin. It can cleave the normal or mutated molecule, and site-directed mutagenesis abolishes this cleavage (Wellington *et al.* 2000). But caspase 3 is only expressed in cells undergoing apoptosis so, in order for it to cleave huntingtin *in vivo*, apoptosis must be occurring. However, if caspases were the only huntingtin-cleaving enzymes then fragments of huntingtin larger than those detected should be deposited in inclusions (DiFiglia *et al.* 1997). Interestingly, caspases themselves are detected in inclusions (Sanchez *et al.* 1999), which may imply that they do interact closely with huntingtin as it aggregates. So, if caspase cleavage of huntingtin occurs, it seems likely to be secondary to whatever is causing cellular dysfunction.

To further investigate the effects of caspases, Kim *et al.* (1999) used a cell culture model in mouse clonal striatal cells and found a dissociation of inclusion formation from neuronal survival using caspase inhibitors. In their cultures, expanded huntingtin formed cytoplasmic and nuclear inclusions. Each consisted of truncated huntingtin fragments, but the cytoplasmic inclusions generally had longer sections of more C-terminal protein within them. They observed apoptosis induced by overexpression of wild-type or mutant huntingtin, but more in response to mutant huntingtin. Their most interesting finding was that Z-VAD-FMK, an inhibitor of caspases 1 and 3, did not alter inclusion formation, but did increase cell survival and prevented the accumulation of at least one molecular species of N-terminally truncated huntingtin. In contrast, Z-DEVD-FMK, a caspase 3 inhibitor, decreased inclusion formation in both the cytoplasm and nucleus, but did not affect cell survival. This implies that inhibiting caspase 1 can prevent cell death due to mutant huntingtin whereas inhibiting caspase 3 cannot, although it affects aggregation of huntingtin. Further studies have also implicated caspase 1 in ameliorating huntingtin toxicity.

The antibiotic minocyline, which is a caspase 1 and 3 inhibitor, delays the onset of the motor phenotype in the R6/2 mouse model of HD (Chen *et al.* 2000) as does the expression of a dominant negative mutant of caspase 1 (Ona *et al.* 1999). Minocyline inhibition delays, but does not prevent, the behavioural changes normally seen in this mouse model and this is consistent with apoptosis being a downstream effect of some initiating toxic event. Mitochondrial metabolism is altered in HD and this may be a trigger for an apoptotic pathway, as suggested by the work of Sanchez *et al.* (1999), or a downstream effect of apoptosis—the role of mitochondrial metabolism in HD is discussed in Chapter 10. In PC12 cells intranuclear huntingtin upregulates expression of caspase 1, with concomitant activation of caspase 3 and release of cytochrome c from the mitochondria, although no direct relationship between these observations was established (Li *et al.* 1999c).

However, anything that potentiates the apoptotic pathway is likely to activate caspases that at this point may cleave huntingtin and lead to the appearance of truncated huntingtin fragments in the cell. An initial proteolytic event mediated by caspases may cause parts of the remaining protein to be vulnerable to other cellular proteases. This argument is supported by the results of Wellington *et al.* (2000) who showed that caspase-resistant huntingtin has reduced toxicity in cultured cells and forms aggregates much less readily. An important caveat, however, is that the culture in which the study was carried out had apoptosis induced by the addition of tamoxifen and thus it cannot be established what the precipitating pathogenic event was in these cells; the tamoxifen may have initiated a downstream pathway normally initiated by other stimuli in HD.

Another recent study has demonstrated that huntingtin containing expanded polyglutamine inhibits proteasomal function and that several characteristic events of apoptosis ensue (Jana *et al.* 2001). These include disrupted mitochondrial function with the release of cytochrome c into the cytosol, a classical marker of early apoptotic events, and activation of caspase 9 and a caspase 3-like activity. In another cell model when mutated huntingtin was expressed, caspase 1 expression also increased (Li *et al.* 1999c), and this may have led to the observed activation of caspase 3 and release of cytochrome c from the mitochondria in this model. The proteasomal degradation of huntingtin is discussed in detail below.

Caspase 8 has also been found to be necessary for the death of primary rat neurones expressing 79, but not 35 glutamines. These constructs had only 12 amino acids of surrounding huntingtin plus a haemagglutinin tag. Specific inhibition of caspase 8 blocked this polyglutamine-induced toxicity and cell death (Sanchez *et al.* 1999). Caspase 8 is recruited and activated through the Fas pathway, important in the regulation of lymphocytes in the immune system. There is some supporting evidence for increased caspase 8 immunoreactivity in the caudate of HD brains (Sanchez *et al.* 1999).

A few studies have been carried out in peripheral cells derived from HD patients. Increased apoptotic cell death correlated with glutamine repeat length was seen in lymphoblasts derived from juvenile HD cases subjected to proapoptotic stresses and this was associated with caspase 3 activation. A recent study of apoptosis in control and HD lymphocytes showed that both symptomatic- and presymptomatic-derived HD lymphocytes are more susceptible to ultraviolet B (UVB)-irradiation-induced apoptosis. Even more tantalizing is the report that HD patients suffer from fewer cancers than would be expected in an age- and sex-matched control population (Sorensen *et al*. 1999). If all cells are balanced on a threshold between division and death, then the fact that mutated huntingtin presdisposes cells to apoptosis might be shifting the balance to death rather than division, resulting in fewer than expected cancers. This is speculation, but the conclusion of these studies is that the presence of the expanded glutamine tract in huntingtin predisposes all cells, not just neurones, to be more vulnerable to death stimuli, irrespective of whether inclusions have formed in those cells or not. The precipitating factor, however, remains unknown.

In contrast, wild-type huntingtin appears to confer protection from various apoptotic stimuli on cells (Ho *et al*. 2001; Rigamonti *et al*. 2000) with some evidence that this is through inhibition of procaspase 9 processing (Rigamonti *et al*. 2001). The huntingtin interacting protein, HIP1, has recently been shown to possess proapoptotic activity that can be modulated by huntingtin (Hackam *et al*. 2000). Conceivably, sequestration of this protein by huntingtin in the normal cell inhibits apoptosis. The strength of the HIP1 interaction with huntingtin is inversely proportional to polyglutamine repeat length; thus in the disease more HIP1 could exist free in the cell, predisposing that cell to apoptosis. Similar, weaker, evidence exists for the mixed lineage kinase 2 (MLK2) whose interaction with huntingtin is attenuated by the expanded glutamine tract. MLK2 induces C-Jun N-terminal kinase (JNK) activation and thus apoptosis. However, overexpression of wild-type huntingtin can rescue these cells, consistent with the evidence of Rigamonti *et al*. (2000) and Leavitt *et al*. (2001).

Many of the pathways that seem to be altered in HD or models of the disease, and that are discussed below, would be expected to result in apoptosis. The classic hallmark of apoptosis, fragmented DNA as observed by TUNEL staining, has been reported in HD brain (Dragunow *et al*. 1995; Portera-Cailliau *et al*. 1995; Thomas *et al*. 1995) and in some mouse models (Reddy *et al*. 1998). However, other detailed studies in HD brain and in transgenic animal models show no changes characteristic of apoptosis (Turmaine *et al*. 2000). Condensation of neuronal cells into compact dark bodies in the brain seems to be a common observation (Turmaine *et al*. 2000). It is also observed in human HD brain and other mouse models, and this may be accompanied or preceded by apoptosis (Iannicola *et al*. 2000).

Neuronal apoptosis, though, could be caused by many of the other events that the presence of the expanded glutamine tract in huntingtin appears to precipitate. A long-standing explanation for the neurodegeneration in HD is the weak excitotoxic hypothesis (Albin and Greenamyre 1992; Beal *et al*. 1993). The medium spiny neurones most susceptible to degeneration are characterized by the presence of *N*-methyl-D-aspartate (NMDA) receptors in their synapses, which are sensitive to the excitatory amino acid glutamate. Overactivation of these receptors allows increased Ca^{2+} influx into the cell and leads to cell dysfunction and death through apoptosis. Zeron *et al*. (2001) co-expressed NR1A and NR2B subunits of the NMDA receptor along with mutated huntingtin and demonstrated that susceptibility to apoptotic stress in these cells was increased over that seen when wild-type huntingtin was expressed, and Levine *et al*. (1999) demonstrated enhanced sensitivity to NMDA receptor activation in HD mouse models. Mutant huntingtin itself may potentiate oversensitivity of the predominant type of medium spiny neurone NMDA receptor to its ligand, glutamate, thus increasing Ca^{2+} influx. This effect could be modulated by the reduced association of mutant huntingtin to postsynaptic density (PSD) 95 (Savinainen *et al.* 2001) as PSD95 binds to NR2 subunits and controls receptor density at synapses; that is, increased Ca^{2+} influx could reflect increased NMDA receptor density. It is not clear that anyone has measured Ca^{2+} fluxes in any of these cellular systems.

Other alterations in cellular metabolism associated with expression of mutant huntingtin that could lead ultimately to cell death include altered transcription, protein processing through the unfolded protein pathways, and proteasomal insufficiency or changes in neuro-transmission across synapses leading to anteriograde or retrograde signals that will end in apoptosis. The observed decrease of cortical BDNF in HD brain (Zuccato *et al.* 2001) may be just such a precipitating insult. Given the evidence for neuronal dysfunction before death, it may be wise to regard apoptosis as a possible end pathway leading from upstream events in the pathological pathway. Finally, the cell death occurring may demonstrate some, but not all, of the characteristic features of apoptosis.

It is difficult to extrapolate the results, particularly from cellular models, directly to the human disease. Overexpressing proteins for relatively short times can be misleading because of the precipitation of massive cellular stress caused by a large concentration of an even mildly toxic protein. The cell models, however, provide an environment in which specific hypotheses can be tested quickly, but results of these experiments should be interpreted conservatively, and followed up by work in transgenic animal models.

Huntingtin degradation

Apart from possible degradation through caspase activity, there are a number of other cellular proteolysis systems that may play a role in huntingtin degradation. It has emerged over the past decade that huntingtin can be actively degraded by ubiquitination followed by hydrolysis in the proteasome. Proteasomes exist in the nucleus and cytoplasm of cells, and have different characteristics depending on their location (Voges *et al.* 1999). The proteasomal degradation pathway is important for cell viability as demonstrated by the toxicity of proteasome inhibitors (for example, lactacystin). Their primary functions appear to be the coordinated regulation, through active degradation, of proteins such as short-lived signalling mediators and the removal of misfolded proteins (Voges *et al.* 1999). As huntingtin itself is a long-lived protein, it should not normally be targeted for rapid degradation in the proteasome. The ubiquitin-conjugating enzyme, E2–25K (also known as huntingtin-interacting protein 2, HIP2) appears to bind equally to both expanded and wild-type huntingtin (Kalchman *et al.* 1996), implying no preferential labelling of the mutated protein for degradation by this pathway, although other steps in the pathway could confer such specificity. Huntingtin has been demonstrated to interact with proteasomal components (Gusella and MacDonald 1998) as well as the E2-25K ubiquitin-conjugating enzyme (Kalchman *et al.* 1996), and ubiquitin and proteasomal components are found sequestered into inclusions (Waelter *et al.* 2001a). Chaperones, which assist in the correct folding of proteins and can refold improperly folded proteins, particularly Hsp40 and Hsp70, can affect both the aggregation state and toxicity of mutant huntingtin and other polyglutamine proteins (Cummings *et al.* 1998; Krobitsch and Lindquist 2000; Warrick *et al.* 1999; see also Chapter 14). The effects of chaperones on aggregation and toxicity are dealt with in detail in Chapter 11.

Although there is no evidence that mutated huntingtin is preferentially targeted to the pro-teasome, the effects it exerts on proteasome activity when degradation is taking place could be responsible for eventual proteasome dysfunction. The hypothesis that mutant huntingtin might interfere with proteasomal degradation of other cellular proteins by blocking or disrupting its function has recently been tested directly by Bence *et al.* (2001) who found that cells transfected with mutant huntingtin or cystic fibrosis transmembrane conductance regulator (CFTR) failed to degrade a recombinant green fluorescent protein (GFP)-tagged protein that would normally have been degraded by this pathway. This provides strong support for the hypothesis of Jana *et al.* (2001) that expanded polyglutamine inhibits proteasome function. Both transient and inducible cell culture systems expressing *N*-terminal huntingtin and the R6/1 model demonstrated sequestration of the 20S catalytic proteasomal subunit to inclusions (Waelter *et al.* 2001a; Wyttenbach *et al.* 2000). When a proteasomal inhibitor was added to the inducible cell culture model it increased aggregation markedly if the *N*-terminal huntingtin contained 60 glutamines, although this was not the case with 150 glutamines (Waelter *et al.* 2001a). In the latter case aggregation may have been so rapid that no degradation of the soluble protein by any means took place. The rapid dispersal of aggregates seen in primary striatal neurones cultured from the inducible HD94 mouse brain is proteasome-dependent (Martin-Aparicio *et al.* 2001). Further, once the transgene is switched off in the HD94 mice, reversal of aggregation is rapid—5 days—and precedes phenotypic normality by several weeks. In this animal the proteasomal and cellular dysfunction appears to be reversible and, remarkably, the neuronal cells, which never die, can recover (Martin-Aparicio *et al.* 2001). The structural properties of polyglutamine that might lead to its aggregation and aberrant proteasomal processing are discussed in greater detail in Chapter 11.

Circumstantial evidence also supports the notion that huntingtin accumulates and cannot be cleared from cells and that this leads to other proteins being similarly accumulated. There are many individual reports of increased immunoreactivity of proteins such as the nuclear co-repressor (N-CoR), the silencing mediator of retinoic acid and thyroid hormone receptors (SMRT), CA150 (Boutell *et al.* 1999; Jones *et al.*, unpublished; Holbert *et al.* 2001), and huntingtin itself (Sapp *et al.* 1997), seen in HD brain compared with controls. N-CoR and SMRT, like cyclic AMP binding protein response element binding (CREB)-binding protein (CBP), are proteins present at limiting quantities in the cell, tightly regulated to maintain their specific function, and N-CoR is known to be degraded in the proteasome, through mSiah2 (Zhang *et al.* 1998). Overexpression of CBP can overcome huntingtin-induced toxicity in cell culture (Nucifora *et al.* 2001), implying that sequestration of this protein into aggregates can be overcome by increasing CBP activity. These observations could be a result of mutant huntingtin accumulating in the cell and sequestering other proteins, or it could be a reflection of a specific inhibition of protein degradation mechanisms in the cells of HD brain. Interestingly, another protein deposited in a neurodegeneration, α-synuclein, also inhibits proteasome activity in neuronal cells, leading to apoptosis and cell death (Tanaka *et al.* 2001).

It has also been suggested that huntingtin is degraded in lysosomes through autophagy. Kegel *et al.* (2000) found normal and mutated huntingtin in lysosomes and that autophagy within these lysosomes could be producing the *N*-terminal fragments of huntingtin that go on to form aggregates. This degradation was seen in a system overexpressing huntingtin and it is possible that huntingtin is normally degraded by this pathway and that it is only when it is misfolded that the proteasomal pathway is induced, although there is no direct evidence to support this. However, whether the huntingtin cleavage is by the proteasome or autophagy, the amounts of huntingtin and of other proteins detected in HD brain indicate that mutated huntingtin may well overwhelm the cellular systems for dealing with them. Thus the cells reach a point where they can no longer degrade the abnormal protein and it builds up, causing downstream cellular defects that lead to neuronal dysfunction and death. This work has recently been extended by Petersen *et al.* (2001). Using cultures of striatal neurones from R6/2 mice, they found that cells containing the mutant protein were much more susceptible to dopamine exposure than those without. Subsequent to the dopamine exposure the neurones developed autophagic granules and electron-dense lysosomes. Concomitant with these observations was the appearance of cytoplasmic puncta containing high levels of reactive oxygen species (ROS) and ubiquitin; these observations are consistent with previous observations of similar structures in human HD brain (Roizin *et al.* 1979; Sapp *et al.* 1999; Tellez-Nagel *et al.* 1974).

Oxidative damage is another final pathway of neural cell death long suggested to occur in HD. Aconitase activity, a sensitive marker for the presence of ROS, is known to show markedly reduced activity in both HD patient tissue and transgenic mouse brain (Browne *et al.* 1997; Tabrizi *et al.* 1999). Production of ROS is intimately connected to oxidative energy metabolism and is discussed further in Chapter 10.

It remains unclear exactly how huntingtin is processed but there is a difference between processing and degradation of the normal and mutated proteins. It is clear that the mutated protein can aggregate before adequate clearance takes place. Mutated huntingtin is certainly cleaved in a way that the normal protein is not, but this appears to be specific and not to be part of the normal degradative pathway. A parsimonious explanation for the appearance of aggregates is that the concentration of expanded glutamine-containing fragments of huntingtin increases to the point where aggregation can occur—possibly through nucleation (Perutz and Windle 2001). This can occur as a result of mass action—many proteins aggregate with increased concentrations (Samuel *et al.* 1990). The concentration can rise through increased synthesis or reduced degradation of the aggregating molecular species. In the case of huntingtin the current evidence supports altered degradation rather than altered synthesis. Perhaps one final and intriguing insight is that the ubiquitin–proteasome system of yeast is important in transcriptional activity (Ferdous *et al.* 2001; Salghetti *et al.* 2001). Thus it may be that changes in proteasomal function, and the observed transcriptional alterations discussed below, are actually part of the same dysfunctional mechanism.

Huntingtin's role in cellular processes

Transcriptional regulation

Alterations in gene expression have been detected in HD and other polyglutamine diseases (Lin *et al.* 2001; Luthi-Carter *et al.* 2000), implying a dysregulation of transcription. Over the years before and after the cloning of the HD gene, up- or downregulation in expression of various genes early in the disease has been noted (Albin *et al.* 1991; Augood *et al.* 1996; Denovan-Wright and Robertson 2000; Glass *et al.* 2000; Richfield *et al.* 1995; see also Chapter 9). This evidence, whilst intrinsically interesting, has been difficult to attribute to particular mechanisms of polyglutamine action and has been complicated by the lack of clarity surrounding the relationship of neurodegeneration to the appearance of symptoms (Chapters 2, 3, and 15). More recently, however, a number of studies have indicated that huntingtin containing an expanded polyglutamine repeat may be directly involved in altering transcriptional regulatory processes and that this may, therefore, be part of its pathogenic action (Boutell *et al.* 1999; Nucifora *et al.* 2001; Steffan *et al.* 2000).

The first suggestion of a role for transcriptional processes in HD pathogenesis came from the observation by Gerber *et al.* (1994) soon after the gene was cloned that proteins with long polyglutamine and polyproline stretches were often involved in transcriptional processes. The androgen receptor, causing the neurodegeneration in SBMA when its glutamine tract is expanded, is itself a transcription factor. A number of these transcriptionally active proteins, for instance, the TATA-binding protein (TBP), have long polyglutamine stretches. Interestingly, in the case of TBP, the normal range is 25–42 glutamines (Rubinsztein *et al.* 1996), at the upper range enough glutamines to give disease if found in huntingtin. Expansion of these glutamines is now known to occur and to cause disease: a rare neurodegeneration, SCA-17, has been attributed to expansion to 55+ glutamines in this protein (Nakamura *et al.* 2001; Zuhlke *et al.* 2001). However, as huntingtin was thought to reside mainly in the cytoplasm and thus to be excluded from a nuclear role, this observation was not followed up to any great extent until after the observation of intranuclear inclusions in 1997 (Davies *et al.* 1997; DiFiglia *et al.* 1997).

A number of proteins detected as interacting with huntingtin (CBP, CA150, polyglutamine binding protein 1 (PQBP1), TAFII130; see Table 12.1) or found sequestered in intranuclear inclusions (TBP, CBP, TFIID, mSin3a and b) are known to be involved in transcription, and some functional studies indicate that huntingtin can repress transcription in *in vitro* reporter systems (Nucifora *et al.* 2001; Jones, unpublished). Huntingtin represses transcription through a p53 reporter complex (Steffan *et al.* 2000) and is known to alter transcription of various genes (Cha *et al.* 1998; Luthi-Carter *et al.* 2000; Richfield *et al.* 1995; Zuccato *et al.* 2001). p53 transcriptional repression is dependent on mSin3 as mSin3 stabilizes p53 and prevents its degradation by the proteasome (Zilfou *et al.* 2001). As mSin3a is relocalized in HD brain (Boutell *et al.* 1999), this may affect p53 activity and also assist in recruiting mSin3 proteins into inclusions.

CBP is a transcriptional activation protein itself, activated in response to intracellular signalling pathways mediated by growth factors, such as those downstream of epidermal growth factor (EGF) or insulin, which signal through cyclic adenosine monophosphate (cAMP). The 8-bp cAMP-responsive element (CRE) 5′-TGACGTCA-3′, found in regulatory regions upstream of genes, binds CREB, a bZIP transcription factor (Shaywitz and Greenberg 1999). However, CREB activity is modulated not by DNA binding but by a phosphorylation event at Ser133 in CREB, and it is this phosphorylated form to which CBP binds. CBP binding to DNA may modulate transcriptional activity in two ways: first, by acting as a bridge between the cAMP enhancer and RNA polymerase II and, second, through the intrinsic histone acetylase activity of CBP—acetylated histones have an open structure allowing the transcriptional machinery access to promoters (Fig. 12.3(b)). CBP has a wide distribution in the body and many genes have CREs upstream and CRE-signalling is mediated through a number of different cellular pathways (Shaywitz and Greenberg 1999). In the brain, CBP mediates the transcription of a number of important neuronal survival factors, including BDNF (Bonni *et al.* 1999; Riccio *et al.* 1999; Walton and Dragunow 2000). CBP is also recruited to genes containing POU and AP1 response elements.

Mutations in CBP cause Rubinstein–Taybi syndrome, which is associated with severe mental retardation and is generally sporadic because of the severity of the phenotype, so alterations in CBP can have profound neurological consequences. The CBP interacts with huntingtin through the polyglutamine stretch of huntingtin; CBP is also known to interact with atrophin (Nucifora *et al.* 2001; Wood *et al.* 2000) and the androgen receptor (AR; McCampbell *et al.*

2000) through their respective polyglutamine tracts. Overexpression of CBP prevents mutant huntingtin toxicity in neuronal cell cultures and removal of the polyglutamine tract from CBP makes this effect more marked (Nucifora *et al.* 2001), whilst reporter assays indicate that transcription mediated through CRE-responsive sites was repressed by mutant huntingtin. CBP, like many transcriptional regulators, is known to be under tight control in the cell, with total levels controlled by specific expression and degradation pathways; thus small changes in its total level could rapidly lead to transcriptional aberrations. Expression of CBP is ubiquitous, but nevertheless it is an attractive candidate for involvement in huntingtin-mediated cell death. It cannot, however, be the ubiquitous expression pattern of CBP itself that determines the specificity of cell death, but the specificity may reflect the control of expression of cell-type specific factors (Zuccato *et al.* 2001).

PQBP1 is a relatively uncharacterized protein that binds to huntingtin and AR and is a Brn-2 binding protein (Waragai *et al.* 1999). Brn-2 is a POU domain binding transcription factor involved in controlling CNS-specific gene expression in a developmentally regulated fashion (Hagino-Yamagishi *et al.* 1998; Schonemann *et al.* 1995) and thus may alter transcription in HD and SBMA.

A further huntingtin interacting transcriptional activator is the CA150 protein (Holbert *et al.* 2001). This protein contains a glutamine/alanine 38-residue repeat through which its interaction with the polyglutamine of huntingtin is probably mediated, and is detected in intranuclear inclusions in HD brain. It appears to be highly expressed in HD striatum compared with control tissue. The targets of this activator are unknown, although it is known to act in concert with CBP in at least one situation (Ott *et al.* 1999; Sune *et al.* 1997). It also has one rare allele that appears to account for a small proportion of the residual variation in age of onset of HD unaccounted for by the length of the HD glutamine repeat. This, together with its restricted expression pattern, makes it worthy of consideration as a factor involved in HD pathogenesis.

The nuclear receptor co-repressor, N-CoR, has also been detected as interacting with huntingtin (Boutell *et al.* 1999) as has the closely related SMRT (also called N-CoR2). Both are mainly detected in brain in the neurones of the cortex, and hardly at all in the caudate, but are relocalized in HD cortical neurones and occasionally detected in inclusions. N-CoR represses transcription from sequence-specific transcription factors in the absence of cognate ligand, by recruiting a repressor complex that includes the mSin3 proteins and histone deacetylases (Alland *et al.* 1997; see Fig. 12.3(a)). The mSin3 proteins are relocalized in HD brain and detected in a proportion, but not all, huntingtin immunoreactive intranuclear inclusions in HD brain. Amongst the transcription factors known to be repressed by N-CoR are the thyroid hormone receptor (TR) and retinoic acid receptor (RAR), hetero- or homodimers of which are involved in growth and differentiation of cells, as well as the MAD protein, which represses transcription from MYC target genes. These actions were confirmed in a mouse model with disrupted N-CoR where it was involved in long-term repression of neural-specific genes outside the nervous system through the REST sequence (Jepsen *et al.* 2000). Luthi-Carter *et al.* (2000) demonstrated that 25 per cent of genes with altered transcription in the R6/2 mouse were under the control of retinoic acid—these genes were mainly downregulated and sequestration of N-CoR from its normal site of action, as observed in HD brain (Boutell *et al.* 1999), might be expected to activate transcription from genes whose normal repression had been alleviated. However, N-CoR is also essential for activation of one class of RAR response elements (Jepsen *et al.* 2000) and its absence could cause their downregulation as observed.

(a)   (i)

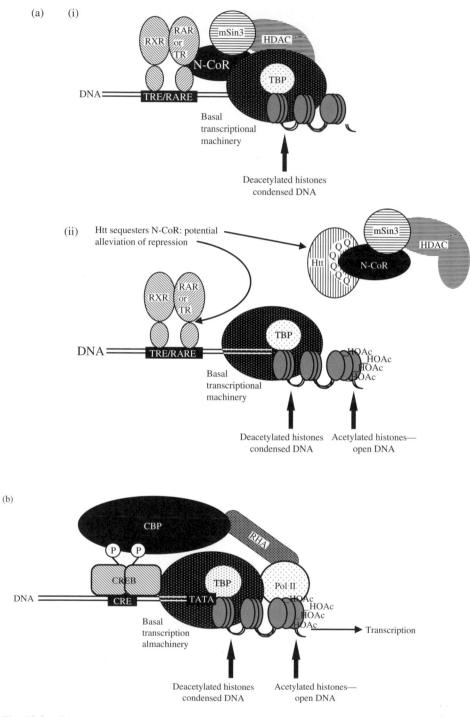

Fig. 12.3 (*Cont.*)

Fig. 12.3 (a) Possible action of huntingtin with respect to N-CoR. Dimeric sequence-specific receptors bind to cognate sites on the DNA upstream of transcriptional start sites. Part(i) shows that, in the absence of ligand, the receptors bind N-CoR, which recruits the repressor proteins, mSin3 and histone deacetylases, to the receptors. The histones remain deacetylated and closed, and transcription is blocked. (ii) If huntingtin can sequester N-CoR away from its normal site of action, then it may physically remove the block and allow transcription to occur. RXR, retinoid X receptor; RAR retinoic acid receptor; TR, thyroid hormone receptor; TRE, thyroid response element; RARE, retinoic acid response element; HDAC, histone deacetylase; TBP, TATA-binding protein; HOAc, acetyl groups. (b) CBP interactions in activating transcription. CREB dimers bind to CREs in the DNA, upstream of TATA boxes, which bind the basal trancriptional machinery including TFIIB, TFIID, and TBP. CBP binds CREB when it is phosphorylated at Ser133. CBP also interacts with RNA helicase (RHA) through which it binds indirectly to PolII. This stabilizes PolII on the promoter of CREB target genes. CBP also has intrinsic histone acetylase activity and thus can acetylate histones and maintain them in the open, transcribable, formation. Huntingtin appears to be able to sequester CBP and thus cAMP-mediated transcriptional activation (Nucifora *et al.* 2001) can be blocked. CRE, cAMP response element; CREB, CRE response element binding protein; CBP, CREB binding protein; RHA, RNA helicase; PolII, RNA polymerase II.

The mechanism proposed for the interference of huntingtin in transcriptional processes is that proteins important in transcriptional events are sequestered by huntingtin and end up in inclusions or sequestered elsewhere in the cell unable to carry out their normal functions. Transcriptional regulation is a finely balanced system with complexes of activators and inhibitors determining expression levels of particular genes in response to cellular signals. These complexes contain general activating and repressing proteins, such as the histone acetyl transferases, whose action opens up chromatin for the transcriptional machinery to enter, and histone deacetylases, which have the opposite effect (Hassig and Schreiber 1997). They also contain cell-specific activators and inhibitors that can be recruited into the complexes and modulate their activity: these proteins are responsible for cell-type-specific gene expression. Changes in the availability of these proteins within the cell could alter the finely balanced regulation of transcription and contribute to HD pathology. The evidence presented by Nucifora *et al.* (2001) is consistent with this hypothesis. It remains unclear whether TBP, the mSin3s, and CBP are the only, or the most important, transcriptionally active proteins to be sequestered in inclusions.

Further work in a *Drosophila* model of polyglutamine disease demonstrates a broad effect of huntingtin on histone acetylation through the polyglutamine interaction with histone acetylase domains. *N*-terminal huntingtin carrying 51 glutamines directly inhibited the acetyl transferase activity of CBP, p300, and P/CAF *in vitro* and, most telling, administration of histone deacetylase inhibitors to the mutant flies slowed or prevented polyglutamine-mediated cell dysfunction or death (Steffan *et al.* 2001). This finding, along with findings in yeast that implicate histone acetylation defects in response to expanded polyglutamine tracts (Hughes *et al.* 2001), implicates a widespread defect in chromatin structure in HD and also suggests a possible therapeutic route. Histone deacetylase inhibitors are already in phase I clinical trials as cancer treatments (Marks *et al.* 2001). These important findings also suggest why most of the transcriptional changes detected in HD are downregulations (Luthi-Carter *et al.* 2000).

More indirect evidence also points to the importance of transcriptional regulation in HD. The aggregation and nuclear localization of huntingtin and AR were found to be altered by the glucocorticoid receptor (GR) in a manner that proved to be dependent on the transcriptional activity of GR (Diamond *et al.* 2000). The mechanism by which this occurs is unknown but it is noteworthy in this context that GR can recruit histone deacetylases and acts as a direct inhibitor of CBP-associated histone acetylase activity (Ito *et al*. 2000). CBP also activates transcription of the ferritin heavy chain gene (Ishitani *et al*. 1999). This is pertinent as a mutation in the ferritin light chain gene has been shown to cause a rare neurodegeneration whose pathology overlaps with that of HD (Curtis *et al*. 2001) and iron metabolism is altered in huntingtin null ES cells (Wang *et al*. 1999b). The mechanism by which huntingtin alters BDNF expression is also unknown but this too may be modulated by CBP (Zuccato *et al*. 2001). The upregulation by wild-type huntingtin and downregulation in the presence of the mutant protein may imply that huntingtin is affecting transcription directly. However, most cortical neuronal cells in HD do not demonstrate nuclear localization of wild-type huntingtin; thus it is more likely that this too is an indirect effect on a signalling pathway leading to a downstream transcriptional defect. In R6/2 mice a downregulation of neuronal tenascin C in regions projecting to the striatum is seen (Kusakabe *et al*. 2001) and a downregulation in protein kinase C (PKC) beta II levels (Harris *et al*. 2001). PKC is involved in long-term potentiation and its downregulation could have effects on learning and memory in HD.

The changes in gene expression known to occur in HD are mostly downregulations. These include decreases in expression of substance P and enkephalin in early-grade HD brain (Albin *et al*. 1991; Augood *et al*. 1996; Richfield *et al*. 1995), although this may simply reflect the loss of medium spiny neurones in the striatum (see Chapter 9). Transgenic mouse models also show a decrease in enkephalin mRNA (Levine *et al*. 1999; Menalled *et al*. 2000). Dopamine D1 and D2 receptor RNA is decreased in the striatum of HD patients even at early disease stages (Augood *et al*. 1997), correlating with loss of activity of these receptors (Lawrence *et al*. 1998); in R6/2 mice an early loss of D1 receptor mRNA was also seen (Cha *et al*. 1998). Consistent with these changes, presymptomatic HD transgenic mice demonstrated severe deficiencies in dopamine signalling (Bibb *et al*. 2000). The NR1 and NR2B subunits of the NMDA receptor are downregulated in human HD brain (Arzberger *et al*. 1997) but not in R6/2 mice (Cha *et al*. 1998, 1999). Cannabinoid receptor mRNAs are also decreased in HD transgenic mice (Denovan-Wright and Robertson 2000), which is consistent with the early loss of cannabinoid receptors seen in HD patients (Richfield and Herkenham 1994). Cha *et al*. (1998, 1999) detected downregulations in specific neurotransmitters in transgenic mice, which correlated with earlier reductions in their mRNAs. These included receptors for glutamate, dopamine, acetylcholine, and adenosine. The R6/2 mice in which this latter study was conducted demonstrate no overt cell death so the downregulation observed must be independent of alteration in neuronal population subtypes.

The problem with huntingtin interacting proteins detected by various systems (Table 12.1) is that huntingtin seems to be relatively reactive and interacts with many proteins in various systems and it has proved difficult to determine which are genuine and significant interactions and which are relatively unimportant or do not occur because of temporal or spatial separation of the putative interactors.

The importance of transcriptional changes in HD is likely to be revealed by analysis of global gene expression using microarray technology in the near future: the ability to analyse the expression of large numbers of genes from particular tissues is one of the first spin-offs from the human genome project. The first such experiments in HD, conducted in the R6/2 mouse model, reported a series of changes in gene expression (Luthi-Carter *et al*. 2000), noting that most expression changes in the transgenic mouse caudate were downregulations, as observed previously in the *in situ* studies reported above, and that 25 per cent of the genes with altered expression were retinoic acid regulated. Some of the changes in gene expression mentioned earlier were also replicated in this initial global gene expression study. Further detailed experiments of this type in transgenic animals and human tissue are likely to reveal the transcriptional changes that occur in HD and, by extrapolation through examining the common regulatory features of such genes, determine whether specific transcriptional complexes are involved in the disease.

Transport processes and events at the synapse

Neuronal cells, with their extended branched systems of axons and dendrites, need to be able to move molecules long distances around the cell. There is evidence not only that RNA species are moved in neurones to allow protein synthesis *in situ* (Eberwine *et al.* 2001; Steward and Worley 2001), but also that there is mass transport of molecules up and down the cellular processes, often over long distances (Silverman *et al.* 2001). Transport takes place along the microtubule lattice and involves a whole series of proteins, including motor components and adaptor molecules, which attach vesicles and individual molecules to the transport mechanisms. The evidence from animal models (Carter *et al.* 1999; Lione *et al.* 1999; Murphy *et al.* 2000) and probably from HD patients too (Kirkwood *et al.* 2000b) indicates that alterations in neurotransmission represent early events in the disease process. Thus the role of huntingtin in transport and synaptic signalling processes has been investigated by many researchers.

Several experimental lines of evidence support a role for huntingtin in vesicle transport processes within the cell. Huntingtin purifies with vesicle fractions from human and rat brain (DiFiglia *et al.* 1995; Gutekunst *et al.* 1995; Sharp *et al.* 1995; Velier *et al.* 1998; Wood *et al.* 1996), associates with microtubules (Bhide *et al.* 1996; DiFiglia *et al.* 1995; Gutekunst *et al.* 1995; Tukamoto *et al.* 1997), and is known to interact with several proteins involved in retrograde transport (from the synapse to the cell body) in cells (Colomer *et al.* 1997; Engelender *et al.* 1997; Hattula and Peranen 2000; Velier *et al.* 1998). Polyglutamine tracts also interact specifically with neurofilament proteins (Nagai *et al.* 1999) and may exert a toxic effect through such aberrant binding, although most evidence indicates that neurofilament disruption is most toxic in motor neurones (Lee and Cleveland 1994). The clearest evidence for involvement of huntingtin in cellular transport comes from studies in rat where huntingtin, full-length and *N*-terminally truncated, accumulated on both sides of a crush injury to rat sciatic nerve along with proteins involved in vesicle transport along the axon terminals (Block-Galarza *et al.* 1997), but there is other, less direct, evidence.

Huntingtin-associated protein 1 (HAP1), the first huntingtin interactor to be discovered (Li *et al.* 1995), is expressed in neurones and binds the p150 subunit of dynactin (Engelender *et al.* 1997; Li *et al.* 1998); huntingtin, p150 and HAP1 co-immunoprecipitate from rat brain homogenates (Li *et al.* 1998). Dynactin is a multisubunit activator protein required by the minus-end motor protein dynein to move vesicles along microtubules and p150 is the largest subunit of this multimolecular complex (Boylan *et al.* 2000; Holleran *et al.* 1998; Valetti *et al.* 1999). Dynein itself appears to have a long rigid tail and an ATPase head, and probably transports vesicles along microtubules using a power stroke mechanism reminiscent of myosin (Allan 1996; see Fig. 12.4). The fast axonal transport observed by Block-Galarza *et al.* (1997) appears to be dependent on this interaction between dynactin and dynein (Waterman-Storer *et al.* 1997) and Li *et al.* (1998) have proposed that HAP1–huntingtin complexes play a role in the formation of this complex. It is also known that dystrophic neurites of the kind seen in

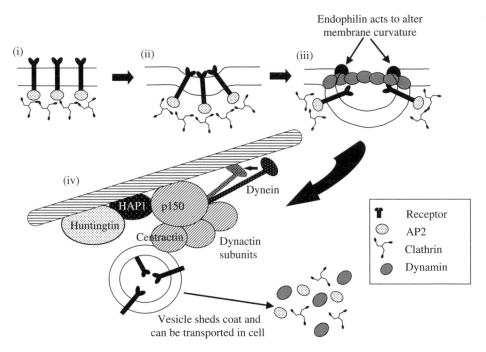

Fig. 12.4 Outline of events with which huntingtin is known to be associated, at the synapse, and in retrogade transport. Clathrin triskelions are recruited to the membrane through α-adaptin, with which huntingtin interacts (i), and the membrane curves inwards to form a coated pit (ii). The dynamin ring forms around the neck of the invaginated coated pit (iii) and endophilin is involved in altering membrane curvature. The endosome is snipped off the membrane and uncoated and can at that point be transported within the cell (iv). Huntingtin is known to interact with dynactin through HAP1 and also interacts with microtubules (see the subsection 'Transport processes and events at the synapse'). It is therefore possible that huntingtin has a role in both these processes.

human HD brain can result from defective retrograde axonal transport in neurones (Sapp *et al.* 1999). Huntingtin also binds FIP2 (Rab8 family interacting protein 2), which is part of a complex involved in regulation of membrane trafficking and cellular morphogenesis (Hattula and Peranen 2000).

The transport of molecules in neurones takes them from the cell body to the ends of processes (plus-end directed) or from processes to the cell body (minus-end directed), where they may be involved in what can be regarded as the function of the neurone: communication. At the ends of axons vesicles are loaded with neurotransmitter and fuse with the membrane, releasing this transmitter into the synaptic cleft, with re-uptake of membrane through endocytosis and recycling of vesicles. This occurs very rapidly with only a small pool of vesicles so recycling is very important to the continued functioning of the synapse (Jarousse and Kelly 2001). Receptors in the postsynaptic membrane bind the transmitter and can respond by depolarizing the membrane and propagating an electric signal (ionotropic receptors), or by signalling through the membrane into the cell (metabotropic receptors). There have been a number of experimental findings that implicate huntingtin in endocytosis. Endocytosis occurs in several places in the cell, most importantly at the plasma membrane where vesicles are pinched off and recycled in the cell, but also in the transGolgi network, where this process allows release of loaded vesicles that can fuse with other organelles or the plasma membrane. Retrograde signalling at the synapse, transducing cellular survival signals back into the signalling neurone, is important to cellular survival and function and, in particular, in neurones, signalling at the synapse can be changed by altering receptor-mediated endocytosis (RME). The process of RME is illustrated diagrammatically in Fig. 12.4.

RME is the process by which many cell surface molecules are recycled into cells and is important in the recycling of synaptic vesicles in neuronal signalling. RME occurs through the recruitment of clathrin to invaginations of the membrane by various accessory proteins, receptor recruitment, coated pit invagination, and vesicle budding (Schmid 1997). Huntingtin associates with clathrin-coated pits and uncoated endosomal vesicles (Velier *et al.* 1998), and the accumulation of mutant huntingtin seen in processes and the presence of huntingtin in pre- and postsynaptic regions in both human and animal studies makes this involvement a possibility.

It was noted when HIP1 was first isolated as a huntingtin interacting protein that mutations in the HIP1 yeast homologue, Sla2p, disrupt endocytosis (Raths *et al.* 1993). Recent evidence reveals that HIP1 binds to clathrin and α-adaptin A and C (Metzler *et al.* 2001; Waelter *et al.* 2001b), is localized to clathrin-coated vesicles, and is almost certainly involved in the mechanisms of RME. Huntingtin itself also binds to α-adaptin C (Faber *et al.* 1999). HAP1 was also shown to interact directly with HIP1 (Waelter *et al.* 2001b) and was enriched in the same fractions as the HIP1 and the α-adaptins (Metzler *et al.* 2001). This adds support to the theory that huntingtin links vesicles to the microtubule transport systems in cells and thus HAP1 may be the protein that links huntingtin to the dynactin/dynein motor components of the cellular transport systems. The major components of this system are illustrated in Fig. 12.4.

Huntingtin also interacts with the protein product of *SH3GL3*, the human homologue of mouse the endophilin 3 gene (Sittler *et al.* 1998). The endophilins are a group of three homologous proteins found in mammals, and endophilin 1 is known to be a lysophosphatidic acyl transferase, which is thought to be instrumental in changing the curvature of the membrane as it invaginates in RME by altering its lipid composition.

Although there is no direct evidence to indicate that huntingtin can alter RME, the internalization of at least one cell surface receptor is altered, that of EGF (Liu *et al.* 1997), and a number of cellular signalling systems mediated through RME are altered. *N*-terminal huntingtin binds synaptic vesicles and inhibits glutamate uptake *in vitro* (Li *et al.* 2000). An association between huntingtin and postsynaptic density 95 (PSD-95) protein has been reported (Sun *et al.* 2001) mediated through an SH3 domain in PSD-95, and this interaction was very markedly reduced in the presence of expanded polyglutamine. PSD-95 is a scaffold protein that binds to the NR2 subunit of the NMDA receptor and the GluR6 subunit of the kainate receptor, regulating long-term potentiation (LTP) and long-term depression (LTD) by modulating receptor density at the postsynaptic membrane and linking the receptors to intracellular signalling cascades (Garcia *et al.* 1998). Receptor-mediated activation of NO synthase and excitotoxicity by NMDA receptor signalling is inhibited if PSD-95 expression is suppressed (Sattler *et al.* 1999; Tezuka *et al.* 1999; Yamada *et al.* 1999) and, furthermore, PSD-95 null mice have severe spatial learning problems (Migaud *et al.* 1998), a notable feature of HD, which is also observed in transgenic mouse models of HD (Lione *et al.* 1999; Murphy *et al.* 2000). The weakening of the PSD-95–huntingtin interaction in the presence of longer glutamine tracts may result in increased NMDA receptor signalling, as increased free PSD-95 should increase such signalling. Cells expressing mutant huntingtin and NMDA receptors, such as the medium spiny neurones of the caudate, which are most vulnerable in HD, might therefore demonstrate increased susceptibility to excitotoxic insults. This interaction might also underlie the observed protective effects of normal huntingtin (Dragatsis *et al.* 2000; Ho *et al.* 2001; Leavitt *et al.* 2001). It is also possible that this finding underlies the observed genetic association of a polymorphic marker in the GluR6 gene with age of onset in HD (see Chapter 5).

Experiments in clonal striatal neurones also implicate huntingtin in endosomal processes. Cells transfected with huntingtin showed an activation of the endosomal–lysosomal system and the appearance of tubulovesicular structures that look remarkably similar to early and recycling endosomes (Kegel *et al.* 2000; Petersen *et al.* 2001). This lends further credence to endocytosis and transport being the normal cellular role of huntingtin, and alterations of this role could be involved in HD pathogenesis.

There is less evidence that huntingtin is involved in exocytosis, but a specific reduction in complexin II has been detected in the R6/2 mice from a relatively early stage. Complexin II is involved in regulating synaptic vesicle release at excitatory synapses and appears to confer calcium sensitivity on the process. Neurones with no complexins have reduced transmitter release and are calcium-insensitive (Reim *et al.* 2001). Aberrant calcium signalling has been implicated previously in HD but it has never been clear whether it is a downstream effect of other processes. The NMDA receptor is a calcium channel and alterations in its function would give rise to changes in calcium fluxes in the cell. This is the molecular basis of the weak excitotoxic hypothesis (Albin and Greenamyre 1992; Coyle and Puttfarcken 1993).

One further effect huntingtin may have on vesicles is to render them more permeable in a rather unselective way. Polyglutamine is reported to induce large non-selective ion channels in lipid bilayers (Hirakura *et al.* 2000) and mutant huntingtin has been observed to bind to vesicles in a polyglutamine-dependent fashion that may result in the observed permeability (Li *et al.* 2000). Prion peptides with amyloid structures bind tightly to membranes (Rymer and Good 2000) and β-amyloid can form channels in bilayers (Lin *et al.* 2001). This effect has remained largely unexplored, but recent evidence indicates that in Alzheimer's disease and parkinsonism the toxic moiety, rather than being the large insoluble aggregate seen in brain tissues of those with these diseases, may be the protofibrils—short flexible structures that precede accumulation into frank, observable aggregations (Conway *et al.* 2000; Harper *et al.* 1999; Harper *et al.* 1997; Nilsberth *et al.* 2001). Further, protofibrillar α-synuclein binds 1999 tightly to synaptic vesicles through its β-sheet structure and permeabilizes these vesicles (Volles *et al.* 2001). Thus it is possible that huntingtin protofibrils may have the same effect.

Conclusion

It is still difficult to come to any firm conclusions about the normal or pathological functions of huntingtin, and to decide how these functions might be related. There is substantial evidence that the pathway to the formation of insoluble protein deposits is important in most, if not all, neurodegenerations (Kopito 2000; Schulz and Dichgans 1999; Sherer *et al.* 2001; Wanker 2000). This would involve a ubiquitous cellular system, which is particularly vulnerable in different sets of neurones in different diseases. Neurones, because of their long life and high oxidative respiratory rates, are vulnerable to toxic insults and aberrant degradative pathways appear the most likely to be involved in disease causation. In particular, the finding that the proteasomally mediated reversal of aggregation can restore function (Martin-Aparicio *et al.* 2001) holds out the promise that interventions before cell death will be effective in treating HD. The intimate relationships between transcriptional control and proteasomal degradation also suggest that perhaps this is where the future efforts to elucidate the molecular mechanisms immediately downstream of the mutated protein should be concentrated. So, although we still have no clear sequence of pathological events subsequent to expression of the mutated protein, perhaps we now have a reasonable guidebook.

References

Albin, R. L. and Greenamyre, J. T. (1992). Alternative excitotoxic hypotheses. *Neurology* **42** (4), 733–738.

—— Qin, Y., Young, A. B., Penney, J. B., and Chesselet, M. F. (1991). Preproenkephalin messenger RNA-containing neurons in striatum of patients with symptomatic and presymptomatic Huntington's disease: an *in situ* hybridization study. *Ann. Neurol.* **30** (4), 542–549.

Allan, V. (1996). Motor proteins: a dynamic duo. *Curr. Biol.* **6** (6), 630–633.

Alland, L., Muhle, R., Hou, H., Jr., Potes, J., Chin, L., Schreiber-Agus, N., and DePinho, R. A. (1997). Role for N-CoR and histone deacetylase in Sin3-mediated transcriptional repression. *Nature* **387** (6628), 49–55.

Ambrose, C. M., Duyao, M. P., Barnes, G., Bates, G. P., Lin, C. S., Srinidhi, J., Baxendale, S., Hummerich, H., Lehrach, H., and Altherr, M. (1994). Structure and expression of the Huntington's disease gene: evidence against simple inactivation due to an expanded CAG repeat. *Somat Cell Mol Genet* **20** (1), 27–38.

Andrade, M. A. and Bork, P. (1995). HEAT repeats in the Huntington's disease protein [letter]. *Nat Genet.* **11** (2), 115–116.

Aronin, N., Kim, M., LaForet, G., and DiFiglia, M. (1999). Are there multiple pathways in the pathogenesis of Huntington's disease? *Philos. Trans. R. Soc. Lond. B Biol. Sci.* **354** (1386), 995–1003.

Arzberger, T., Krampfl, K., Leimgruber, S., and Weindl, A. (1997). Changes of NMDA receptor subunit (NR1, NR2B), and glutamate transporter (GLT1), mRNA expression in Huntington's disease—an *in situ* hybridization study. *J. Neuropathol. Exp. Neurol.* **56** (4), 440–454.

Augood, S. J., Faull, R. L., Love, D. R., and Emson, P. C. (1996). Reduction in enkephalin and substance P messenger RNA in the striatum of early grade Huntington's disease: a detailed cellular *in situ* hybridization study. *Neuroscience* **72** (4), 1023–1036.

—— —— Emson, P. C. (1997). Dopamine D1 and D2 receptor gene expression in the striatum in Huntington's disease. *Ann. Neurol.* **42** (2), 215–221.

Barnes, G. T., Duyao, M. P., Ambrose, C. M., McNeil, S., Persichetti, F., Srinidhi, J., Gusella, J. F., and MacDonald, M. E. (1994). Mouse Huntington's disease gene homolog (Hdh). *Somat. Cell Mol. Genet.* **20** (2), 87–97.

Baxendale, S., Abdulla, S., Elgar, G., Buck, D., Berks, M., Micklem, G., Durbin, R., Bates, G., Brenner, S., and Beck, S. (1995). Comparative sequence analysis of the human and pufferfish Huntington's disease genes [see comments]. *Nat. Genet.* **10** (1), 67–76.

Beal, M. F., Hyman, B. T., and Koroshetz, W. (1993). Do defects in mitochondrial energy metabolism underlie the pathology of neurodegenerative diseases? [see comments]. *Trends Neurosci.* **16** (4), 125–131.

Bence, N. F., Sampat, R. M., and Kopito, R. R. (2001). Impairment of the ubiquitin–proteasome system by protein aggregation. *Science* **292** (5521), 1552–1555.

Bhide, P. G., Day, M., Sapp, E., Schwarz, C., Sheth, A., Kim, J., Young, A. B., Penney, J., Golden, J., Aronin, N., and DiFiglia, M. (1996). Expression of normal and mutant huntingtin in the developing brain. *J. Neurosci.* **16** (17), 5523–5535.

Bibb, J. A., Yan, Z., Svenningsson, P., Snyder, G. L., Pieribone, V. A., Horiuchi, A., Nairn, A. C., Messer, A., and Greengard, P. (2000). Severe deficiencies in dopamine signaling in presymptomatic Huntington's disease mice. *Proc. Natl Acad. Sci., USA* **97** (12), 6809–6814.

Block-Galarza, J., Chase, K. O., Sapp, E., Vaughn, K. T., Vallee, R. B., DiFiglia, M., and Aronin, N. (1997). Fast transport and retrograde movement of huntingtin and HAP 1 in axons. *Neuroreport* **8**, (9–10), 2247–2251.

Bonni, A., Brunet, A., West, A. E., Datta, S. R., Takasu, M. A., and Greenberg, M. E. (1999). Cell survival promoted by the Ras-MAPK signaling pathway by transcription-dependent and -independent mechanisms. *Science* **286** (5443), 1358–1362.

Boutell, J. M., Thomas, P., Neal, J. W., Weston, V. J., Duce, J., Harper, P. S., and Jones, A. L. (1999). Aberrant interactions of transcriptional repressor proteins with the Huntington's disease gene product, huntingtin. *Hum. Mol. Genet.* **8** (9), 1647–1655.

Boutell, J. M., Wood, J. D., Harper, P. S., Jones, A. L. (1998). Huntingtin interacts with cystathionine β-synthase. *Hum. Mol. Genet.* **7** (3), 371–378.

Boylan, K., Serr, M., and Hays, T. (2000). A molecular genetic analysis of the interaction between the cytoplasmic dynein intermediate chain and the glued (dynactin) complex. *Mol. Biol. Cell* **11** (11), 3791–3803.

Browne, S. E., Bowling, A. C., MacGarvey, U., Baik, M. J., Berger, S. C., Muqit, M. M., Bird, E. D., and Beal, M. F. (1997). Oxidative damage and metabolic dysfunction in Huntington's disease: selective vulnerability of the basal ganglia. *Ann. Neurol.* **41** (5), 646–653.

Canals, J. M., Checa, N., Marco, S., Akerud, P., Michels, A., Perez-Navarro, E., Tolosa, E., Arenas, E., and Alberch, J. (2001). Expression of brain-derived neurotrophic factor in cortical neurons is regulated by striatal target area. *J. Neurosci.* **21** (1), 117–124.

Carter, R. J., Lione, L. A., Humby, T., Mangiarini, L., Mahal, A., Bates, G. P., Dunnett, S. B., and Morton, A. J. (1999). Characterization of progressive motor deficits in mice transgenic for the human Huntington's disease mutation. *J. Neurosci.* **19** (8), 3248–3257.

Cha, J. H., Kosinski, C. M., Kerner, J. A., Alsdorf, S. A., Mangiarini, L., Davies, S. W., Penney, J. B., Bates, G. P., and Young, A. B. (1998). Altered brain neurotransmitter receptors in transgenic mice expressing a portion of an abnormal human huntington disease gene. *Proc. Natl Acad. Sci., USA* **95** (11), 6480–6485.

—— Frey, A. S., Alsdorf, S. A., Kerner, J. A., Kosinski, C. M., Mangiarini, L., Penney, J. B., Jr., Davies, S. W., Bates, G. P., and Young, A. B. (1999). Altered neurotransmitter receptor expression in transgenic mouse models of Huntington's disease. *Philos. Trans. R. Soc. Lond. B Biol. Sci.* **354** (1386), 981–989.

Chen, M., Ona, V. O., Li, M., Ferrante, R. J., Fink, K. B., Zhu, S., Bian, J., Guo, L., Farrell, L. A., Hersch, S. M., Hobbs, W., Vonsattel, J. P., Cha, J. H., and Friedlander, R. M. (2000). Minocycline inhibits caspase-1 and caspase-3 expression and delays mortality in a transgenic mouse model of Huntington disease. *Nat. Med.* **6** (7), 797–801.

Coles, R., Caswell, R., and Rubinsztein, D. C. (1998). Functional analysis of the Huntington's disease (HD), gene promoter. *Hum. Mol. Genet.* **7** (5), 791–800.

Colomer, V., Engelender, S., Sharp, A. H., Duan, K., Cooper, J. K., Lanahan, A., Lyford, G., Worley, P., and Ross, C. A. (1997). Huntingtin-associated protein 1 (HAP1), binds to a Trio-like polypeptide, with a rac1 guanine nucleotide exchange factor domain. *Hum. Mol. Genet.* **6** (9), 1519–1525.

Conway, K. A., Harper, J. D., and Lansbury, P. T., Jr (2000). Fibrils formed *in vitro* from alpha-synuclein and two mutant forms linked to Parkinson's disease are typical amyloid. *Biochemistry* **39** (10), 2552–2563.

Cooper, J. K., Schilling, G., Peters, M. F., Herring, W. J., Sharp, A. H., Kaminsky, Z., Masone, J., Khan, F. A., Delanoy, M., Borchelt, D. R., Dawson, V. L., Dawson, T. M., and Ross, C. A. (1998). Truncated N-terminal fragments of huntingtin with expanded glutamine repeats form nuclear and cytoplasmic aggregates in cell culture. *Hum. Mol. Genet.* **7** (5), 783–790.

Coyle, J. T. and Puttfarcken, P. (1993). Oxidative stress, glutamate, and neurodegenerative disorders. *Science* **262** (5134), 689–695.

Cummings, C. J., Mancini, M. A., Antalffy, B., DeFranco, D. B., Orr, H. T., and Zoghbi, H. Y. (1998). Chaperone suppression of aggregation and altered subcellular proteasome localization imply protein misfolding in SCA1. *Nat. Genet.* **19** (2), 148–154.

Curtis, A. R., Fey, C., Morris, C. M., Bindoff, L. A., Ince, P. G., Chinnery, P. F., Coulthard, A., Jackson, M. J., Jackson, A. P., McHale, D. P., Hay, D., Barker, W. A., Markham, A. F., Bates, D., Curtis, A., and Burn, J. (2001). Mutation in the gene encoding ferritin light polypeptide causes dominant adult-onset basal ganglia disease. *Nat. Genet.* **28** (4), 350–354.

Davies, S. W., Turmaine, M., Cozens, B. A., DiFiglia, M., Sharp, A. H., Ross, C. A., Scherzinger, E., Wanker, E. E., Mangiarini, L., and Bates, G. P. (1997). Formation of neuronal intranuclear inclusions underlies the neurological dysfunction in mice transgenic for the HD mutation. *Cell* **90** (3), 537–548.

De Rooij, K. E., Dorsman, J. C., Smoor, M. A., den Dunnen, J. T., and Van Ommen, G. J. (1996). Subcellular localization of the Huntington's disease gene product in cell lines by immunofluorescence and biochemical subcellular fractionation. *Hum. Mol. Genet.* **5** (8), 1093–1099.

Denovan-Wright, E. M. and Robertson, H. A. (2000). Cannabinoid receptor messenger RNA levels decrease in a subset of neurons of the lateral striatum, cortex and hippocampus of transgenic Huntington's disease mice. *Neuroscience* **98** (4), 705–713.

Diamond, M. I., Robinson, M. R., and Yamamoto, K. R. (2000). Regulation of expanded polyglutamine protein aggregation and nuclear localization by the glucocorticoid receptor. *Proc. Natl Acad. Sci., USA* **97** (2), 657–661.

DiFiglia, M., Sapp, E., Chase, K., Schwarz, C., Meloni, A., Young, C., Martin, E., Vonsattel, J. P., Carraway, R., and Reeves, S. A. (1995). Huntingtin is a cytoplasmic protein associated with vesicles in human and rat brain neurons. *Neuron* **14** (5), 1075–1081.

—— —— Chase, K. O., Davies, S. W., Bates, G. P., Vonsattel, J. P., and Aronin, N. (1997). Aggregation of huntingtin in neuronal intranuclear inclusions and dystrophic neurites in brain. *Science* **277** (5334), 1990–1993.

Dragatsis, I., Dietrich, P., and Zeitlin, S. (2000). Expression of the Huntingtin-associated protein 1 gene in the developing and adult mouse. *Neurosci. Lett.* **282**, (1–2), 37–40.

Dragunow, M., Faull, R. L., Lawlor, P., Beilharz, E. J., Singleton, K., Walker, E. B., and Mee, E. (1995). *In situ* evidence for DNA fragmentation in Huntington's disease striatum and Alzheimer's disease temporal lobes. *Neuroreport* **6** (7), 1053–1057.

Dure, L. S., Landwehrmeyer, G. B., Golden, J., McNeil, S. M., Ge, P., Aizawa, H., Huang, Q., Ambrose, C. M., Duyao, M. P., and Bird, E. D. (1994). IT15 gene expression in foetal human brain. *Brain Res.* **659**, (1–2), 33–41.

Durr, A., Hahn-Barma, V., Brice, A., Pecheux, C., Dode, C., and Feingold, J. (1999). Homozygosity in Huntington's disease. *J. Med. Genet.* **36** (2), 172–173.

Duyao, M. P., Auerbach, A. B., Ryan, A., Persichetti, F., Barnes, G. T., McNeil, S. M., Ge, P., Vonsattel, J. P., Gusella, J. F., and Joyner, A. L. (1995). Inactivation of the mouse Huntington's disease gene homolog Hdh. *Science* **269** (5222), 407–410.

Eberwine, J., Miyashiro, K., Kacharmina, J. E., and Job, C. (2001). Local translation of classes of mRNAs that are targeted to neuronal dendrites. *Proc. Natl Acad. Sci., USA* **98** (13), 7080–7085.

Engelender, S., Sharp, A. H., Colomer, V., Tokito, M. K., Lanahan, A., Worley, P., Holzbaur, E. L., and Ross, C. A. (1997). Huntingtin-associated protein 1 (HAP1), interacts with the p150Glued subunit of dynactin. *Hum. Mol. Genet.* **6** (13), 2205–2212.

Faber, P. W., Alter, J. R., MacDonald, M. E., and Hart, A. C. (1999). Polyglutamine-mediated dysfunction and apoptotic death of a *Caenorhabditis elegans* sensory neuron. *Proc. Natl Acad. Sci., USA* **96** (1), 179–184.

Faber, P. W., Barnes, G. T., Srinidhi, J., Chen, J., Gusella, J. F., and MacDonald, M. E. (1998). Huntingtin interacts with a family of ww domain proteins. *Hum. Mol. Genet.* **7** (9), 1463–1474.

Ferdous, A., Gonzalez, F., Sun, L., Kodadek, T., and Johnston, S. A. (2001). The 19S regulatory particle of the proteasome is required for efficient transcription elongation by RNA polymerase II. *Mol. Cell* **7** (5), 981–991.

Garcia, E. P., Mehta, S., Blair, L. A., Wells, D. G., Shang, J., Fukushima, T., Fallon, J. R., Garner, C. C., and Marshall, J. (1998). SAP90 binds and clusters kainate receptors causing incomplete desensitization. *Neuron* **21** (4), 727–739.

Gellera, C., Meoni, C., Castellotti, B., Zappacosta, B., Girotti, F., Taroni, F., and DiDonato, S. (1996). Errors in Huntington disease diagnostic test caused by trinucleotide deletion in the IT15 gene. *Am. J. Hum. Genet.* **59** (2), 475–477.

Gerber, H. P., Seipel, K., Georgiev, O., Hofferer, M., Hug, M., Rusconi, S., and Schaffner, W. (1994). Transcriptional activation modulated by homopolymeric glutamine and proline stretches. *Science* **263** (5148), 808–811.

Glass, M., Dragunow, M., and Faull, R. L. (2000). The pattern of neurodegeneration in Huntington's disease: a comparative study of cannabinoid, dopamine, adenosine and GABA(A) receptor alterations in the human basal ganglia in Huntington's disease. *Neuroscience* **97** (3), 505–519.

Goldberg, Y. P., Nicholson, D. W., Rasper, D. M., Kalchman, M. A., Koide, H. B., Graham, R. K., Bromm, M., Kazemi-Esfarjani, P., Thornberry, N. A., Vaillancourt, J. P., and Hayden, M. R. (1996). Cleavage of huntingtin by apopain, a proapoptotic cysteine protease, is modulated by the polyglutamine tract [see comments]. *Nat. Genet.* **13** (4), 442–449.

Gomez-Tortosa, E., MacDonald, M. E., Friend, J. C., Taylor, S. A., Weiler, L. J., Cupples, L. A., Srinidhi, J., Gusella, J. F., Bird, E. D., Vonsattel, J. P., and Myers, R. H. (2001). Quantitative neuropathological changes in presymptomatic Huntington's disease. *Ann. Neurol.* **49** (1), 29–34.

Gusella, J. F. and MacDonald, M. E. (1998). Huntingtin: a single bait hooks many species. *Curr. Opin. Neurobiol.* **8** (3), 425–430.

Gutekunst, C. A., Levey, A. I., Heilman, C. J., Whaley, W. L., Yi, H., Nash, N. R., Rees, H. D., Madden, J. J., and Hersch, S. M. (1995). Identification and localization of huntingtin in brain and human lymphoblastoid cell lines with anti-fusion protein antibodies. *Proc. Natl Acad. Sci., USA* **92** (19), 8710–8714.

—— Li, S. H., Yi, H., Ferrante, R. J., Li, X. J., and Hersch, S. M. (1998). The cellular and subcellular localization of huntingtin- associated protein 1 (HAP1): comparison with huntingtin in rat and human. *J. Neurosci.* **18** (19), 7674–7686.

—— —— —— Mulroy, J. S., Kuemmerle, S., Jones, R., Rye, D., Ferrante, R. J., Hersch, S. M., and Li, X. J. (1999). Nuclear and neuropil aggregates in Huntington's disease: relationship to neuropathology. *J. Neurosci.* **19** (7), 2522–2534.

Hackam, A. S., Singaraja, R., Wellington, C. L., Metzler, M., McCutcheon, K., Zhang, T., Kalchman, M., and Hayden, M. R. (1998). The influence of huntingtin protein size on nuclear localization and cellular toxicity. *J. Cell Biol.* **141** (5), 1097–1105.

—— Yassa, A. S., Singaraja, R., Metzler, M., Gutekunst, C. A., Gan, L., Warby, S., Wellington, C. L., Vaillancourt, J., Chen, N., Gervais, F. G., Raymond, L., Nicholson, D. W., and Hayden, M. R. (2000). Huntingtin interacting protein 1 induces apoptosis via a novel caspase-dependent death effector domain. *J. Biol. Chem.* **275** (52), 41299–41308.

Hagino-Yamagishi, K., Saijoh, Y., Yamazaki, Y., Yazaki, K., and Hamada, H. (1998). Transcriptional regulatory region of Brn-2 required for its expression in developing olfactory epithelial cells. *Brain Res. Dev. Brain Res.* **109** (1), 77–86.

Harper, J. D., Wong, S. S., Lieber, C. M., and Lansbury, P. T. (1997). Observation of metastable Abeta amyloid protofibrils by atomic force microscopy. *Chem. Biol.* **4** (2), 119–125.

—— —— —— Lansbury, P. T., Jr. Assembly of A beta amyloid protofibrils: an *in vitro* model for a possible early event in Alzheimer's disease. *Biochemistry* **38** (28), 8972–8980.

Harris, A. S., Denovan-Wright, E. M., Hamilton, L. C., and Robertson, H. A. (2001). Protein kinase C beta II mRNA levels decrease in the striatum and cortex of transgenic Huntington's disease mice. *J. Psychiatry Neurosci.* **26** (2), 117–122.

Hassig, C. A. and Schreiber, S. L. (1997). Nuclear histone acetylases and deacetylases and transcriptional regulation: HATs off to HDACs. *Curr. Opin. Chem. Biol.* **1** (3), 300–308.

Hattula, K. and Peranen, J. (2000). FIP-2, a coiled-coil protein, links Huntingtin to Rab8 and modulates cellular morphogenesis. *Curr. Biol.* **10** (24), 1603–1606.

Hirakura, Y., Azimov, R., Azimova, R., and Kagan, B. L. (2000). Polyglutamine-induced ion channels: a possible mechanism for the neurotoxicity of Huntington and other CAG repeat diseases. *J. Neurosci. Res.* **60** (4), 490–494.

Ho, L. W., Brown, R., Maxwell, M., Wyttenbach, A., and Rubinsztein, D. C. (2001). Wild type huntingtin reduces the cellular toxicity of mutant huntingtin in mammalian cell models of Huntington's disease. *J. Med. Genet.* **38** (7), 450–452.

Holbert, S., Denghien, I., Kiechle, T., Rosenblatt, A., Wellington, C., Hayden, M. R., Margolis, R. L., Ross, C. A., Dausset, J., Ferrante, R. J., and Neri, C. (2001). The Gln–Ala repeat transcriptional activator CA150 interacts with huntingtin: neuropathologic and genetic evidence for a role in Huntington's disease pathogenesis. *Proc. Natl Acad. Sci., USA* **98** (4), 1811–1816.

Holleran, E. A., Karki, S., and Holzbaur, E. L. (1998). The role of the dynactin complex in intracellular motility. *Int. Rev. Cytol.* **182**, 69–109.

Holzmann, C., Schmidt, T., Thiel, G., Epplen, J. T., and Riess, O. (2001). Functional characterization of the human Huntington's disease gene promoter. *Brain Res. Mol. Brain Res.* **92**, (1–2), 85–97.

Hughes, R. E., Lo, R. S., Davis, C., Strand, A. D., Neal, C. L., Olson, J. M., and Fields, S. (2001). Altered transcription in yeast expressing expanded polyglutamine. *Proc. Natl Acad. Sci., USA* **98** (23), 13201–13206.

Huntington's Disease Collaborative Research Group (1993). A novel gene containing a trinucleotide repeat that is expanded and unstable on Huntington's disease chromosomes. The Huntington's Disease Collaborative Research Group [see comments]. *Cell* **72** (6), 971–983.

Iannicola, C., Moreno, S., Oliverio, S., Nardacci, R., Ciofi-Luzzatto, A., and Piacentini, M. (2000). Early alterations in gene expression and cell morphology in a mouse model of Huntington's disease. *J. Neurochem.* **75** (2), 830–839.

Ishitani, T., Ninomiya-Tsuji, J., Nagai, S., Nishita, M., Meneghini, M., Barker, N., Waterman, M., Bowerman, B., Clevers, H., Shibuya, H., and Matsumoto, K. (1999). The TAK1–NLK–MAPK-related pathway antagonizes signalling between beta-catenin and transcription factor TCF. *Nature* **399** (6738), 798–802.

Ito, K., Barnes, P. J., and Adcock, I. M. (2000). Glucocorticoid receptor recruitment of histone deacetylase 2 inhibits interleukin-1beta-induced histone H4 acetylation on lysines 8 and 12. *Mol. Cell Biol.* **20** (18), 6891–6903.

Jana, N. R., Zemskov, E. A., Wang, G., and Nukina, N. (2001). Altered proteasomal function due to the expression of polyglutamine-expanded truncated N-terminal huntingtin induces apoptosis by caspase activation through mitochondrial cytochrome c release. *Hum. Mol. Genet.* **10** (10), 1049–1059.

Jarousse, N. and Kelly, R. B. (2001). Endocytotic mechanisms in synapses. *Curr. Opin. Cell Biol.* **13** (4), 461–469.

Jepsen, K., Hermanson, O., Onami, T. M., Gleiberman, A. S., Lunyak, V., McEvilly, R. J., Kurokawa, R., Kumar, V., Liu, F., Seto, E., Hedrick, S. M., Mandel, G., Glass, C. K., Rose, D. W., and Rosenfeld, M. G. (2000). Combinatorial roles of the nuclear receptor corepressor in transcription and development. *Cell* **102** (6), 753–763.

Kalchman, M. A., Graham, R. K., Xia, G., Koide, H. B., Hodgson, J. G., Graham, K. C., Goldberg, Y. P., Gietz, R. D., Pickart, C. M., and Hayden, M. R. (1996). Huntingtin is ubiquitinated and interacts with a specific ubiquitin-conjugating enzyme. *J. Biol. Chem.* **271** (32), 19385–19394.

Kalchman, M. A., Koide, H. B., McCutchton, K., Graham, R. K., Nichol, K., Nishiyama, K., Kazomi-Esfarjani, P., Lynn, F. C., Wellington, C., Metzler, M, Goldberg, Y. P., Kanazawa, I., Gietz, R. D., Hayden, M. R. (1997). HIP1, a human homologue of *S. Cerevisiae* Sla2p, interacts with membrane-associated huntingtin in the brain. *Nat. Genet.* **16** (1), 44–53.

Kazantsev, A., Preisinger, E., Dranovsky, A., Goldgaber, D., and Housman, D. (1999). Insoluble detergent-resistant aggregates form between pathological and nonpathological lengths of polyglutamine in mammalian cells. *Proc. Natl Acad. Sci., USA* **96** (20), 11404–11409.

Kegel, K. B., Kim, M., Sapp, E., McIntyre, C., Castano, J. G., Aronin, N., and DiFiglia, M. (2000). Huntingtin expression stimulates endosomal–lysosomal activity, endosome tubulation, and autophagy. *J. Neurosci.* **20** (19), 7268–7278.

Kennedy, L. and Shelbourne, P. F. (2000). Dramatic mutation instability in HD mouse striatum: does polyglutamine load contribute to cell-specific vulnerability in Huntington's disease? *Hum. Mol. Genet.* **9** (17), 2539–2544.

Kim, M., Lee, H. S., LaForet, G., McIntyre, C., Martin, E. J., Chang, P., Kim, T. W., Williams, M., Reddy, P. H., Tagle, D., Boyce, F. M., Won, L., Heller, A., Aronin, N., and DiFiglia, M. (1999). Mutant huntingtin expression in clonal striatal cells: dissociation of inclusion formation and neuronal survival by caspase inhibition. *J. Neurosci.* **19** (3), 964–973.

Kirkwood, S. C., Siemers, E., Bond, C., Conneally, P. M., Christian, J. C., and Foroud, T. (2000a). Confirmation of subtle motor changes among presymptomatic carriers of the Huntington disease gene. *Arch. Neurol.* **57** (7), 1040–1044.

—— —— Hodes, M. E., Conneally, P. M., Christian, J. C., and Foroud, T. (2000b). Subtle changes among presymptomatic carriers of the Huntington's disease gene. *J. Neurol. Neurosurg. Psychiatry* **69** (6), 773–779.

Kopito, R. R. (2000). Aggresomes, inclusion bodies and protein aggregation. *Trends Cell Biol.* **10** (12), 524–530.

Kosinski, C. M., Cha, J. H., Young, A. B., Persichetti, F., MacDonald, M., Gusella, J. F., Penney, J. B., Jr, and Standaert, D. G. (1997). Huntingtin immunoreactivity in the rat neostriatum: differential accumulation in projection and interneurons. *Exp. Neurol.* **144** (2), 239–247.

Krobitsch, S. and Lindquist, S. (2000). Aggregation of huntingtin in yeast varies with the length of the polyglutamine expansion and the expression of chaperone proteins. *Proc. Natl. Acad. Sci., USA* **97** (4), 1589–1594.

Kusakabe, M., Mangiarini, L., Laywell, E. D., Bates, G. P., Yoshiki, A., Hiraiwa, N., Inoue, J., and Steindler, D. A. (2001). Loss of cortical and thalamic neuronal tenascin-C expression in a transgenic mouse expressing exon 1 of the human Huntington disease gene. *J. Comp. Neurol.* **430** (4), 485–500.

Landwehrmeyer, G. B., McNeil, S. M., Dure, L. S. 4., Ge, P., Aizawa, H., Huang, Q., Ambrose, C. M., Duyao, M. P., Bird, E. D., and Bonilla, E. (1995). Huntington's disease gene: regional and cellular expression in brain of normal and affected individuals. *Ann. Neurol.* **37** (2), 218–230.

Lawrence, A. D., Weeks, R. A., Brooks, D. J., Andrews, T. C., Watkins, L. H., Harding, A. E., Robbins, T. W., and Sahakian, B. J. (1998). The relationship between striatal dopamine receptor binding and cognitive performance in Huntington's disease. *Brain* **121**, (7), 1343–1355.

Leavitt, B. R., Guttman, J. A., Hodgson, J. G., Kimel, G. H., Singaraja, R., Vogl, A. W., and Hayden, M. R. (2001). Wild-type huntingtin reduces the cellular toxicity of mutant huntingtin *in vivo*. *Am. J. Hum. Genet.* **68** (2), 313–324.

Lee, M. K. and Cleveland, D. W. (1994). Neurofilament function and dysfunction: involvement in axonal growth and neuronal disease. *Curr. Opin. Cell Biol.* **6** (1), 34–40.

Levine, M. S., Klapstein, G. J., Koppel, A., Gruen, E., Cepeda, C., Vargas, M. E., Jokel, E. S., Carpenter, E. M., Zanjani, H., Hurst, R. S., Efstratiadis, A., Zeitlin, S., and Chesselet, M. F. (1999). Enhanced sensitivity to N-methyl-D-aspartate receptor activation in transgenic and knockin mouse models of Huntington's disease. *J. Neurosci. Res.* **58** (4), 515–532.

Li, H., Li, S. H., Cheng, A. L., Mangiarini, L., Bates, G. P., and Li, X. J. (1999b). Ultrastructural localization and progressive formation of neuropil aggregates in Huntington's disease transgenic mice. *Hum. Mol. Genet.* **8** (7), 1227–1236.

—— —— Johnston, H., Shelbourne, P. F., and Li, X. J. (2000). Amino-terminal fragments of mutant huntingtin show selective accumulation in striatal neurons and synaptic toxicity. *Nat. Genet.* **25** (4), 385–389.

Li, S. H., Gutckunst, C. A., Hersch, S. M., and Li, X. J. (1998). Interaction of huntingtin-associated protein with dynactin P150Glued. *J. Neurosci.* **18** (4), 1261–1269.

—— Cheng, A. L., Li, H., and Li, X. J. (1999c). Cellular defects and altered gene expression in PC12 cells stably expressing mutant huntingtin. *J. Neurosci.* **19** (13), 5159–5172.

Li, X. J., Li, S. H., Sharp, A. H., Nucifora, F. C., Jr., Schilling, G., Lanahan, A., Worley, P., Snyder, S. H., and Ross, C. A. (1995). A huntingtin-associated protein enriched in brain with implications for pathology. *Nature* **378** (6555), 398–402.

Li, Z., Karlovich, C. A., Fish, M. P., Scott, M. P., and Myers, R. M. (1999a). A putative *Drosophila* homolog of the Huntington's disease gene. *Hum. Mol Genet.* **8** (9), 1807–1815.

Lin, B., Rommens, J. M., Graham, R. K., Kalchman, M., MacDonald, H., Nasir, J., Delaney, A., Goldberg, Y. P., and Hayden, M. R. (1993). Differential 3′ polyadenylation of the Huntington disease gene results in two mRNA species with variable tissue expression. *Hum. Mol. Genet.* **2** (10), 1541–1545.

—— Nasir, J., Kalchman, M. A., McDonald, H., Zeisler, J., Goldberg, Y. P., and Hayden, M. R. (1995). Structural analysis of the 5′ region of mouse and human Huntington disease genes reveals conservation of putative promoter region and di- and trinucleotide polymorphisms. *Genomics* **25** (3), 707–715.

Lin, C. H., Tallaksen-Greene, S., Chien, W. M., Cearley, J. A., Jackson, W. S., Crouse, A. B., Ren, S., Li, X. J., Albin, R. L., and Detloff, P. J. (2001). Neurological abnormalities in a knock-in mouse model of Huntington's disease. *Hum. Mol. Genet.* **10** (2), 137–144.

Lione, L. A., Carter, R. J., Hunt, M. J., Bates, G. P., Morton, A. J., and Dunnett, S. B. (1999). Selective discrimination learning impairments in mice expressing the human Huntington's disease mutation. *J Neurosci.* **19** (23), 10428–10437.

Liu, Y. F. (1998). Expression of polyglutamine-expanded Huntingtin activates the SEK1–JNK pathway and induces apoptosis in a hippocampal neuronal cell line. *J. Biol. Chem.* **273** (44), 28873–28877.

—— Deth, R. C., and Devys, D. (1997). SH3 domain-dependent association of huntingtin with epidermal growth factor receptor signaling complexes. *J. Biol. Chem.* **272** (13), 8121–8124.

Lunkes, A. and Mandel, J. L. (1998). A cellular model that recapitulates major pathogenic steps of Huntington's disease. *Hum. Mol. Genet.* **7** (9), 1355–1361.

Luthi-Carter, R., Strand, A., Peters, N. L., Solano, S. M., Hollingsworth, Z. R., Menon, A. S., Frey, A. S., Spektor, B. S., Penney, E. B., Schilling, G., Ross, C. A., Borchelt, D. R., Tapscott, S. J., Young, A. B., Cha, J. H., and Olson, J. M. (2000). Decreased expression of striatal signaling genes in a mouse model of Huntington's disease. *Hum. Mol. Genet.* **9** (9), 1259–1271.

Mangiarini, L., Sathasivam, K., Seller, M., Cozens, B., Harper, A., Hetherington, C., Lawton, M., Trottier, Y., Lehrach, H., Davies, S. W., and Bates, G. P. (1996). Exon 1 of the HD gene with an expanded CAG repeat is sufficient to cause a progressive neurological phenotype in transgenic mice. *Cell* **87** (3), 493–506.

Marks, P. A., Richon, V. M., Breslow, R., and Rifkind, R. A. (2001). Histone deacetylase inhibitors as new cancer drugs. *Curr. Opin. Oncol.* **13** (6), 477–483.

Marsh, J. L., Walker, H., Theisen, H., Zhu, Y. Z., Fielder, T., Purcell, J., and Thompson, L. M. (2000). Expanded polyglutamine peptides alone are intrinsically cytotoxic and cause neurodegeneration in *Drosophila. Hum. Mol. Genet.* **9** (1), 13–25.

Martin-Aparicio, E., Yamamoto, A., Hernandez, F., Hen, R., Avila, J., and Lucas, J. J. (2001). Proteasomal-dependent aggregate reversal and absence of cell death in a conditional mouse model of Huntington's disease. *J. Neurosci.* **21** (22), 8772–8781.

Martindale, D., Hackam, A., Wieczorek, A., Ellerby, L., Wellington, C., McCutcheon, K., Singaraja, R., Kazemi-Esfarjani, P., Devon, R., Kim, S. U., Bredesen, D. E., Tufaro, F., and Hayden, M. R. (1998). Length of huntingtin and its polyglutamine tract influences localization and frequency of intracellular aggregates. *Nat. Genet.* **18** (2), 150–154.

McCampbell, A., Taylor, J. P., Taye, A. A., Robitschek, J., Li, M., Walcott, J., Merry, D., Chai, Y., Paulson, H., Sobue, G., and Fischbeck, K. H. (2000). CREB-binding protein sequestration by expanded polyglutamine. *Hum. Mol. Genet.* **9** (14), 2197–2202.

Menalled, L., Zanjani, H., MacKenzie, L., Koppel, A., Carpenter, E., Zeitlin, S., and Chesselet, M. F. (2000). Decrease in striatal enkephalin mRNA in mouse models of Huntington's disease. *Exp. Neurol.* **162** (2), 328–342.

Metzler, M., Chen, N., Helgason, C. D., Graham, R. K., Nichol, K., McCutcheon, K., Nasir, J., Humphries, R. K., Raymond, L. A., and Hayden, M. R. (1999). Life without huntingtin: normal differentiation into functional neurons. *J. Neurochem.* **72** (3), 1009–1018.

—— Legendre-Guillemin, V., Gan, L., Chopra, V., Kwok, A., McPherson, P. S., and Hayden, M. R. (2001). HIP1 functions in clathrin-mediated endocytosis through binding to clathrin and adaptor protein 2. *J. Biol. Chem.* **276** (42), 39271–39276.

Migaud, M., Charlesworth, P., Dempster, M., Webster, L. C., Watabe, A. M., Makhinson, M., He, Y., Ramsay, M. F., Morris, R. G., Morrison, J. H., O'Dell, T. J., and Grant, S. G. (1998). Enhanced long-term potentiation and impaired learning in mice with mutant postsynaptic density-95 protein. *Nature* **396** (6710), 433–439.

Miyashita, T., Matsui, J., and Ohtsuka, Y. (1999). Expression of extended polyglutamine sequentially activates initiator and effector caspases. *Biochem. Biophys. Res. Commun.* **257** (3), 724–730.

Morton, A. J., Lagan, M. A., Skepper, J. N., and Dunnett, S. B. (2000). Progressive formation of inclusions in the striatum and hippocampus of mice transgenic for the human Huntington's disease mutation. *J. Neurocytol.* **29** (9), 679–702.

Moulder, K. L., Onodera, O., Burke, J. R., Strittmatter, W. J., and Johnson, E. M. Jr. (1999). Generation of neuronal intranuclear inclusions by polyglutamine-GFP: analysis of inclusion clearance and toxicity as a function of polyglutamine length. *J. Neurosci.* **19** (2), 705–715.

Murphy, K. P., Carter, R. J., Lione, L. A., Mangiarini, L., Mahal, A., Bates, G. P., Dunnett, S. B., and Morton, A. J. (2000). Abnormal synaptic plasticity and impaired spatial cognition in mice transgenic for exon 1 of the human Huntington's disease mutation. *J. Neurosci.* **20** (13), 5115–5123.

Myers, R. H., Leavitt, J., Farrer, L. A., Jagadeesh, J., McFarlane, H., Mastromauro, C. A., Mark, R. J., and Gusella, J. F. (1989). Homozygote for Huntington disease. *Am. J. Hum. Genet.* **45** (4), 615–618.

Nagai, Y., Onodera, O., Chun, J., Strittmatter, W. J., and Burke, J. R. (1999). Expanded polyglutamine domain proteins bind neurofilament and alter the neurofilament network. *Exp. Neurol.* **155** (2), 195–203.

Nakamura, K., Jeong, S. Y., Uchihara, T., Anno, M., Nagashima, K., Nagashima, T., Ikeda, S., Tsuji, S., and Kanazawa, I. (2001). SCA17, a novel autosomal dominant cerebellar ataxia caused by an expanded polyglutamine in TATA-binding protein. *Hum. Mol. Genet.* **10** (14), 1441–1448.

Narain, Y., Wyttenbach, A., Rankin, J., Furlong, R. A., and Rubinsztein, D. C. (1999). A molecular investigation of true dominance in Huntington's disease. *J. Med. Genet.* **36** (10), 739–746.

Nasir, J., Floresco, S. B., O'Kusky, J. R., Diewert, V. M., Richman, J. M., Zeisler, J., Borowski, A., Marth, J. D., Phillips, A. G., and Hayden, M. R. (1995). Targeted disruption of the Huntington's disease gene results in embryonic lethality and behavioral and morphological changes in heterozygotes. *Cell* **81** (5), 811–823.

Nilsberth, C., Westlind-Danielsson, A., Eckman, C. B., Condron, M. M., Axelman, K., Forsell, C., Stenh, C., Luthman, J., Teplow, D. B., Younkin, S. G., Naslund, J., and Lannfelt, L. (2001). The 'Arctic' APP mutation (E693G), causes Alzheimer's disease by enhanced $A\beta$ protofibril formation. *Nat. Neurosci.* **4** (9), 887–893.

Nucifora, F. C., Jr., Sasaki, M., Peters, M. F., Huang, H., Cooper, J. K., Yamada, M., Takahashi, H., Tsuji, S., Troncoso, J., Dawson, V. L., Dawson, T. M., and Ross, C. A. (2001). Interference by huntingtin and atrophin-1 with cbp-mediated transcription leading to cellular toxicity. *Science* **291** (5512), 2423–2428.

O'Kusky, J. R., Nasir, J., Cicchetti, F., Parent, A., and Hayden, M. R. (1999). Neuronal degeneration in the basal ganglia and loss of pallido-subthalamic synapses in mice with targeted disruption of the Huntington's disease gene. *Brain Res.* **818** (2), 468–479.

Ona, V. O., Li, M., Vonsattel, J. P., Andrews, L. J., Khan, S. Q., Chung, W. M., Frey, A. S., Menon, A. S., Li, X. J., Stieg, P. E., Yuan, J., Penney, J. B., Young, A. B., Cha, J. H., and Friedlander, R. M. (1999). Inhibition of caspase-1 slows disease progression in a mouse model of Huntington's disease [see comments]. *Nature* **399** (6733), 263–267.

Ordway, J. M., Tallaksen-Greene, S., Gutekunst, C. A., Bernstein, E. M., Cearley, J. A., Wiener, H. W., Dure, L. S. 4., Lindsey, R., Hersch, S. M., Jope, R. S., Albin, R. L., and Detloff, P. J. (1997). Ectopically expressed CAG repeats cause intranuclear inclusions and a progressive late onset neurological phenotype in the mouse. *Cell* **91** (6), 753–763.

Ott, M., Schnolzer, M., Garnica, J., Fischle, W., Emiliani, S., Rackwitz, H. R., and Verdin, E. (1999). Acetylation of the HIV-1 Tat protein by p300 is important for its transcriptional activity. *Curr. Biol.* **9** (24), 1489–1492.

Persichetti, F., Carlee, L., Faber, P. W., McNeil, S. M., Ambrose, C. M., Srinidhi, J., Anderson, M., Barnes, G. T., Gusella, J. F., and MacDonald, M. E. (1996). Differential expression of normal and mutant Huntington's disease gene alleles. *Neurobiol. Dis.* **3** (3), 183–190.

Perutz, M. F. and Windle, A. H. (2001). Cause of neural death in neurodegenerative diseases attributable to expansion of glutamine repeats. *Nature* **412** (6843), 143–144.

Peters, M. F., Nucifora, F. C., Jr., Kushi, J., Seaman, H. C., Cooper, J. K., Herring, W. J., Dawson, V. L., Dawson, T. M., and Ross, C. A. (1999). Nuclear targeting of mutant Huntingtin increases toxicity. *Mol. Cell Neurosci.* **14** (2), 121–128.

Petersen, A., Larsen, K. E., Behr, G. G., Romero, N., Przedborski, S., Brundin, P., and Sulzer, D. (2001). Expanded CAG repeats in exon 1 of the Huntington's disease gene stimulate dopamine-mediated striatal neuron autophagy and degeneration. *Hum. Mol. Genet.* **10** (12), 1243–1254.

Philipsen, S. and Suske, G. (1999). A tale of three fingers: the family of mammalian Sp/XKLF transcription factors. *Nucl. Acids Res.* **27** (15), 2991–3000.

Portera-Cailliau, C., Hedreen, J. C., Price, D. L., and Koliatsos, V. E. (1995). Evidence for apoptotic cell death in Huntington disease and excitotoxic animal models. *J. Neurosci.* **15** (5, pt. 2), 3775–3787.

Raths, S., Rohrer, J., Crausaz, F., and Riezman, H. (1993). end3 and end4: two mutants defective in receptor-mediated and fluid-phase endocytosis in *Saccharomyces cerevisiae*. *J. Cell Biol.* **120** (1), 55–65.

Reddy, P. H., Williams, M., Charles, V., Garrett, L., Pike-Buchanan, L., Whetsell, W. O., Jr., Miller, G., and Tagle, D. A. (1998). Behavioural abnormalities and selective neuronal loss in HD transgenic mice expressing mutated full-length HD cDNA. *Nat. Genet.* **20** (2), 198–202.

Reim, K., Mansour, M., Varoqueaux, F., McMahon, H. T., Sudhof, T. C., Brose, N., and Rosenmund, C. (2001). Complexins regulate a late step in Ca2+-dependent neurotransmitter release. *Cell* **104** (1), 71–81.

Riccio, A., Ahn, S., Davenport, C. M., Blendy, J. A., and Ginty, D. D. (1999). Mediation by a CREB family transcription factor of NGF-dependent survival of sympathetic neurons. *Science* **286** (5448), 2358–2361.

Richfield, E. K. and Herkenham, M. (1994). Selective vulnerability in Huntington's disease: preferential loss of cannabinoid receptors in lateral globus pallidus. *Ann. Neurol.* **36** (4), 577–584.

—— Maguire-Zeiss, K. A., Cox, C., Gilmore, J., and Voorn, P. (1995). Reduced expression of preproenkephalin in striatal neurons from Huntington's disease patients. *Ann. Neurol.* **37** (3), 335–343.

Rigamonti, D., Bauer, J. H., De Fraja, C., Conti, L., Sipione, S., Sciorati, C., Clementi, E., Hackam, A., Hayden, M. R., Li, Y., Cooper, J. K., Ross, C. A., Govoni, S., Vincenz, C., and Cattaneo, E. (2000). Wild-type huntingtin protects from apoptosis upstream of caspase-3. *J. Neurosci.* **20** (10), 3705–3713.

—— Sipione, S., Goffredo, D., Zuccato, C., Fossale, E., and Cattaneo, E. (2001). Huntingtin's neuroprotective activity occurs via inhibition of procaspase-9 processing. *J. Biol. Chem.* **276** (18), 14545–14548.

Roizin, L., Stellar, S., and Lui, J. C. 1979). Neuronal nuclear-cytoplasmic inclusions in Huntington's disease: electron microscopic investigations. *Advan. Neurol.* **23**, 95–122.

Rubinsztein, D. C., Leggo, J., Coles, R., Almqvist, E., Biancalana, V., Cassiman, J. J., Chotai, K., Connarty, M., Crauford, D., Curtis, A., Curtis, D., Davidson, M. J., Differ, A. M., Dode, C., Dodge, A., Frontali, M., Ranen, N. G., Stine, O. C., Sherr, M., Abbott, M. H., Franz, M. L., Graham, C. A., Harper, P. S., Hedreen, J. C., and Hayden, M. R. (1996). Phenotypic characterization of individuals with 30–40 CAG repeats in the Huntington disease (HD), gene reveals HD cases with 36 repeats and apparently normal elderly individuals with 36–39 repeats. *Am. J. Hum. Genet.* **59** (1), 16–22.

Rymer, D. L. and Good, T. A. (2000). The role of prion peptide structure and aggregation in toxicity and membrane binding. *J. Neurochem.* **75** (6), 2536–2545.

Salghetti, S. E., Caudy, A. A., Chenoweth, J. G., and Tansey, W. P. (2001). Regulation of transcriptional activation domain function by ubiquitin. *Science* **293** (5535), 1651–1653.

Samuel, R. E., Salmon, E. D., and Briehl, R. W. (1990). Nucleation and growth of fibres and gel formation in sickle cell haemoglobin. *Nature* **345** (6278), 833–835.

Sanchez, I., Xu, C. J., Juo, P., Kakizaka, A., Blenis, J., and Yuan, J. (1999). Caspase-8 is required for cell death induced by expanded polyglutamine repeats [see comments]. *Neuron* **22** (3), 623–633.

Sapp, E., Schwarz, C., Chase, K., Bhide, P. G., Young, A. B., Penney, J., Vonsattel, J. P., Aronin, N., and DiFiglia, M. (1997). Huntingtin localization in brains of normal and Huntington's disease patients. *Ann. Neurol.* **42** (4), 604–612.

—— Penney, J., Young, A., Aronin, N., Vonsattel, J. P., and DiFiglia, M. (1999). Axonal transport of N-terminal huntingtin suggests early pathology of corticostriatal projections in Huntington disease. *J. Neuropathol. Exp. Neurol.* **58** (2), 165–173.

Sattler, R., Xiong, Z., Lu, W. Y., Hafner, M., MacDonald, J. F., and Tymianski, M. (1999). Specific coupling of NMDA receptor activation to nitric oxide neurotoxicity by PSD-95 protein. *Science* **284** (5421), 1845–1848.

Saudou, F., Finkbeiner, S., Devys, D., and Greenberg, M. E. (1998). Huntingtin acts in the nucleus to induce apoptosis but death does not correlate with the formation of intranuclear inclusions. *Cell* **95** (1), 55–66.

Scherzinger, E., Lurz, R., Turmaine, M., Mangiarini, L., Hollenbach, B., Hasenbank, R., Bates, G. P., Davies, S. W., Lehrach, H., and Wanker, E. E. (1997). Huntingtin-encoded polyglutamine expansions form amyloid-like protein aggregates *in vitro* and *in vivo*. *Cell* **90** (3), 549–558.

Schilling, G., Becher, M. W., Sharp, A. H., Jinnah, H. A., Duan, K., Kotzuk, J. A., Slunt, H. H., Ratovitski, T., Cooper, J. K., Jenkins, N. A., Copeland, N. G., Price, D. L., Ross, C. A., and Borchelt, D. R. (1999). Intranuclear inclusions and neuritic aggregates in transgenic mice expressing a mutant N-terminal fragment of huntingtin. *Hum. Mol. Genet.* **8** (3), 397–407.

Schmid, S. L. (1997). Clathrin-coated vesicle formation and protein sorting: an integrated process. *Annu. Rev. Biochem.* **66**, 511–48.

Schmitt, I., Bachner, D., Megow, D., Henklein, P., Hameister, H., Epplen, J. T., and Riess, O. (1995a). Expression of the Huntington disease gene in rodents: cloning the rat homologue and evidence for downregulation in non-neuronal tissues during development. *Hum. Mol. Genet.* **4** (7), 1173–1182.

—— Epplen, J. T., and Riess, O. (1995b). Predominant neuronal expression of the gene responsible for dentatorubral-pallidoluysian atrophy (DRPLA), in rat. *Hum. Mol. Genet.* **4** (9), 1619–1624.

Schonemann, M. D., Ryan, A. K., McEvilly, R. J., O'Connell, S. M., Arias, C. A., Kalla, K. A., Li, P., Sawchenko, P. E., and Rosenfeld, M. G. (1995). Development and survival of the endocrine hypothalamus and posterior pituitary gland requires the neuronal POU domain factor Brn-2. *Genes Dev.* **9** (24), 3122–3135.

Schulz, J. B. and Dichgans, J. (1999). Molecular pathogenesis of movement disorders: are protein aggregates a common link in neuronal degeneration? *Curr. Opin. Neurol.* **12** (4), 433–439.

Sharp, A. H., Loev, S. J., Schilling, G., Li, S. H., Li, X. J., Bao, J., Wagster, M. V., Kotzuk, J. A., Steiner, J. P., and Lo, A. (1995). Widespread expression of Huntington's disease gene (IT15) protein product. *Neuron* **14** (5), 1065–1074.

Shaywitz, A. J. and Greenberg, M. E. (1999). CREB: a stimulus-induced transcription factor activated by a diverse array of extracellular signals. *Annu. Rev. Biochem.* **68**, 821–861.

Shearwin-Whyatt, L. M. and Kumar, S. (1999). Caspases in developmental cell death. *IUBMB Life* **48** (2), 143–150.

Shelbourne, P. F., Killeen, N., Hevner, R. F., Johnston, H. M., Tecott, L., Lewandoski, M., Ennis, M., Ramirez, L., Li, Z., Iannicola, C., Littman, D. R., and Myers, R. M. (1999). A Huntington's disease CAG expansion at the murine hdh locus is unstable and associated with behavioural abnormalities in mice. *Hum. Mol. Genet.* **8** (5), 763–774.

Sherer, T. B., Betarbet, R., and Greenamyre, J. T. (2001). Pathogenesis of Parkinson's disease. *Curr. Opin. Invest. Drugs* **2** (5), 657–662.

Sieradzan, K. A. and Mann, D. M. (1998). On the pathological progression of Huntington's disease [letter; comment]. *Ann. Neurol.* **44** (1), 148–149.

—— Mechan, A. O., Jones, L., Wanker, E. E., Nukina, N., and Mann, D. M. (1999). Huntington's disease intranuclear inclusions contain truncated, ubiquitinated huntingtin protein. *Exp. Neurol.* **156** (1), 92–99.

Silverman, M. A., Kaech, S., Jareb, M., Burack, M. A., Vogt, L., Sonderegger, P., and Banker, G. (2001). Sorting and directed transport of membrane proteins during development of hippocampal neurons in culture. *Proc. Natl Acad. Sci., USA* **98** (13), 7051–7057.

Sittler, A., Walter, S., Wedemeyer, N., Hasenbank, R., Scherzinger, E., Eickhoff, H., Bates, G. P., Lehrach, H., and Wanker, E. E. (1998). SH3GL3 associates with the Huntingtin exon 1 protein and promotes the formation of polygln-containing protein aggregates. *Mol. Cell* **2** (4), 427–436.

Sorensen, S. A., Fenger, K., and Olsen, J. H. (1999). Significantly lower incidence of cancer among patients with Huntington disease: an apoptotic effect of an expanded polyglutamine tract? *Cancer* **86** (7), 1342–1346.

Steffan, J. S., Kazantsev, A., Spasic-Boskovic, O., Greenwald, M., Zhu, Y. Z., Gohler, H., Wanker, E. E., Bates, G. P., Housman, D. E., and Thompson, L. M. (2000). The Huntington's disease protein interacts with p53 and CREB-binding protein and represses transcription. *Proc. Natl Acad. Sci., USA* **97** (12), 6763–6768.

—— Bodai, L., Pallos, J., Poelman, M., McCampbell, A., Apostol, B. L., Kazantsev, A., Schmidt, E., Zhu, Y. Z., Greenwald, M., Kurokawa, R., Housman, D. E., Jackson, G. R., Marsh, J. L., and Thompson, L. M. (2001). Histone deacetylase inhibitors arrest polyglutamine-dependent neurodegeneration in *Drosophila. Nature* **413** (6857), 739–743.

Steward, O. and Worley, P. F. (2001). A cellular mechanism for targeting newly synthesized mRNAs to synaptic sites on dendrites. *Proc. Natl Acad. Sci., USA* **98** (13), 7062–7068.

Strong, T. V., Tagle, D. A., Valdes, J. M., Elmer, L. W., Boehm, K., Swaroop, M., Kaatz, K. W., Collins, F. S., and Albin, R. L. (1993). Widespread expression of the human and rat Huntington's disease gene in brain and nonneural tissues. *Nat. Genet.* **5** (3), 259–265.

Sun, Y., Savanenin, A., Reddy, P. H., and Liu, Y. F. (2001). Polyglutamine-expanded huntingtin promotes sensitization of N-methyl-D-aspartate receptors via post-synaptic density 95. *J. Biol. Chem.* **276** (27), 24713–24718.

Sune, C., Hayashi, T., Liu, Y., Lane, W. S., Young, R. A., and Garcia-Blanco, M. A. (1997). CA150, a nuclear protein associated with the RNA polymerase II holoenzyme, is involved in Tat-activated human immunodeficiency virus type 1 transcription. *Mol. Cell Biol.* **17** (10), 6029–6039.

Tabrizi, S. J., Cleeter, M. W., Xuereb, J., Taanman, J. W., Cooper, J. M., and Schapira, A. H. (1999). Biochemical abnormalities and excitotoxicity in Huntington's disease brain. *Ann. Neurol.* **45** (1), 25–32.

Tanaka, Y., Engelender, S., Igarashi, S., Rao, R. K., Wanner, T., Tanzi, R. E., Sawa, A., Dawson, L., Dawson, T. M., and Ross, C. A. (2001). Inducible expression of mutant alpha-synuclein decreases proteasome activity and increases sensitivity to mitochondria-dependent apoptosis. *Hum. Mol. Genet.* **10** (9), 919–926.

Tellez-Nagel, I., Johnson, A. B., and Terry, R. D. (1974). Studies on brain biopsies of patients with Huntington's chorea. *J. Neuropathol. Exp. Neurol.* **33** (2), 308–332.

Tezuka, T., Umemori, H., Akiyama, T., Nakanishi, S., and Yamamoto, T. (1999). PSD-95 promotes Fyn-mediated tyrosine phosphorylation of the N-methyl-D-aspartate receptor subunit NR2A. *Proc. Natl Acad. Sci., USA* **96** (2), 435–440.

Thomas, L. B., Gates, D. J., Richfield, E. K., O'Brien, T. F., Schweitzer, J. B., and Steindler, D. A. (1995). DNA end labeling (TUNEL) in Huntington's disease and other neuropathological conditions. *Exp. Neurol.* **133** (2), 265–272.

Trettel, F., Rigamonti, D., Hilditch-Maguire, P., Wheeler, V. C., Sharp, A. H., Persichetti, F., Cattaneo, E., and MacDonald, M. E. (2000). Dominant phenotypes produced by the HD mutation in STHdh(Q111) striatal cells. *Hum. Mol. Genet.* **9** (19), 2799–2809.

Trojanowski, J. Q. and Lee, V. M. (2000). 'Fatal attractions' of proteins. A comprehensive hypothetical mechanism underlying Alzheimer's disease and other neurodegenerative disorders. *Ann. NY Acad. Sci.* **924**, 62–67.

Tukamoto, T., Nukina, N., Ide, K., and Kanazawa, I. (1997). Huntington's disease gene product, huntingtin, associates with microtubules *in vitro*. *Brain Res. Mol. Brain Res.* **51** (1–2), 8–14.

Turmaine, M., Raza, A., Mahal, A., Mangiarini, L., Bates, G. P., and Davies, S. W. (2000). Nonapoptotic neurodegeneration in a transgenic mouse model of Huntington's disease. *Proc. Natl Acad. Sci., USA* **97** (14), 8093–8097.

Valetti, C., Wetzel, D. M., Schrader, M., Hasbani, M. J., Gill, S. R., Kreis, T. E., and Schroer, T. A. (1999). Role of dynactin in endocytic traffic: effects of dynamitin overexpression and colocalization with CLIP-170. *Mol. Biol. Cell* **10** (12), 4107–4120.

Velier, J., Kim, M., Schwarz, C., Kim, T. W., Sapp, E., Chase, K., Aronin, N., and DiFiglia, M. (1998). Wild-type and mutant huntingtins function in vesicle trafficking in the secretory and endocytic pathways. *Exp. Neurol.* **152** (1), 34–40.

Voges, D., Zwickl, P., and Baumeister, W. (1999). The 26S proteasome: a molecular machine designed for controlled proteolysis. *Annu. Rev. Biochem.* **68**, 1015–1068.

Volles, M. J., Lee, S. J., Rochet, J. C., Shtilerman, M. D., Ding, T. T., Kessler, J. C., and Lansbury, P. T., Jr. (2001). Vesicle permeabilization by protofibrillar alpha-synuclein: implications for the pathogenesis and treatment of Parkinson's disease. *Biochemistry* **40** (26), 7812–7819.

Waelter, S., Boeddrich, A., Lurz, R., Scherzinger, E., Lueder, G., Lehrach, H., and Wanker, E. E. (2001a). Accumulation of mutant huntingtin fragments in aggresome-like inclusion bodies as a result of insufficient protein degradation. *Mol. Biol. Cell* **12** (5), 1393–1407.

—— Scherzinger, E., Hasenbank, R., Nordhoff, E., Lurz, R., Goehler, H., Gauss, C., Sathasivam, K., Bates, G. P., Lehrach, H., and Wanker, E. E. (2001b). The huntingtin interacting protein HIP1 is a clathrin and alpha-adaptin-binding protein involved in receptor-mediated endocytosis. *Hum. Mol. Genet.* **10** (17), 1807–1817.

Walton, M. R. and Dragunow, I. (2000). Is CREB a key to neuronal survival? *Trends Neurosci.* **23** (2), 48–53.

Wang, G. H., Mitsui, K., Kotliarova, S., Yamashita, A., Nagao, Y., Tokuhiro, S., Iwatsubo, T., Kanazawa, I., and Nukina, N. (1999a). Caspase activation during apoptotic cell death induced by expanded polyglutamine in N2a cells. *Neuroreport* **10** (12), 2435–2438.

Wang, V., Yeh, T. P., Chen, C. M., Yan, S. H., and Soong, B. W. (1999b). Usefulness of molecular testing in Huntington's disease. *Chung Hua I. Hsueh Tsa Chih (Taipei)* **62** (9), 586–590.

Wanker, E. E. (2000). Protein aggregation and pathogenesis of Huntington's disease: mechanisms and correlations. *Biol. Chem.* **381**, (9–10), 937–942.

Wanker, E. E., Rovira, C., Scherzinger, E., Hasenbank, R., Walter, S., Tait, D., Colichelli, J., and Lerach, H. (1997). HIP-I: a huntingtin interacting protein isolated by the yeast two-hybrid system. *Hum. Mol. Genet.* **6** (3), 487–495.

Waragai, M., Lammers, C. H., Takeuchi, S., Imafuku, I., Udagawa, Y., Kanazawa, I., Kawabata, M., Mouradian, M. M., and Okazawa, H. (1999). PQBP-1, a novel polyglutamine tract-binding protein, inhibits transcription activation by Brn-2 and affects cell survival. *Hum. Mol. Genet.* **8** (6), 977–987.

Warrick, J. M., Chan, H. Y., Gray-Board, G. L., Chai, Y., Paulson, H. L., and Bonini, N. M. (1999). Suppression of polyglutamine-mediated neurodegeneration in *Drosophila* by the molecular chaperone HSP70. *Nat. Genet.* **23** (4), 425–428.

Waterman-Storer, C. M., Karki, S. B., Kuznetsov, S. A., Tabb, J. S., Weiss, D. G., Langford, G. M., and Holzbaur, E. L. (1997). The interaction between cytoplasmic dynein and dynactin is required for fast axonal transport. *Proc. Natl Acad. Sci., USA* **94** (22), 12180–12185.

Wellington, C. L., Ellerby, L. M., Hackam, A. S., Margolis, R. L., Trifiro, M. A., Singaraja, R., McCutcheon, K., Salvesen, G. S., Propp, S. S., Bromm, M., Rowland, K. J., Zhang, T., Rasper, D., Roy, S., Thornberry, N., Pinsky, L., Kakizuka, A., Ross, C. A., Nicholson, D. W., Bredesen, D. E., and Hayden, M. R. (1998). Caspase cleavage of gene products associated with triplet expansion disorders generates truncated fragments containing the polyglutamine tract. *J. Biol. Chem.* **273** (15), 9158–9167.

—— Singaraja, R., Ellerby, L., Savill, J., Roy, S., Leavitt, B., Cattaneo, E., Hackam, A., Sharp, A., Thornberry, N., Nicholson, D. W., Bredesen, D. E., and Hayden, M. R. (2000). Inhibiting caspase cleavage of huntingtin reduces toxicity and aggregate formation in neuronal and nonneuronal cells. *J. Biol. Chem.* **275** (26), 19831–19838.

Wexler, N. S., Young, A. B., Tanzi, R. E., Travers, H., Starosta-Rubinstein, S., Penney, J. B., Snodgrass, S. R., Shoulson, I., Gomez, F., and Ramos Arroyo, M. A. (1987). Homozygotes for Huntington's disease. *Nature* **326** (6109), 194–197.

Wheeler, V. C., Auerbach, W., White, J. K., Srinidhi, J., Auerbach, A., Ryan, A., Duyao, M. P., Vrbanac, V., Weaver, M., Gusella, J. F., Joyner, A. L., and MacDonald, M. E. (1999). Length-dependent gametic CAG repeat instability in the Huntington's disease knock-in mouse. *Hum. Mol. Genet.* **8** (1), 115–122.

—— White, J. K., Gutekunst, C. A., Vrbanac, V., Weaver, M., Li, X. J., Li, S. H., Yi, H., Vonsattel, J. P., Gusella, J. F., Hersch, S., Auerbach, W., Joyner, A. L., and MacDonald, M. E. (2000). Long glutamine tracts cause nuclear localization of a novel form of huntingtin in medium spiny striatal neurons in HdhQ92 and HdhQ111 knock-in mice. *Hum. Mol. Genet.* **9** (4), 503–513.

White, J. K., Auerbach, W., Duyao, M. P., Vonsattel, J. P., Gusella, J. F., Joyner, A. L., and MacDonald, M. E. (1997). Huntingtin is required for neurogenesis and is not impaired by the Huntington's disease CAG expansion. *Nat. Genet.* **17** (4), 404–410.

Wood, J. D., MacMillan, J. C., Harper, P. S., Lowenstein, P. R., and Jones, A. L. (1996). Partial characterisation of murine huntingtin and apparent variations in the subcellular localisation of huntingtin in human, mouse and rat brain. *Hum. Mol. Genet.* **5** (4), 481–487.

—— Nucifora, F. C., Jr., Duan, K., Zhang, C., Wang, J., Kim, Y., Schilling, G., Sacchi, N., Liu, J. M., and Ross, C. A. (2000). Atrophin-1, the dentato-rubral and pallido-luysian atrophy gene product, interacts with ETO/MTG8 in the nuclear matrix and represses transcription. *J. Cell Biol.* **150** (5), 939–948.

Wyttenbach, A., Carmichael, J., Swartz, J., Furlong, R. A., Narain, Y., Rankin, J., and Rubinsztein, D. C. (2000). Effects of heat shock, heat shock protein 40 (HDJ-2), and proteasome inhibition on protein aggregation in cellular models of Huntington's disease. *Proc. Natl Acad. Sci., USA* **97** (6), 2898–2903.

Yamada, Y., Chochi, Y., Takamiya, K., Sobue, K., and Inui, M. (1999). Modulation of the channel activity of the epsilon2/zeta1-subtype N-methyl D-aspartate receptor by PSD-95. *J. Biol. Chem.* **274** (10), 6647–6652.

Yamamoto, A., Lucas, J. J., and Hen, R. (2000). Reversal of neuropathology and motor dysfunction in a conditional model of Huntington's disease [see comments]. *Cell* **101** (1), 57–66.

Zeitlin, S., Liu, J. P., Chapman, D. L., Papaioannou, V. E., and Efstratiadis, A. (1995). Increased apoptosis and early embryonic lethality in mice nullizygous for the Huntington's disease gene homologue. *Nat. Genet.* **11** (2), 155–163.

Zeron, M. M., Chen, N., Moshaver, A., Lee, A. T., Wellington, C. L., Hayden, M. R., and Raymond, L. A. (2001). Mutant huntingtin enhances excitotoxic cell death. *Mol. Cell Neurosci.* **17** (1), 41–53.

Zhang, J., Guenther, M. G., Carthew, R. W., and Lazar, M. A. (1998). Proteasomal regulation of nuclear receptor corepressor-mediated repression. *Genes Dev.* **12** (12), 1775–1780.

Zilfou, J. T., Hoffman, W. H., Sank, M., George, D. L., and Murphy, M. (2001). The corepressor mSin3a interacts with the proline-rich domain of p53 and protects p53 from proteasome-mediated degradation. *Mol. Cell Biol.* **21** (12), 3974–3985.

Zuccato, C., Ciammola, A., Rigamonti, D., Leavitt, B. R., Goffredo, D., Conti, L., MacDonald, M. E., Friedlander, R. M., Silani, V., Hayden, M. R., Timmusk, T., Sipione, S., and Cattaneo, E. (2001). Loss of huntingtin-mediated BDNF gene transcription in Huntington's disease. *Science* **293** (5529), 493–498.

Zuhlke, C., Hellenbroich, Y., Dalski, A., Kononowa, N., Hagenah, J., Vieregge, P., Riess, O., Klein, C., and Schwinger, E. (2001). Different types of repeat expansion in the TATA-binding protein gene are associated with a new form of inherited ataxia. *Eur. J. Hum. Genet.* **9** (3), 160–164.

13 Mouse models of Huntington's disease

Gillian P. Bates and Kerry P.S.J. Murphy

Introduction

The isolation of the Huntington's disease (HD) gene in 1993 (Huntington's Disease Collaborative Research Group 1993) made it possible to generate *in vivo* genetic models of HD. The availability of a genetic model is of fundamental importance for two reasons. First, it permits the early stages of the disease to be studied in order that the primary events in the disease pathogenesis might be unravelled. It is only by understanding the very first molecular events in the disease process that curative therapeutic targets can be identified. It is impossible to pinpoint the first stages of a neurodegenerative disease such as HD from the study of patient tissue as most of the brain material that becomes available is from end-stage disease. Second, the genetic models provide a resource that can be used for testing therapeutic interventions as they are developed. The ease with which the mouse genome can be manipulated has made this the mammalian model of choice and nine HD mouse models have been published. The research community is therefore in the fortunate position of having a range of models that are specifically useful for complementary applications. HD has also been modelled in the fruit fly *Drosophila melanogaster* and in the nematode *Caenorhabditis elegans*. The sophistication with which the genetics of these organisms can be manipulated permits the easy identification of genes that modify aspects of the phenotype. The invertebrate models of HD and the other polyglutamine (polyQ) diseases are described collectively in Chapter 14.

Mouse models of HD are already fulfilling their promise. They have provided major insights into the neuropathology of this disease and are beginning to shed light on early molecular events. Pharmaceutical compounds that have caused an improvement in the HD phenotype of transgenic mice are already entering phase II clinical trials. This chapter begins by summarizing the results of knocking out the mouse HD (*Hdh*) locus. This did not model the disease but instead showed that huntingtin is essential for development as its absence results in embryonic lethality. It discusses the limitations of generating a mouse model of a late-onset human disease and the methods that have been employed to overcome these limitations. The behavioural and neuropathological features of the models and the approaches that have been successful in slowing down or reversing these phenotypes are presented.

Huntingtin knock-outs

Mice that do not express the mouse HD gene (*Hdh*) were generated independently by three research groups using knock-out strategies (Duyao *et al*. 1995; Nasir *et al*. 1995; Zeitlin *et al*. 1995). This demonstrated that huntingtin plays a crucial role in embryogenesis because, in all cases, nullizygous mouse embryos died at approximately embryonic day E7.5. Heterozygous mice expressing one allele (*Hdh/−*) were reported to be indistinguishable from wild-type mice in two cases (Duyao *et al.* 1995; Zeitlin *et al.* 1995), indicating that HD is not caused by haploinsufficiency. This is consistent with human studies, as an individual who carries a balanced translocation disrupting one HD gene allele shows no sign of neurological disease (Ambrose *et al.* 1994). In contrast, heterozygous mice resulting from a targeting strategy that disrupts exon 5 were reported to show neuronal loss in the subthalamic nucleus and the globus pallidus, and some behavioural changes (Nasir *et al.* 1995; O'Kusky *et al.* 1999). The cause of this discrepancy is unknown. It has been speculated that targeting exon 5 was unsuccessful in generating a true null allele and instead produced an *N*-terminal fragment. However, the presence of such a fragment could not be detected on Western blots (Nasir *et al.* 1995) and mice expressing *N*-terminal fragments containing repeats in the normal range are indistinguishable from wild type mice (Cha *et al.* 1999; Mangiarini *et al.* 1996; Schilling *et al.* 1999a).

The generation of *Hdh* knock-outs has contributed minimally to our understanding of the function of huntingtin at the cellular level because of the severity of the phenotype. However, chimeric analysis of wild-type (*Hdh/Hdh*) and nullizygous (*−/−*) embryos that were each injected with either knock-out (*−/−*) or wild-type (*Hdh/Hdh*) embryonic stem (ES) cells, has shown that embryonic lethality results from a primary defect in the extra-embryonic tissues (Dragatsis *et al.* 1998). Gene targeted mice that express <50 per cent of normal huntingtin do show extensive mid- and hind-brain abnormalities at embryonic day E18.5 and die at or shortly after birth (White *et al.* 1997), indicating that huntingtin has a role in brain development. A comparison of organelle morphology between *Hdh −/−* and wild-type (*Hdh/Hdh*) ES cell cultures revealed that huntingtin function is essential for the normal morphology of nuclear (nucleoli and transcription factor-speckles) and perinuclear membrane (mitochondria, endoplasmic reticulum, Golgi, and recycling endosomes) organelles, and a role in iron pathway regulation was also implicated (Hilditch-Maguire *et al.* 2000).

The analysis of huntingtin gene function in the context of ES-cell-derived neuronal differentiation, however, has shown that the generation of neurotransmitter-responsive postmitotic neurones is not inhibited by lack of huntingtin. *Hdh −/−* neurones develop synaptic currents, demonstrating that signal transduction events necessary at the pre- and postsynaptic membrane can occur in the absence of huntingtin (Metzler *et al.* 1999). More recently, adult chimeric mice generated by injecting wild-type blastocysts with *Hdh −/−* ES cells were found to have *Hdh −/−* neurones throughout the brain (Reiner *et al.* 2001). The *Hdh −/−* cells were 5–10 times more common in the hypothalamus, midbrain, and hindbrain than in the telencephalon and thalamus. Chimeric animals tended to be smaller than wild-type littermates, and chimeric mice rich in *Hdh −/−* cells showed some motor abnormalities although no brain malformations or pathologies were apparent (Reiner *et al.* 2001).

Mouse models of HD

HD is autosomal dominant and most probably caused by a gain of function mechanism. Therefore, the introduction of the HD mutation into the mouse germline could be predicted to generate a phenotype irrespective of the presence of two copies of the mouse gene. This has been achieved by the introduction of transgenes expressing truncated or full-length versions of huntingtin in the form of genomic or cDNA constructs. An alternative approach to using transgenics is to introduce the mutation into the mouse HD gene via a knock-in gene targeting strategy.

One concern when attempting to model a mid-life onset disease is that a phenotype will not occur within the lifetime of the laboratory mouse (approximately 2 years). However, because HD manifests in childhood when the CAG repeat is at the upper end of the mutant range, it could be predicted that the use of very long repeats might sufficiently accelerate the onset of the phenotype in order to generate useful mouse models. A further reduction in the age of onset is likely to be possible by increasing the level of mutant protein by the use of a strong promoter, although it cannot be discounted that additional phenotypes might be caused by overexpression. Finally, there is now considerable evidence to indicate that one of the first steps in the pathogenesis of HD is the processing of huntingtin to generate N-terminal fragments and the use of truncated constructs might bypass this initiating event. However, this approach would be predicted to widen the pathology and phenotype. Therefore, the knock-in strategy would be expected to generate the most faithful model of HD, although this is the least flexible approach with respect to generating a mouse with an early onset to the phenotype.

Transgenic and gene targeting strategies
To date, nine mouse models of HD have been described in the literature. The details with respect to the type of HD construct used, the length of the CAG/polyQ repeats, the promoter under which the mutant protein is expressed, and the mouse strain background are summarized in Table 13.1.

Table 13.1 Mouse models of Huntington's disease—details concerning construction

Mouse model	Reference	Strain background	Promoter	Glutamine repeat size*	Construct
R6 lines	Mangiarini *et al.* 1996	C57BL/6 × CBA	Human HD[†]	20, 115, 150	Human exon 1 (1–90)[‡]
171 lines	Schilling *et al.* 1999	C57BL/6 × C3H	Prion	18, 44, 82	Human 1–171[‡]
HD lines	Laforet *et al.* 2001	C57BL/6 × SJL	Rat NSE	10, 46, 102	Human 1–~1000 (5′ FLAG tag)
cDNA lines	Reddy *et al.* 1998	FVB	CMV	18, 50, 91	Human full-length cDNA
YAC lines	Hodgson *et al.* 1999	FVB	Human HD	18, 46, 72	Human full-length genomic
Knock-in	Shelbourne *et al.* 1999	129Sv × C57BL/6	Mouse HD	72, 80	Mouse full-length genomic
Knock-in	Wheeler *et al.* 2000	129Sv × CD1	Mouse HD	20, 50, 92, 111	Mouse full-length genomic[§]
Knock-in	Levine *et al.* 1999	129Sv × C57BL/6	Mouse HD	73, 96	Mouse full-length genomic[§]
Knock-in	Lin *et al.* 2001	129Ola × C57BL/6	Mouse HD	80, 150	Mouse full-length genomic

*The length of the glutamine tract is (CAG repeat + 2) as the CAG repeat is followed by a CAACAG sequence encoding two more glutamines.
[†]Under the control of approximately 1 kb of promoter sequences.
[‡]The nomenclature refers to a huntingtin protein with 21 glutamines.
[§]The targeted gene is a hybrid in which mouse exon 1 has been replaced with mutant human exon 1.
NSE, neurone specific enolase; CMV, cytomegalovirus.

Expression of truncated constructs as transgenes

The R6 lines contain exon 1 of the human HD gene (90 amino acids with a $(CAG)_{21}$) as a genomic fragment under the control of human HD promoter sequences (Mangiarini *et al.* 1996). It is expressed ubiquitously at less than endogenous levels in five lines—three lines carrying expanded repeats, namely, R6/1 $((CAG)_{115})$, R6/2 $((CAG)_{150})$, and R6/5 $((CAG)_{128-156})$, and two lines, Hdex6 and Hdex27, with $(CAG)_{18}$ repeats in the normal human range. All three R6 lines develop the same neurological phenotype with an onset, on the basis of home cage behaviour, of 2 months in R6/2 hemizygotes, 4–5 months in R6/1 hemizygotes, and 9 months in line R6/5 (when bred to homozygosity). The mouse lines developed by Schilling *et al.* (1999a), express a slightly larger *N*-terminal fragment (171 amino acids with $(CAG)_{21}$) carrying 18 (N171–18Q), 44 (N171–44Q), or 82 (N171–82Q) glutamines. Expression was at less than endogenous levels under the control of the prion promoter, which drives expression in almost all neurones within the central nervous system (CNS) (with the exception of cerebellar Purkinje cells). Lines expressing the 171–82Q construct developed a phenotype with age of onset from 2 months. Life-span varied from 2.5 months to 5–6 months to 8–11 months, presumably dependent on the expression level of the transgene. Similarly, expression was at less than endogenous levels in the lines transgenic for the first 1 kb of the human HD gene (Laforet *et al.* 2001). The CT18 lines carrying 18 CAG repeats were indistinguishable from wild-type mice in all phenotypic tests conducted. The HD46 and HD100 lines, which carry 46 and 100 CAG repeats, respectively, were more likely to develop a neurological impairment during their lifespan. This was defined as the detection of impairment in at least one of the following: clasping; gait; activity; and rotarod performance (Laforet *et al.* 2001).

Both the R6 and Schilling lines develop a progressive neurological phenotype that includes a failure to gain weight, tremors, a lack of co-ordination, hypokinesis, abnormal gait, hind limb clasping on tail suspension, and a reduced response to stimuli. The life span is shortened and the cause of death is unclear. A small number of the R6 mice have seizures, which might be the cause of death in some cases; however, seizures were not observed in the Schilling mice. In contrast the phenotype that develops in the Laforet mice is much more benign with onset at a comparable time to that of mice expressing the full-length gene with 100 CAG repeats (Laforet *et al.* 2001). Therefore, the use of the larger 1 kb construct (which codes for approximately one-third huntingtin) does not accelerate the mouse phenotype in the same manner as the more dramatic truncations and has possibly not bypassed early steps in the pathogenic process.

Expression of full-length constructs as transgenes

The first mice to express the mutant form of the entire human huntingtin gene were generated by Dan Tagle and co-workers (Reddy *et al.* 1998). These mice are transgenic for the human HD cDNA under the control of the cytomegalovirus (CMV) promoter and express huntingtin carrying 16, 48, or 89 CAG repeats (HD16, HD48, and HD89). The lines showed different patterns of widespread expression on Western blots, the levels of which varied from being equivalent to that of the endogenous mouse huntingtin protein to fivefold overexpression. A progressive neurological phenotype was observed in mice expressing both HD48 (higher expressers) and HD89. This manifested as an initial hyperactive phase (unidirectional rotations, backflips, and excessive grooming) seen in 37 per cent of animals, progressing to hypokinetic and akinetic phases close to end-stage. A failure to gain weight was coincident with the hyperactive phase. The second approach to the generation of transgenic mice expressing the full-length protein has been to introduce a human yeast artificial chromosome (YAC) carrying 18, 46, or 72Q (Hodgson *et al.* 1999) into the mouse germline. A single YAC72 founder (2498) in which the transgene was expressed at 2–3-fold endogenous levels could not be bred and therefore a line could not be established. This mouse showed a marked behavioural phenotype by 9 months including unidirectional circling and gait ataxia, and was sacrificed at 12 months at which point there was a 50 per cent reduction in body weight. In contrast, it was possible to establish a line from a second YAC72 founder (2511) that expressed the transgene at 0.33 to 0.5 times the level of endogenous huntingtin. By 12 months of age, these mice showed no change in body weight. There was no overt neurological phenotype (one mouse showed unidirectional circling); however, the mice showed a statistically significant ($p=0.05$) mild dark-phase hyperkinesia by 7 months of age. The YAC46 lines were identical in behaviour compared with the YAC18 mice (observed up to 20 months).

The 'knock-in' approach

Gene-targeted mice have been independently generated by four research groups to replace the sequence in exon 1 of the *Hdh* gene ($(CAG)_2CAA(CAG)_4$) with a CAG repeat that is pathogenic in humans (Table 13.1). In two cases, the mouse sequence was directly replaced with an expanded CAG repeat (Lin *et al.* 2001; Shelbourne *et al.* 1999). The strategy used by the other two groups was to generate a hybrid gene in which exon 1 of the mouse gene had been replaced with exon 1 from the human HD gene carrying an expanded CAG repeat (Levine *et al.* 1999; Wheeler *et al.* 2000). Overall, these knock-in lines express mouse huntingtin carrying pathogenic polyglutamine repeats ranging from 50Q to 150Q. The only clear indication of the development of a progressive neurological phenotype has been reported recently in the 150Q line. These mice showed a progressive tendency to inactivity, hindlimb clasping on tail suspension, impairment on the rotarod test, and gait disturbance (Lin *et al.* 2001). Prior to this, the only phenotype that had been reported in knock-in mice was an increase in male aggression from 3 months of age ($p<0.05$) (Shelbourne *et al.* 1999). This has not been reported in any of the other knock-in lines (or transgenic lines) and cannot be a consistent consequence of the expression of an expanded CAG repeat in the mouse.

CAG repeat instability

In humans, the CAG expansion in the HD gene is unstable on 80 per cent of transmissions irrespective of whether it has been inherited through the male or female line (Myers *et al.* 1998). In general, in human HD when the HD gene is inherited from a female, the instability is in the form of small expansions or contractions of the order of ± three repeat units. In contrast, transmission through the male line is more likely to result in expansions, some of which can be very large (Myers *et al.* 1998; see Chapter 5, this volume). A modest degree of somatic instability has been described in human HD CNS and non-CNS tissue (Telenius *et al.* 1994). Within the brain, the largest degree of expansion was observed in caudate/putamen and the smallest repeats were in the cerebellum, whilst, outside the CNS, the most instability occurred in liver and kidney (Telenius *et al.* 1994). CAG repeat instability has been documented in two of the knock-in models (Shelbourne *et al.* 1999; Wheeler *et al.* 1999) and in the R6 lines (Bates *et al.* 1997; Mangiarini *et al.* 1997).

Gametic instability

In the mouse, as in human HD, increases in the size of the CAG repeat are generally seen when it is inherited from a male and decreases when inherited from a female (Mangiarini *et al.* 1997; Shelbourne *et al.* 1999; Wheeler *et al.* 1999). For a given repeat size, the frequency with which instability occurs is comparable for male and female transmissions (Shelbourne *et al.* 1999). However, the likelihood of instability increases with the size of the CAG expansion in the parent, increasing from approximately 4 per cent for $(CAG)_{48}$, to 50 per cent for $(CAG)_{90}$, to 73 per cent for $(CAG)_{109}$ (Wheeler *et al.* 1999). As a rule, the magnitude of the changes in repeat size are comparatively small ($\pm$ <5 CAG) irrespective of the sex of the parent. Although larger changes are occasionally seen, the large expansions that occur on male transmission in humans are not found. For line R6/2, an increase in the magnitude of the repeat change was seen to occur with the increase in the age of the transmitting founder (Mangiarini *et al.* 1997). The mechanism that underlies the propensity for repeats to expand on male transmission but decrease on female transmission is not known. However, it is unlikely to be related to position effects, as this is general feature of the behaviour of CAG/CTG repeats in mouse models of many triplet repeat diseases (Gourdon *et al.* 1997; Kaytor *et al.* 1997; Monckton *et al.* 1997). A more recent study of CAG repeat instability in line R6/1 has found that the CAG repeat size is different in male (mostly expansions) and female (mostly contractions) progeny from identical fathers (Kovtun *et al.* 2000). However, these findings are not replicated in the Bates colony at King's College London (unpublished data).

Somatic instability

Extensive, progressive somatic instability was reported in the R6 lines in both CNS and non-CNS tissues (Fig. 13.1). Within the brain, this was pronounced in most brain regions except the cerebellum in which it was relatively stable (Bates *et al.* 1997; Mangiarini *et al.* 1997). Outside of the brain, instability was most prominent in the liver, kidney, and to some extent the adrenals. This pattern of instability was supported by a limited study in the knock-in $(CAG)_{90}$ and $(CAG)_{109}$ mice in which a tendency to expansion was noted in striatum and liver (Wheeler *et al.* 1999). More recently, the application of small-pool polymerase chain reaction (PCR) (Jeffreys *et al.* 1994) to this analysis has shown that the degree of somatic instability is greater than previously appreciated from the analysis of genescan traces (Kennedy and Shelbourne 2000). A progressive and expansion-biased instability was greater in the striatum than the cortex or cerebellum of knock-in mice with $(CAG)_{72-80}$ (Fig. 13.2). In the striatum of 24-month-old mice >80 per cent cells demonstrated an increased allele length (>5 repeats) with 5 per cent having >150 repeats and ~0.5 per cent increasing to >250 repeats. These mice develop a striatal specific aggregate pathology (Li *et al.* 2000) and it is possible that the repeat expansion has a direct effect on reaching a polyQ threshold necessary for aggregate formation. Critical to this interpretation is the identification of the cell types, neurones or glia, in which the expansions are occurring.

Expression of the mismatch repair gene, msh2, is necessary for somatic instability

To investigate the mechanism underlying the somatic instability, Manley *et al.* (1999) crossed R6/1 mice to mice nullizygous for the mismatch repair gene, *msh2*. Surprisingly, they found that expansion was curtailed in all tissues studied on the *msh2*−/− background (Fig. 13.3). They found a statistically significant difference in the level of stability of the CAG repeat between both *msh2* +/− and *msh2* +/+ and the *msh2*−/− genotypes. This data shows that *msh2* is necessary for CAG repeat instability in the R6/1 mice and was an unexpected result

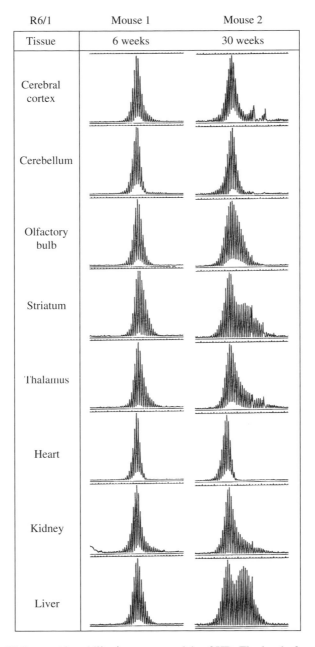

Fig. 13.1 Somatic CAG repeat instability in mouse models of HD. The level of somatic mosaicism in CAG repeat size is compared for a range of CNS and non-CNS tissue from R6/1 mice at 6 and 30 weeks of age (CAG repeat, ~115). (Reprinted from Mangiarini *et al.* (1997) with the permission of Oxford University Press.)

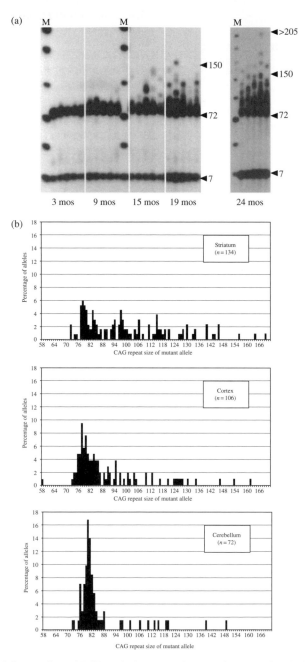

Fig. 13.2 (a) Use of the small pool PCR technique reveals a much greater level of instability than was previously appreciated. Small pool PCR on striatal DNA from knock-in mice (CAG repeat =72) at 3, 9, 15, and 19 months (~20 amplifiable mutant molecules) and 24 months of age (~50 amplifiable mutant molecules). M indicates the size markers and the numbers on the right side of each panel indicate the estimated number of triplet repeats. (b) A comparison of the CAG repeat copy number on individual mutant alleles within the striatum, cerebral cortex, and cerebellum of the 24-month-old heterozygous HD mouse shown in (a). (Reprinted from Kennedy and Shelbourne (2000) with the permission of Oxford University Press.)

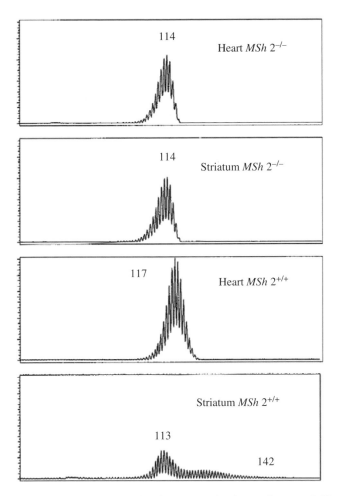

Fig. 13.3 Comparison of the CAG repeat size in heart and striatum from an R6/1 transgene (CAG repeat, ~115) on an *Msh2⁺/⁺* or *Msh2⁻/⁻* background. The *Msh2* gene product is necessary for CAG repeat instability. (Reprinted from Manley *et al.* (1999) with the permission of Oxford University Press.)

because *Msh2* loss predisposes to colon and other cancers as it enhances dinucleotide instability (de Wind *et al.* 1995). The high proportion of non-mitotic cells in the brain tissues that show the most instability suggests that repair or some other non-mitotic synthesis is most likely the mechanism of expansion in these mouse lines.

Phenotype presentation, onset, and progression

A motor disorder has been described in transgenic mice expressing the R6 (exon 1) and 171–82Q truncated huntingtin constructs (Mangiarini *et al.* 1996; Schilling *et al.* 1999a), the mice that express 1 kb of the HD gene (HD46, HD100) (Laforet *et al.* 2001), full-length cDNA (HD48, HD89) (Reddy *et al.* 1998), and YAC (YAC72) (Hodgson *et al.* 1999) constructs and the knock-in (CAG)₁₅₀ mice (Lin *et al.* 2001). Breeding to homozygosity routinely resulted in an earlier onset and more rapid progression of the phenotype. Failure to gain weight is a consistent feature and has been reported in the R6 lines (Mangiarini *et al.* 1996), the 171–82Q mice (Schilling *et al.* 1999a), the HD48 and HD89 (full-length) mice (Reddy *et al.* 1998), the YAC72 2498 mouse (Hodgson *et al.* 1999), and the $(CAG)_{150}$ knock-in mice (Lin *et al.* 2001). There are also many features of the motor disorder that are common to most, if not all, of the models. They all develop hindlimb clasping when suspended by the tail and gait impairment (Carter *et al.* 1999; Hodgson *et al.* 1999; Laforet *et al.* 2001; Lin *et al.* 2001; Mangiarini *et al.* 1996; Reddy *et al.* 1998; Schilling *et al.* 1999a). A decline in rotarod performance was noted in the R6, 171–82Q, HD100 (1 kb) mice, and knock-in $(CAG)_{150}$ lines (Carter *et al.* 1999; Laforet *et al.* 2001; Lin *et al.* 2001; Schilling *et al.* 1999a) and progression to a hypokinetic state was reported for lines R6, 171–82Q, HD46 and HD89 (full-length), and knock-in $(CAG)_{150}$ mice (Carter *et al.* 1999; Lin *et al.* 2001; Mangiarini *et al.* 1996; Schilling *et al.* 1999a). A hyperactive circling stereotypy was described for the HD46 and HD89 (full-length) lines and the YAC72 2498 and 2511 mouse lines. In both instances this was incompletely penetrant (37 per cent cDNA mice and one of the YAC72 2511 mice) and may be related to the FVB/N strain background.

The most detailed characterization of the progression of both the motor and cognitive components of the phenotype has been conducted for line R6/2. Female mice were subjected to a variety of behavioural tests designed to measure the motor aspects of swimming, fore- and hindlimb co-ordination, balance, and sensorimotor gating (Carter *et al.* 1999). R6/2 mice do not show an overt behavioural phenotype until around 8 weeks of age. However, as early as 5–6 weeks they had significant difficulty in swimming, traversing the narrowest square raised beam, and maintaining balance on the rotarod. A reduction in prepulse inhibition, also seen in HD patients, could be seen by 8–9 weeks. The R6/2 mice show progressive motor deficits, which begin subtly, and the time at which they can first be detected is dependent on the nature and difficulty of the task in question (Carter *et al.* 1999). Cognitive performance was measured on R6/2 mice and their wild-type littermates between 3 and 14.5 weeks of age using separate groups of mice for each of four tests: Morris water maze; visual cliff avoidance; two-choice swim tank; and the T-maze (Lione *et al.* 1999). They showed progressive deterioration in specific aspects of learning for all of these tasks between 3.5 and 8 weeks of age. Mice had a spatial learning deficit in the Morris water maze at 3.5 weeks (consistent with a striatal lesion) and were deficient in their ability to alternate in the T-maze between 5 and 6 weeks. The Morris water maze deficits could not result from impaired vision as R6/2 did not show a progressive avoidance of a visual cliff or altered behaviour on a plus maze (File *et al.* 1998) until after 7 weeks. In addition, in the two-choice swim task, mice could perceive a visual cue until at least 8.5 weeks. These cognitive changes were seen before subtle (5–6 weeks) and overt (8–9 weeks) motor symptoms appeared (Carter *et al.* 1999). Thus, as seen in HD patients, R6/2 mice show progressive learning impairments on cognitive tasks that are sensitive to frontostriatal and hippocampal function (Lione *et al.* 1999).

Outside of the CNS, diabetes is the only phenotype to be identified and was initially described in R6/2 mice at 12 weeks (Hurlbert *et al.* 1999). However, there are discrepancies in the percentage of R6/2 mice that develop overt diabetes. Fain *et al.* (2001) have found no evidence of diabetes in their R6/2 colony, even in those fed a high-fat and -sugar diet, whilst Hickey and Morton (2000) found a frequency of 30 per cent and Luesse *et al.* (2001) a frequency of 26 per cent. R6/2 mice may all possess a latent diabetes, which manifests as raised serum levels to varying degrees in different mouse colonies (Luesse *et al.* 2001). R6/2 mice with manifest or latent diabetes showed no differences in survival, weight loss, motor coordination, or spontaneous exploration behaviour (Luesse *et al.* 2001). A 600 per cent increase in the level of glucose in the 12-week R6/2 brain has been measured by nuclear magnetic resonance (NMR) spectroscopy (Jenkins *et al.* 2000). However, despite this, expression microarrays indicated that there were no differences in the expression levels of genes associated with glucose metabolism in either 6-week (prior to the onset of diabetes) or 12-week brains (Luthi-Carter *et al.* 2000). PolyQ aggregates are present in the R6/2 pancreatic islets by 6 weeks (Sathasivam *et al.* 1999) and immunohistochemical staining showed dramatic reductions in glucagon in the α-cells and insulin in the β-cells in the absence of cell death (Hurlbert *et al.* 1999). Whether the diabetes is caused by the presence of the nuclear aggregates is not known as aggregates form in the pancreas of R6/1 mice and yet diabetes has not been found in this line (Hansson *et al.* 1999; van Dellen *et al.* 2000a).

Aggregate pathology

PolyQ aggregate pathology has been described in HD autopsy brains in the form of nuclear inclusions, dystrophic neurites, and neuropil aggregates (Becher *et al.* 1998; DiFiglia *et al.* 1997; Gutekunst *et al.* 1999; see Chapter 8, this volume). These structures can be identified by immunohistochemistry using antibodies raised against the *N*-terminus of huntingtin or ubiquitin but cannot be seen by standard histological stains. They are most prevalent in the cerebral cortex, less frequent in the striatum, and have also been detected in the globus pallidus, substantia nigra, hippocampus, red nucleus, amygdala, hypothalamic nuclei, thalamus, brainstem nuclei, and white matter (Becher *et al.* 1998; DiFiglia *et al.* 1997; Gutekunst *et al.* 1999; Sapp *et al.* 1999; Sieradzan *et al.* 1999). In adult-onset brains, the vast majority of polyQ aggregation occurs outside the nucleus, whereas the frequency of nuclear inclusions increases in brains from juvenile-onset cases (DiFiglia *et al.* 1997; Gutekunst *et al.* 1999). Neuropil aggregates have been detected in the cerebral cortex of autopsy brains from two presymptomatic individuals indicating that they are present in the brain prior to the development of neurological symptoms (DiFiglia *et al.* 1997; Gutekunst *et al.* 1999). Several lines of evidence suggest these structures contain an *N*-terminal huntingtin fragment and that huntingtin truncation may be a requirement for the aggregation process (DiFiglia *et al.* 1997; Gutekunst *et al.* 1999; Martindale *et al.* 1998; Scherzinger *et al.* 1997).

PolyQ aggregate pathology has been described in all HD mouse models. It is most extensive in those expressing the very truncated *N*-terminal fragments of huntingtin and shows a more restricted distribution in the full-length models. Different *N*-terminal huntingtin antibodies can show varying affinities for the aggregated form of the protein and therefore some caution must be employed when comparing the aggregate pathology that has been detected with different antibodies. Fortunately, the recent widespread use of the EM48 antibody (Li and Li 1998) allows a direct comparison between the aggregate pathology in the majority of the mouse models.

Extent and distribution of the nuclear aggregates
The parameter that has the most effect on the extent and distribution of the polyQ aggregate pathology is the length of the mutant huntingtin protein that is expressed. Mice transgenic for constructs that express very truncated *N*-terminal fragments show an extremely widespread pathology, supportive of the hypothesis that the processing of huntingtin is an early event in the molecular pathogenesis of HD. The cellular and subcellular distributions of aggregates are

likely to be determined by local concentrations of the aggregate precursor, which will be influenced in part by the promoter that drives the transgene. Therefore, although nuclear aggregates are present in the vast majority of neurones in the R6/2 brain by 8 weeks, there is a prescribed sequence to their appearance (Morton *et al.* 2000; Smith *et al.* 2001). For example, they appear in the cortex and hippocampus prior to the striatum and within the hippocampus appear in the CA1 before the CA3 and dentate gyrus. This sequence is maintained even when brains are removed at postnatal day 7 (P7) and hippocampal slices are cultured for several weeks (Smith *et al.* 2001). The distribution of aggregates in the Schilling mice, whilst extensive, differs from that in the R6 lines. This is mostly because of the use of the prion rather than HD promoter (for example, aggregates do not form in Purkinje cells where there is no expression) but is possibly also because the 171–82Q protein undergoes further processing (Schilling *et al.* 1999a). PolyQ aggregation in the form of nuclear inclusions has also been detected in a number of postmitotic cells outside of the CNS of the R6 lines (Sathasivam *et al.* 1999), but has not been described for other models.

The aggregate pathology in the mice expressing the 1 kb transgene and in the full-length models is more restricted. This may reflect the cellular specificity of factors necessary for huntingtin processing, but will also be determined by the promoter under which the mutant protein is expressed. As an example, the extent of EM48 staining in the cerebral cortex, striatum, and lateral globus pallidus is compared in Fig. 13.4 where an R6/2 brain at 8 weeks and the brain from a Shelbourne knock-in mouse at 19 months of age are shown. It would be expected that the 'knock-in' models should mirror most closely the progression of the aggregate pathology as it occurs in HD patient brains, presupposing that the expression and processing of huntingtin in mouse is the same as that in man. Nuclear aggregate pathology was restricted to the striatum in the Shelbourne 'knock-in' mice carrying $(CAG)_{70-80}$ (Li *et al.* 2000) and was predominant in the striatum of the Wheeler $(CAG)_{111}$ and the Lin $(CAG)_{150}$ knock-ins, although in the $(CAG)_{111}$ lines it was also documented in the olfactory tubule and piriform cortex and in the $(CAG)_{150}$ lines in the layers III and IV of the somatosensory cortex, the piriform cortex, hippocampus, and cerebellum. Therefore, there is some discrepancy in the distribution of aggregate pathology between knock-in mice and patient brains. A striatal localization predominates in the mice, whereas in autopsy brains most aggregation appears in the cerebral cortex, and striatal aggregates are comparatively rare (DiFiglia *et al.* 1997; Gutekunst *et al.* 1999).

This was not the case in the lines expressing the 1 kb transgene (HD46 and HD100) driven under the control of the rat neurone-specific enolase (NSE) promoter (Laforet *et al.* 2001). In these, neurones with inclusions were more frequent in the cortex and striatum of HD100 mice than in the cortex and striatum of HD46 mice. Inclusions were significantly more frequent in the cortex than the striatum and were occasionally seen in a few cells in one or more of the cerebellum, hippocampus, substantia nigra, and brainstem (Laforet *et al.* 2001). The CMV-promoter-driven cDNA mice (HD48 and HD89) (Reddy *et al.* 1998) developed nuclear aggregates in the cerebral cortex, striatum, hippocampus, thalamus, and cerebellum, the number in the striatum being comparatively infrequent.

Nuclear and neuropil aggregates—structure and composition
Use of the EM48 antibody has revealed a comparable sequence in the formation of nuclear aggregates in all of the models studied. A weak nuclear staining is first detected, followed by more intense nuclear staining and the appearance of small puncta. The puncta increase in size,

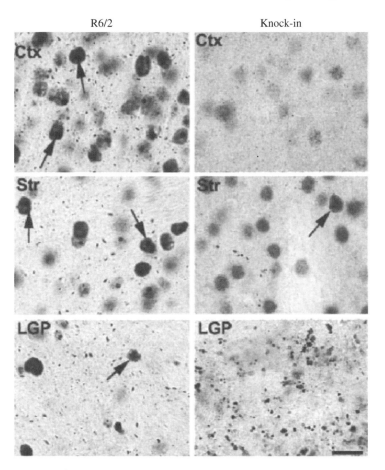

Fig. 13.4 Comparison of huntingtin aggregation in the R6/2 mice and the Selbourne knock-in mice. EM48 immunostaining of the cerebral cortex, striatum, and lateral globus pallidus (LGP) from R6/2 mice at 8 weeks of age (left) and the Shelbourne knock-in mice at 19 months of age (right). Nuclear aggregates appear as arrows and neuropil aggregates appear as punctuate staining. Scale bar, 10 μm. (Reproduced from Li *et al.* (2000) with the permission of Oxford University Press.)

frequently resolving into a single nuclear inclusion. With the formation of a single aggregate the diffuse nuclear staining clears. This chain of events has been described in detail in the R6/2 mice (Li *et al.* 1999; Morton *et al.* 2000) and three of the knock-in models (Li *et al.* 2000; Lin *et al.* 2001; Wheeler *et al.* 2000) and examples of the various types of nuclear pathology are illustrated in Fig. 13.4. A diffuse nuclear staining was also described, albeit with a different antibodies, in the full-length cDNA mice (Reddy *et al.* 1998) and the 1 kb transgenic mice (Laforet *et al.* 2001). In the 1 kb HD46 and HD100 mice, the proportion of neurones with diffuse staining was significantly greater in the striatum than in the cortex. The diffuse staining may represent an alternative conformation or early aggregated form of the *N*-terminus of huntingtin. In support of this, EM48 does not readily detect the soluble exon 1 huntingtin protein on Western blots. The appearance of the diffuse staining in the nucleus may correlate with a translocation of either full-length huntingtin or an *N*-terminal fragment of this protein to the nucleus, or the retention of an altered conformer of huntingtin within the nucleus. Immunogold labelling with EM48 has detected clusters of gold particles that have been termed microaggregates in the neuronal nuclei of the Shelbourne knock-in mice (Li *et al*. 2000) and YAC mice (Hodgson *et al*. 1999).

Nuclear inclusions were first described in the R6 lines (Davies *et al*. 1997). They are apparent at ultrastructure in the absence of immunostaining as granular and fibrillar structures that are devoid of a membrane and are slightly larger than the nucleolus (Fig. 13.5). An identical structure was present at ultrastructure in biopsy material prepared from HD striatum

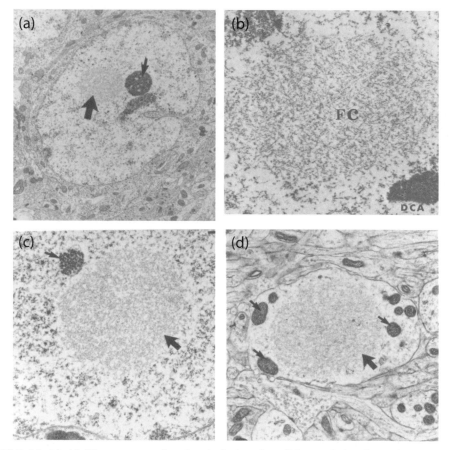

Fig. 13.5 (a), (c), (d) Ultrastructure of nuclear inclusions from R6 transgenic mice and (b) HD patient brain. (a) Neuronal intranuclear inclusion (NII; small arrow) adjacent to the nucleolus (large arrow) in the nucleus of a striatal neurone. Note the invagination of the nuclear membrane. (b) Comparison to NII in striatal biopsy material from an individual with HD. In this plate the NII was labelled as FC (filaments and fine granules). DCA, Dense chromatin aggregates. (c) Ultrastructure of NII (large arrow) adjacent to the much smaller and darkly stained coiled body (small arrow). (d) Rarely, an inclusion of a similar structure can be found in a dystrophic neurite (large arrow) surrounded by mitochondria (small arrows). (Panels (a), (c), (d) reprinted from Bates *et al*. (1998) with the permission of the Internationl Society of Neuropathology and panel (b) from Roizin *et al*. (1979) with the permission of Lippincott–Raven Publishers.)

(Roizin *et al.* 1979; see Fig. 13.5). The nuclei in which these structures form invariably have frequent and dramatic invaginations of the nuclear membrane and an apparent increase in the number and clustering of nuclear pores (Davies *et al.* 1997). Nuclear inclusions are always ubiquitinated and recruit other proteins including: components of the proteasome; the heat shock response (Jana *et al.* 2000; Levine *et al.* 1999); the transcription factors, CREB-binding protein (CBP) (Nucifora *et al.* 2001; Steffan *et al.* 2000) and Sin3b (unpublished data); and the presynaptic SNARE-complex associated protein, complexin II (Morton and Edwardson 2001).

In adult-onset HD brains, most aggregated huntingtin occurs outside of the nucleus. Extensive neuropil aggregation has been documented for the R6 lines (Li *et al.* 1999) and the 171–82Q lines (Schilling *et al.* 1999a), in which the expression of a huntingtin fragment is driven by the prion promoter. Interestingly, neuropil aggregates do not form in the brains of mice transgenic for a full-length dentatorubro-pallidoluysian atrophy (DRPLA) cDNA construct, which is also under the control of the prion promoter (Schilling *et al.* 1999b). In the R6/2 mice, neuropil aggregates were studied in the cerebral cortex and striatum where the majority are localized to axons or axon terminals of predominantly excitatory synapses (Li *et al.* 1999; see Fig. 13.6). In the Shelbourne knock-in mice, neuropil aggregates are

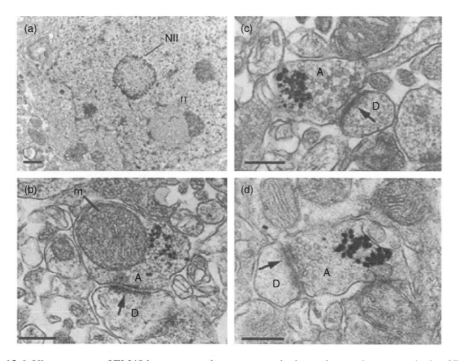

Fig. 13.6 Ultrastructure of EM48 immunoreactive aggregates in the nucleus and axon terminals of R6/2 mice at 12 weeks of age. (a) A huntingtin aggregate (NII) in the nucleus (n) of a cortical neuron is revealed by EM48 immunogold labelling. There are also many diffuse immunogold particles in the nucleus but not in the cytoplasm. (b)–(d) Three micrographs showing that immunogold particles are clustered in axon terminals (a) in (b),(c) cortex and (d) striatum. Postsynaptic densities and the dendrite (D) are indicated. A mitochondrion (m) is within the axon terminal in (b). (c) In a longitudinal axon terminal, immunogold particles are clearly associated with synaptic vesicles in the terminal. Note that axonal huntingtin aggregates are much smaller than NIIs. Scale bars: (a) 0.5 μm; ((b)–(d)) 0.25 μm. (Reprinted from Li *et al.* (1999) with the permission of Oxford University Press.)

enriched in the globus pallidus, where they are found in the inhibitory synapses (Fig. 13.7), which would be consistent with a location in the striatal projection neurones (Li *et al.* 2000). In contrast to the nuclear inclusions, neuropil aggregates cannot easily be detected by immunostaining with ubiquitin (Li *et al.* 1999, 2000) and do not have a recognizable ultra-structure (Li *et al.* 1999).

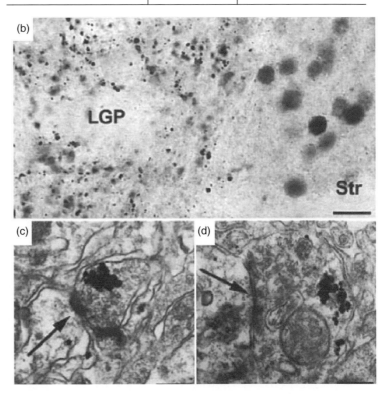

(a)   Aggregates in striata and LGP of HD-repeat mutant mice

EM48 staining	Brain region	Age (month)		
		4	11	21-27
Diffuse nuclear	Striatum	+	++	+++
nuclear aggregates	Striatum	−	++	+++
Neuropil aggregates	LGP	−	+/−	++

(b) LGP Str

(c)   (d)

Fig. 13.7 Age dependence of intranuclear and neuropil aggregates in the Shelbourne knock-in mice. (a) The progressive formation of intranuclear aggregates in the striatum and the late formation of neuropil aggregates in the lateral globus pallidus (LGP) in mice at different ages. (+), Relatively high density of aggregates; (−), negative for aggregates. (b) EM48 immunostaining showing intranuclear aggregates in the striatum (Str) and neuropil aggregates in the LGP of the knock-in mouse at 27 months of age. Electron microscopy shows EM48-immunogold particles clustered in axon terminals in (c) the striatum and (d) LGP. Arrows indicate postsynaptic density. Scale bars: (b) 10 μm; (c), (d) 0.25 μm. (Reprinted from Li *et al.* (2000) with the permission of Oxford University Press.)

Laforet *et al.* (2001) reported that huntingtin immunostaining was markedly increased in the somatodendritic cytoplasm of cortical and striatal neurones in the HD46 and HD100 mice (1 kb transgene). Cortical pyramidal neurones of the HD mice had dysmorphic dendrites that were characterized by marked retraction and disorientation of the apical dendrite and were especially prevalent in the frontal and cingulate cortices. Intracytoplasmic vacuoles and plasma membrane blebs were present in the cell bodies and dendrites of some of the HD neurones that had a cytoplasmic accumulation of huntingtin. These dysmorphic dendrites were not evident in other brain regions despite the presence of increased somatodendritic cytoplasmic labelling for huntingtin.

Huntingtin processing

The failure to detect both nuclear or neuropil aggregates with antibodies raised against regions of huntingtin other than the *N*-terminus (Becher *et al.* 1998; DiFiglia *et al.* 1997; Gutekunst *et al.* 1999) has suggested that the *N*-terminus is released by a processing event prior to aggregation. This interpretation is supported by the relative increase in the rate of aggregate formation by truncated *N*-terminal fragments (Martindale *et al.* 1998; Scherzinger *et al.* 1997). *N*- terminal fragments of approximately 40 kDa have been resolved on Western blots of the nuclear fraction of lysates from juvenile-onset autopsy brains (DiFiglia *et al.* 1997). The relationship of these fragments to the molecular pathogenesis of HD has yet to be determined. It has been expected that mice expressing full-length mutant huntingtin constructs will provide insights into huntingtin processing. An *N*-terminal huntingtin fragment has been detected as a prominent band (~43 kDa) on Western blots containing the nuclear fraction from striatal lysates of knock-in mice carrying $(CAG)_{70-80}$ repeats (Li *et al.* 2000) (Fig. 13.8). This band was not seen in the cytoplasmic fraction or in wild-type mouse brain. Evidence of proteolysis was also seen in mice that expressed a truncated huntingtin fragment, 171–82Q, –44Q, and –18Q, irrespective of whether the CAG repeat was in the mutant or normal range (Schilling *et al.* 1999a) (Fig. 13.8). In each case, the *N*-terminal processed fragment was detected on Western blots and was approximately 10 kDa smaller than the 171 amino acid transgene. The processed fragments identified in lysates from the knock-in mice and from the 82Q transgene were both remarkably similar in size to those detected in the lysates from the juvenile-onset patient brains (DiFiglia *et al.* 1997).

The R6 lines indicate that production of an *N*-terminal fragment cannot alone be toxic (as these mice only express an *N*-terminal fragment and still develop a late-onset disease) and therefore a second event must occur. It is possible that a truncation event is necessary to allow translocation to the nucleus. Wheeler *et al.* (2000), however, have presented evidence to indicate that the full-length protein can cross the nuclear membrane. It is most likely that a truncation is necessary to initiate the aggregation pathway (Martindale *et al.* 1998; Scherzinger *et al.* 1997), although, once it has started, it is likely that huntingtin proteins of a range of sizes containing both normal and expanded repeats can be recruited into the aggregates (see Chapter 14).

Neuronal degeneration

Selective neuronal loss in HD (see Chapter 8) is most prominent in the striatum (Vonsattel *et al.* 1985). It is also frequently reported in the cerebral cortex, affecting all but the medial temporal lobe (Halliday *et al.* 1998; Macdonald *et al.* 1997) with a rate that correlates with CAG repeat number. Atrophy has also been variably reported in other brain regions including

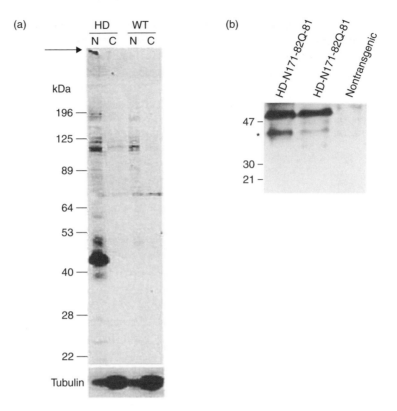

Fig. 13.8 Evidence for huntingtin processing. (a) Western blot showing that an EM48-immunoreactive band (43 kDa) is specific in the nuclear fraction of the striatum from a knock-in mouse (Shelbourne) at 18 months of age. The arrow indicates huntingtin aggregates in the stacking gel. The antibody was subsequently probed with an antibody specific to tubulin (bottom). N, Nuclear fraction; C, cytosolic fraction; WT, wild-type mouse; HD, knock-in mouse. (Reprinted from Li *et al.* (2000) with the permission of Oxford University Press.) (b) Detection of the N171–82Q cleavage product with the antibody 1C2 that preferentially detects expanded polyQ tracts on Western blots. Immunoblots of whole-brain homogenates from two N171–82Q mice and one non-transgenic animal were probed with the 1C2 antibody. The signal of the N171–82Q product can be detected in both animals. In addition, a cleavage product, ~10 kDa smaller, was readily visible in both brains (marked with an asterisk). The 1C2 antibody does not detect a signal in the homogenate of the non-transgenic mouse. This confirms that the N171–82Q fragment is *C*-terminally truncated and that the cleavage product includes the polyglutamine stretch. (Reprinted from Schilling *et al.* (1999) with the permission of Oxford University Press.)

the thalamus (Halliday *et al.* 1998), hippocampus (Spargo *et al.* 1993), and frontal white matter (Halliday *et al.* 1998; Macdonald *et al.* 1997). The early-onset forms of the polyglutamine disorders have a more widespread and less distinct pathology and, in juvenile HD, the cerebellar Purkinje cells frequently degenerate (Young 1998).

Neurodegeneration has been documented in the R6 lines (Turmaine *et al.* 2000), the 1 kb transgenic lines (Laforet *et al.* 2001), the full-length cDNA transgenics (Reddy *et al.* 1998), and the YAC transgenic mice (Hodgson *et al.* 1999). It is not apparent until close to end-stage disease in both the R6 and the Reddy mice indicating that, in these lines, the behavioural phenotype is not caused by the death of neurones but rather by a neuronal dysfunction.

Neurodegeneration has been described in the R6 lines with the appearance of dark degenerating neurones at ultrastructure (Davies *et al.* 1997; Iannicola *et al.* 2000; Turmaine *et al.* 2000). In line R6/2, there is no evidence of cell death within the CNS until 14 weeks of age. This is supported by an absence of marked astrogliosis (Mangiarini *et al.* 1996) and by the absence of neuronal loss as determined from the comparison of striatal neuronal counts between R6/2 and wild-type mice at 6 and 12 weeks of age (Jenkins *et al.* 2000). At 14 weeks an extremely selective neurodegeneration, restricted to the anterior cingulate cortex, dorsal striatum, and the Purkinje cells of the cerebellar vermis, becomes apparent and increases in frequency up to 17 weeks of age (Turmaine *et al.* 2000). Similar dark degenerating cells are also present in post-mortem HD brains (Turmaine *et al.* 2000; Vonsattel and DiFiglia 1998). Figure 13.9 shows a comparison of degenerating cells in the anterior cingulate cortex of a juvenile HD autopsy brain with those in the R6/2 mouse. The dark degenerating neurones do not appear to be dying by apoptosis in that they show no TUNEL staining and there is no fragmentation or blebbing of either the nucleus or cytoplasm. The same ultrastructural features have been described for degenerating photoreceptor neurones in a *Drosophila* model of HD expressing an *N*-terminal fragment of huntingtin with 120Q (Jackson *et al.* 1998; see also Chapter 14, this volume).

In the Reddy mice (HD48 and HD89), neuronal loss and accompanying astrogliosis were detected in the cerebral cortex, striatum, hippocampus, and thalamus and were most evident in the mice that had entered the hypokinetic and akinetic end stage of the disease. Degenerating neurones appeared as scattered dark shrunken cells with pyknotic or small densely staining nuclei and an eosinophilic cytoplasm. In this case, neurones were positive for TUNEL

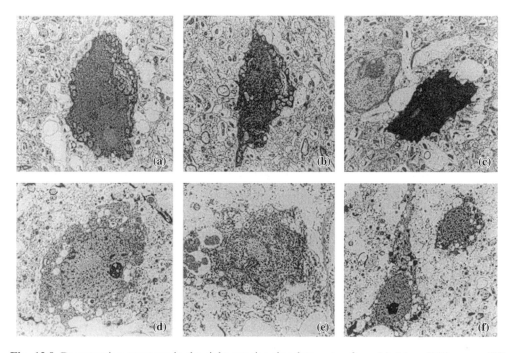

Fig. 13.9 Degenerating neurones in the right anterior cingulate cortex from (a)–(c) an R6/2 mouse (17 weeks, ~150 CAG repeats) and (d)–(f) HD patient (an 11 years old, 100 CAG repeats). Nuclear aggregates are present within all of these neurones. (Magnifications: (a)–(c) 1250×; (d)–(e) 2250×; (f) 1000×. (Reprinted with permission from Turmaine *et al.* (2000) ©National Academy of Sciences, USA.)

labelling suggesting that these cells might be dying via an apoptotic process (Reddy *et al.* 1998). However, the ultrastructure of these neurones was not shown.

Neurodegeneration that occurred in the absence of reactive astrogliosis has also been reported in the YAC mice (Hodgson *et al.* 1999). In this case it was assessed in toluidine blue semi-thin sections from striatum cerebral cortex, hippocampus, and cerebellum. Degenerating neurones were present in the YAC72 2498 mouse and in the YAC72 2511 line and then only in the striatum (Fig. 13.10). In mouse 2498 striatum (at 1 year), there was a degeneration gradient

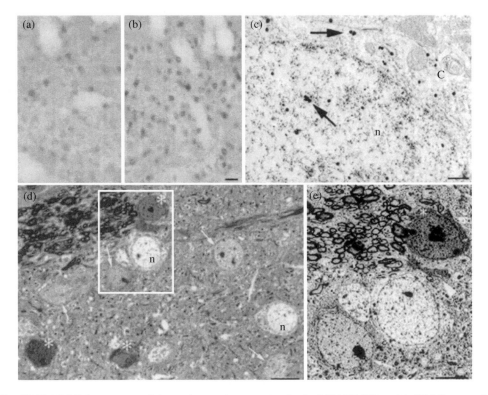

Fig. 13.10 EM48 immunoreactivity and neurodegeneration in the 2511 YAC line. (a), (b) Micrographs of representative striatal sections from (a) a 1-year-old wild-type control and (b) an age-matched YAC72 mouse from line 2511 stained with EM48. As compared with the wild-type control, many more neuronal nuclei were EM48-positive in the striatum of the YAC72 2511 line. (c) An electron micrograph showing a striatal neurone containing many EM48 immunogold particles in the nucleas (n), and to a lesser extent, in the cytoplasm (C). Particles were found singly or in clusters of no more than three particles (arrows). (d) A light micrograph of a representative toluidine blud-stained 1.5 μm semithin section from the lateral portion of the striatum of a YAC 2511 mouse. Many shrunken and hyperchromatic degenerating neurones are present (asterisks). In addition, neurones with abnormal morphological changes, including hyperchromasia, can also be seen (arrows) adjacent to normal neurones (n). (e) An electron micrograph showing the morphological features of the normal and the abnormal (arrow), and the neurodegenerated (asterisk) neurones shown in (d) (inset). A degenerating dendrite can also be seen in the neuropil (arrow). Scale bar: (a), (b) 60 μm; (c) 350 nm; (d) 20 μm; and (e) 10 μm. (Reprinted from Hodgson *et al.* (1999) © (1999) with permission from Elsevier Science.)

of 4 per cent of cells medially to 80 per cent laterally. In line 2511 the degeneration could be detected at 12 months when there was a striatal gradient of 4 per cent of cells medially to 40 per cent laterally but this was absent at 8 months. The degenerative features of these cells at ultrastructure were similar to those described for the R6 lines. The neurodegeneration described in the YAC72 2511 line occurs at a time when an overt behavioural phenotype has yet to develop and is not therefore an end-stage phenomenon as found in the R6 lines and Reddy mice. However, using the same criteria, toluidine blue-stained semithin sections from R6/2 brain sections taken at 6.5 weeks show evidence of pronounced neurodegeneration (Gutekunst *et al.* 2000). As complementary data would indicate that cell death has not occurred at this time point (Jenkins *et al.* 2000; Turmaine *et al.* 2000), it is currently unclear what this increased affinity to toluidine blue represents.

Huntingtin immunoreactive neurones appeared smaller or reduced in number in the striatum and in layer 6 of the cortex in the majority of HD mice expressing the 1 kb construct (Laforet *et al.* 2001). Cell counts of striatal neurones in cresyl violet sections of HD46 and HD100 mice showed the density of neurones to be significantly lower than in controls and therefore neuronal cell loss has occurred in this model.

Neuronal shrinkage and dysmorphic neurites are also recognized neuropathological features of HD patient brains (Vonsattel and DiFiglia 1998). A decrease in cross-sectional somatic area in striatal and cortical neurones from both the HD100 mice (Laforet *et al.* 2001) and from symptomatic R6/2 mice (Klapstein *et al.* 2001; Levine *et al.* 1999) have been reported. Biocytin injection and Golgi impregnation have identified dystrophic neurites in the R6/2 mice, the full-length cDNA mice, and those carrying the 1 kb transgene. Cortical and hippocampal pyramidal neurones and medium-sized spiny neurones from the striatum of symptomatic R6/2 mice have thinner dendrites and reduced dendritic spines compared to those from age-matched controls (Klapstein *et al.* 2001). These morphological changes most probably account for the decrease in weight that occurs in R6 mouse brains (Davies *et al.* 1997). Golgi staining of cortical and striatal neurones in the brains from full-length cDNA mice uncovered morphological abnormalities that included a significant decrease in the number of dendritic spines and a thickening of the proximal dendrites (Guidetti *et al.* 2001). In contrast, biocytin injection of medium-sized striatal neurones from HD100 mice (1 kb transgene) had spine densities relatively similar to those of wild-type mice. However, the HD100 mice had significantly more dendrites with endings that curved back towards the soma (J-dendrites) and/or had sharp bends (wavy dendrites) (Laforet *et al.* 2001). Cortical neurones from HD100 mice also displayed dendritic abnormalities including beading, small sharp bends, and misaligned and markedly bifurcated apical dendrites that were consistent with the changes seen with huntingtin labelling (Laforet *et al.* 2001).

Neuropathological changes and behavioural phenotypes

An overt behavioural phenotype has been described in only a few lines in which there is also sufficient data to allow the comparison of the appearance of aggregate pathology with the onset of the phenotype. This includes the R6 lines (Carter *et al.* 1999; Davies *et al.* 1997; Li *et al.* 1999; Lione *et al.* 1999; Morton *et al.* 2000), the 1 kb cDNA lines (Laforet *et al.* 2001), the full-length cDNA lines (Reddy *et al.* 1998), and the knock-in line with $(CAG)_{150}$ (Lin *et al.* 2001). In these models, polyQ aggregation is present in neurones prior to the onset of the phenotype. Despite an aggregate pathology, the onset of a progressive behavioural phenotype has not occurred within the time-scale of the analysis of the knock-in lines carrying CAG tracts of up to 111 repeats (Levine *et al.* 1999; Shelbourne *et al.* 1999; Wheeler *et al.* 2000).

Only the study by Laforet *et al.* (2001) has attempted to dissect out the relationship between the presence of the various neuropathological changes in the cortex and striatum with the behavioural phenotype that occurs in their mice. They found that the dysmorphic dendritic score and the prevalence of diffuse nuclear labelling in the cortex correlated with a poor rotarod score and with a relatively higher number of neurological defects. In contrast, diffuse nuclear labelling in striatal neurones did not predict neurological impairments. The frequency of nuclear inclusions was not associated with worse rotarod scores in either brain region but in cortex was correlated with a better rotarod performance. Neuronal loss in the striatum bore no relationship to lower rotarod scores (Laforet *et al.* 2001). Therefore, in this model, the extent of dendritic abnormalities revealed by extensive cytoplasmic labelling and diffuse nuclear localization of huntingtin in cortical neurones was most predictive of the degree of neurological impairment. In contrast, they found that the presence of huntingtin-positive nuclear inclusions or loss of neurones had no predictive value.

Electrophysiology

Changes in hippocampal electrophysiological properties have been reported for R6/2 (Murphy *et al.* 2000), YAC (Hodgson *et al.* 1999), and the Shelbourne knock-in mice (Usdin *et al.* 1999) as summarized in Table 13.2. In the hippocampus, basal neurotransmission at CA1 and granule cell synapses is normal. However, analysis of presynaptic function, postsynaptic responsiveness, and synaptic plasticity has revealed marked differences. Striatal electrophysiological changes have also been documented for R6/2 mice (Klapstein *et al.* 2001; Levine *et al.* 1999), Levine knock-ins (Levine *et al.* 1999), and 1 kb HD100 mice (Laforet *et al.* 2001) as summarized in Table 13.3.

Table 13.2 Synaptic transmission and plasticity at hippocampal synapses

	Membrane properties	Synaptic transmission	Input/ output	PPF	PTP	LTP	LTD	NMDA receptor	Age-dependent
R6/2 (Murphy *et al.* 2000)	Normal	Normal	Normal	Normal	Reduced*	Reduced[†]	Enhanced	Normal	Yes
Shelbourne knock-in (Usdin *et al.* 1999)	—	Normal	Normal	Reduced	Reduced	Reduced[†]	—	Normal	—
YAC46 (Hodgson *et al.* 1999)	—	Normal	—	Normal	Reduced	Reduced[‡]	?[§]	?[¶]	Yes

PPF, paired-pulse facilitation; PTP, Post-tetanic potentiation.
*But normal when NMDA receptors are pharmacologically blocked.
[†]Can be rescued by increasing the conditioning intensity.
[‡]LTP enhanced in YAC72 at 6 months, reduced at 10 months (all experiments done in zero magnesium).
[§]Not assessed, but YAC72 exhibited slow-onset depression after high-frequency stimulation.
[¶]Difficult to assess as experiments performed in magnesium-free ACSF. NMDA receptor-mediated potentials are augmented in the YAC72 line.

Table 13.3 Corticostriatal transmission and cellular properties of medium-sized spiny striatal neurones

	Resting membrane potential	Input resistence	Membrane time constant	Action potential	EPSP	Input/output/	PPF	NMDA receptor	Age-dependent
R6/2 (Klapstein 2001) *et al.*	Depolarized	Increased	Decreased	Altered	Smaller	Shifted right	Reduced	Increased current	Yes
Levine knock-in (Levine *et al.* 1999)	Depolarized*	Normal	—	Normal	—	—	—	Increased current	—
1 kb HD100 (Laforet *et al.* 2001)	Normal	Reduced	—	Normal	Smaller	Shifted right	—	Increased current	Yes

EPSP, Excitatory postsynaptic potential; PPF, Paired-pulse facilitation.
*Subpopulation only.

Presynaptic function

The discovery that polyQ aggregates are present in neuropil and presynaptic terminals of human and transgenic mouse brain (Gutekunst *et al.* 1999; Li *et al.* 1999; Sapp *et al.* 1999) fuelled the suggestion that abnormal transmitter release might be implicated in the disease process underlying HD. This view was strengthened by functional studies of synaptic transmission in the emerging mouse models. In all mice studied thus far, low-frequency transmission at hippocampal synapses appears to be normal. Measures of the efficiency of transmitter release, such as paired-pulse facilitation (PPF), are also largely unaffected in that they are normal in the R6/2 and YAC lines, although reduced in the Shelbourne knock-in mouse. In contrast, post-tetanic potentiation (PTP), a measure of presynaptic function during intense synaptic activity, is reduced in all three of these mouse models. These data suggest an impairment in transmitter release, but one that is only apparent during periods of intense synaptic activity. Further evidence supporting this view comes from the comparison of MK-801 use-dependent blockade at *N*-methyl-D-aspartate (NMDA) receptors in the knock-in mouse (Usdin *et al.* 1999). At low rates of afferent stimulation, the rate of block is similar for both wild-type and mutant synapses. At higher stimulation frequencies, the rate of NMDA receptor blockade at mutant synapses is slower, suggesting a rate-dependent decrease in the release of neurotransmitter.

Morton and Edwardson (2001) have recently reported that the presynaptic SNARE-complex-associated protein, complexin II, is progressively lost in R6/2 mice. Normal neurones lacking complexins show a dramatic reduction in the efficiency of transmitter release (Reim *et al.* 2001). The electrophysiological synaptic properties of R6/2 and complexin II knock-out mice are similar (Murphy *et al.* 2000; Takahashi *et al.* 1999), suggesting that depletion of complexin contributes to the altered synaptic function observed in R6/2 mice.

Postsynaptic function

HD is associated with changes in the distribution of postsynaptic receptors. Similar changes have been reported in the striatum and cortex of the R6/2 mouse (Cha *et al.* 1998, 1999).

Furthermore, injection of full-length mutant huntingtin into cells expressing NMDA receptors shows a selective enhancement of receptors containing the NMDA receptor 2B (NR2B) subunit (Chen *et al.* 1999). Analysis of postsynaptic sensitivity has revealed considerable differences between the mouse models. Input/output analysis of synaptic transmission at CA1 synapses is normal in the R6/2 mouse and the Shelbourne knock-in line. NMDA receptors are augmented in the YAC72 mouse but appear to be unaffected in both the R6/2 and Shelbourne knock-in models. Interestingly, R6/2 striatal medium-sized spiny neurones appear to be more sensitive to the excitotoxic effects of NMDA (Levine *et al.* 1999), presumably because, unlike the hippocampal neurones, which express both NR2A and NR2B subunits, striatal cells only express the NR2B form. A similar sensitivity to NMDA within the striatum has also been reported for the Levine knock-in mice (Levine *et al.* 1999) and the 1 kb HD100 mice (Laforet *et al.* 2001).

Another hippocampal postsynaptic function altered in mutant mice is a weakening of the coupling between synaptic current and the initiation of the action potential in the R6/2 line (Murphy *et al.* 2000). A reduction in the ability of synaptic current to generate an action potential will have a profound effect on information flow within a polysynaptic neural circuit. Indeed, a reduction in neural efficiency could account, in part, for the early neurological and motor phenotype seen in the R6/2 line. In addition, deficits in neural processing have been reported in the corticostriatal pathway in both R6/2 mice (Klapstein *et al.* 2001) and 1 kb HD100 mice (Laforet *et al.* 2001). Both lines display a marked decrease in the ability of cortical afferents to elicit excitatory postsynaptic potentials in medium-sized spiny striatal neurones.

Synaptic plasticity

It is widely believed that changes in synaptic strength underlie the cellular mechanisms of learning and memory (Bliss and Collingridge 1993). Abnormalities in synaptic plasticity might contribute to the early cognitive deficit reported in some presymptomatic HD patients. The development of progressive mouse models of HD has, for the first time, made it possible to study learning-related forms of synaptic plasticity, such as long-term potentiation (LTP) and long-term depression (LTD), in a time- and phenotype-dependent manner. The most conspicuous finding is that the R6/2, Shelbourne knock-in, and YAC lines all show an impairment of LTP at hippocampal synapses. Furthermore, the impairment in LTP precedes the development of an overt phenotype, suggesting that altered synaptic plasticity might indeed contribute to the early cognitive deficit seen in HD. A study of hippocampal synaptic plasticity and spatial cognition in R6/2 mice (Table 13.2) showed marked alterations in synaptic plasticity at both CA1 and granule cell synapses, and impaired spatial cognitive performance in the Morris water maze (Murphy *et al.* 2000). CA1 synapses showed a marked reduction in LTP that was fully apparent from 5 weeks of age. Unexpectedly, these synapses also exhibited a pronounced form of NMDA-receptor-dependent LTD that was also present at 5 weeks, but absent in age-matched control synapses. This form of LTD is believed to be important during brain development and declines as dendrites mature. Its presence in adult R6/2 mice suggests that the process of synaptic maturation is altered in R6/2 hippocampus.

In contrast to CA1 synapses, impairment of LTP at granule cell synapses is not fully evident until 10–12 weeks of age. The temporal difference between these populations of synapses was also mirrored by the appearance of intranuclear inclusions in CA1 neurones and granule cells (Murphy *et al.* 2000), suggesting that impaired synaptic function is associated with the nuclear aggregation of mutant protein.

LTP and hippocampal synaptic function has also been studied in the reversible HD mouse model (see the eponymous section for full details on this line). These mice display an electrophysiological and synaptic phenotype that is very similar to that seen in the R6/2 line. They also show a deficit in working memory similar to the cognitive impairment seen in the R6/2 mouse. Remarkably, both synaptic and cognitive function recover on inactivation of the HD transgene (Ottavio Arancio, personal communication), suggesting that certain aspects of HD pathogenesis can be reversed (see the section 'The reversible HD mouse' for a fuller discussion).

The corticostriatal synapses also support synaptic plasticity, a mechanism that modulates the weighting of glutamatergic cortical input to the basal ganglia and is believed to be important in motor learning and for certain forms of cognition. Changes in the electrophysiological properties of striatal neurones in R6/2 mice (Klapstein *et al.* 2001; Levine *et al.* 1999) and 1 kb HD100 mice (Laforet *et al.* 2001) are associated with an apparent reduction in the efficacy of transmission at corticostriatal synapses, a deficit that is also correlated with the development of abnormal dendritic morphology (Klapstein *et al.* 2001; Laforet *et al.* 2001) and changes in receptor expression (Cha *et al.* 1998, 1999). Whilst a study of LTP and LTD at corticostriatal synapses has yet to be published, preliminary data suggest that, in contrast to the hippocampal findings, the incidence of LTP is enhanced in R6/2 mice, possibly due to the augmentation of striatal NMDA receptor function (Murphy, unpublished data).

Changes in gene expression occurring as a consequence of the HD mutation

Overwhelming evidence indicates that the behavioural phenotype seen in mouse models of HD is caused by neuronal dysfunction and is present prior to any evidence of neuronal cell death (with the possible exception of the YAC mice (Hodgson *et al.* 1999)). Insights into the possible molecular basis of this have arisen from gene expression studies (see also Chapters 9, 12, and 14, this volume). A decrease in the expression (mRNA and protein) of selective neurotransmitter receptors was found to occur in the R6/2, R6/1, and R6/5 lines but not the HDex lines carrying a normal $(CAG)_{18}$ repeat (Cha *et al.* 1998, 1999). These changes primarily involved the G-protein coupled receptors, including mGluR1, mGluR3, dopamine D1 and D2, adenosine A2a (Cha *et al.* 1998, 1999), and the cannabinoid CB1 (Denovan-Wright and Robertson 2000). Significant decreases in expression could be detected early, in some cases prior to 4 weeks of age for line R6/2 (Cha *et al.* 1998, 1999). Perturbations in these neurotransmitter receptor levels, which are important for striatal function, might be predicted to be responsible for some of the motor abnormalities that develop. Similarly, such changes could also account for the reduction in the ability of hippocampal synapses to support LTP (Murphy *et al.* 2000). A decrease in the mRNA levels of CB1, A2a, and the dopamine receptors D1 and D2 has also been reported in early-grade HD autopsy brains (Glass *et al.* 2000). In both the mouse and human brains, these changes cannot be attributed to the degeneration of a specific subpopulation of cells but rather to the downregulation of a specific set of genes (Cha *et al.* 1998; Denovan-Wright and Robertson 2000). The fact that these changes may also occur early in HD patients is consistent with positron emission tomography (PET) studies that show a decrease in D1 and D2 dopamine receptor binding in 'HD mutation-positive' presymptomatic individuals (Weeks *et al.* 1996). The mRNA level of the neuropeptide met-enkephalin is also reduced in both the R6 and Levine knock-in mice and HD autopsy brains (Augood *et al.* 1996; Menalled *et al.* 2000).

The consequences of the HD mutation on striatal gene expression levels were extended by a more global approach using gene expression microarrays (Luthi-Carter *et al.* 2000). The levels of striatal mRNA species in R6/2 mice were compared with those of littermate controls at 6 and 12 weeks of age. RNA samples were analysed using Affymetrix murine expression arrays, which assessed close to 6000 known genes. The expression level of 1.2 or 1.7 per cent of these genes was changed in the R6/2 striata at 12 weeks and 6 weeks, respectively; 75 per cent of the expression changes were decreases. A subset of these changes were also found in the 171–82Q mice indicating that the gene expression changes might be characteristic of HD pathogenesis (Luthi-Carter *et al.* 2000). Messenger RNAs encoding mitochondrial proteins, caspases, and other apoptosis-related molecules were relatively unaffected, consistent with the absence of TUNEL staining and ultrastructural morphology (Menalled *et al.* 2000; Turmaine *et al.* 2000). Increases were largely restricted to mRNAs associated with inflammatory or cell cycle function, whereas decreases were observed primarily in signal transduction pathways, ion channels, transcription, metabolism, and cell structure. The previously reported decrease in the expression of G-protein-coupled neurotransmitter receptors was confirmed. However, the microarray analysis showed that not only were the receptors downregulated but also that the mRNAs of many components of their signalling pathways were decreased, which has been confirmed by independent studies (Bibb *et al.* 2000; van Dellen *et al.* 2000b), as were their target genes. Therefore, the mice are impaired in the transduction of neurone-specific signals. The abnormal expression of multiple genes involved in calcium signalling suggests a disruption in calcium homeostasis. This study also produced the first evidence to suggest that impaired retinoid signalling might contribute to HD pathophysiology. Not only is the retinoic acid receptor (RXRγ) downregulated, but retinoic acid signalling regulates at least 22/104 genes that showed decreased expression in R6/2 mice. This may have arisen due to the diminished activity of the dopamine-signalling pathway in the R6/2 striata or through the interaction with nuclear receptor co-repressor (N-CoR), which binds both mutant huntingtin and the retinoic acid receptor (Boutell *et al.* 1999; Horlein *et al.* 1995). In general, whether these changes arise as a result of direct interactions with the transcriptional machinery, through the recruitment of transcription factors into aggregates (Nucifora *et al.* 2001; Steffan *et al.* 2000), or through adaptive neuronal responses is yet to be determined (Cha 2000; see also Chapters 9, 12, and 14).

Excitotoxicity and oxidative damage

Studies measuring the concentrations of brain metabolites that looked for evidence of oxidative damage or examined the susceptibility of HD mouse models to excitotoxic and mitochondrial toxins have been almost exclusively conducted in the R6 models.

R6/1 mice were shown to be totally resistant to striatal lesions caused by the NMDA receptor agonist quinolinic acid (QA) at 18 weeks of age (Hansson *et al.* 1999). This neuroprotection developed gradually over time in both the R6/1 and the R6/2 mice and occurred earlier in the R6/2 than in the R6/1 line (Hansson *et al.* 2001b). The development of the resistance coincided with the appearance of nuclear inclusions and with the onset of motor deficits. The hippocampal neurones were also found to be resistant to QA, especially in the CA1 regions. There was no change in the susceptibility to QA in the HDex lines carrying a normal CAG repeat. R6/1 mice were also found to be resistant to NMDA but not to α-amino-3-hydroxy-5-methyl-4-isoxazolepropionic acid (AMPA)-induced striatal damage (Hansson *et al.* 2001b). The same authors showed that there was no decrease in the QA-induced current and calcium influx in the striatal R6/2 neurones. However, in R6/2 they found that the neurones had a better capacity to handle cytoplasmic calcium overload following QA administration and could avoid calcium deregulation and cell lysis (Hansson *et al.* 2001b). In addition, basal calcium levels were increased fivefold in striatal R6/2 neurones. This might result in an upregulation of protective mechanisms, including an increased capacity to handle calcium overload. In addition, the increased level of basal calcium in the R6 mice might perturb intracellular signalling in striatal neurones and thereby cause neuronal dysfunction and behavioural deficits (Hansson *et al.* 2001b).

What evidence is there that the striatal neurones might be adapting to an excitotoxic insult? High-performance liquid chromatography (HPLC) analysis of frozen brain tissue (Reynolds *et al.* 1999) and magnetic resonance spectroscopy (MRS) (Jenkins *et al.* 2000) did not find any difference in the levels of glutamate between the R6/2 mice and their non-transgenic littermate controls. In contrast, *in vivo* microdialysis following depolarization with KCl produced an enhanced local glutamate release in the R6/1 mice above that observed in controls (Nicniocaill *et al.* 2001). This is suggestive of an impairment in glutamate clearance, and is consistent with the downregulation of the expression of the major astroglial transporter (GLT1) and the decreased glutamate and aspartate uptake that has been demonstrated in the R6/2 and R6/1 lines (Lievens *et al.* 2001). Therefore, it is possible that local, transient increases in glutamate concentration take place within the R6/2 striatum.

Alternatively, the increased resistance could be explained by the loss of dendritic spines and decrease in excitatory input to the cortex (Klapstein *et al.* 2001). There is evidence that the generation of excitotoxicity *in vivo* requires an intact glutamatergic input to the target structure that is the subject of the excitatory challenge. Therefore, if the corticostriatal pathway is partially disconnected, striatal neurones might display protection from excitotoxicity (Klapstein *et al.* 2001). However, measurement of glutamate release from synaptosomes found no difference between those prepared from R6/1 brains and those of wild-type littermates at 18 weeks under basal or evoked conditions (Hansson *et al.* 2001a).

In addition to quinolinate and NMDA, R6/2 mice have also been shown to be comparatively resistant to the excitotoxin kainate at 3–9 weeks (Morton and Leavens 2000) and to the mitochondrial toxin 3-nitropropionic acid (3-NP) at 7–10 weeks (Hickey and Morton 2000). However, increased sensitivity to 3-NP was found in R6/2 mice at 12 weeks (Bogdanov *et al.* 1998), possibly suggesting a breakdown in the mechanism that affords resistance to the inhibition of mitochondrial function. Hansson *et al.* (2001a) looked more closely at the susceptibility of striatal neurones to this class of toxin. They found a partial resistance to malonate infusion at 6 and 12 weeks in R6/2 mice and at 18 weeks but not at 6 weeks in R6/1 mice. Therefore, a partial resistance to malonate-induced striatal cell death (Hansson *et al.* 2001a) follows the same pattern as resistance to QA (Hansson *et al.* 1999, 2001b) in that an early susceptibility precedes the development of resistance. More recently, R6/1 and R6/2 mice have been shown to develop a partial resistance to dopamine and to 6-hydroxydopamine-mediated toxicity (Petersen *et al.* 2001).

There is substantial evidence to indicate that mitochondrial impairment forms a component of HD pathogenesis. Consistent with this, *N*-acetyl aspartate (NAA) is decreased in HD patient brains (Jenkins *et al.* 1993). MRS has shown a nonlinear decrease in NAA levels in R6/2 striatum with respect to wild-type controls from 6 weeks of age (Jenkins *et al.* 2000). However, a decrease in mitochondrial complex IV activity was only detectable at 12 weeks of age in the cortex and striatum of the R6/2 mice, and the activities of complexes II/III were unchanged (Tabrizi *et al.* 2000). Similarly, measurement of the mitochondrial electron transport complexes I–IV did not reveal changes in the striatum or cortex of mice transgenic for the full-length mutant protein (Guidetti *et al.* 2001). Pathological grade I cases also showed no change in the activity of mitochondrial complexes I–IV and, therefore, a decrease in mitochondrial function is likely to be a consequence rather than a cause of early neuropathological changes (Guidetti *et al.* 2001).

Analysis of markers of oxidative stress in the R6 lines indicates that neuronal damage occurs disproportionately in the striatum despite the widespread distribution of polyQ aggregation. A significant reduction in striatal but not cortical aconitase has been detected in R6/2 brains at 12 weeks (Tabrizi *et al.* 2000). This is accompanied by an increase in immunostaining for inducible nitric oxide synthase (iNOS) and nitrotyrosine. The decrease in aconitase activity and increased nitrotyrosine residues may be caused by the excitotoxic activation of free radicals (Tabrizi *et al.* 2000). Similarly, striatal-specific lipid peroxidation has been documented in R6/1 mice at 24 weeks of age (Perez-Severiano *et al.* 2000). Two of the metabolites of the kynurenine pathway of tryptophan degradation, the free radical generator 3-hydroxykynurenine (3HK) and the neuroprotectant kynurenate (KYNA), were both found to be increased in grade 1 HD brains and in brains from mice transgenic for full-length mutant huntingtin (Guidetti *et al.* 2000). In both cases, the elevation of 3HK was more pronounced, resulting in significant increases in the 3HK/KYNA ratios, which may result in an increase in oxidative damage (Guidetti *et al.* 2000).

The reversible HD mouse

An HD mouse model expressing exon 1 huntingtin under the control of an inducible promoter has shown that the behavioural phenotype can be reversed (Yamamoto *et al.* 2000). A bidirectional tetO operator/CMV promoter (Gossen and Bujard 1992) was used to express an exon 1 HD construct with $(CAG)_{94}$ in one direction (HD94) and a β-galactosidase reporter gene in the other, thereby allowing direct visualization of the cells in which the promoter was active. The HD94 mice were crossed to mice expressing the tetracycline-regulated transactivator (tTA) under the control of the CamKII α-promoter, which is necessary for transcription from tetO/CMV and restricts expression to the forebrain. The double transgenic mice developed a progressive movement disorder with onset at 4 weeks as measured by the appearance of a progressive dystonic clasping posture induced upon tail suspension; at 20 weeks they had developed a mild tremor and by 36 weeks were clearly hypoactive. Neuropathological examination revealed that the HD94 brains were smaller and that striatal size had decreased with the accompanying enlargement of the lateral ventricles. Reactive astrocytosis was present in the striatum suggestive of neuronal loss, although there was no significant decrease in striatal cell number. A diffuse nuclear staining was apparent upon immunohistochemistry with anti-huntingtin antibodies and aggregate pathology in the form of nuclear and extranuclear aggregates. Consistent with previous studies, reduced binding at the D1 receptor was detected.

A set of transgenic mice was monitored until 18 weeks of age, when the mice clearly displayed a neurological phenotype, and were then divided into two groups. Half of the mice were given a tetracycline derivative (doxycycline) to switch off the exon 1 protein (gene off) and in the other half expression of the transgene was allowed to continue (gene on). The groups of mice were compared after a further 16 weeks. In the gene-off mice, doxycycline had abolished expression of the transgene (Fig. 13.11). Remarkably, the diffuse nuclear staining and intranuclear and extranuclear aggregates had disappeared from the striatum and were

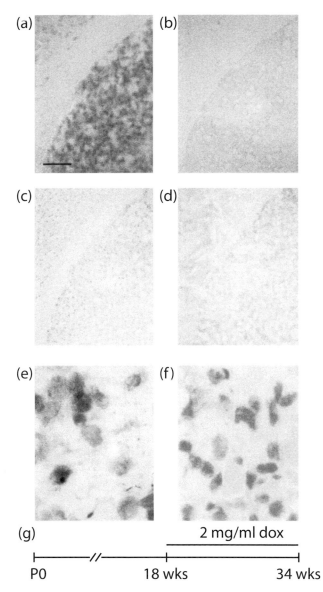

Fig. 13.11 LacZ and huntingtin aggregate staining after the 16-week 'gene-off' period. HD94 mice at 18 weeks of age were given either 2 mg/ml dox ('gene-off') or vehicle ('gene-on') for 16 weeks (see (g) for schematic). (a), (b) LacZ expression was abolished in gene-off HD94 mice and maintained in age-matched HD94 gene-on mice. (c), (d) Immunopositive staining with an *N*-terminal huntingtin antibody is present in the cortex and striatum of gene-on mice. In age-matched gene-off mice, the staining in the striatum was undetectable, whilst staining in the cortex was confined to scattered cells. (e), (f) Higher magnification of striatum counterstained with cresyl violet revealed that the lack of immunoreactivity in gene-off mice corresponds to a disappearance of both intra- and extra-nuclear aggregates. Scale bars: (a)–(d) 500 μm; (e)–(f) 100 μm. (Reprinted from Yamamoto *et al.* (2000) © (2000) with permission from Elsevier Science.)

much decreased in the cortex (Fig. 13.11). This finding was unexpected given the insoluble properties of these structures (Kazantsev *et al.* 1999; Scherzinger *et al.* 1997). The gene-off mice showed no further reduction in striatal size, the extent of reactive astrocytosis had decreased, and the progressive loss in D1 receptor binding was halted and a slight reversal observed (Fig. 13.12). Finally, the progression of the dystonic clasping phenotype was reversed to that generally seen in HD94 mice at 8 weeks of age (Fig. 13.12) and, more recently, a reversal of electrophysiological changes has been observed (see the section 'Electrophysiology').

This study has demonstrated that the progression of the disease depends on the continuous expression of the mutant protein. Suppression of mutant huntingtin between the ages of 18 and 34 weeks either halted or reversed all aspects of the phenotype. Despite the difficulty in biochemically dissolving or denaturing the aggregated form of huntingtin, neurones are capable of dispelling these structures. The motor recovery indicates that plastic changes can occur when the toxic insult ceases and that irreversible changes that commit the cell to neurodysfunction or cell death have not occurred. This suggests that it might be possible to treat HD after the onset of symptoms and that the disease may not be irreversible.

Strategies employed to modify phenotype progression in HD mouse models

The therapeutic effects of creatine

Several lines of evidence have suggested that mitochondrial impairment might be secondary to the gene defect in HD. These include: an elevation of lactate in HD striatum and cerebral

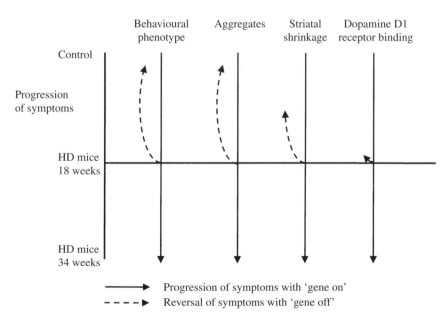

Fig. 13.12 Illustration of the extent to which phenotypic characteristics are halted and reversed in the gene-off mice. The solid black lines represent the progression of the respective phenotypes over a 34-week period. The dashed line indicates the extent to which the phenotype was reversed in the gene-off mice after switching off expression of the transgene at 18 weeks. (Reprinted from Bates (2000) with the permission of Oxford University Press.)

cortex; a reduction in phosphocreatine/inorganic phosphate in resting muscle of HD patients; the induction of HD-like pathology in the striatum of animals that have been given mitochondrial toxins; and a reduction in the mitochondrial electron transport enzymes in HD postmortem tissue (Brouillet *et al.* 1995; Browne *et al.* 1997; Gu *et al.* 1996; Jenkins *et al.* 1993; Koroshetz *et al.* 1997). Although the evidence of mitochondrial impairment in the R6 mice is not compelling, a decrease in complex IV activity has been measured in brains from R6/2 mice at 12 weeks of age (Tabrizi *et al.* 2000). Also, there is a marked decrease in NAA levels in the R6/2 brains from 5 weeks, which can be interpreted as a consequence of mitochondrial dysfunction (Jenkins *et al.* 2000).

Creatine kinase and its substrates, creatine and phosphocreatine, provide a cellular energy buffering and transport system, connecting sites of energy production with those of energy consumption (Ferrante *et al.* 2000; Hemmer and Wallimann 1993). R6/2 mice were given dietary supplements of creatine to determine whether this could have beneficial effects. Remarkably, all aspects of the phenotype were improved. Mice were given chow supplemented with 1, 2, or 3 per cent creatine; the beneficial effects were most pronounced at the 2 per cent dose and 1 per cent was better than 3 per cent. Creatine supplementation at 2 per cent led to a 17.5 per cent increase in survival, a significant increase in body weight at all points in the trial, and delayed motor impairment as measured by performance on the rotarod. Interestingly, it also delayed the onset of diabetes. Two per cent creatine dramatically improved all aspects of R6/2 neuropathology causing delays in brain weight decrease, lateral ventricle enlargement, and the shrinkage of striatal neurones. Unexpectedly, it also decreased the formation of aggregates in the striatum and cortex in the brain and in the islets of Langerhan in pancreas. The ability of creatine to delay the formation of huntingtin aggregates in the brains of R6/2 mice has independently been demonstrated in an organotypic cell culture system (Smith *et al.* 2001). MRS showed that 2 per cent creatine significantly increased brain creatine concentrations by 21 per cent and attenuated the early decrease in the concentration of NAA (Ferrante *et al.* 2000). The beneficial effects of creatine have more recently been confirmed in the N171–82 mouse model of HD (Andreassen *et al.* 2001).

Creatine administration has several potential neuroprotective effects including the buffering of intracellular energy reserves, stabilizing intracellular calcium, and inhibiting activation of the mitochondrial permeability transition pore. The mechanism by which it exerts beneficial effects in the R6/2 mice is currently unclear, although an increase in intracellular energy reserves might aid in the clearance of misfolded and/or aggregated forms of mutant huntingtin.

Targeting caspase 1 activation
To investigate a possible role for caspases in the pathogenesis that occurs in the R6/ mice, line R6/2 was crossed to mice that express a dominant negative caspase 1 transgene (NSE M17Z) (Ona *et al.* 1999). As with creatine, this had the unexpected effect of alleviating all aspects of the phenotype. In the double transgenics (R6/2-NSE M17Z), aggregate formation, motor dysfunction, weight loss, and neurotransmitter changes were all delayed. The appearance of nuclear inclusions was postponed from 3 weeks until after 9 weeks in the CA1 region of the hippocampus (Ona *et al.* 1999). As caspase 1 activation, as detected by interleukin 1β (IL-1β) cleavage, is not detected until 8 weeks of age, the mechanism by which inhibiting caspase 1 activity delays this very early and aggressive process of aggregation is not understood.

Following on from the work of Ona *et al.* (1999), Chen and colleagues (2000) assessed the effects of the administration of the antibiotic minocycline to the R6/2 mice. Minocycline inhibits caspase 1 and iNOS activation and decreases infarct size after experimental ischaemia. Minocycline was administered to R6/2 mice by the intraparenteral (IP) injection of 5 mg/kg and was found to delay disease progression as measured by a decline in rotarod performance, and to extend survival by 14 per cent. Minocycline inhibited activation of caspase 1 as measured by IL-1β processing and reduced iNOS induction by 72 per cent. However, in contrast to creatine, it had no effect on loss of body weight, the elevation of blood glucose, the formation of polyglutamine aggregates, or the decrease in neurotransmitter receptor binding.

Dietary arginine modulates the phenotype in R6/1 mice

Nitric oxide (NO) is produced when dietary arginine is converted to citrilline via the action of nitric oxide synthase (NOS) (Bredt and Snyder 1990). In pathological states, NO can combine with superoxide to generate peroxynitrite (Strijbos 1998), which in turn causes neuronal cell death due to its ability to form nitrotyrosine products, oxidize proteins, fragment DNA, and deplete cells of NAD$^+$ by activation of pol-ADP-ribose synthetase (Scott *et al.* 1999). Both NO and peroxinitrite can have a profound effect on cerebral blood flow (CBF), and complex changes in the CBF in early-stage HD have recently been uncovered by imaging techniques (Deckel *et al.* 2000b). Deckel and colleagues (2000a) tested the effects of altering the levels of NO on the phenotype of the R6/1 mice by manipulating dietary arginine. Mice were assigned at 12 weeks of age to one of three isocaloric diets that varied only in their content of arginine, that is, 0, 1.2 (that found in typical mouse chow), or 5 per cent. The 5 per cent arginine diets resulted in an earlier onset of body weight loss and motor impairments and increased CBF in R6/1 compared with those on the 1.2 per cent diet. For the 0 per cent arginine group, body weight gain was the same in R6/1 as controls and in both cases was decreased compared with the mice on the 1.2 per cent arginine diet. CBF did not differ between R6/1 and control mice in the 0 per cent group but the transgenic mice showed significant motor deficits. There was a greater deposition of nitrotyrosine in the cortex and vasculature of R6/1 mice on the 5 and 1.2 per cent diets than in those on the 0 per cent diet. Therefore, the dietary consumption of arginine has a measurable but complex effect on symptom progression in the R6/1 mice (Deckel *et al.* 2000a).

Environmental stimulation delays onset of symptoms

Exposure of R6/1 mice to a stimulating enriched environment from an early age helped to prevent the loss of cerebral volume and delayed the onset of the motor disorder (van Dellen *et al.* 2000a). In addition to the provision of normal feed and bedding, the cages of the environmentally enriched groups also contained cardboard, paper, and plastic objects that were changed every 2 days from the age of 4 weeks. The enrichment did not have an effect on body mass or spontaneous motor activity and blood and urine glucose levels were normal in all mice. The onset of the motor tasks, a 'turning task' and hindlimb clasping when suspended by the tail, were both delayed (van Dellen *et al.* 2000a). A further study assessed the effects of different degrees of enrichment on the phenotype of the R6/2 mice (Hockly *et al.* 2002). It was found that even the limited enrichment of adding a cardboard toilet roll to the cage and placing food pellets on the floor slowed the decline in rotarod performance to the same extent as maximal levels of enrichment. In contrast, in normal littermates, maximal levels of enrichment were required to induce a marked improvement in behavioural tests (Hockly *et al.* 2002).

Quantitative histology showed an increase in the 'peristriatal cerebral volume' in the environmentally enriched mice as compared to the non-enriched controls, whereas enrichment did not affect the peristriatal cerebral volume of enriched wild-type mice (Hockly *et al.* 2002;

van Dellen *et al.* 2000a). An enlargement in the striatal volume in the enriched HD mice was not significant and enrichment had no detectable effects on aggregate formation in either study. Therefore, the environmental enrichment delays the degenerative loss of cerebral volume in HD mice and indicates that the corticostriatal pathway plays a role in HD pathogenesis. Environmental enrichment might overcome deficiencies of synaptic plasticity, particularly at the intracortical and corticostriatal synapses, and help to improve the defects in HD mice. The demonstration that monozygotic twins with HD and identical CAG repeat lengths can display different clinical symptoms and behavioural abilities (Georgiou *et al.* 1999) indicates that environmental differences might alter disease onset and progression in humans (Hockly *et al.* 2002; van Dellen *et al.* 2000a).

Concluding remarks

The generation of mouse models of HD has been extraordinarily successful. It has been possible to model the disease in all of the organisms that are amenable to powerful and sophisticated genetic manipulation. The characteristic aggregations common to HD and the other polyglutamine diseases were first recognized in mouse models of HD with their detection in human HD following the mouse findings. Mouse models have thus led to major insights into the neuropathology of HD and are beginning to elucidate the very early molecular events in its pathogenesis. Work in other model organisms such as *Drosophila* has also begun to yield the identity of genes that can modify polyglutamine aggregation and neurodegeneration and will be increasingly used in the testing of therapeutic compounds: these models are discussed in the next chapter. Pharmaceutical trials in mouse models are already exerting an influence in the clinic and compounds are moving to phase II clinical trials. These advances have all occurred in the space of less than 5 years and there is every reason to be optimistic about the development of effective therapeutics, through trials in animal models, that will have a major impact on HD in the near future.

References

Ambrose, C. M., Duyao, M. P., Barnes, G., Bates, G. P., Lin, C. S., Srinidhi, J., Baxendale, S., Hummerich, H., Lehrach, H., Altherr, M., *et al.* (1994). Structure and expression of the Huntington's disease gene: evidence against simple inactivation due to an expanded CAG repeat. *Somat Cell Mol Genet* **20**, 27–38.

Andreassen, O. A., Dedeoglu, A., Ferrante, R. J., Jenkins, B. G., Ferrante, K. L., Thomas, M., Friedlich, A., Browne, S. E., Schilling, G., Borchelt, D. R., Hersch, S. M., Ross, C. A., and Beal, M. F. (2001). Creatine increase survival and delays motor symptoms in a transgenic animal model of Huntington's disease. *Neurobiol Dis* **8**, 479–91.

Augood, S. J., Faull, R. L., Love, D. R., and Emson, P. C. (1996). Reduction in enkephalin and substance P messenger RNA in the striatum of early grade Huntington's disease: a detailed cellular *in situ* hybridization study. *Neuroscience* **72**, 1023–36.

Bates, G. P., Mangiarini, L., Mahal, A., and Davies, S. W. (1997). Transgenic models of Huntington's disease. *Hum Mol Genet* **6**, 1633–7.

Becher, M. W., Kotzuk, J. A., Sharp, A. H., Davies, S. W., Bates, G. P., Price, D. L., and Ross, C. A. (1998). Intranuclear neuronal inclusions in Huntington's disease and dentatorubral and pallidoluysian atrophy: correlation between the density of inclusions and IT15 CAG triplet repeat length. *Neurobiol Dis* **4**, 387–97.

Bibb, J. A., Yan, Z., Svenningsson, P., Snyder, G. L., Pieribone, V. A., Horiuchi, A., Nairn, A. C., Messer, A., and Greengard, P. (2000). Severe deficiencies in dopamine signaling in presymptomatic Huntington's disease mice. *Proc Natl Acad Sci, USA* **97**, 6809–14.

Bliss, T. V. and Collingridge, G. L. (1993). A synaptic model of memory: long-term potentiation in the hippocampus. *Nature* **361**, 31–9.

Bogdanov, M. B., Ferrante, R. J., Kuemmerle, S., Klivenyi, P., and Beal, M. F. (1998). Increased vulnerability to 3-nitropropionic acid in an animal model of Huntington's disease. *J Neurochem* **71**, 2642–4.

Boutell, J. M., Thomas, P., Neal, J. W., Weston, V. J., Duce, J., Harper, P. S., and Jones, A. L. (1999). Aberrant interactions of transcriptional repressor proteins with the Huntington's disease gene product, huntingtin. *Hum Mol Genet* **8**, 1647–55.

Bredt, D. S. and Snyder, S. H. (1990). Isolation of nitric oxide synthetase, a calmodulin-requiring enzyme. *Proc Natl Acad Sci, USA* **87**, 682–5.

Brouillet, E., Hantraye, P., Ferrante, R. J., Dolan, R., Leroy-Willig, A., Kowall, N. W., and Beal, M. F. (1995). Chronic mitochondrial energy impairment produces selective striatal degeneration and abnormal choreiform movements in primates. *Proc Natl Acad Sci, USA* **92**, 7105–9.

Browne, S. E., Bowling, A. C., MacGarvey, U., Baik, M. J., Berger, S. C., Muqit, M. M., Bird, E. D., and Beal, M. F. (1997). Oxidative damage and metabolic dysfunction in Huntington's disease: selective vulnerability of the basal ganglia. *Ann Neurol* **41**, 646–53.

Carter, R. J., Lione, L. A., Humby, T., Mangiarini, L., Mahal, A., Bates, G. P., Dunnett, S. B., and Morton, A. J. (1999). Characterization of progressive motor deficits in mice transgenic for the human Huntington's disease mutation. *J Neurosci* **19**, 3248–57.

Cha, J. H. (2000). Transcriptional dysregulation in Huntington's disease. *Trends Neurosci* **23**, 387–92.

—— Kosinski, C. M., Kerner, J. A., Alsdorf, S. A., Mangiarini, L., Davies, S. W., Penney, J. B., Bates, G. P., and Young, A. B. (1998). Altered brain neurotransmitter receptors in transgenic mice expressing a portion of an abnormal human huntington disease gene. *Proc Natl Acad Sci, USA* **95**, 6480–5.

—— Frey, A. S., Alsdorf, S. A., Kerner, J. A., Kosinski, C. M., Mangiarini, L., Penney, J. B., Jr., Davies, S. W., Bates, G. P., and Young, A. B. (1999). Altered neurotransmitter receptor expression in transgenic mouse models of Huntington's disease. *Philos Trans R Soc Lond B Biol Sci* **354**, 981–9.

Chen, M., Ona, V. O., Li, M., Ferrante, R. J., Fink, K. B., Zhu, S., Bian, J., Guo, L., Farrell, L. A., Hersch, S. M., Hobbs, W., Vonsattel, J. P., Cha, J. H., and Friedlander, R. M. (2000). Minocycline inhibits caspase-1 and caspase-3 expression and delays mortality in a transgenic mouse model of Huntington disease. *Nat Med* **6**, 797–801.

Chen, N., Luo, T., Wellington, C., Metzler, M., McCutcheon, K., Hayden, M. R., and Raymond, L. A. (1999). Subtype-specific enhancement of NMDA receptor currents by mutant huntingtin. *J Neurochem* **72**, 1890–8.

Davies, S. W., Turmaine, M., Cozens, B. A., DiFiglia, M., Sharp, A. H., Ross, C. A., Scherzinger, E., Wanker, E. E., Mangiarini, L., and Bates, G. P. (1997). Formation of neuronal intranuclear inclusions underlies the neurological dysfunction in mice transgenic for the HD mutation. *Cell* **90**, 537–48.

Deckel, A. W., Volmer, P., Weiner, R., Gary, K. A., Covault, J., Sasso, D., Schmerler, N., Watts, D., Yan, Z., and Abeles, I. (2000a). Dietary arginine alters time of symptom onset in Huntington's disease transgenic mice(1). *Brain Res* **875**, 187–95.

—— Weiner, R., Szigeti, D., Clark, V., and Vento, J. (2000b). Altered patterns of regional cerebral blood flow in patients with Huntington's disease: a SPECT study during rest and cognitive or motor activation. *J Nucl Med* **41**, 773–80.

Denovan-Wright, E. M. and Robertson, H. A. (2000). Cannabinoid receptor messenger RNA levels decrease in a subset of neurons of the lateral striatum, cortex and hippocampus of transgenic Huntington's disease mice. *Neuroscience* **98**, 705–13.

de Wind, N., Dekker, M., Berns, A., Radman, M., and te Riele, H. (1995). Inactivation of the mouse Msh2 gene results in mismatch repair deficiency, methylation tolerance, hyperrecombination, and predisposition to cancer. *Cell* **82**, 321–30.

DiFiglia, M., Sapp, E., Chase, K. O., Davies, S. W., Bates, G. P., Vonsattel, J. P., and Aronin, N. (1997). Aggregation of huntingtin in neuronal intranuclear inclusions and dystrophic neurites in brain. *Science* **277**, 1990–3.

Dragatsis, I., Efstratiadis, A., and Zeitlin, S. (1998). Mouse mutant embryos lacking huntingtin are rescued from lethality by wild-type extraembryonic tissues. *Development* **125**, 1529–39.

Duyao, M. P., Auerbach, A. B., Ryan, A., Persichetti, F., Barnes, G. T., McNeil, S. M., Ge, P., Vonsattel, J. P., Gusella, J. F., Joyner, A. L., and MacDonald M. E. (1995). Inactivation of the mouse Huntington's disease gene homolog Hdh. *Science* **269**, 407–10.

Fain, J. N., Del Mar, N. A., Meade, C. A., Reiner, A., and Goldowitz, D. (2001). Abnormalities in the functioning of adipocytes from R6/2 mice that are transgenic for the Huntington's disease mutation. *Hum Mol Genet* **10**, 145–52.

Ferrante, R. J., Andreassen, O. A., Jenkins, B. G., Dedeoglu, A., Kuemmerle, S., Kubilus, J. K., Kaddurah-Daouk, R., Hersch, S. M., and Beal, M. F. (2000). Neuroprotective effects of creatine in a transgenic mouse model of Huntington's disease. *J Neurosci* **20**, 4389–97.

File, S. E., Mahal, A., Mangiarini, L., and Bates, G. P. (1998). Striking changes in anxiety in Huntington's disease transgenic mice. *Brain Res* **805**, 234–40.

Georgiou, N., Bradshaw, J. L., Chiu, E., Tudor, A., O'Gorman, L., and Phillips, J. G. (1999). Differential clinical and motor control function in a pair of monozygotic twins with Huntington's disease. *Mov Disord* **14**, 320–5.

Glass, M., Dragunow, M., and Faull, R. L. (2000). The pattern of neurodegeneration in Huntington's disease: a comparative study of cannabinoid, dopamine, adenosine and GABA(A) receptor alterations in the human basal ganglia in Huntington's disease. *Neuroscience* **97**, 505–19.

Gossen, M. and Bujard, H. (1992). Tight control of gene expression in mammalian cells by tetracycline-responsive promoters. *Proc Natl Acad Sci, USA* **89**, 5547–51.

Gourdon, G., Radvanyi, F., Lia, A. S., Duros, C., Blanche, M., Abitbol, M., Junien, C., and Hofmann-Radvanyi, H. (1997). Moderate intergenerational and somatic instability of a 55-CTG repeat in transgenic mice [see comments]. *Nat Genet* **15**, 190–2.

Gu, M., Gash, M. T., Mann, V. M., Javoy-Agid, F., Cooper, J. M., and Schapira, A. H. (1996). Mitochondrial defect in Huntington's disease caudate nucleus. *Ann Neurol* **39**, 385–9.

Guidetti, P., Reddy, P. H., Tagle, D. A., and Schwarcz, R. (2000). Early kynurenergic impairment in Huntington's disease and in a transgenic animal model. *Neurosci Lett* **283**, 233–5.

—— Charles, V., Chen, E. Y., Reddy, P. H., Kordower, J. H., Whetsell, W. O., Jr., Schwarcz, R., and Tagle, D. A. (2001). Early degenerative changes in transgenic mice expressing mutant huntingtin involve dendritic abnormalities but no impairment of mitochondrial energy production. *Exp Neurol* **169**, 340–50.

Gutekunst, C. A., Li, S. H., Yi, H., Mulroy, J. S., Kuemmerle, S., Jones, R., Rye, D., Ferrante, R. J., Hersch, S. M., and Li, X. J. (1999). Nuclear and neuropil aggregates in Huntington's disease: relationship to neuropathology. *J Neurosci* **19**, 2522–34.

—— Norflus, F., C., D., Yi, H., Schilling, G., Borchelt, D. R., Ross, C. A., Woodman, B., Bates, G., Ferrante, R. J., and Hersch, S. (2000). Neuropathology in transgenic mouse models of Huntington's disease. *Soc Neurosci Abstr* **26**, 1029.

Halliday, G. M., McRitchie, D. A., Macdonald, V., Double, K. L., Trent, R. J., and McCusker, E. (1998). Regional specificity of brain atrophy in Huntington's disease. *Exp Neurol* **154**, 663–72.

Hansson, O., Peters n, A., Leist, M., Nicotera, P., Castilho, R. F., and Brundin, P. (1999). Transgenic mice expressing a Huntington's disease mutation are resistant to quinolinic acid-induced striatal excitotoxicity. *Proc Natl Acad Sci, USA* **96**, 8727–32.

—— Castilho, R. F., Korhonen, L., Lindholm, D., Bates, G. P., and Brundin, P. (2001a). Partial resistance to malonate-induced striatal cell death in transgenic mouse models of Huntington's disease is dependent on age and CAG repeat length. *J Neurochem* **78**, 694–703.

—— Guatteo, E., Mercuri, N. B., Bernardi, G., Li, X. J., Castilho, R. F., and Brundin, P. (2001b). Resistance to NMDA toxicity correlates with appearance of nuclear inclusions, behavioural deficits and changes in calcium homeostasis in mice transgenic for exon 1 of the huntingtin gene. *Eur J Neurosci* **14**, 1492–504.

Hemmer, W. and Wallimann, T. (1993). Functional aspects of creatine kinase in brain. *Dev Neurosci* **15**, 249–60.

Hickey, M. A. and Morton, A. J. (2000). Mice transgenic for the Huntington's disease mutation are resistant to chronic 3-nitropropionic acid-induced striatal toxicity. *J Neurochem* **75**, 2163–71.

Hilditch-Maguire, P., Trettel, F., Passani, L. A., Auerbach, A., Persichetti, F., and MacDonald, M. E. (2000). Huntingtin: an iron-regulated protein essential for normal nuclear and perinuclear organelles. *Hum Mol Genet* **9**, 2789–97.

Hockly, E., Cordery, P. M., Woodman, B., Mahal, A., van Dellen, A., Blakemore, C., Lewis, C. M., Hannan, A. J., and Bates, G. P. (2002). Environmental enrichment slows disease progression in R6/2 Huntington's disease mice. *Ann Neurol*, **51**, 235–42.

Hodgson, J. G., Agopyan, N., Gutekunst, C. A., Leavitt, B. R., LePiane, F., Singaraja, R., Smith, D. J., Bissada, N., McCutcheon, K., Nasir, J., Jamot, L., Li, X. J., Stevens, M. E., Rosemond, E., Roder, J. C., Phillips, A. G., Rubin, E. M., Hersch, S. M., and Hayden, M. R. (1999). A YAC mouse model for Huntington's disease with full-length mutant huntingtin, cytoplasmic toxicity, and selective striatal neurodegeneration. *Neuron* **23**, 181–92.

Horlein, A. J., Naar, A. M., Heinzel, T., Torchia, J., Gloss, B., Kurokawa, R., Ryan, A., Kamei, Y., Soderstrom, M., Glass, C. K., *et al.* (1995). Ligand-independent repression by the thyroid hormone receptor mediated by a nuclear receptor co-repressor. *Nature* **377**, 397–404.

Huntington's Disease Collaborative Research Group (1993). A novel gene containing a trinucleotide repeat that is expanded and unstable on Huntington's disease chromosomes. The Huntington's Disease Collaborative Research Group. *Cell* **72**, 971–83.

Hurlbert, M. S., Zhou, W., Wasmeier, C., Kaddis, F. G., Hutton, J. C., and Freed, C. R. (1999). Mice transgenic for an expanded CAG repeat in the Huntington's disease gene develop diabetes. *Diabetes* **48**, 649–51.

Iannicola, C., Moreno, S., Oliverio, S., Nardacci, R., Ciofi-Luzzatto, A., and Piacentini, M. (2000). Early alterations in gene expression and cell morphology in a mouse model of Huntington's disease. *J Neurochem* **75**, 830–9.

Jackson, G. R., Salecker, I., Dong, X., Yao, X., Arnheim, N., Faber, P. W., MacDonald, M. E., and Zipursky, S. L. (1998). Polyglutamine-expanded human huntingtin transgenes induce degeneration of *Drosophila* photoreceptor neurons. *Neuron* **21**, 633–42.

Jana, N. R., Tanaka, M., Wang, G., and Nukina, N. (2000). Polyglutamine length-dependent interaction of Hsp40 and Hsp70 family chaperones with truncated N-terminal huntingtin: their role in suppression of aggregation and cellular toxicity. *Hum Mol Genet* **9**, 2009–18.

Jeffreys, A. J., Tamaki, K., MacLeod, A., Monckton, D. G., Neil, D. L., and Armour, J. A. (1994). Complex gene conversion events in germline mutation at human minisatellites. *Nat Genet* **6**, 136–45.

—— Koroshetz, W. J., Beal, M. F., and Rosen, B. R. (1993). Evidence for impairment of energy metabolism *in vivo* in Huntington's disease using localized 1H NMR spectroscopy. *Neurology* **43**, 2689–95.

Jenkins, B. G., Klivenyi, P., Kustermann, E., Andreassen, O. A., Ferrante, R. J., Rosen, B. R., and Beal, M. F. (2000). Nonlinear decrease over time in N-acetyl aspartate levels in the absence of neuronal loss and increases in glutamine and glucose in transgenic Huntington's disease mice. *J Neurochem* **74**, 2108–19.

Kaytor, M. D., Burright, E. N., Duvick, L. A., Zoghbi, H. Y., and Orr, H. T. (1997). Increased trinucleotide repeat instability with advanced maternal age. *Hum Mol Genet* **6**, 2135–9.

Kazantsev, A., Preisinger, E., Dranovsky, A., Goldgaber, D., and Housman, D. (1999). Insoluble detergent-resistant aggregates form between pathological and nonpathological lengths of polyglutamine in mammalian cells. *Proc Natl Acad Sci, USA* **96**, 11404–9.

Kennedy, L. and Shelbourne, P. F. (2000). Dramatic mutation instability in HD mouse striatum: does polyglutamine load contribute to cell-specific vulnerability in Huntington's disease? *Hum Mol Genet* **9**, 2539–44.

Klapstein, G. J., Fisher, R. S., Zanjani, H., Cepeda, C., Jokel, E. S., Chesselet, M. F., and Levine, M. S. (2001). Age-related electrophysiological and morphological changes in medium-sized striatal spiny neurons in R6/2 Huntington's disease transgenic mice. *J Neurophysiol* **6**, 2667–77.

Koroshetz, W. J., Jenkins, B. G., Rosen, B. R., and Beal, M. F. (1997). Energy metabolism defects in Huntington's disease and effects of coenzyme Q10. *Ann Neurol* **41**, 160–5.

Kovtun, I. V., Therneau, T. M., and McMurray, C. T. (2000). Gender of the embryo contributes to CAG instability in transgenic mice containing a Huntington's disease gene. *Hum Mol Genet* **9**, 2767–75.

Laforet, G. A., Sapp, E., Chase, K., McIntyre, C., Boyce, F. M., Campbell, M., Cadigan, B. A., Warzecki, L., Tagle, D. A., Reddy, P. H., Cepeda, C., Calvert, C. R., Jokel, E. S., Klapstein, G. J., Ariano, M. A., Levine, M. S., DiFiglia, M., and Aronin, N. (2001). Changes in cortical ans striatal neurons predict behavioural and electrophysiological abnormalities in a transgenic murine model of Huntington's disease. *J Neurosci* **21**, 9112–23.

Levine, M. S., Klapstein, G. J., Koppel, A., Gruen, E., Cepeda, C., Vargas, M. E., Jokel, E. S., Carpenter, E. M., Zanjani, H., Hurst, R. S., Efstratiadis, A., Zeitlin, S., and Chesselet, M. F. (1999). Enhanced sensitivity to N-methyl-D-aspartate receptor activation in transgenic and knockin mouse models of Huntington's disease. *J Neurosci Res* **58**, 515–32.

Li, H., Li, S. H., Cheng, A. L., Mangiarini, L., Bates, G. P., and Li, X. J. (1999). Ultrastructural localization and progressive formation of neuropil aggregates in Huntington's disease transgenic mice. *Hum Mol Genet* **8**, 1227–36.

—— Johnston, H., Shelbourne, P. F., and Li, X. J. (2000). Amino-terminal fragments of mutant huntingtin show selective accumulation in striatal neurons and synaptic toxicity. *Nat Genet* **25**, 385–9.

Li, S. H. and Li, X. J. (1998). Aggregation of N-terminal huntingtin is dependent on the length of its glutamine repeats. *Hum Mol Genet* **7**, 777–82.

Lievens, J. C., Woodman, B., Mahal, A., Spasic-Boscovic, O., Samuel, D., Kerkerian-Le Goff, L., and Bates, G. P. (2001). Impaired glutamate uptake in the r6 huntington's disease transgenic mice. *Neurobiol Dis* **8**, 807–21.

Lin, C. H., Tallaksen-Greene, S., Chien, W. M., Cearley, J. A., Jackson, W. S., Crouse, A. B., Ren, S., Li, X. J., Albin, R. L., and Detloff, P. J. (2001). Neurological abnormalities in a knock-in mouse model of Huntington's disease. *Hum Mol Genet* **10**, 137–44.

Lione, L. A., Carter, R. J., Hunt, M. J., Bates, G. P., Morton, A. J., and Dunnett, S. B. (1999). Selective discrimination learning impairments in mice expressing the human Huntington's disease mutation. *J Neurosci* **19**, 10428–37.

Luesse, H. G., Schiefer, J., Spruenken, A., Puls, C., Block, F., and Kosinski, C. M. (2001). Evaluation of R6/2 HD transgenic mice for therapeutic studies in Huntington's disease: behavioral testing and impact of diabetes mellitus. *Behav Brain Res* **126**, 185–95.

Luthi-Carter, R., Strand, A., Peters, N. L., Solano, S. M., Hollingsworth, Z. R., Menon, A. S., Frey, A. S., Spektor, B. S., Penney, E. B., Schilling, G., Ross, C. A., Borchelt, D. R., Tapscott, S. J., Young, A. B., Cha, J. H., and Olson, J. M. (2000). Decreased expression of striatal signaling genes in a mouse model of Huntington's disease. *Hum Mol Genet* **9**, 1259–71.

Macdonald, V., Halliday, G. M., Trent, R. J., and McCusker, E. A. (1997). Significant loss of pyramidal neurons in the angular gyrus of patients with Huntington's disease. *Neuropathol Appl Neurobiol* **23**, 492–5.

Mangiarini, L., Sathasivam, K., Seller, M., Cozens, B., Harper, A., Hetherington, C., Lawton, M., Trottier, Y., Lehrach, H., Davies, S. W., and Bates, G. P. (1996). Exon 1 of the HD gene with an expanded CAG repeat is sufficient to cause a progressive neurological phenotype in transgenic mice. *Cell* **87**, 493–506.

Mangiarini, L., Sathasivam, K., Mahal, A., Mott, R., Seller, M., and Bates, G. P. (1997). Instability of highly expanded CAG repeats in mice transgenic for the Huntington's disease mutation. *Nat Genet* **15**, 197–200.

Manley, K., Shirley, T. L., Flaherty, L., and Messer, A. (1999). Msh2 deficiency prevents *in vivo* somatic instability of the CAG repeat in Huntington disease transgenic mice. *Nat Genet* **23**, 471–3.

Martindale, D., Hackam, A., Wieczorek, A., Ellerby, L., Wellington, C., McCutcheon, K., Singaraja, R., Kazemi-Esfarjani, P., Devon, R., Kim, S. U., Bredesen, D. E., Tufaro, F., and Hayden, M. R. (1998). Length of huntingtin and its polyglutamine tract influences localization and frequency of intracellular aggregates. *Nat Genet* **18**, 150–4.

Menalled, L., Zanjani, H., MacKenzie, L., Koppel, A., Carpenter, E., Zeitlin, S., and Chesselet, M. F. (2000). Decrease in striatal enkephalin mRNA in mouse models of Huntington's disease. *Exp Neurol* **162**, 328–42.

Metzler, M., Chen, N., Helgason, C. D., Graham, R. K., Nichol, K., McCutcheon, K., Nasir, J., Humphries, R. K., Raymond, L. A., and Hayden, M. R. (1999). Life without huntingtin: normal differentiation into functional neurons. *J Neurochem* **72**, 1009–18.

Monckton, D. G., Coolbaugh, M. I., Ashizawa, K. T., Siciliano, M. J., and Caskey, C. T. (1997). Hypermutable myotonic dystrophy CTG repeats in transgenic mice. *Nat Genet* **15**, 193–6.

Morton, A. J. and Edwardson, J. M. (2001). Progressive depletion of complexin II in a transgenic mouse model of Huntington's disease. *J Neurochem* **76**, 166–72.

—— Leavens, W. (2000). Mice transgenic for the human Huntington's disease mutation have reduced sensitivity to kainic acid toxicity. *Brain Res Bull* **52**, 51–9.

—— Lagan, M. A., Skepper, J. N., and Dunnett, S. B. (2000). Progressive formation of inclusions in the striatum and hippocampus of mice transgenic for the human Huntington's disease mutation. *J Neurocytol* **29**, 679–702.

Murphy, K. P., Carter, R. J., Lione, L. A., Mangiarini, L., Mahal, A., Bates, G. P., Dunnett, S. B., and Morton, A. J. (2000). Abnormal synaptic plasticity and impaired spatial cognition in mice transgenic for exon 1 of the human Huntington's disease mutation. *J Neurosci* **20**, 5115–23.

Myers, R. H., Marans, K. S., and MacDonald, M. E. (1998) In *Genetic instabilities and hereditary neurological diseases* (ed. R. D. Wells and S. T. Warren), pp. 301–23. Academic Press, San Diego.

Nasir, J., Floresco, S. B., O'Kusky, J. R., Diewert, V. M., Richman, J. M., Zeisler, J., Borowski, A., Marth, J. D., Phillips, A. G., and Hayden, M. R. (1995). Targeted disruption of the Huntington's disease gene results in embryonic lethality and behavioral and morphological changes in heterozygotes. *Cell* **81**, 811–23.

Nicniocaill, B., Haraldsson, B., Hansson, O., O'Connor, W. T., and Brundin, P. (2001). Altered striatal amino acid neurotransmitter release monitored using microdialysis in R6/1 Huntington transgenic mice. *Eur J Neurosci* **13**, 206–10.

Nucifora, F. C., Jr., Sasaki, M., Peters, M. F., Huang, H., Cooper, J. K., Yamada, M., Takahashi, H., Tsuji, S., Troncoso, J., Dawson, V. L., Dawson, T. M., and Ross, C. A. (2001). Interference by huntingtin and atrophin-1 with cbp-mediated transcription leading to cellular toxicity. *Science* **291**, 2423–8.

O'Kusky, J. R., Nasir, J., Cicchetti, F., Parent, A., and Hayden, M. R. (1999). Neuronal degeneration in the basal ganglia and loss of pallido- subthalamic synapses in mice with targeted disruption of the Huntington's disease gene. *Brain Res* **818**, 468–79.

Ona, V. O., Li, M., Vonsattel, J. P., Andrews, L. J., Khan, S. Q., Chung, W. M., Frey, A. S., Menon, A. S., Li, X. J., Stieg, P. E., Yuan, J., Penney, J. B., Young, A. B., Cha, J. H., and Friedlander, R. M. (1999). Inhibition of caspase-1 slows disease progression in a mouse model of Huntington's disease. *Nature* **399**, 263–7.

Perez-Severiano, F., Rios, C., and Segovia, J. (2000). Striatal oxidative damage parallels the expression of a neurological phenotype in mice transgenic for the mutation of Huntington's disease. *Brain Res* **862**, 234–7.

Petersen, A., Hansson, O., Puschban, Z., Sapp, E., Romero, N., Castilho, R. F., Sulzer, D., Rice, M., DiFiglia, M., Przedborski, S., and Brundin, P. (2001). Mice transgenic for exon 1 of the Huntington's disease gene display reduced striatal sensitivity to neurotoxicity induced by dopamine and 6-hydroxy-dopamine. *Eur J Neurosci* **14**, 1425–35.

Reddy, P. H., Williams, M., Charles, V., Garrett, L., Pike-Buchanan, L., Whetsell, W. O. Jr., Miller, G., and Tagle, D. A. (1998). Behavioural abnormalities and selective neuronal loss in HD transgenic mice expressing mutated full-length HD cDNA. *Nat Genet* **20**, 198–202.

Reim, K., Mansour, M., Varoqueaux, F., McMahon, H. T., Sudhof, T. C., Brose, N., and Rosenmund, C. (2001). Complexins regulate a late step in Ca2+-dependent neurotransmitter release. *Cell* **104**, 71–81.

Reiner, A., Del Mar, N., Meade, C. A., Yang, H., Dragatsis, I., Zeitlin, S., and Goldowitz, D. (2001). Neurons lacking huntingtin differentially colonize brain and survive in chimeric mice. *J Neurosci* **21**, 7608–19.

Reynolds, G. P., Dalton, C. F., Tillery, C. L., Mangiarini, L., Davies, S. W., and Bates, G. P. (1999). Brain neurotransmitter deficits in mice transgenic for the Huntington's disease mutation. *J Neurochem* **72**, 1773–6.

Roizin, L., Stellar, S., and Liu, J. C. (1979). In *Advances in neurology*, Vol. 23 (ed. T. N. Chase, N. S. Wexler, and A. Barbeau), pp. 95–122. Raven Press, New York.

Sapp, E., Penney, J., Young, A., Aronin, N., Vonsattel, J. P., and DiFiglia, M. (1999). Axonal transport of N-terminal huntingtin suggests early pathology of corticostriatal projections in Huntington disease. *J Neuropathol Exp Neurol* **58**, 165–73.

Sathasivam, K., Hobbs, C., Turmaine, M., Mangiarini, L., Mahal, A., Bertaux, F., Wanker, E. E., Doherty, P., Davies, S. W., and Bates, G. P. (1999). Formation of polyglutamine inclusions in non-CNS tissue. *Hum Mol Genet* **8**, 813–22.

Scherzinger, E., Lurz, R., Turmaine, M., Mangiarini, L., Hollenbach, B., Hasenbank, R., Bates, G. P., Davies, S. W., Lehrach, H., and Wanker, E. E. (1997). Huntingtin-encoded polyglutamine expansions form amyloid-like protein aggregates *in vitro* and *in vivo*. *Cell* **90**, 549–58.

Schilling, G., Becher, M. W., Sharp, A. H., Jinnah, H. A., Duan, K., Kotzuk, J. A., Slunt, H. H., Ratovitski, T., Cooper, J. K., Jenkins, N. A., Copeland, N. G., Price, D. L., Ross, C. A., and Borchelt, D. R. (1999a). Intranuclear inclusions and neuritic aggregates in transgenic mice expressing a mutant N-terminal fragment of huntingtin [published erratum appears in *Hum Mol Genet* 1999, **8** (5), 943]. *Hum Mol Genet* **8**, 397–407.

—— Wood, J. D., Duan, K., Slunt, H. H., Gonzales, V., Yamada, M., Cooper, J. K., Margolis, R. L., Jenkins, N. A., Copeland, N. G., Takahashi, H., Tsuji, S., Price, D. L., Borchelt, D. R., and Ross, C. A. (1999b). Nuclear accumulation of truncated atrophin-1 fragments in a transgenic mouse model of DRPLA. *Neuron* **24**, 275–86.

Scott, G. S., Jakeman, L. B., Stokes, B. T., and Szabo, C. (1999). Peroxynitrite production and activation of poly (adenosine diphosphate- ribose) synthetase in spinal cord injury. *Ann Neurol* **45**, 120–4.

Shelbourne, P. F., Killeen, N., Hevner, R. F., Johnston, H. M., Tecott, L., Lewandoski, M., Ennis, M., Ramirez, L., Li, Z., Iannicola, C., Littman, D. R., and Myers, R. M. (1999). A Huntington's disease CAG expansion at the murine Hdh locus is unstable and associated with behavioural abnormalities in mice. *Hum Mol Genet* **8**, 763–74.

Sieradzan, K. A., Mechan, A. O., Jones, L., Wanker, E. E., Nukina, N., and Mann, D. M. (1999). Huntington's disease intranuclear inclusions contain truncated, ubiquitinated huntingtin protein. *Exp Neurol* **156**, 92–9.

Smith, D. L., R., P., Woodman, B., E., H., Mahal, A., Klunk, W. E., J., L. X., Wanker, E. E., D., M. K., and Bates, G. P. (2001). Inhibition of polyglutamine aggregation in R6/2 HD brain slices—complex dose response profiles. *Neurobiol Dis*, 8, 1017–26.

Spargo, E., Everall, I. P., and Lantos, P. L. (1993). Neuronal loss in the hippocampus in Huntington's disease: a comparison with HIV infection. *J Neurol Neurosurg Psychiatry* **56**, 487–91.

Steffan, J. S., Kazantsev, A., Spasic-Boskovic, O., Greenwald, M., Zhu, Y. Z., Gohler, H., Wanker, E. E., Bates, G. P., Housman, D. E., and Thompson, L. M. (2000). The Huntington's disease protein interacts with p53 and CREB-binding protein and represses transcription. *Proc Natl Acad Sci, USA* **97**, 6763–8.

Strijbos, P. J. (1998). Nitric oxide in cerebral ischemic neurodegeneration and excitotoxicity. *Crit Rev Neurobiol* **12**, 223–43.

Tabrizi, S. J., Workman, J., Hart, P. E., Mangiarini, L., Mahal, A., Bates, G., Cooper, J. M., and Schapira, A. H. (2000). Mitochondrial dysfunction and free radical damage in the Huntington R6/2 transgenic mouse. *Ann Neurol* **47**, 80–6.

Takahashi, S., Ujihara, H., Huang, G. Z., Yagyu, K. I., Sanbo, M., Kaba, H., and Yagi, T. (1999). Reduced hippocampal LTP in mice lacking a presynaptic protein: complexin II. *Eur J Neurosci* **11**, 2359–66.

Telenius, H., Kremer, B., Goldberg, Y. P., Theilmann, J., Andrew, S. E., Zeisler, J., Adam, S., Greenberg, C., Ives, E. J., Clarke, L. A., *et al.* (1994). Somatic and gonadal mosaicism of the Huntington disease gene CAG repeat in brain and sperm [published erratum appears in *Nat Genet* 1994 ; **7** (1), 113]. *Nat Genet* **6**, 409–14.

Turmaine, M., Raza, A., Mahal, A., Mangiarini, L., Bates, G. P., and Davies, S. W. (2000). Nonapoptotic neurodegeneration in a transgenic mouse model of Huntington's disease. *Proc Natl Acad Sci, USA* **97**, 8093–97.

Usdin, M. T., Shelbourne, P. F., Myers, R. M., and Madison, D. V. (1999). Impaired synaptic plasticity in mice carrying the Huntington's disease mutation. *Hum Mol Genet* **8**, 839–46.

van Dellen, A., Blakemore, C., Deacon, R., York, D., and Hannan, A. J. (2000a). Delaying the onset of Huntington's in mice. *Nature* **404**, 721–2.

van Dellen, A., Welch, J., Dixon, R. M., Cordery, P., York, D., Styles, P., Blakemore, C., and Hannan, A. J. (2000b). N-Acetylaspartate and DARPP-32 levels decrease in the corpus striatum of Huntington's disease mice. *Neuroreport* **11**, 3751–7.

Vonsattel, J. P. and DiFiglia, M. (1998). Huntington disease. *J Neuropathol Exp Neurol* **57**, 369–84.

—— Myers, R. H., Stevens, T. J., Ferrante, R. J., Bird, E. D., and Richardson, E. P., Jr. (1985). Neuropathological classification of Huntington's disease. *J Neuropathol Exp Neurol* **44**, 559–77.

Weeks, R. A., Piccini, P., Harding, A. E., and Brooks, D. J. (1996). Striatal D1 and D2 dopamine receptor loss in asymptomatic mutation carriers of Huntington's disease. *Ann Neurol* **40**, 49–54.

Wheeler, V. C., Auerbach, W., White, J. K., Srinidhi, J., Auerbach, A., Ryan, A., Duyao, M. P., Vrbanac, V., Weaver, M., Gusella, J. F., Joyner, A. L., and MacDonald, M. E. (1999). Length-dependent gametic CAG repeat instability in the Huntington's disease knock-in mouse. *Hum Mol Genet* **8**, 115–22.

—— White, J. K., Gutekunst, C. A., Vrbanac, V., Weaver, M., Li, X. J., Li, S. H., Yi, H., Vonsattel, J. P., Gusella, J. F., Hersch, S., Auerbach, W., Joyner, A. L., and MacDonald, M. E. (2000). Long glutamine tracts cause nuclear localization of a novel form of huntingtin in medium spiny striatal neurons in HdhQ92 and HdhQ111 knock-in mice. *Hum Mol Genet* **9**, 503–13.

White, J. K., Auerbach, W., Duyao, M. P., Vonsattel, J. P., Gusella, J. F., Joyner, A. L., and MacDonald, M. E. (1997). Huntingtin is required for neurogenesis and is not impaired by the Huntington's disease CAG expansion. *Nat Genet* **17**, 404–10.

Yamamoto, A., Lucas, J. J., and Hen, R. (2000). Reversal of neuropathology and motor dysfunction in a conditional model of Huntington's disease. *Cell* **101**, 57–66.

Young, A. B. (1998) In *Molecular neurology* (ed. J. B. Martin), pp. 35–54. Scientific American Inc., New York.

Zeitlin, S., Liu, J. P., Chapman, D. L., Papaioannou, V. E., and Efstratiadis, A. (1995). Increased apoptosis and early embryonic lethality in mice nullizygous for the Huntington's disease gene homologue. *Nat Genet* **11**, 155–63.

Section 5 Other polyglutamine diseases

14 The polyglutamine diseases

Gillian P. Bates and Caroline Benn

Introduction

In 1991, the first triplet repeat mutation was identified as the CGG repeat expansion that causes fragile X syndrome (Verkerk *et al*. 1991). That same year, La Spada *et al*. (1991) identified the mutation that causes spinal and bulbar muscular atrophy (SBMA), also known as Kennedy's disease, and found it to be a $(CAG)_n$ expansion in the gene that encodes the androgen receptor (AR). The mutation lay within the coding region of the gene leading to an increase in the length of a stretch of polyglutamine (polyQ) residues in the androgen receptor protein. Since then, a further eight late-onset neurodegenerative diseases have been found to be caused by an increased number of CAG repeat residues, which in each case leads to the expansion of a polyQ tract in the protein in question. These disorders include Huntington's disease (HD; Huntington's Disease Collaborative Research Group 1993), dentatorubral-pallidoluysian atrophy (DRPLA; Koide *et al*. 1994; Nagafuchi *et al*. 1994), and the spinocerebellar ataxias (SCAs) types 1 (Orr *et al*. 1993), 2 (Imbert *et al*. 1996; Pulst *et al*. 1996; Sanpei *et al*. 1996), 3 (also known as Machado–Joseph disease; Kawaguchi *et al*. 1994), 6 (Zhuchenko *et al*. 1997), 7 (David *et al*. 1997), and 17 (Fujigasaki *et al*. 2001; Koide *et al*. 1999; Nakamura *et al*. 2001; Zuhlke *et al*. 2001). This chapter describes and compares the major features of the clinical course, genetics, and neuropathology of these diseases and attempts to distil common pathways of their molecular pathogenesis from recent insights.

Clinical manifestations

The polyQ diseases present a wide spectrum of clinical profiles. In all cases the disease is progressive and unfailingly leads to death over a period of 10–30 years. As a rule, onset is in midlife, although most of the polyQ disorders may also present with a distinct set of symptoms during childhood or adolescence. These early-onset cases have generally inherited the mutation from their father.

SBMA is a mild motor neurone disease that causes proximal muscle weakness and atrophy, dysarthria, dysphagia, fasciculations of the tongue, lips, or perioral region of the face, and, frequently, a subclinical sensory neuropathy (Lieberman and Fischbeck 2000). Affected males may also show signs of androgen insensitivity including gynaecomastia, testicular atrophy, and reduced fertility. As SBMA is X-linked, it predominantly affects males, although female carriers have been reported to exhibit mild symptoms of the disease (Belsham *et al*. 1992; Ferlini *et al*. 1995). The other polyQ disorders are autosomal dominant. The clinical presentation of HD has been described in detail in Chapters 2 and 3. Symptoms are variable and complex comprising psychiatric, motor, and cognitive components and the first presentation may be either psychiatric or motor in nature. The movement disorder seen in adult-onset individuals includes chorea, dystonia, ataxia, bradykinesia, dysphagia, and dysarthria and often progresses to an akinetic state. In contrast, juvenile HD patients may never exhibit chorea but instead develop rigidity, seizures, tremor, and/or myoclonus. Prior to mutation detection, a diagnosis of HD was sometimes mistakenly given to individuals carrying the DRPLA mutation, because the adult forms of these diseases can present with similar signs. The cardinal features of DRPLA are ataxia and dementia and, if onset is after the age of 20, patients may additionally exhibit choreoathetosis and psychiatric symptoms, whereas before 20 the additional signs are epilepsy and myoclonus (corresponding to the progressive myoclonus epilepsy phenotype) (Tsuji 2000). DRPLA shows marked heterogeneity in the clinical presentation, which may even occur within the same family.

Prior to the impact of genetics, classification of the autosomal dominant spinocerebellar ataxias (ADCAs, now known as spinocerebellar ataxias, SCAs) proved extraordinarily difficult. The most useful system, devised by Harding (1984), divided these diseases into three categories based on clinical criteria. This system has turned out to be vastly oversimplified and reflects the wide variation and overlap in the symptoms of the different SCA diseases. Genetic analysis has now defined 17 SCA mutations, a number set to increase further. Of these, 8 have been cloned. SCA1, SCA2, SCA3, SCA6, SCA7, and SCA17 are caused by a CAG repeat expansion in the coding region of the gene in question and are polyQ expansion diseases. In contrast, SCA8 (Koob *et al.* 1999) and SCA12 (Holmes *et al.* 1999) associated with CTG and CAG expansions, respectively, are located in non-coding regions, and therefore do not result in polyQ expansions; they will not be discussed in this chapter.

As with HD and DRPLA, the SCAs can show a large degree of clinical heterogeneity within each disease and even between members of the same family, which in the past often made clinical diagnosis difficult. The frequency of signs associated with five of the SCA mutations is illustrated in Table 14.1 (taken from a review by Stevanin *et al.* 2000). SCAs 1, 2, 3, 4, and 12 were initially categorized as ADCA type I by Harding, in that they exhibit cerebellar ataxia and, variably, ophthalmoplegia, optic atrophy, dementia, extrapyramidal signs, and amyotrophy. SCA7 falls into ADCA type II, in that it also presents with progressive macular dystrophy. It accounts for almost all of the ADCA type II families as only one family with this phenotype does not segregate the SCA7 mutation (Stevanin *et al.* 2000). ADCA type III encompasses the pure cerebellar syndrome (SCA5, SCA6, SCA8, and SCA11). Several families have recently been described in which the CAG repeat lies in the reading frame of TBP (TATA-binding protein), denoted SCA17 (Fujigasaki *et al.* 2001; Koide *et al.* 1999; Nakamura *et al.* 2001; Zuhlke *et al.* 2001). SCA10 and SCA17 families develop cerebellar ataxia with epilepsy. Dementia, psychosis, hyperreflexia, bradykinesia, and, in some cases, dystonia or chorea have also been described in SCA17.

The juvenile forms of these diseases may present very differently from those that initiate in midlife. For example, retinitis pigmentosa has been described in an infant with an SCA2 expansion of greater than 200 CAGs (Babovic-Vuksanovic *et al.* 1998) and the juvenile form of SCA7 also affects nonneuronal tissue (heart) (Benton *et al.* 1998; David *et al.* 1998). A juvenile case of HD presenting with progressive myoclonic epilepsy was recently described (Gambardella *et al.* 2001).

The identification of the mutation underlying the polyQ disorders has provided new opportunities for diagnostic and predictive testing. One consequence of this is that the variability of

Table 14.1 Frequency of neurological signs associated with SCA mutations (reproduced with permission from Stevanin *et al.* 2000)

	SCA1	SCA2	SCA3	SCA6	SCA7
Mean age at onset (years)	34	35	38	45	30
Onset after 55 years	−	−	±	++	−
Cerebellar syndrome	+++	+++	+++	+++	+++
Dysarthria	+++	+++	+++	++	+++
Babinski sign	++	+	++	0	++
Brisk reflexes	++	+	++	+	+++
Diminished or abolished reflexes	+	++	++	++	0
Spasticity in lower limbs	++	±	++	±	++
Amyotrophy	+	+	++	−	++
Extrapyramidal syndrome/dystonia	±	±	+	0	+
Myoclonus	−	++	±	−	
Nystagmus	++	+	+++	++	+
Ophthalmoplegia	++	++	++	0	++
Decreased saccade velocity	+	++	+	0	+++
Decreased visual acuity	0	0	0	0	+++
Bulging eyes	+	+	+	0	+
Myokymia	+	++	+	0	+
Decreased vibration sense	++	++	+	++	++
Dysphagia	++	++	++	++	++
Sphincter disturbances	++	++	++	++	++
Dementia	+	+	+	0	+
Tremor	−	+	±	±	+
Axonal neuropathy	++	+++	++	0	+
Decreased hearing acuity	0	0	0	0	+

Frequency of neurological signs ranging from rare (−) to frequent (+++). O=no association with disease.

symptoms for a given disorder grows wider as individuals are given an accurate diagnosis based on mutation analysis, which may not correspond to the previously defined clinical criteria for that disease. For example, recent reports include a family in which SCA3 phenotypically resembles parkinsonism and is levodopa-responsive (Gwinn-Hardy *et al.* 2001) and a disorder, similar both clinically and neuropathologically to multiple system atrophy (MSA), that segregates with the SCA1 mutation (Gilman *et al.* 1996).

Genetics, epidemiology, and the CAG repeat mutation

The distribution of normal and expanded CAG alleles

The size distribution of the normal and expanded CAG alleles for all of the polyQ disorders is collated in Table 14.2. In general, the normal alleles are highly polymorphic although the degree of polymorphism varies between loci. It is lowest in the case of SCA2 and SCA7, for which the heterozygosity rates are only 24 and 35 per cent, respectively, because allele frequencies approach 80 per cent for alleles with 22 and 10 CAG repeats at the SCA2 and SCA7 loci, respectively (Stevanin *et al.* 2000). Normal alleles are composed of pure CAG repeat tracts in all of the diseases except SCA1, in which most are interrupted by 1–3 CAT triplets (Chong *et al.* 1995), and SCA2 and SCA17, where the interrupting triplet is CAA (Imbert

Table 14.2 Summary of the normal and pathogenic CAG repeat ranges for the polyQ diseases

Disease	Gene location	CAG repeat range*	
		Normal	Mutant
HD	4p16.3	6–39	36– >200
DRPLA	12p13.31	3–35	49–88
SBMA	Xq11–12	9–33	38–65
SCA1	6p23	6–44	39–83
SCA2	12q24.1	13–33	32– >200
SCA3/MJD	14q32.1	3–40	54–89
SCA6	19p13.1	4–19	20–33
SCA7	3p12–13	4–35	37–306
SCA17	6q27	25–44	46–63

*Repeat sizes were collated from a wide literature reporting repeat sizes for these diseases.

et al. 1996; Koide *et al.* 1999; Pulst *et al.* 1996; Sanpei *et al.* 1996). SCA1 and SCA2 interrupted repeats can reach a size corresponding to small pathological alleles in rare cases. The interruptions have been proposed to stabilize the normal alleles, which are transmitted without changing size, even when in the pathological size range. For SCA17 the sequence of the repeat is more complex, with all pathogenic alleles harbouring at least two distinct CAA interruptions (Fujigasaki *et al.* 2001; Nakamura *et al.* 2001; Zuhlke *et al.* 2001).

Pathological alleles translate into polyQ repeats of a length beyond a certain size threshold. The normal and pathogenic repeat ranges overlap in three of the diseases, HD, SCA1, and SCA2 (Table 14.2). In HD the repeats that fall within the region of overlap (36–39) are incompletely penetrant, the risk of developing HD increasing with size (Myers *et al.* 1998; see Chapters 5 and 7, this volume). This region of overlap may be caused by the influence of modifier genes on the onset of the disease. The overlap in SCA1 could reflect a different amino acid repeat composition, as the CAT interruptions in the DNA translate to histidine interruptions in the ataxin-1 protein, which results in a reduced pathogenicity as compared to that of a pure polyQ tract of an equivalent size (Matsuyama *et al.* 1999). The CAA interruptions in SCA2 and SCA17 could not reduce pathogenicity in the same way, because CAA, like CAG, encodes the amino acid glutamine. In keeping with this, two SCA2 patients have been found to carry interrupted 34-CAG repeat pathogenic alleles (Costanzi-Porrini *et al.* 2000) and all SCA17 pathogenic alleles are interrupted repeats (Fujigasaki *et al.* 2001; Nakamura *et al.* 2001; Zuhlke *et al.* 2001).

The slight overlap in the normal and pathogenic ranges and the closeness in size of the largest normal and smallest pathogenic alleles in HD, SBMA, SCA1, SCA2, SCA6, SCA7, and SCA17 suggest that the pathogenic mechanism is caused by a threshold effect. The diseases can be roughly sorted into clusters in which the smallest mutant alleles are comparable: 32–39 for HD, SBMA, SCA1, SCA2, and SCA7 and 47–54 for DRPLA, SCA3, and SCA17. These differences most probably reflect the influence of the protein context on the polyQ toxicity in each of these diseases. The pathogenic range of SCA6 differs most, in that it completely overlaps with the normal range for all of the other diseases. Whether this reflects a different pathogenic mechanism or merely a more dramatic influence of the protein context in which the repeat is located is currently unknown and is discussed further in the subsection

'Gain of function/loss of function'. In all cases, relatively few expansions exceed 100 repeats and, when they do occur, these are always associated with infantile forms of the disease.

Genetics and epidemiology

The overall prevalence of all of the SCAs is estimated to be less than 10/100 000 (Stevanin *et al.* 2000). DRPLA occurs most frequently in Japan (Inazuki *et al.* 1990), where it has a prevalence of approximately 0.2 to 0.7/100 000 (corresponding to the prevalence of HD in Japan), and SBMA is extremely rare. These compare with a prevalence of 4–7/100 000 for HD (see Chapter 6). The relative frequencies of the polyQ repeat diseases can vary widely depending upon the ethnic and/or geographical origin of the families. Although DRPLA occurs predominantly in Japan, mutation analysis has now identified a number of families in Caucasian populations (Becher *et al.* 1997; Warner *et al.* 1995; Norremolle *et al.* 1995) and shown that DRPLA is also segregating in the African–American family with Haw River syndrome (Burke *et al.* 1994). In most countries, SCA3 represents the major SCA locus, but the frequency varies widely (Durr *et al.* 1996; Leggo *et al.* 1997; Mizushima *et al.* 1998; Riess *et al.* 1997a; Schols *et al.* 1997; Silveira *et al.* 1996, 1998; Stevanin *et al.* 2000; Takano *et al.* 1998; Zhou *et al.* 1998) with SCA3 representing 80 per cent of ADCA families in Portugal, 30 per cent in France, 40 per cent in Germany, and 39 per cent in Japan, whilst it has yet to be detected in Italy (Pareyson *et al.* 1999). Similarly, the frequency of SCA6 varies considerably accounting for 1–15 per cent of SCAs in White ethnic subgroups (Geschwind *et al.* 1997; Moseley *et al.* 1998; Pujana *et al.* 1999; Schols *et al.* 1998; Silveira *et al.* 1998; Stevanin *et al.* 1997a) compared with 5.9–30 per cent in Japan (Matsumura *et al.* 1997; Matsuyama *et al.* 1997; Nagai *et al.* 1998; Takano *et al.* 1998; Watanabe *et al.* 1998).

These regional differences most probably result from founder effects, in support of which linkage disequilibrium has been detected with flanking or intragenic markers at the loci for HD (see Chapters 5 and 6), SMBA (Tanaka *et al.* 1996a), and SCA1 (Wakisaka *et al.* 1995) in Japan; SCA2 in northern Europe (Didierjean *et al.* 1999); SCA3/MJD in France, Portugal, and Japan (Endo *et al.* 1996; Gaspar *et al.* 1996; Stevanin *et al.* 1995, 1997b; Takiyama *et al.* 1995); SCA6 in Germany (Dichgans *et al.* 1999) and Japan (Yabe *et al.* 2001); and SCA7 in Korea, north Africa, continental Europe, and Anglo-Saxon populations (Stevanin *et al.* 1999). On the other hand, linkage disequilibrium with intragenic polymorphisms in the SCA3 gene has shown that several different founders existed in Portugal, where this locus is responsible for nearly all SCAs (Stevanin *et al.* 1997b). It has also established that SCA3 mutations have arisen independently in Black African and Jewish populations and so were not introduced by Portuguese sailors or travellers as had previously been proposed (Stevanin *et al.* 1997b, 2000).

Mutation analysis has also provided insights into the mechanism of mutation. New mutations have been reported in HD (Myers *et al.* 1993; see Chapters 5 and 7, this volume), SCA2 (Schols *et al.* 1997), SCA6 (Shimazaki *et al.* 2001; Shizuka *et al.* 1998), and SCA7 (Stevanin *et al.* 1998). In all cases these have arisen as expansions from alleles at the high end of the normal range, sometimes termed intermediate alleles. These are $(CAG)_{27-35}$ in the case of HD, $(CAG)_{34}$ for SCA2, $(CAG)_{14/17-19}$ for SCA6, and $(CAG)_{28-35}$ for SCA7. With the exception of the SCA6 expansions, which occurred on maternal alleles, the new mutations all occurred in alleles transmitted from the father. Therefore, a degree of instability has been observed in alleles at the high end of the normal range and almost exclusively occurs on paternal chromosomes. These large normal alleles may act as a reservoir for new mutations, which would occur in a recurrent but random manner. In the case of SCA7 this might explain the persistence of the disease despite the great anticipation (~20 years/generation) (Stevanin *et al.* 1998). If this were the case, the relative frequency of a polyQ disease should correlate with the frequency of large normal alleles in a given population. In support of this, the proportion of large normal alleles (>17 repeats) at the DRPLA locus is significantly higher in the Japanese than in Caucasians and reflects the relative disease frequency of 20 per cent and less than 1 per cent, respectively, in these populations (Takano *et al.* 1998). It would also be expected that the haplotype of pathogenic and large normal alleles might correspond. Indeed, the haplotype segregating in all French SCA3 families is present on only 25 per cent of normal alleles but in all large normal alleles over 33 repeats (Stevanin *et al.* 1997b).

CAG repeat size and age at onset

In all cases, the polyQ diseases show an inverse relationship between the age of onset of the disorder and CAG repeat size (see review by Gusella and MacDonald 2000). However, in all cases, there is a wide variation in the age of onset for any given repeat size (David *et al.* 1997; Fujigasaki *et al.* 2001; Igarashi *et al.* 1992; Imbert *et al.* 1996; Ishikawa *et al.* 1997; Kawaguchi *et al.* 1994; Koide *et al.* 1994; Nagafuchi *et al.* 1994; Nakamura *et al.* 2001; Orr *et al.* 1993; Pulst *et al.* 1996; Riess *et al.* 1997b; Sanpei *et al.* 1996; see Chapter 5, this volume), indicating that other factors are also important in determining onset and progression. These other factors are likely to be both genetic, in the form of modifying genes (see Chapter 5), and environmental (Georgiou *et al.* 1999).

Homozygosity and its impact on disease manifestation

Individuals who are homozygous for the mutations that cause HD (Wexler *et al.* 1987; see Chapter 5, this volume), DRPLA (Goldfarb *et al.* 1996; Kurohara *et al.* 1997), SCA3 (Kawakami *et al.* 1995; Lang *et al.* 1994), and SCA6 (Geschwind *et al.* 1997; Kato *et al.* 2000; Matsumura *et al.* 1997; Matsuyama *et al.* 1997; Takiyama *et al.* 1998) have been described. The consequences of homozygosity are not consistent between the polyQ diseases. HD and SCA1 are similar in that the disease onset and clinical manifestation correspond to those observed in individuals heterozygous for the larger of the two expanded alleles (Goldfarb *et al.* 1996; see Chapter 5, this volume). In contrast, homozygosity for SCA3 and DRPLA results in a dramatic reduction in the age of onset and clinical course (Kawakami *et al.* 1995; Lang *et al.* 1994; Sato *et al.* 1995). Unexpectedly, homozygosity for an intermediate DRPLA allele (40 or 41 CAGs) causes autosomal recessive spastic paraplegia, a disease quite distinct from DRPLA (Kurohara *et al.* 1997). Overall, SCA6 homozygotes have been reported to show a more severe phenotype (Geschwind *et al.* 1997; Kato *et al.* 2000; Matsumura *et al.* 1997; Matsuyama *et al.* 1997), although in one case (23/23), the disease onset corresponded to the earliest observed for SCA6 heterozygotes with a mutant allele of 23 repeats (Matsuyama *et al.* 1997).

CAG repeat instability

Instability is a cardinal feature of pathogenic triplet repeats and can be detected both on propagation through the germline and also in the form of somatic mosaicism. Repeats that fall well within the normal range are stable, although their highly polymorphic nature indicates that instability must occur, but at a frequency too low to observe when monitoring the inheritance of repeats through families. CAG repeats that fall at the high end of the normal range (also known as intermediate alleles) have been observed to change in size. This usually manifests as an expansion on a paternal chromosome and may produce an allele in the pathogenic range thereby constituting a new mutation.

Gametic instability

All CAG repeat expansions in the pathogenic range can exhibit instability on transmission from one generation to the next, but the extent to which this occurs can vary widely (Table 14.3). In all cases, instability is more pronounced upon inheritance of a paternal allele and there is an overall tendency for the repeats to increase when passed through successive generations. The SCA7 mutation exhibits by far the greatest instability with a mean increase of 18.5 repeats on transmission through the male line compared with only 1.3 repeats for SCA3. This relative degree of instability cannot be a function of repeat size and is most probably related to flanking sequences. In contrast, repeats at the SCA6 locus are comparatively stable and have only rarely been observed to change in size (Shimazaki *et al.* 2001). Changes in repeat size upon transmission are a consequence of gametic instability, which can easily be detected by analysis of whole (Cancel *et al.* 1995; Duyao *et al.* 1993; David *et al.* 1998) or single sperm samples (Monckton *et al.* 1999; Zhang *et al.* 1995).

Gametic instability is the molecular basis of anticipation, a predictive feature of triplet repeat diseases. Due to the strong negative correlation of CAG repeat size and age of disease onset, the tendency of repeats to increase on transmission leads to an earlier age of onset in

Table 14.3 Comparison of the instability of CAG repeats on maternal and paternal transmission and between the polyQ diseases (adapted with permission from Stevanin *et al.* 2000)

Disease	Gender of transmitting parent		References
	Male	Female	
HD	+6.4 (−3 to +41, n=78)	+0.25 (−6 to +12, n=70)	Duyao *et al.* 1993; Ranen *et al.* 1995
DRPLA	+6.6 (0 to +28, n=38)	+0.06 (−4 to +4, n=11)	Koide *et al.* 1994; Ikeuchi *et al.* 1995; Komure *et al.* 1995
SBMA	+1.8 (−2 to +5, n=11)	+0.2 (−4 to +2, n=20)	La Spada *et al.* 1992; Biancalana *et al.* 1992; Watanabe *et al.* 1996
SCA1	+2.7 (−4 to +28, n=43)	−0.04 (−6 to +4, n=46)	Chung *et al.* 1993; Goldfarb *et al.* 1996; Stevanin *et al.* 2000
SCA2	+3.8 (−8 to +17, n=42)	+1.1 (−4 to +8, n=30)	Cancel *et al.* 1997; Sanpei *et al.* 1996; Filla *et al.* 1999
SCA3/ MJD*	+1.3 (−5 to +9, n=57)	+0.7 (−8 to +3, n=63)	Cancel *et al.* 1995; Maruyama *et al.* 1995; Maciel *et al.* 1995; Stevanin *et al.* 1995
SCA6	+0.8 (0 to +6, n=10)	+0.07 (0 to +1, n=15)	Matsuyama *et al.* 1997; Geschwind *et al.* 1997; Shimazaki *et al.* 2001; Reiss *et al.* 1997b
SCA7	+18.5 (−6 to +166, n=49)	+4.2 (−13 to +17, n=66)	David *et al.* 1998; Giunti *et al.* 1999; Gouw *et al.* 1998

*MJD, Machado–Joseph disease.

successive generations. The degree of anticipation observed in any given disease correlates with the level of instability detected at the corresponding gene locus. Therefore, the greatest anticipation is seen in SCA7 families in which the repeat is most unstable. Small pool polymerase chain reaction (PCR) showed that the SCA7 repeat is extremely unstable in the male germline and biased towards massive increases. Most of the mutant sperm of two SCA7 males had repeats so large that many of the resultant offspring would have had at best a severe infantile disease. The underrepresentation of such alleles in patients suggests that a significant proportion of these alleles would be associated with embryonic lethality or dysfunctional sperm (Monckton *et al.* 1999). This is in keeping with the report that the most of the transmitting parents of SCA7 patients are females (Gouw *et al.* 1998). Such an extreme anticipation should lead to the extinction of the disorder because the disease is no longer transmitted by juvenile or infantile patients (Stevanin *et al.* 2000). New mutations, as have been detected for SCA7 (Giunti *et al.* 1999; Stevanin *et al.* 1998), would be essential to maintain a pool of mutant alleles. Surprisingly, anticipation has also been reported in some SCA6 families (Ikeuchi *et al.* 1997; Matsuyama *et al.* 1997; Schols *et al.* 1998), whilst in others it could not be proven (Ishikawa *et al.* 1997). As almost no instability has been detected for the repeat at the SCA6 locus, it is possible that these reports of anticipation are due to ascertainment bias (Stevanin *et al.* 2000). This phenomenon most probably accounted for the discrepancy in the observed and expected levels of anticipation for SCA2 (Cancel *et al.* 1997) and SCA3 (Durr *et al.* 1996), which differed by 8 and 7 years, respectively (Stevanin *et al.* 2000).

Somatic instability

A degree of somatic CAG repeat mosaicism has been reported between different brain regions for HD, DRPLA, SCA1, and SCA3. In all cases, mosaicism was generally higher in the central nervous system (CNS) than the peripheral tissues. The repeat detected in the cerebellar cortex was consistently lower than in other brain regions (Cancel *et al.* 1998; Chong *et al.* 1995; Hashida *et al.* 1997; Lopes-Cendes *et al.* 1996; Takano *et al.* 1996; Tanaka *et al.* 1996b; Telenius *et al.* 1994; Ueno *et al.* 1995). In contrast, CAG instability has not been found in the tissues of SBMA patients or SBMA fibroblast cultures (Spiegel *et al.* 1996; Tanaka *et al.* 1996b).

In an attempt to determine comparative levels of CAG repeat instability at the cellular levels, Watanabe *et al.* (2000) have employed a laser capture dissection approach. In DRPLA they found that the repeats in cerebellar granule cells were smaller than those in cerebellar glial cells and that those in cerebral neuronal cells were smaller than in cerebral glial cells. This is supportive of a previous report showing that cerebellar and hippocampal granule cells have comparatively low levels of CAG repeat instability (Hashida *et al.* 1997). Similarly, it has been shown that more instability can be detected in the cerebral and cerebellar white matter than in the cerebral and cerebellar cortex, respectively (Takano *et al.* 1996).

The proteins containing polyQ repeat expansions

The polyQ expansions that cause SBMA (La Spada *et al.* 1991), SCA6 (Zhuchenko *et al.* 1997), and SCA17 (Koide *et al.* 1999) are located in genes of known function, namely, the androgen receptor (AR; Chang *et al.* 1988), the α_{1A} voltage-dependent calcium channel (CACNA1A), and the TATA-binding protein (TBP; Kao *et al.* 1990), a component of the basal transcription complex. By contrast, the genes that cause HD, DRPLA, SCA1, SCA2,

SCA3, and SCA7 were found to encode proteins of unknown function, identified by positional cloning strategies. These proteins are unrelated except for their polyQ tracts and their major characteristics are summarized in Table 14.4. In all cases these proteins have a very wide or ubiquitous expression profile in both the brain and peripheral tissues that extends far beyond the documented pathology of the diseases with which they are associated.

Although most of the disease proteins have been detected in the nucleus and cytoplasm, TBP function is nuclear and ataxin-2 and the α_{1A} voltage-dependent calcium channel have so far been detected only in the cytoplasm. The AR is a ligand-activated transcription factor that is located predominantly in the cytoplasm of neurones and predominantly in the nuclei of non-neuronal tissue (Li *et al.* 1998a). There are six isoforms of the human α_{1A} voltage-dependent calcium channel and the polyQ tract is present in three of these (Zhuchenko *et al.* 1997). The polyQ-containing isoforms are localized to the cytoplasm and show a higher level of expression in Purkinje cells than other brain regions (Ishikawa *et al.* 1999). Atrophin 1, the ataxins-1, -2, -3, and -7, and huntingtin remain novel proteins and experiments designed to determine subcellular localization and identify interacting partners are being conducted in order to elucidate their functions. The cell biology of huntingtin is described in detail in Chapter 12.

Atrophin 1 is predominantly cytoplasmic but also present in the nuclear compartments of neurones (Schilling *et al.* 1999; Yazawa *et al.* 1995). It has a granular appearance in the cytoplasm and is enriched in the membrane-rich fraction suggestive of a location in the endoplasmic reticulum or transport vesicles (Yazawa *et al.* 1995). It has thus far been found to interact with ETO/MTG8, a component of nuclear receptor co-repressor complexes (Wood *et al.* 2000), with the SH3 domain of an insulin receptor tyrosine kinase substrate (Okamura-Oho *et al.* 1999), two families of WW domain-containing proteins (Wood *et al.* 1998), and with RERE, a homologue of atrophin 1 (Yanagisawa *et al.* 2000).

Ataxin-1 has a nuclear localization in most neurones, except Purkinje cells, where it is found in the cytoplasm and the nucleus; it has also been detected in the cytoplasm in peripheral tissues (Banfi *et al.* 1994; Servadio *et al.* 1995). It contains a self-association domain (Burright *et al.* 1997) and has RNA binding activity (Yue *et al.* 2001). It associates with the

Table 14.4 Major characteristics of the proteins containing pathogenic polyglutamine repeats

Disease	Gene product	Molecular weight (kDa)	Position of polyQ (amino acids)	Intracellular localization	Reference
HD	Huntingtin	348	18/3144	Cytoplasm/nucleus	HDCRG 1993*
DRPLA	Atrophin 1	190	474/1184	Cytoplasm/nucleus	Yazawa *et al.* 1995
SBMA	AR	104	58/918	Cytoplasm/nucleus	Chang *et al.* 1988
SCA1	Ataxin-1	87	197/816	Cytoplasm/nucleus	Banfi *et al.* 1994
SCA2	Ataxin-2	145	166/1313	Cytoplasm	Pulst *et al.* 1996; Sanpei *et al.* 1996; Imbert *et al.* 1996
SCA3	Ataxin-3	46	292/359	Cytoplasm/nucleus	Kawaguchi *et al.* 1994
SCA6	CACNA1A	280	2328/2410	Cytoplasm	Zhuchenko *et al.* 1997
SCA7	Ataxin-7	95	30/893	Cytoplasm/nucleus	David *et al.* 1997
SCA17	TBP	38	58/339	Nucleus	Kao *et al.* 1990

*HDCRG, Huntington's Disease Collaborative Research Group.

nuclear matrix-associated subnuclear structures: promyelocytic leukaemia (PML) bodies in Purkinje cells (Skinner *et al.* 1997), where it co-localizes with the cerebellar leucine-rich acidic nuclear protein (LANP) (Matilla *et al.* 1997). It has also been found to interact with A1UP, a novel protein that contains an *N*-terminal ubiquitin-like region (Davidson *et al.* 2000).

Ataxin-2 is a basic protein with two domains that implicate it in RNA splicing and protein interaction (Huynh *et al.* 1999; Kiehl *et al.* 2001) and is found predominantly in the cytoplasm (Huynh *et al.* 1999; Koyano *et al.* 1999). It has been localized to the trans-Golgi network (Shibata *et al.* 2000) where it co-localizes with A2BP1, a novel protein with RNA-binding motifs with which it interacts (Shibata *et al.* 2000). Both ataxin-2 and A2BP1 have orthologues in *C. elegans*, in which ATX-2, the orthologue of ataxin-2, is essential for early embryonic patterning (Kiehl *et al.* 2000).

Ataxin-3 has been detected in both cytoplasmic and nuclear compartments (Paulson *et al.* 1997a; Tait *et al.* 1998; Wang *et al.* 1997) and interacts with the nuclear matrix (Perez *et al.* 1999; Tait *et al.* 1998). In most neurones it is found to have a cytoplasmic, dendritic, and axonal localization (Trottier *et al.* 1998). There are four different mRNA transcripts arising from the SCA3 gene as a result of differential splicing and polyadenylation (Ichikawa *et al.* 2001). These most probably correspond to the isoforms of ataxin-3 found to be expressed in HeLa cells, only one of which is found in brain where it occurs at an equivalent level in all brain regions (Trottier *et al.* 1998). More recently, ataxin-3 has been found to interact with two human homologues of the yeast DNA repair protein (RAD23) (Wang *et al.* 2000).

Although some ataxin-7 is found in the nucleus in neurones, it is predominantly located in the cell body and processes (Cancel *et al.* 2000; Lindenberg *et al.* 2000) where it co-localizes with BiP, a marker for the endoplasmic reticulum, and not with markers of mitochondria or the trans-Golgi network (Cancel *et al.* 2000). Ataxin-7 interacts with products of the SH3P12 gene (Lebre *et al.* 2001), which may be involved in the regulation, ubiquitination, and degradation of ataxin-7. It has also been found to interact with cone–rod homeobox protein (CRX) and can suppress its transactivation (La Spada *et al.* 2001). In SCA7 transgenic mice, CRX binding activity was reduced, as was the expression of CRX-regulated genes, which may account for the retinal degeneration that occurs in SCA7 (La Spada *et al.* 2001).

Neuropathology of the polyQ diseases

Neurodegeneration

The polyQ disorders each display a characteristic neuropathology. The major sites of neuronal loss occurring in these diseases are summarized in Table 14.5, and a more detailed comparison of the neuropathology occurring in the spinocerebellar ataxias can be found in Stevanin *et al.* (2000). In most cases, a more widespread pathology occurs in individuals carrying CAG expansions at the higher end of the disease range (Fig. 14.1) (Young 1998). For example, expansions that cause juvenile onset lead to extensive involvement of the cerebellum, globus pallidus, and cerebral cortex in HD; striatal, cortical, and white matter pathology in DRPLA; and basal ganglia pathology in SCA3. In juvenile SCA7, in addition to a wider CNS pathology, nonneuronal tissues (heart) are also affected (Benton *et al.* 1998; David *et al.* 1998). The appearance of more extensive, widespread, and overlapping pathologies in individuals carrying large CAG expansions in many of these genes suggests that common mechanisms underlie the neuronal degeneration occurring in these diseases.

Table 14.5 Brain regions showing the major pathology for each of the polyQ disorders

Disease	Typical neuropathology of the adult disease
HD	Atrophy of the caudate-putamen, deep layers of the cerebral cortex, thalamus, globus pallidus, hippocampus, and occasionally the cerebellum; see Chapter 8
DRPLA	Marked neuronal loss in the cerebral cortex, cerebellar cortex, globus pallidus, striatum, and the dentate nucleus and subthalamic and red nuclei; intense gliosis and severe demyelination at many of the sites of neuronal degeneration and in some families, calcification of the basal ganglia
SBMA	Loss of anterior horn cells in the spinal cord, sensory neurones in the dorsal root ganglia, brainstem nuclei, lower motor neurones in the spinal cord
SCA1	Cerebellar atrophy with severe loss of Purkinje cells (vermis), dentate nucleus and neurones of the inferior olive, and cranial nerve nuclei III, IV, IX, X, and XII; gliosis of the cerebellar molecular layer
SCA2	Loss of Purkinje cells and granule cells from the cerebellum; atrophy of the frontotemporal lobes; degeneration of the substantia nigra; gliosis of the inferior olive and pons
SCA3	Lesions of the basal ganglia (internal pallidum, subthalamic nucleus, and substantia nigra), brainstem motor nuclei, spinal cord, and dentate nucleus; Purkinje cell loss is mild and the inferior olives are typically spared
SCA6	Marked cerebellar atrophy with loss of Purkinje cells, and moderate loss of cerebellar granule cells, dentate nucleus neurones, and neurones of the inferior olive
SCA7	Primary cell loss in the cerebellum, inferior olive, and some cranial nerve nuclei; hypomyelination of the optic tract and gliosis of the lateral geniculate body and loss of photoreceptors and some epithelial pigment cells in the visual cortex
SCA17	Neuronal loss in the caudate nucleus and putamen, thalamus, frontal cortex, temporal cortex, Purkinje cells and increase in Bergmann glia. Only two patients have been described: in one the loss of Purkinje cells was the major lesion; in the other Purkinje cell loss was mild

Whilst the proteins that harbour the polyQ expansions have extensively overlapping expression patterns, expression levels are likely to be partially responsible for the differing pathological profiles. SBMA retains a relatively selective neurodegeneration even at the higher repeat numbers, probably because of the low level of expression of the AR in neurones other than the anterior horn cells and brainstem nuclei (Young 1998). In the case of SCA3, only a small population of interneurones in the striatum express ataxin-3, which may account for the absence of striatal pathology and the sparing of the GABAergic projection neurones that are most vulnerable in HD (Paulson *et al.* 1997a). In keeping with this, expression of the same truncated AR transgene under either the neurofilament light chain or prion promoters in transgenic mice resulted in different neurological phenotypes (Abel *et al.* 2001). Similarly, expression of a polyQ tract under the control of the AR promoter produced a distribution of polyQ aggregates that resembled that in SBMA, but yet was more widespread (Adachi *et al.* 2001). Of course, expression levels are only one factor that distinguishes the molecular pathogenesis of these disorders, and the protein context in which the mutation resides is also clearly important. This is nicely illustrated by the comparison of mouse models in which mutant versions of either truncated huntingtin or full-length atrophin transgenes are expressed under the control of the prion promoter. Although cell death was not seen in either model, nuclear aggregates form in both models, but extranuclear aggregates are only present in the HD mice and tremors and seizures are only seen in the DRPLA mice (Schilling *et al.* 2001).

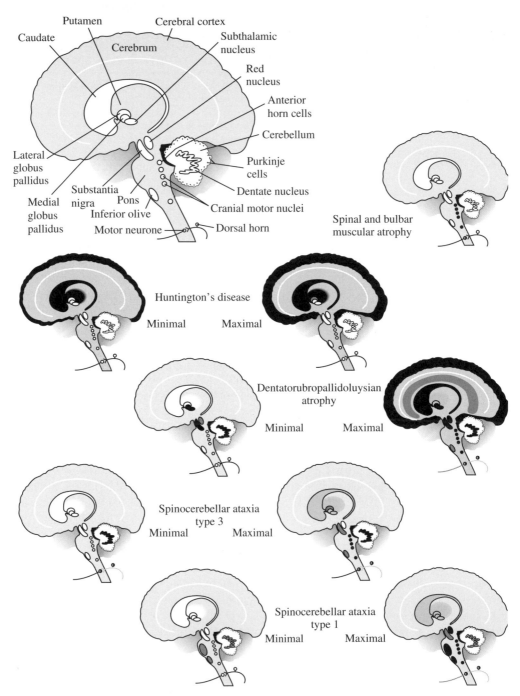

Fig. 14.1 Illustration of the brain pathology in five of the polyQ diseases. Both minimal pathology as seen with CAG repeats at the lower end of the mutant range and maximal pathology as seen with larger expansions are shown. Areas that are shaded darkly depict severe pathology and the lighter shades indicate different degrees of intermediate pathology. (Reproduced from Young 1998 with permission of WebMO Corporation.)

Polyglutamine aggregation and the formation of inclusion bodies

PolyQ aggregates or inclusion bodies are present in neuronal nuclei for all of the polyQ diseases (Table 14.6). They can be detected with antibodies to the protein that harbours the polyQ expansion, ubiquitin, and the 1C2 antibody (Trottier *et al.* 1995). In some cases, they cannot be identified with antibodies raised against all regions of the protein in question, possibly because of epitope masking or, alternatively, because aggregates contain only a fragment of the disease protein. This is true for huntingtin (DiFiglia *et al.* 1997) and for the AR (Li *et al.* 1998a), in which aggregates are not recognized by *C*-terminal antibodies, which detect epitopes physically distant from the polyQ tracts in the proteins. In general, antibodies to ubiquitin detect fewer nuclear aggregates than those raised against the disease protein (DiFiglia *et al.* 1997; Duyckaerts *et al.* 1999; Holmberg *et al.* 1998; Mauger *et al.* 1999), although this is not always the case (Hayashi *et al.* 1998). This may indicate that not all aggregates are ubiquitinated or may reflect differences in antibody affinities. The 1C2 antibody was initially raised against TBP and selectively recognized pathogenic polyQ stretches on Western blots (Trottier *et al.* 1995). However, 1C2 is often less successful than antibodies raised against the disease protein at identifying nuclear aggregates and studies that have only used 1C2 are likely to have underestimated the frequency with which these inclusion bodies occur (Mauger *et al.* 1999). At the ultrastructural level, nuclear inclusions appear as granular and filamentous structures that are devoid of a membrane (DiFiglia *et al.* 1997; Hayashi *et al.* 1998; Mauger *et al.* 1999; Takahashi *et al.* 2001) and are frequently associated with nuclear indentations (Davies *et al.* 1997; Takahashi *et al.* 2001).

Nuclear aggregates are generally found in regions associated with neurodegeneration (Becher *et al.* 1998; DiFiglia *et al.* 1997; Duyckaerts *et al.* 1999; Fujigasaki *et al.* 2001; Gutekunst *et al.* 1999; Hayashi *et al.* 1998; Holmberg *et al.* 1998; Ishikawa *et al.* 2001; Koyano *et al.* 1999; Li *et al.* 1998a; Mauger *et al.* 1999; Nakamura *et al.* 2001; Paulson *et al.* 1997b; Skinner *et al.* 1997), including the retina in SCA7 (Mauger *et al.* 1999), although one notable exception is the absence of nuclear inclusions in the cerebellum in SCA2 (Huynh *et al.* 1999; Koyano *et al.* 1999, 2000). A wider distribution for nuclear aggregates than for the classical neurodegenerative pathology has been described for HD (Becher *et al.* 1998), DRPLA (Hayashi *et al.* 1998), SCA1 (Duyckaerts *et al.* 1999), SCA3 (Paulson *et al.* 1997b), SCA7 (Holmberg *et al.* 1998), and SCA17 (Fujigasaki *et al.* 2001), and a wider distribution has been described in juvenile DRPLA than in the adult-onset form of the disease (Hayashi *et al.* 1998). Nuclear aggregates are not restricted to neurones and have been identified in glial cells in DRPLA (Hayashi *et al.* 1998). In SBMA, they have been described in a range of peripheral tissues including scrotal skin, dermal skin, kidney, heart, and testis (Li *et al.* 1998b).

Cytoplasmic aggregates have been detected in HD (DiFiglia *et al.* 1997; Gutekunst *et al.* 1999), SCA2 (Huynh *et al.* 2000), and SCA6 (Ishikawa *et al.* 1999, 2001; see Table 14.6). In adult-onset HD brains, extranuclear aggregates in the form of dystrophic neurites and neuropil aggregates are more extensive than nuclear aggregates (DiFiglia *et al.* 1997; Gutekunst *et al.* 1999), although the frequency of nuclear aggregates increases in brains from juvenile patients (DiFiglia *et al.* 1997). Cytoplasmic microaggregates have been described in SCA2 (Huynh *et al.* 2000). In SCA6 both nuclear and cytoplasmic aggregates are found exclusively in Purkinje cells (Ishikawa *et al.* 1999, 2001). Immunostaining with either 1C2 or a Ca^{2+} channel-specific antibody detected aggregates in both locations but double labelling showed that they do not often co-localize and those staining with the Ca^{2+} channel-specific antibody are typically larger (Ishikawa *et al.* 2001). An SCA1 patient has also been described with

Table 14.6 The location of polyQ aggregates and detection of cleavage products in the polyQ diseases

Disease	Protein	Location of polyQ aggregates	Possible cleavage product*
HD	Huntingtin	Nuclear/cytoplasmic	+
DRPLA	Atrophin 1	Nuclear	+
SBMA	AR	Nuclear	+
SCA1	Ataxin-1	Nuclear	−
SCA2	Ataxin-2	Nuclear/cytoplasmic	+
SCA3	Ataxin-3	Nuclear	−
SCA6	CACNA1A	Nuclear/cytoplasmic	NS
SCA7	Ataxin-7	Nuclear	+
SCA17	TBP	Nuclear	NS

*NS, Not studied.

neuropathological findings similar to those of MSA with glial cytoplasmic inclusions (Gilman *et al.* 1996).

The accumulation of a diffuse staining pattern in neuronal nuclei and cytoplasm has also been described as an additional pathological feature. This has taken the form of diffuse ataxin-2 staining in the nuclei and cytoplasm of cerebellar neurones in SCA2 brains (Huynh *et al.* 1999; Koyano *et al.* 2000). Atrophin 1 staining was present in the neuronal and some glial nuclei in DRPLA brains (Yamada *et al.* 2000) and in neuronal nuclei in a mouse model of DRPLA (Schilling *et al.* 1999). 1C2 immunostaining has also been seen in the cytoplasm of neurones from an SCA7 brain (Holmberg *et al.* 1998) and in the nuclei from HD, SCA3, SBMA (Yamada *et al.* 2000), and SCA17 brains (Nakamura *et al.* 2001). In DRPLA, SCA3, and SBMA, the diffuse intranuclear accumulation of mutant disease proteins occurred much more frequently than nuclear inclusions and involved a much wider distribution (Yamada *et al.* 2000).

In certain cases, a complete correlation between the relative distributions of the aggregated form of the mutant proteins and neuronal cell death has not been observed. For example, in HD huntingtin aggregates predominate in the cerebral cortex and can be comparatively sparse in the striatum (Gutekunst *et al.* 1999; see Chapter 8, this volume). This has been used to argue that polyQ aggregates are not causative in the molecular pathogenesis of these diseases. However, for a polyQ aggregate to lead to the death of a neurone, it is not a prerequisite that it is located in the neurone that dies. Recent neuropathological studies suggest that, in the earlier stages of HD, accumulation of *N*-terminal huntingtin in the cytoplasm is associated with the degeneration of the corticostriatal pathway (Sapp *et al.* 1999). In support of this principle it has been found recently that, in mice transgenic for mutant ataxin-7 expressed under the control of highly specific promoters, neuronal degeneration occurs postsynaptic to neurones that express ataxin-7 and contain ataxin-7 aggregates (Yvert *et al.* 2000).

In vivo models of polyQ disease

Without exception polyQ expansions cause late-onset neurodegenerative diseases; therefore, it might seem surprising that it has been possible to model polyQ disease in organisms as

Table 14.7 Mouse models of the polyQ diseases for which a progressive neurological disorder has been described*

Disease	Strain background	Promoter	Protein	Repeat size	Aggregates	Reference
DRPLA	C57BL/6 × C3H	Prion	Atrophin 1	65Q	Nuclear	Schilling *et al.* 1999
SBMA	C57BL/6 × SJL	Prion	AR (t)	112Q	Nuclear	Abel *et al.* 2001
SBMA	C57BL/6 × SJL	NFL	AR (t)	112Q	Nuclear	Abel *et al.* 2001
SBMA	C57BL/6 × (C57BL/6 × SJL)	AR	polyQ	239Q	Nuclear	Adachi *et al.* 2001
SCA1	FVB/N	Pcp2	Ataxin-1	82Q	Nuclear[†]	Burright *et al.* 1995
SCA1	FVB/N	Pcp2	Ataxin-1Δ77[‡]	82Q	Nuclear	Klement *et al.* 1998
SCA1	C57BL/6 × 129	Endogenous	Ataxin-7	78Q[§]	Not detected	Lorenzetti *et al.* 2000
SCA2	C57BL/6 × DBA	Pcp2	Ataxin-2	58Q	Cytoplasmic[¶]	Huynh *et al.* 2000
SCA3	NR	Pcp2	Ataxin-3 (t)	79Q	NR	Ikeda *et al.* 1996
SCA7	C57BL/6 × (C57BL/6 × SJL)	Pcp2	Ataxin-7	90Q	Nuclear	Yvert *et al.* 2000
	C57BL/6 × (C57BL/6 × SJL)	Rhodopsin	Ataxin-7	90Q	Nuclear[∥]	Yvert *et al.* 2000
SCA7	C57BL/6 × (C57BL/6 × SJL)	PDGF-B	Ataxin-7	128Q	Nuclear	Yvert *et al.* 2001
SCA7	C57BL/6 × (C57BL/6 × C3H)	Prion	Ataxin-7	92Q	Nuclear	La Spada *et al.* 2001

*Abbreviations: AR, androgen receptor; (t), truncated protein; NFL, neurofilament light chain; Pcp2, Purkinje cell-specific promoter 2; NR, not reported; PDGF-B, platelet-derived growth factor B chain.
[†]Subsequently reported in Skinner *et al.* (1997).
[‡]Deletion of self-association domain.
[§]Knocked-in to the mouse ataxin-1 gene.
[¶]1C2 immunostained microaggregates.
[∥]Cytoplasmic aggregates seen early in the course of the phenotype.

diverse as *Saccharomyces cerevisiae*, *Caenorhabditis elegans*, *Drosophila melanogaster*, and the mouse. The mouse models of HD were discussed in Chapter 13. This section presents the mouse models that have been generated for the other polyQ disorders (Table 14.7), along with the invertebrate models that have been developed for all polyQ diseases, including HD (Tables 14.8 and 14.9). Together these provide an extraordinarily rich resource for identifying the common and distinct molecular pathways that cause these diseases and will be invaluable for comparing the efficacy of a variety of therapeutic strategies.

Mouse models

Mouse models of HD have been generated by a wide variety of gene targeting and transgenic approaches as discussed in detail in Chapter 13. In comparison, there have been fewer models generated for each of the other polyQ diseases. Those reported to develop a neurological pheno-type are all transgenic mice expressing cDNA constructs under the control of a variety of promoters except for one gene-targeted model in which 78 CAG repeats have been knocked into the mouse ataxin-1 gene (Lorenzetti *et al.* 2000). The predominant molecular and genetic characteristics of each of these models are listed in Table 14.7. Without exception, the observed phenotypes have arisen as a result of neuronal dysfunction rather than neurodegen-eration (Abel *et al.* 2001; Adachi *et al.* 2001; Burright *et al.* 1995; Clark *et al.* 1997; Huynh *et al.* 1999; Ikeda *et al.* 1996; Klement *et al.* 1998; La Spada *et al.* 2001; Lorenzetti *et al.* 2000; Schilling *et al.* 1999; Yvert *et al.* 2000, 2001). Other than for one SCA1 model (Burright *et al.* 1995), each of these mice has only been described in a single publication and this section serves to direct the reader to these reports. Dramatic differences in phenotype onset and

Table 14.8 *Drosophila* models of polyQ disease

Construct*	Driver	Target cells	Repeat size[†]	Aggregates	Phenotype	Reference
UAS ataxin-3 (t)[‡]	gmr-GAL4	Eye retina	78Q	Nuclear	Retinal degeneration	Warrick *et al.* 1998
UAS ataxin-3 (t)[‡]	elav-GAL4	All neurones	78Q	Nuclear	Premature death[§]	Warrick *et al.* 1998
UAS ataxin-3 (t)[‡]	24B	Muscle	78Q	Not reported	Lethal[§]	Warrick *et al.* 1998
GMR huntingtin (t)[¶]	Not used	Eye retina	75Q, 120Q	Nuclear	Retinal degeneration	Jackson *et al.* 1998
UAS polyQ HA[‖]	gmr-GAL4	Eye retina	127Q	Nuclear/ cytoplasmic	Retinal degeneration	Kazemi-Esfarjani and Benzer 2000
UAS polyQ**	elav-GAL4	All neurones	108Q	Not reported	80% lethal	Marsh *et al.* 2000[††]
UAS polyQ**	sev-GAL4	Photoreceptor/ cones	108Q	Not reported	100% lethal	Marsh *et al.* 2000
UAS polyQ**	gmr-GAL4	Eye retina	108Q	Not reported	50% lethal	Marsh *et al.* 2000
UAS polyQ**	dpp[blk]-GAL4	Imaginal discs	108Q	Not reported	100% lethal	Marsh *et al.* 2000
UAS ataxin-1	gmr-GAL4	Eye retina	82Q	Nuclear	Retinal degeneration	Fernandez-Funez *et al.* 2000
UAS ataxin-1	gmr-GAL4	Eye retina	30Q[‡‡]	Nuclear	Retinal degeneration	Fernandez-Funez *et al.* 2000
UAS ataxin-1	ap[VNC]-GAL4	Ventral nerve cord	82Q	Nuclear	Neurodegeneration	Fernandez-Funez *et al.* 2000
UAS huntingtin (t)[§§]	gmr-GAL4	Eye retina	93Q	Not reported	Retinal degeneration/ lethality	Steffan *et al.* 2001
UAS polyQ	gmr-GAL4	Eye retina	46Q	Not reported	Retinal degeneration	Steffan *et al.* 2001

*See the subsection 'Invertebrate models' for a description of the UAS::GAL4 transcriptional activation system.
[†]Models expressing expanded repeat sizes are given.
[‡]C-terminal fragment of ataxin-3.
[§]Weak and moderate expression causes early adult death; strong expression is lethal.
[¶]N-terminal 171 amino acids of huntingtin.
[‖]PolyQ repeat attached to a haemagglutinin tag.
**The toxicity of the polyQ was reduced considerably by the addition of myc and FLAG tags.
[††]This paper also described flies in which a polyQ tract has been introduced into the *Drosophila* Dishevelled protein.
[‡‡]This model also develops a phenotype when a non-pathogenic allele is expressed.
[§§]N-terminal 90 amino acids of huntingtin (exon 1 protein).

Table 14.9 *C. elegans* models of polyglutamine disease

Construct	Promoter	Target cells	Repeat size	Aggregates	Phenotype	Reference
Huntingtin (t)[†]	*osm-10*	ASH sensory neurones	Q150, Q95	Cytoplasmic	Touch response defect	Faber *et al.* 1999
GFP polyQ	*unc-54*	Body wall muscle	Q82	Cytoplasmic	Growth retardation	Satyal *et al.* 2000
GFP polyQ	*myo-2*	Pharyngeal wall muscle	Q82	Cytoplasmic	Not reported	Satyal *et al.* 2000
Huntingtin (t)–GFP[‡]	*mec3*	Touch receptor neurones	Q128, Q88	Cytoplasmic	Touch response defect	Parker *et al.* 2001

*Abbreviations: GFP, green fluorescent protein; ASH, class of bilateral sensory neurons.
[†]N-terminal 121 amino acids of huntingtin.
[‡]N-terminal 57 amino acids of huntingtin fused to GFP.

progression can occur between models even when the same promoter and full-length transgenes carrying comparable repeat expansions are used. This is illustrated by the use of the Pcp2 promoter to drive ataxin-1 or ataxin-7 in the SCA1 and SCA7 transgenic mice (Burright *et al*. 1995; Clark *et al*. 1997; Yvert *et al*. 2000). The reason for this dramatic difference is not clear but could be due to the nature of the mutant proteins, possible differences in expression levels, or the influence of the different genetic background. The models are not presented in detail here, but rather the contribution that each has made to our understanding of the molecular pathogenesis of polyQ disease is discussed in the relevant sections elsewhere in this chapter.

The SCA1 model in which full-length mutant ataxin-1 is overexpressed in Purkinje cells under the control of the Pcp2 promoter (Burright *et al*. 1995; Clark *et al*. 1997) has been characterized extensively. An early downregulation in genes involved in signal transduction and calcium homeostasis has been reported (Lin *et al*. 2000) as well as downregulation of calcium-binding proteins (Vig *et al*. 1998, 2000). However, despite the dramatic alteration in morphology and the downregulation of Ca^{2+} handling molecules, the basic physiological properties of the wild-type and mutant Purkinje cells proved to be similar (Inoue *et al*. 2001). A molecular analysis of the cytoplasmic vacuoles that form in the Purkinje cells of the SCA1 transgenic mice indicated that altered somatodendritic membrane trafficking and loss of proteins including PKCγ (protein kinase C) might contribute to the neuronal dysfunction (Skinner *et al*. 2001). The SCA1 transgenic mice have been crossed to mice constitutively expressing the inducible form of hsp70 (Cummings *et al*. 2001) and to mice that do not express the ubiquitin ligase E3-A6 in Purkinje cells (Cummings *et al*. 1999; see the subsection 'Misfolding and aggregation' in this chapter). Supplementation with creatine was found to extend Purkinje cell survival but not to prevent the ataxic phenotype (Kaemmerer *et al*. 2001).

Invertebrate models

The polyQ diseases have been modelled successfully in the fruit fly, *D. melanogaster*. Constructs that have been used to introduce the polyQ expansions include *N*-terminal fragments of huntingtin (Jackson *et al*. 1998; Steffan *et al*. 2001), *C*-terminal fragments of ataxin-3 (Warrick *et al*. 1998), naked polyQ tracts (Marsh *et al*. 2000), epitope-tagged polyQ tracts (Kazemi-Esfarjani and Benzer 2000; Marsh *et al*. 2000), and the full-length ataxin-1 gene (Fernandez-Funez *et al*. 2000; see Table 14.8). In all cases but one (Jackson *et al*. 1998), the polyQ-containing transgene protein was placed under the control of the upstream activating sequence (UAS). This is not expressed until crossed to strains of flies that express the yeast GAL4 transcriptional activator. This therefore facilitates expression of the transgene in many cell types dependent on the promoter that drives transcription of the GAL4 activator. The polyQ protein expression level, in any given line, is influenced by the transgene site of integration, with the result that a single experiment can generate several lines exhibiting different levels of expression. Aggregate formation, neurodegeneration, a behavioural phenotype, and lethality have all been described. Expression of naked polyQ suggested that polyQ tracts are intrinsically toxic in a strongly cell-type-dependent manner that is not restricted to neurones as both neuronal and nonneuronal tissues showed cell death (Marsh *et al*. 2000).

These models have been used to identify genes that modify the phenotype induced by a polyQ expansion (see the subsections 'Misfolding and aggregation' and 'Transcriptional dysregulation' below) either by crossing to candidate genes (Chan *et al*. 2000; Steffan *et al*. 2001; Warrick *et al*. 1999) or by conducting modifier screens (Fernandez-Funez *et al*. 2000;

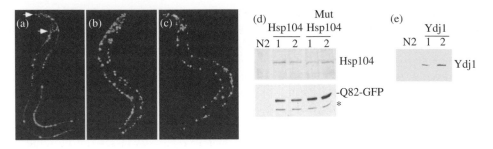

Fig. 14.2 Expression of wild-type Hsp 104 diminishes aggregation of Q82-GFP (GFP, green fluorescent protein). To assess the effects of chaperone expression on polyQ aggregates, wild-type or mutant Hsp104 or Ydj1 (dnaJ/Hsp40 chaperone) was co-expressed with Q82-GFP in body wall muscle cells (*unc-54* promoter), whereas only Q82-GFP was expressed in the pharyngeal cells (*myo-2* promoter) (see Table 14.9). (a) Overexpression of Hsp104 reduced Q82-GFP aggregates in body wall muscle cells but not in the pharyngeal cells (between the arrows). In animals expressing (b) mutant Hsp104 or (c) Ydj1, Q82 aggregates were unaffected. (d),(e) Immunoblot analysis of extracts of wild-type N2 or chaperone-expressing animals for: (d) two lines, each expressing Hsp104 and mutant Hsp104 by using anti-Hsp104 and anti-GFP antibodies (asterisk corresponds to mobility of free GFP); (e) Ydj-1 levels in wild-type N2 animals and two lines expressing Ydj1. (Reproduced with permission from Satyal *et al.* 2000 © (2000) National Academy of Sciences, USA.)

Kazemi-Esfarjani and Benzer 2000), and their potential for screening potential therapeutic compounds is starting to be exploited (Steffan *et al.* 2001). The development and application of *C. elegans* models of polyQ disease (Faber *et al.* 1999; Parker *et al.* 2001; Satyal *et al.* 2000; see Table 14.9) is at a more preliminary stage than those using *Drosophila* but they hold the same potential for the rapid identification of modifier genes and conducting high-throughput drug screens. Figure 14.2 illustrates the suppression of aggregate formation in a *C. elegans* model by co-expression with the yeast heat shock protein hsp104 (Satyal *et al.* 2000; see the subsection 'Misfolding and aggregation' below).

Molecular mechanisms underlying the pathogenesis

Gain of function/loss of function

It is generally accepted that the mechanism by which a polyQ expansion causes disease is to impart a toxic gain of function to the protein in which it is located. In 1997, Ordway *et al.* (1997) demonstrated that the ectopic expression of a $(CAG)_{150}$ repeat within the context of the *hprt* protein caused a late-onset, progressive, neurodegenerative disorder. It is thus likely that the insertion of a sufficiently long stretch of glutamines into any protein expressed in neurones would have the same consequence. Therefore, the protein context of the repeat is irrelevant to the induction of a neurological disease *per se*, but acts to restrict the pattern of neuronal dysfunction and neurodegeneration.

In the case of HD, it has recently been suggested that the molecular pathology may also arise as consequence of loss of function of the huntingtin protein (Cattaneo *et al.* 2001; see Chapter 12, this volume). To what extent might loss of function be contributing to the other polyQ disorders? Loss of function of the AR is certainly apparent in SBMA because patients exhibit signs of androgen insensitivity including gynaecomastia, testicular atrophy, and reduced fertility (Lieberman and Fischbeck 2000). However, this loss of function probably does not contribute to the neurological disorder as loss of AR function leads to testicular feminization and does not cause motor neurone disease (La Spada *et al*. 1991). The mechanism by which the CAG expansion in SBMA results in mild androgen insensitivity has not been resolved. Evidence has been presented to support both a decreased efficiency in the transactivation of target genes (Chamberlain *et al*. 1994; MacLean *et al*. 1995; Mhatre *et al*. 1993) and also a reduced expression of the AR (Brooks *et al*. 1997; Choong *et al*. 1996). Because SBMA is X-linked, a loss of function is more likely to be expressed than in the other polyQ diseases for which a normal copy of the protein in question is expressed in each cell. In the case of the other diseases, the mutation would have to have a dominant negative action in order to compromise the function of the normal protein. Proteins containing polyQ tracts in the non-expanded range are recruited into polyQ aggregates (Chen *et al*. 2001; Kazantsev *et al*. 1999; Martindale *et al*. 1998; Paulson *et al*. 1997b; Perez *et al*. 1998), which presents one mechanism by which this could occur. However, knock-outs of the SCA1 gene do not develop ataxia (Matilla *et al*. 1998), suggesting that loss of function does not contribute to SCA1 pathogenesis and it is likely that this is not a prominent mechanism in the aetiology of the polyQ diseases.

The polyQ expansion that causes SCA6 lies in the cytoplasmic tail of the α_{1A} subunit of the P/Q type voltage-dependent calcium channel (CACNA1A). Mutations in CACNA1A also cause familial hemiplegic migraine (FHM) and episodic ataxia type 2 (EA2) (Ophoff *et al*. 1996). These diseases are associated with missense mutations in the transmembrane domains and deletions and splice variants leading to a truncated protein. There is a rough genotype–phenotype correlation in that CAG expansions are associated with progressive ataxia, missense mutations with hemiplegic migraine, and nonsense mutations with episodic ataxia. However, the clinical overlap between the phenotypes produced by the different mutations is considerable and the same mutation may lead to variable clinical expression in a single family (Klockgether *et al*. 2000). The fact that the repeat expansions that cause SCA6 are much smaller than for the other diseases and, in all cases, completely overlap with the normal range (Zhuchenko *et al*. 1997) has raised the question as to whether the mechanism underlying SCA6 differs from that causing the other polyQ diseases. The SCA6 expansion could cause disease by perturbing the gating of the P/Q-type channels, which is supported by the phenotypic overlap caused by the different mutations. Alternatively, it may operate by imparting a toxic property to the tail of the α_{1A} subunit, and the identification of nuclear and cytoplasmic aggregates in SCA6 (Ishikawa *et al*. 2001) indicates that this is also a viable possibility. The lower CAG repeat threshold may arise because the amino acids flanking the repeat have a propensity to beta-sheet formation. Alternatively, as part of the cytoplasmic tail of a densely packed membrane protein, this domain of the α_{1A} subunit may occur in a more ordered or locally concentrated environment than do the other cytoplasmic polyQ proteins (Gomez 2001), which is more likely to induce aggregation. The relative contribution of these two mechanistic possibilities to the molecular pathogenesis of SCA6 remains to be determined.

Processing as an event in the pathogenic process

There is compelling evidence to indicate that the first step in the pathogenesis of HD might be the processing of huntingtin to generate toxic N-terminal fragments, which have been shown to accumulate in the nucleus (DiFiglia *et al*. 1997; Hodgson *et al*. 1999; Li *et al*. 2000;

Chapter 12, this volume). The processing of huntingtin might be a factor that restricts the pathology to specific neuronal populations. This is supported by the observation that the aggregate pathology is more restricted in transgenic and knock-in mice expressing full-length huntingtin under the control of ubiquitous promoters than in mice that express only an N-terminal fragment (see Chapter 13). This is in turn consistent with the fact that exon 1 huntingtin proteins expressing polyQ expansions *in vitro* remain soluble until removal of the glutathione S-transferase (GST) tag causes self-assembly into amyloid fibrils (Scherzinger *et al.* 1997, 1999; see Chapter 11 this volume).

The evidence that a processing step might similarly take place in the other polyQ disorders is summarized in Table 14.6. A 120 kDa truncated product of atrophin 1 has been detected in brain lysates from DRPLA transgenic mice and autopsy brain tissue (Schilling *et al.* 1999). This processing event separates a C-terminal NES (nuclear export signal) away from the part of the protein containing the polyQ repeat, possibly allowing the latter to translocate to the nucleus. Similarly, processed fragments of ataxin-7 have been identified on Western blots of SCA7 transgenic mouse brains (Yvert *et al.* 2000) and N-terminal fragments have been shown to accumulate in nuclei by immunohistochemistry (Yvert *et al.* 2000, 2001). Arguing against the hypothesis that truncation restricts the pathology, a similar pattern of processing was observed in all brain regions in mice in which ataxin-7 was expressed under the control of the PDGF-B (platelet derived growth factor B chain) promoter, and did not parallel the selective neurodegeneration observed in SCA7 patients (Yvert *et al.* 2001). However, this could be a function of the high expression levels driven by the exogenous promoter. Therefore, comparable molecular pathways may be operating in HD, DRPLA, and SCA7. Nuclear aggregates are only detected by antibodies recognizing the N-terminus of the AR (Li *et al.* 1998a, b) and so it is possible that a cleavage event is also important in SBMA. Although cleavage products have been detected on Western blots, there is no consensus as to the size of the fragments that are generated (Abdullah *et al.* 1998; Butler *et al.* 1998; Ellerby *et al.* 1999; Merry *et al.* 1998). Antibodies to SCA2 have been shown to detect three cleavage products on Western blots of lysates from SCA2 and control brains (Huynh *et al.* 1999). An absence of cleavage products has been reported for ataxin-1 (Servadio *et al.* 1995) and ataxin-3 (Perez *et al.* 1999). The possibility that cleavage products of the CACNA1A calcium channel or of TBP are important for the pathogenesis of SCA6 or SCA17 has not been investigated.

Misfolding and aggregation

It is generally accepted that the molecular pathogenesis of the polyQ disorders is linked to protein misfolding initiated by polyQ tracts that are expanded into the mutant range. Chaperone proteins, which are known to assist in folding proteins into their native conformation, refold abnormally folded proteins, and rescue previously aggregated proteins, are frequently found as components of polyQ aggregates. Immunohistochemical studies have shown that proteins in polyQ aggregates are ubiquitinated (Davies *et al.* 1997; DiFiglia *et al.* 1997; Paulson *et al.* 1997b), indicating that the mutant proteins have been marked for degradation by the proteasome. This process requires the conjugation of proteins with multiple ubiquitin molecules (Bonifacino and Weissman 1998), which are then recognized and hydrolysed by the 26S proteasome (Voges *et al.* 1999).

The proteasome is composed of two major subcomplexes: the 20S proteasome core, a barrel-shaped multicatalytic protease and associated with it the 19S (PA700) regulatory complex which is required for the recognition of ubiquitinated proteins. In addition to the 19S complex, a second regulator of the 20S proteasome has been described. This is a ring-shaped structure, termed 11S or PA28, which binds to the 20S proteasome in an orientation similar to that of 19S and is mainly required for the degradation of short peptides rather than large ubiquitinated proteins. The formation of ubiquitinated aggregates suggests that mutant protein is either resistant to degradation or that the rate of accumulation exceeds the rate of degradation. The latter is more likely as intranuclear aggregates that have formed in a transgenic mouse model expressing an inducible exon 1 mutant huntingtin transgene were found to disappear when the expression of the transgene was switched off. This demonstrates that polyQ aggregates are dynamic structures that are amenable to degradation (Yamamoto *et al.* 2000).

There is some evidence to suggest that proteins containing polyQ expansions are more resistant to degradation than their wild-type counterparts. Cummings *et al.* (1999) found that ataxin-1 with 2Q and with 92Q were polyubiquitinated equally well *in vitro* but that the mutant form was three times more resistant to degradation. Similarly, transgenic mice expressing ataxin-7 had higher levels of protein in the expanded lines even though transgenic mRNA was present at a higher level in the normal lines. It seemed that normal ataxin-7 could not be detected because of a rapid turn-over and that detection of the mutant protein was due to stabilization by the expanded repeat (Yvert *et al.* 2001).

There is a rich literature documenting the co-localization of chaperone proteins or components of the proteasome with polyQ aggregates and demonstrating that aggregation and toxicity can be modulated by controlling chaperone expression levels. PolyQ aggregates in SCA1 patient brains and transgenic mice contain the 20S proteasome and the chaperone HDJ-2 (Cummings *et al.* 1998) and in SCA3 brains the chaperones HDJ-1, HDJ-2, and, less frequently, Hsp70 (Chai *et al.* 1999). A more comprehensive study of ataxin-7 aggregates in transgenic mice found co-localization with the 20S proteasome, HDJ-2 but not HDJ-1, the proteasomal subunit 5a (the putative recognition site of poly-ubiquitinated proteins), a set of ATPase activity containing 19S subunits, and, in some cases, the 11S complex (Yvert *et al.* 2000).

PolyQ aggregates that form in a variety of mammalian cell lines transfected with ataxin-1 (Cummings *et al.* 1998), ataxin-3 (Chai *et al.* 1999), or huntingtin (Waelter *et al.* 2001; Wyttenbach *et al.* 2000, 2001) co-localize with the core 20S proteasome and the Hsp40 chaperone, HDJ-2. Ataxin-3 aggregates were also found to co-localize with HDJ-1 (Hsp40) and Hsp70 but not Hsp27, Hsp60, Hsp90, or Hsp110 (Chai *et al.* 1999) and huntingtin aggregates with Hsp70, Hsc 70 (the constitutive form of Hsp 70), HDJ1, and HDJ2 (Waelter *et al.* 2001; Wyttenbach *et al.* 2000, 2001); the 20S, 19S, and 11S subunits of the proteasome; and the chaperone BiP/GRP78 (Waelter *et al.* 2001; Wyttenbach *et al.* 2001). The expanded AR recruited Hsp70, Hsp90, NEDD8 (60 per cent identical and 80 per cent similar to ubiquitin), and the 19S proteasome cap but not the 20S core or Hsp 25, 27, or 110 (Stenoien *et al.* 1999).

Overexpression of HDJ-2 was found to decrease the frequency of aggregates formed by ataxin-1 (Cummings *et al.* 1998) and the AR (Stenoien *et al.* 1999), and HDJ-1 and HDJ-2 suppressed aggregation of ataxin-3, which correlated with a decrease in toxicity (Chai *et al.* 1999). Similarly, fragments of the bacterial chaperone GroEL and the full-length yeast Hsp104 were found to reduce both aggregate formation and cell death in mammalian cell models of HD, although in this case co-localization was not detected (Carmichael *et al.* 2000). In contrast, Wyttenbach *et al.* (2000) found that overexpression of HDJ-2 did not modify inclusion formation in PC12 or SH-SY5Y cells but increased inclusion formation in COS-7 cells (Wyttenbach *et al.* 2000). The ability of molecular chaperones to promote refolding or ubiquitin-dependent degradation could be exploited in the development of therapeutic interventions. Geldanamycin is a benzoquinone ansamycin that binds to Hsp90 and activates the heat shock response in mammalian cells. Sittler *et al.* (2001) showed that treatment of mammalian cells with geldanamycin at nanomolar concentrations induces the expression of Hsp40, Hsp70, and Hsp90 and inhibits HD exon 1 protein aggregation in a dose-dependent manner.

Experiments both *in vitro* and in yeast have demonstrated that chaperones alter the biochemical properties of aggregates. *In vitro*, Hsp70 and its co-chaperone Hsp40 suppressed the assembly of the exon 1 huntingtin protein into detergent-insoluble amyloid-like fibrils in an adenosine triphosphate (ATP)-dependent manner and caused the formation of amorphous, detergent-soluble aggregates instead (Muchowski *et al.* 2000). The chaperones were most active in preventing fibrillization when added during the lag phase of the polymerization reaction. Similarly in yeast, co-expression of Hsp40 and Hsp70 with the exon 1 huntingtin protein inhibited the formation of large, detergent-insoluble polyQ aggregates resulting in the accumulation of detergent-soluble inclusions (Muchowski *et al.* 2000). In a separate study (Krobitsch and Lindquist 2000), overexpression of Sis1 (the yeast homologue of Hsp40), Hsp70, and the yeast chaperone Hsp104 decreased the number of aggregates formed with exon 1 huntingtin proteins containing 72 or 103 glutamines and also increased their solubility. Deletion of Hsp104 virtually eliminated the formation of cytoplasmic aggregates and only the soluble form of exon-1 huntingtin could be detected on Western blots (Krobitsch and Lindquist 2000; Cao *et al.* 2001); however, this had no effect on the formation of nuclear aggregates (Cao *et al.* 2001). Therefore, chaperones may act to direct polyQ proteins into soluble, amorphous structures instead of fibrillar aggregates. In addition, changes in the concentration of chaperones may have complex effects on aggregate formation (Cao *et al.* 2001; Krobitsch and Lindquist 2000; Wyttenbach *et al.* 2000).

In vivo models have been more informative in establishing a link between the modulation of misfolding and aggregation and the rescue of cellular dysfunction and degeneration. Expression of polyQ tracts as EGFP (enhanced green fluorescent protein) fusion proteins in the body wall muscle cells of *C. elegans* causes discrete cytoplasmic aggregates that appear early in embryogenesis and correlate with the delay in larval to adult development. Co-expression of the yeast chaperone Hsp104 reversed both the formation of aggregates and the associated developmental delay (Fig. 14.2; Satyal *et al.* 2000). Warrick *et al.* (1999) showed that the direct expression of Hsp70 in a *D. melanogaster* model of polyQ disease suppressed polyQ-induced neurodegeneration and that this occurred without a visible effect on aggregate formation. This study was extended to demonstrate that Hsp40 and Hsp70 act synergistically in their suppression of neurotoxicity and that, as *in vitro* and in yeast, the chaperones had the effect of altering the solubility properties of the aggregated protein (Chan *et al.* 2000). Therefore the chaperone modulation of neurodegeneration in this *D. melanogaster* model is associated with altered biochemical properties of the mutant polyQ protein.

Using a less direct approach, *D. melanogaster* models have been used to screen for dominant modifiers of polyQ toxicity (Fernandez-Funez *et al.* 2000; Kazemi-Esfarjani and Benzer 2000). In one such experiment, *D. melanogaster* expressing 127Q in the eye were crossed with approximately 7000 P-element insertion strains. Two lines that suppress neurodegeneration both contained a chaperone-related J domain that stimulates the ATP activity of Hsp70, namely, the lines, dHDJ1 (HDJ-1 homologue) and dTPR2 (homologous to the human tetratricopeptide repeat protein 2). In both cases, the deterioration of the eye structure was inhibited but aggregate formation was not suppressed, although aggregate solubility was not studied (Kazemi-Esfarjani and Benzer 2000). Similarly, modifier screens for flies expressing the full-length mutant ataxin-1 gene identified several proteins that have roles in protein folding and clearance (Fernandez-Funez *et al.* 2000). Overexpression of the inducible form of Hsp70 has also been shown to protect against neurodegeneration in mice that overexpress ataxin-1 in Purkinje cells (Cummings *et al.* 2001), although effects on aggregate solubility were not reported.

Treatment with lactacystin, a proteasome inhibitor, leads to an increase in polyQ aggregation in a number of cell culture models (Cummings *et al.* 1999; Waelter *et al.* 2001; Wyttenbach *et al.* 2000). Attempts have also been made to prevent the proteasome degradation of polyQ proteins by blocking ubiquitin ligases (Cummings *et al.* 1999; Saudou *et al.* 1998). In cell culture, the transient co-transfection of a dominant interfering mutant of the ubiquitin-conjugating enzyme hCdc34p(CL-S) resulted in a decrease in the number of huntingtin aggregates, whereas the extent of cell death was increased (Saudou *et al.* 1998). However, ubiquitination of huntingtin was not blocked in this experiment. The results are more likely to have arisen due to an overall effect on cell function than through a direct manipulation of mutant huntingtin processing.

In mice, Purkinje cells that express mutant ataxin-1 and not a ubiquitin protein ligase (E6-AP) have significantly fewer nuclear aggregates than those expressing ataxin-1 on an otherwise wild-type background. However, the Purkinje cell pathology was markedly worse than that in SCA1 mice. There are many possible interpretations of this experiment. The interpretation of the authors is that nuclear aggregates are not necessary for neurodegeneration, but impaired proteasomal degradation of mutant ataxin-1 may contribute to SCA1 pathogenesis (Cummings *et al.* 1999). However, no evidence is presented to show that E6-AP ubiquitinates ataxin-1. The decrease in aggregation may reflect increased proteasomal degradation of ataxin-1, which is still ubiquitinated by a U3 ligase(s). The E6-AP gene has tissue-specific imprinting and thus a unique expression pattern, and the paternal allele is silenced in Purkinje cells and hippocampal neurones (Albrecht *et al.* 1997). Mice with a maternal deficiency of E6-AP are a model of Angelman syndrome and display learning deficits, impaired performance on the rotating rod, and inducible seizures. It is possible that the enhanced cerebellar pathology in mice expressing mutant ataxin-1 in Purkinje cells deficient for E6-AP arises from the overexpression of an expanded polyQ in neurones that are already dysfunctional.

The deletion of the self-association domain in a mutant ataxin-1 transgene led to mice that developed ataxia and Purkinje cell pathology similar to those of mutant ataxin-1 mice but the formation of nuclear aggregates was much delayed. However, the phenotype in these mice was not progressive and mice containing the wild-type version of this mutant construct were not reported (Klement *et al.* 1998).

Transcriptional dysregulation

The first indication that transcriptional dysregulation might be important in the pathogenesis of HD was that selective neurotransmitter receptors were downregulated at the RNA level in the HD R6/2 mouse brain (Cha *et al.* 1998, 1999). These findings were consistent with limited studies that have been performed in low-grade HD patient brains (Glass *et al.* 2000). This analysis was extended by the use of microarrays to generate expression profiles of R6/2 striata as compared to controls (Luthi-Carter *et al.* 2000). The genes whose expression levels were altered (decreased in 75 per cent of cases) were limited to several key molecular systems including neurotransmitter receptors, intracellular signalling mechanisms, retinoic acid receptor machinery, and maintenance of calcium homeostasis (Cha 2000; Luthi-Carter *et al.* 2000). A more limited study in ataxin-1 transgenic mice also found that genes involved in signal transduction and calcium homeostasis were downregulated. These decreases in gene transcription occurred before detectable pathology and were also present in SCA1 patients' brains (Lin *et al.* 2000).

A more recent study has generated a yeast model of polyQ disease in which the expanded polyQ was directed to the nucleus or cytoplasm by appropriate localization signals (Hughes *et al.* 2001). Microarray analysis was used to identify changes in gene expression levels in response to the presence of the polyQ repeat tract. Expanded polyQ in either the nucleus or the cytoplasm caused the induction of genes encoding chaperones and heat shock factors. Transcriptional repression was most prominent in yeast expressing nuclear expanded polyQ, and was similar to profiles of yeast strains deleted for components of the histone acetyltransferase complex SAGA (Hughes *et al.* 2001). It is possible that altered gene expression may be the earliest mediator of polyQ toxicity.

Kazantsev *et al.* (1999) were the first to show that CREB-binding protein (CBP), an acetyl transferase, can be recruited into polyQ aggregates and that this is dependent on a stretch of 18 glutamine residues in the CBP protein. Since then, a wide range of transcription factors has been found to co-localize with polyQ aggregates. In DRPLA, SCA3, and HD patient brains, they have been found to contain one or more of the following transcription factors: TATA binding protein (TBP), TBP-associated factor (TAF$_{II}$130), cAMP-response-element-binding protein (CREB), CREB binding protein (CBP), Sp1, and the transcriptional co-activator, CA150 (Holbert *et al.* 2001; Huang *et al.* 1998; Nucifora *et al.* 2001; Perez *et al.* 1998; Shimohata *et al.* 2000). Transcription factors that have been found to co-localize in cellular and mouse models of polyQ disease include the steroid receptor co-activator 1 (SRC-1), which interacts with AR to enhance transcriptional activity (Stenoien *et al.* 1999), and the cone–rod homeobox protein (CRX), which is suppressed by interaction with ataxin-7 (La Spada *et al.* 2001). In addition, p53 (Steffan *et al.* 2000; Suhr *et al.* 2001), TAF$_{II}$30, TFIIEα, TFIIFβ, SNF5 (a component of the SWI/SNF chromatin remodelling complex), and the p89 (XPB) subunit of TFIIH (Yvert *et al.* 2001) have been found to co-localize with nuclear aggregates.

Whilst not all of these proteins contain polyQ domains they often exist in transcription factor complexes with proteins that do and could be recruited in a piggy-back fashion. A reduction in CRE-mediated transcription has been reported in an inducible PC12 model of HD (Wyttenbach *et al.* 2001) and it has been shown in transfection assays of HD, DRPLA, and SBMA that replenishment of CBP or TAFII$_{130}$ can rescue toxicity (McCampbell *et al.* 2000; Nucifora *et al.* 2001; Shimohata *et al.* 2000). Therefore, it is possible that neuronal dysfunction and degeneration in polyQ disease may result from the nuclear depletion of transcription factors. In support of this, cells are known to be exquisitely sensitive to levels of CBP and loss of function mutations in the acetyl transferase domain are dominant and cause the congenital malformation syndrome known as Rubinstein–Taybi syndrome (Murata *et al.* 2001).

PolyQ-containing proteins have also been found to interact with transcriptional activators and repressors in the absence of large aggregation complexes. Huntingtin was found to bind directly to the nuclear co-repressor N-CoR in a polyQ repeat length dependent manner (Boutell *et al.* 1999). N-CoR is part of a complex that represses transcription in combination with several specific DNA-binding transcriptional repressors including the thyroid hormone receptor, retinoic acid receptors, Mad:Max dimers, and some of the orphan nuclear receptors. N-CoR and mSin3 proteins link specific DNA binding proteins to proteins with histone deacetylase activity (Cha 2000). In HD patient brains, Boutell *et al.* (1999) found the location of N-CoR and Sin3A to be exclusively cytoplasmic in patient brain material, whereas in control brains these proteins were also present in the nucleus. Sin3A also co-localized to some intranuclear inclusions. More recently, atrophin 1 has been found to interact with ETO/MTG8, which is also a component of nuclear receptor core repressor complexes and, in a cell-transfection based assay, atrophin 1 was found to repress transcription (Wood *et al.* 2000). Therefore, atrophin 1 represses transcription and interacts with ETO/MTG8 in nuclear matrix-associated structures that contain mSin3A and histone deacetylases.

Nuclear receptors such as the retinoic acid receptor (RARα) and the retinoid X receptor (RXRα) can associate with PML (promyelocytic leukaemia) bodies. The function of PML bodies remains unclear, although they have been linked to gene transcription and cell death. The SCA1, SCA3, and DRPLA gene products have all been found to have an effect on the PML protein or PML bodies. Mutant ataxin-1 has been shown to sequester PML and alter its normal distribution (Skinner *et al.* 1997), ataxin-3 aggregates co-localize with PML bodies (Chai *et al.* 1999; Yasuda *et al.* 1999), and overexpression of atrophin 1 and ETO-MTG8 with PML causes the redistribution of PML (Wood *et al.* 2000). In DRPLA and SCA3 patient brains, PML protein is redistributed around nuclear inclusions forming a single capsular structure (Yamada *et al.* 2001).

The exon 1 huntingtin protein has also been shown to directly interact with the acetyl transferase domains of CBP and p300/CBP associated factor (P/CAF) (Steffan *et al.* 2001). In cell-free systems it inhibited the acetyltransferase activity of at least three enzymes, CBP, p300, and P/CAF, and in cultured cells reduced the acetylation of histones H3 and H4, a reduction that could be reversed by administering histone deacetylase (HDAC) inhibitors (Steffan *et al.* 2001). *In vivo*, Steffan *et al.* (2001) showed that HDAC inhibitors arrest on-going progressive neuro-degeneration and reduce lethality in *Drosophila* models of polyQ disease. As would be predicted, crossing the polyQ flies with those with a partial loss of Sin3A function (a co-repressor protein that is a component of HDAC complexes) also led to a partial reversal of neurodegeneration and lethality (Steffan *et al.* 2001). It is not yet clear why, when a similar cross was performed with flies expressing mutant ataxin-1, the severity of the phenotype was enhanced rather than alleviated (Fernandez-Funez *et al.* 2000).

At first, it might seem unlikely that a pathogenic mechanism involving the impairment of transcription factors that are expressed ubiquitously from early development could cause late-onset neurodegenerative disease. However, the recent discovery that polyQ expansions in TBP, a component of the basal transcription machinery, cause SCA17 demonstrates that such concerns are unfounded (Koide *et al.* 1999; Nakamura *et al.* 2001). The late onset and specificity of the disease is likely to be governed by transcription factor interactions with mis-folded, aggregated, or relocated mutant proteins. Therefore, although the molecular basis of transcriptional dysregulation in polyQ disease requires further dissection, the net result of dysregulation appears to be transcriptional repression. In an invertebrate model at least, this can be rescued by the administration of HDAC inhibitors (Steffan *et al.* 2001).

Recruitment of cellular proteins by polyQ aggregates

One mechanism by which polyQ expansion could result in cellular dysfunction and cell death is by depleting the cell of essential proteins (Kazantsev *et al.* 1999; Perez *et al.* 1998). This will not be discussed at length in this section because aspects of this topic have been covered elsewhere in this chapter. This section will serve to summarize the classes of molecules that are recruited to polyQ aggregates.

It has been demonstrated in a number of cellular models (Kazantsev *et al.* 1999; Perez *et al.* 1998) as well as *Drosophila* (Perez *et al.* 1998) and *C. elegans* systems (Satyal *et al.* 2000) that, once aggregates have been seeded by an expanded polyQ tract, they can recruit proteins containing non-pathological polyQ stretches. One such protein (except in the case of SBMA) could be the normal counterpart of the protein carrying the polyQ expansion. This could cause a dominant negative effect by which loss of function of the mutated protein could potentially contribute to the disease phenotype (see the subsection 'Gain of function/loss of function' above). Other proteins that contain polyQ tracts are frequently transcription factors (Preisinger *et al.* 1999) and the mechanism by which polyQ expansions can perturb the transcription of specific genes has been discussed at length in the previous subsection. Components of the proteasome and molecular chaperones also frequently co-localize with polyQ aggregates (see the subsection 'Misfolding and aggregation' above), most probably remnants of attempts by the cell to remove the misfolded or aggregated proteins. This might have an effect on the ability of the cell to process other misfolded proteins efficiently, either by depletion of essential components or by effectively blocking the entrance to the proteasome with elongated polyQ peptides. It has recently emerged that ubiquitin and components of the proteasome also play a role in transcriptional regulation (Ferdous *et al.* 2001; Salghetti *et al.* 2001; see Chapter 12, this volume) and so might conceivably contribute to the transcriptional dysregulation in polyQ disease.

Structural molecules that have been purified from aggregates include neurofilament light chain (NLF), actin, and components of the nuclear pore complex (Suhr *et al.* 2001). Caspase 8 recruitment was reported in aggregates from both cell models and in lysates from HD patient brains in one paper (Sanchez *et al.* 1999), whereas a second failed to find caspase 8 but did detect caspase 3 (Suhr *et al.* 2001).

The importance of the nucleus in polyQ pathogenesis

There are several lines of evidence to indicate that a nuclear location of the mutant polyQ-containing protein is essential for pathogenesis. Consistent with this, a relocation of mutant polyQ proteins to the nucleus, either in the form of a diffuse nuclear staining or as nuclear aggregates, has been reported for all mouse models of HD (see Chapter 13), DRPLA (Schilling *et al.* 1999), SBMA (Abel *et al.* 2001; Adachi *et al.* 2001), SCA1 (Skinner *et al.* 1997), and SCA7 (Yvert *et al.* 2000, 2001). Nuclear aggregates are also detected in autopsy brains from patients with each of the polyQ disorders (see the subsection 'Polyglutamine aggregation and the formation of inclusion bodies' above) and a nuclear diffuse staining has also been reported in many cases (Yamada *et al.* 2000). Mice transgenic for an ataxin-1 construct in which the nuclear localization signal (NLS) has been mutated do not develop disease (Klement *et al.* 1998). However, inconsistent with this hypothesis, a nuclear location was not found to be important for the pathogenic mechanism operating in SCA2 transgenic mice (Huynh *et al.* 2000).

Cell culture models have also pointed to the importance of a nuclear location (Saudou *et al.* 1998; Yasuda *et al.* 1999). Yasuda *et al.* (1999) found that the formation of nuclear but not cytoplasmic ataxin-3 aggregates in PC12 cells resulted in the activation of SEK1 *in situ*, which triggered cell death. It was possible to rescue this lethality by dominant negative SEK-1 but not by caspase inhibitors. Interestingly, cell-death-resistant cells that arose spontaneously contained cytoplasmic but not nuclear polyQ aggregates (Yasuda *et al.* 1999). It has been suggested that the diffuse staining often identified in neuronal nuclei represents a unique conformation of the polyQ protein in question (Perez *et al.* 1999; Wheeler *et al.* 2000). Ataxin-3 was found to adopt a unique conformation when expressed within the nucleus of transfected cells thereby exposing the glutamine domain of the full-length non-pathological protein, allowing it to bind to the antibody 1C2. This altered conformation is not due to proteolysis and might arise from nuclear-specific protein interactions and represent an early event in SCA3 pathogenesis that exposes the polyQ domain (Perez *et al.* 1999). The translocation of the polyQ-containing soluble proteins to the nucleus, the altered conformers of these proteins, and the formation of polyQ aggregates might all contribute to the mechanism underlying transcriptional dysregulation in polyQ disease.

Cell death

The molecular events that result in cell death in polyQ disease are not well established. A detailed discussion of the experiments that have been conducted to address cell death mechanisms in cellular models of HD has been presented in Chapter 12. In this last section the discussion will be limited to what we might have learned from *in vivo* models of polyQ disease. Consistent with the mouse models of HD (see Chapter 13), cell death, when described in mouse models of other polyQ disease, is a late event that occurs considerably after the onset of a neurological phenotype. Directing expression to specific neurones has shown that neurodegeneration need not be restricted to the cells in which the mutant protein is expressed. In both SCA7 models in which mutant ataxin-7 is expressed specifically in Purkinje cells or in the eye under the control of the rhodopsin promoter, morphological alterations were identified in neurones postsynaptic to those expressing the mutant protein (Yvert *et al.* 2000). The molecular basis of neurodegeneration in the mouse models is not known.

To date, neurodegeneration has not been observed in any of the *C. elegans* models (Faber *et al.* 1999; Parker *et al.* 2001; Satyal *et al.* 2000), but has been successfully generated by expressing polyQ expansions in the *Drosophila* eye. It was shown in the first *Drosophila* model to be reported, that this neurodegeneration could be mitigated by the co-expression of the viral anti-apoptotic gene P35 (Warrick *et al.* 1998), suggesting that an apoptotic cell death process had been activated. In contrast, ultrastructural analysis of the neurodegeneration induced in the *Drosophila* model expressing an *N*-terminal fragment of huntingtin (Jackson *et al.* 1998) appeared as nuclear and cytoplasm condensation, chromatin clumping, and an increased affinity for osmium. Although these cells showed features of apoptosis, DNA fragmentation and phagocytosis by adjacent cells were both absent (Fig. 14.3). In this case crossing the HD flies to flies expressing P35 did not rescue the polyQ-induced neurodegeneration, indicating that the cells are not dying by apoptosis and that the cell death might be proceeding by a novel pathway. The morphological neurodegenerative characteristics in this fly model are remarkably similar to those described for the R6 HD mouse model (Turmaine *et al.* 2000; see Chapter 13, this volume).

Concluding remarks

CAG/polyQ expansion has been identified as the causative mutation for nine late-onset neurodegenerative diseases, a number that is set to increase. In recent years, detailed information concerning the behaviour of these mutations has enabled us to explain the molecular basis of

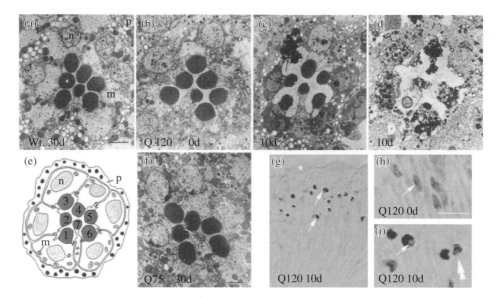

Fig. 14.3 Electron microscopic analysis of polyQ-induced degeneration of photoreceptor neurones in *Drosophila*. (a), (e) Morphology of ommatidia in wild type at 30 days is normal. Sections of ommatidia were analysed at a level at which seven of the eight photoreceptor neurones are seen. Asterisk, rhabdomere; m, mitochondrion; n, nucleus; p, processes of pigment cells surrounding photoreceptor neurones in each ommatidium. (b) Normal morphology of Q120 ommatidia is seen at eclosion. (c) Degeneration with some ultrastructural features of apoptosis is evident in Q120 at 10 days. Arrowhead, nucleus with aggregation of condensed chromatin; arrow, shrunken cell with highly osmiophillic cytoplasm. (d) Severely affected ommatidium in Q120. Some photoreceptor cells are missing, as are the majority of the rhabdomeres in remaining cells. (f) Mild degeneration is observed in Q75 Ommatidia at 30 days. (g) Huntington immunoreactivity in Q120 photoreceptor neurones at 10 days is largely nuclear (arrows). The morphology of the retina is disrupted reflecting degeneration of photoreceptor neurones visible by Normarski optics. (h),(i) High-magnification views of nuclei in Q120 photoreceptor neurones. Huntingtin immunoreactivity is evenly distributed throughout nuclei at 0 days (arrow). At 10 days the protein is highly concentrated in the nucleus but is excluded from the nucleolus (arrow). In some nuclei, the distribution of the protein has a more punctate appearance with multiple spots of high immunoreactivity (double arrowhead). (Reproduced from Jackson *et al.* (1998) © (1998) with permission from Elsevier Science.)

anticipation. We have developed very accurate predictive tests and have gained much experience in genetic counselling for these disorders so that, as new CAG repeat diseases are uncovered, we are in a position to understand the genetics of the disorder in question very quickly. Enormous advances have been made in unravelling the molecular events that are triggered by the mutations that lead to cellular dysfunction and eventually cell death. A wide variety of complementary disease models, which include *in vitro*, yeast, mammalian cell culture, *C. elegans*, *Drosophila*, and mouse systems, have been generated and the pace of discovery can only increase. In the last 3 to 4 years a set of completely new therapeutic targets has been identified and in some cases large-scale screens are already in place to identify effective therapeutic approaches. The challenge of the next few years will be to determine how these new therapeutics can be evaluated in a systematic and informative set of screening protocols, first in mouse models and then in patient trials.

References

Abdullah, A., Trifiro, M. A., Panet-Raymond, V., Alvarado, C., de Tourreil, S., Frankel, D., Schipper, H. M., and Pinsky, L. (1998). Spinobulbar muscular atrophy: polyglutamine-expanded androgen receptor is proteolytically resistant *in vitro* and processed abnormally in transfected cells. *Hum Mol Genet* **7**, 379–84.

Abel, A., Walcott, J., Woods, J., Duda, J., and Merry, D. E. (2001). Expression of expanded repeat androgen receptor produces neurologic disease in transgenic mice. *Hum Mol Genet* **10**, 107–16.

Adachi, H., Kume, A., Li, M., Nakagomi, Y., Niwa, H., Do, J., Sang, C., Kobayashi, Y., Doyu, M., and Sobue, G. (2001). Transgenic mice with an expanded CAG repeat controlled by the human AR promoter show polyglutamine nuclear inclusions and neuronal dysfunction without neuronal cell death. *Hum Mol Genet* **10**, 1039–48.

Albrecht, U., Sutcliffe, J. S., Cattanach, B. M., Beechey, C. V., Armstrong, D., Eichele, G., and Beaudet, A. L. (1997). Imprinted expression of the murine Angelman syndrome gene, Ube3a, in hippocampal and Purkinje neurons. *Nat Genet* **17**, 75–8.

Babovic-Vuksanovic, D., Snow, K., Patterson, M. C., and Michels, V. V. (1998). Spinocerebellar ataxia type 2 (SCA 2) in an infant with extreme CAG repeat expansion. *Am J Med Genet* **79**, 383–7.

Banfi, S., Servadio, A., Chung, M. Y., Kwiatkowski, T. J., Jr., McCall, A. E., Duvick, L. A., Shen, Y., Roth, E. J., Orr, H. T., and Zoghbi, H. Y. (1994). Identification and characterization of the gene causing type 1 spinocerebellar ataxia. *Nat Genet* **7**, 513–20.

Becher, M. W., Kotzuk, J. A., Sharp, A. H., Davies, S. W., Bates, G. P., Price, D. L., and Ross, C. A. (1998). Intranuclear neuronal inclusions in Huntington's disease and dentatorubral and pallidoluysian atrophy: correlation between the density of inclusions and IT15 CAG triplet repeat length. *Neurobiol Dis* **4**, 387–97.

—— Rubinsztein, D. C., Leggo, J., Wagster, M. V., Stine, O. C., Ranen, N. G., Franz, M. I., Abbott, M. H., Sherr, M., MacMillan, J. C., Barron, L., Porteous, M., Harper, P. S., and Ross, C. A. (1997). Dentatorubral and pallidoluysian atrophy (DRPLA). Clinical and neuropathological findings in genetically confirmed North American and European pedigrees. *Mov Disord* **12**, 519–30.

Belsham, D. D., Yee, W. C., Greenberg, C. R., and Wrogemann, K. (1992). Analysis of the CAG repeat region of the androgen receptor gene in a kindred with X-linked spinal and bulbar muscular atrophy. *J Neurol Sci* **112**, 133–8.

Benton, C. S., de Silva, R., Rutledge, S. L., Bohlega, S., Ashizawa, T., and Zoghbi, H. Y. (1998). Molecular and clinical studies in SCA-7 define a broad clinical spectrum and the infantile phenotype. *Neurology* **51**, 1081–6.

Biancalana, V., Serville, F., Pommier, J., Julien, J., Hanauer, A., and Mandel, J. L. (1992). Moderate instability of the trinucleotide repeat in spino bulbar muscular atrophy. *Hum Mol Genet* **1**, 255–8.

Bonifacino, J. S. and Weissman, A. M. (1998). Ubiquitin and the control of protein fate in the secretory and endocytic pathways. *Annu Rev Cell Dev Biol* **14**, 19–57.

Boutell, J. M., Thomas, P., Neal, J. W., Weston, V. J., Duce, J., Harper, P. S., and Jones, A. L. (1999). Aberrant interactions of transcriptional repressor proteins with the Huntington's disease gene product, huntingtin. *Hum Mol Genet* **8**, 1647–55.

Brooks, B. P., Paulson, H. L., Merry, D. E., Salazar-Grueso, E. F., Brinkmann, A. O., Wilson, E. M., and Fischbeck, K. H. (1997). Characterization of an expanded glutamine repeat androgen receptor in a neuronal cell culture system. *Neurobiol Dis* **3**, 313–23.

Burke, J. R., Wingfield, M. S., Lewis, K. E., Roses, A. D., Lee, J. E., Hulette, C., Pericak-Vance, M. A., and Vance, J. M. (1994). The Haw River syndrome: dentatorubropallidoluysian atrophy (DRPLA) in an African-American family. *Nat Genet* **7**, 521–4.

Burright, E. N., Clark, H. B., Servadio, A., Matilla, T., Feddersen, R. M., Yunis, W. S., Duvick, L. A., Zoghbi, H. Y., and Orr, H. T. (1995). SCA1 transgenic mice: a model for neurodegeneration caused by an expanded CAG trinucleotide repeat. *Cell* **82**, 937–48.

—— Davidson, J. D., Duvick, L. A., Koshy, B., Zoghbi, H. Y., and Orr, H. T. (1997). Identification of a self-association region within the SCA1 gene product, ataxin-1. *Hum Mol Genet* **6**, 513–8.

Butler, R., Leigh, P. N., McPhaul, M. J., and Gallo, J. M. (1998). Truncated forms of the androgen receptor are associated with polyglutamine expansion in X-linked spinal and bulbar muscular atrophy. *Hum Mol Genet* **7**, 121–7.

Cancel, G., Abbas, N., Stevanin, G., Durr, A., Chneiweiss, H., Neri, C., Duyckaerts, C., Penet, C., Cann, H. M., Agid, Y., *et al.* (1995). Marked phenotypic heterogeneity associated with expansion of a CAG repeat sequence at the spinocerebellar ataxia 3/Machado–Joseph disease locus. *Am J Hum Genet* **57**, 809–16.

—— Durr, A., Didierjean, O., Imbert, G., Burk, K., Lezin, A., Belal, S., Benomar, A., Abada-Bendib, M., Vial, C., Guimaraes, J., Chneiweiss, H., Stevanin, G., Yvert, G., Abbas, N., Saudou, F., Lebre, A. S., Yahyaoui, M., Hentati, F., Vernant, J. C., Klockgether, T., Mandel, J. L., Agid, Y., and Brice, A. (1997). Molecular and clinical correlations in spinocerebellar ataxia 2: a study of 32 families. *Hum Mol Genet* **6**, 709–15.

—— Gourfinkel-An, I., Stevanin, G., Didierjean, O., Abbas, N., Hirsch, E., Agid, Y., and Brice, A. (1998). Somatic mosaicism of the CAG repeat expansion in spinocerebellar ataxia type 3/Machado–Joseph disease. *Hum Mutat* **11**, 23–7.

—— Duyckaerts, C., Holmberg, M., Zander, C., Yvert, G., Lebre, A. S., Ruberg, M., Faucheux, B., Agid, Y., Hirsch, E., and Brice, A. (2000). Distribution of ataxin-7 in normal human brain and retina. *Brain* **123** (pt. 12), 2519–30.

Cao, F., Levine, J. J., Li, S., and Li, X. (2001). Nuclear aggregation of huntingtin is not prevented by deletion of chaperone Hsp104. *Biochim Biophys Acta* 1**537**, 158–66.

Carmichael, J., Chatellier, J., Woolfson, A., Milstein, C., Fersht, A. R., and Rubinsztein, D. C. (2000). Bacterial and yeast chaperones reduce both aggregate formation and cell death in mammalian cell models of Huntington's disease. *Proc Natl Acad Sci, USA* **97**, 9701–5.

Cattaneo, E., Rigamonti, D., Goffredo, D., Zuccato, C., Squitieri, F., and Sipione, S. (2001). Loss of normal huntingtin function: new developments in Huntington's disease research. *Trends Neurosci* **24**, 182–8.

Cha, J. H. (2000). Transcriptional dysregulation in Huntington's disease. *Trends Neurosci* **23**, 387–92.

—— Kosinski, C. M., Kerner, J. A., Alsdorf, S. A., Mangiarini, L., Davies, S. W., Penney, J. B., Bates, G. P., and Young, A. B. (1998). Altered brain neurotransmitter receptors in transgenic mice expressing a portion of an abnormal human huntington disease gene. *Proc Natl Acad Sci, USA* **95**, 6480–5.

—— Frey, A. S., Alsdorf, S. A., Kerner, J. A., Kosinski, C. M., Mangiarini, L., Penney, J. B., Jr., Davies, S. W., Bates, G. P., and Young, A. B. (1999). Altered neurotransmitter receptor expression in transgenic mouse models of Huntington's disease. *Philos Trans R Soc Lond B Biol Sci* **354**, 981–9.

Chai, Y., Koppenhafer, S. L., Bonini, N. M., and Paulson, H. L. (1999). Analysis of the role of heat shock protein (Hsp) molecular chaperones in polyglutamine disease. *J Neurosci* **19**, 10338–47.

Chamberlain, N. L., Driver, E. D., and Miesfeld, R. L. (1994). The length and location of CAG trinucleotide repeats in the androgen receptor N-terminal domain affect transactivation function. *Nucl Acids Res* **22**, 3181–6.

Chan, H. Y., Warrick, J. M., Gray-Board, G. L., Paulson, H. L., and Bonini, N. M. (2000). Mechanisms of chaperone suppression of polyglutamine disease: selectivity, synergy and modulation of protein solubility in *Drosophila*. *Hum Mol Genet* **9**, 2811–20.

Chang, C. S., Kokontis, J., and Liao, S. T. (1988). Structural analysis of complementary DNA and amino acid sequences of human and rat androgen receptors. *Proc Natl Acad Sci, USA* **85**, 7211–5.

Chen, S., Berthelier, V., Yang, W., and Wetzel, R. (2001). Polyglutamine aggregation behavior *in vitro* supports a recruitment mechanism of cytotoxicity. *J Mol Biol* **311**, 173–82.

Chong, S. S., McCall, A. E., Cota, J., Subramony, S. H., Orr, H. T., Hughes, M. R., and Zoghbi, H. Y. (1995). Gametic and somatic tissue-specific heterogeneity of the expanded SCA1 CAG repeat in spinocerebellar ataxia type 1. *Nat Genet* **10**, 344–50.

Choong, C. S., Kemppainen, J. A., Zhou, Z. X., and Wilson, E. M. (1996). Reduced androgen receptor gene expression with first exon CAG repeat expansion. *Mol Endocrinol* **10**, 1527–35.

Chung, M.-Y., Ranum, L. P. W., Duvick, L. A., Servadio, A., Zoghbi, H. Y., and Orr, H. T. (1993). Evidence for a mechanism predisposing to intergenerational CAG repeat instability in spinocerebellar ataxia type 1. *Nat Genet* **5**, 254–8.

Clark, H. B., Burright, E. N., Yunis, W. S., Larson, S., Wilcox, C., Hartman, B., Matilla, A., Zoghbi, H. Y., and Orr, H. T. (1997). Purkinje cell expression of a mutant allele of SCA1 in transgenic mice leads to disparate effects on motor behaviors, followed by a progressive cerebellar dysfunction and histological alterations. *J Neurosci* **17**, 7385–95.

Costanzi-Porrini, S., Tessarolo, D., Abbruzzese, C., Liguori, M., Ashizawa, T., and Giacanelli, M. (2000). An interrupted 34-CAG repeat SCA-2 allele in patients with sporadic spinocerebellar ataxia. *Neurology* **54**, 491–3.

Cummings, C. J., Mancini, M. A., Antalffy, B., DeFranco, D. B., Orr, H. T., and Zoghbi, H. Y. (1998). Chaperone suppression of aggregation and altered subcellular proteasome localization imply protein misfolding in SCA1. *Nat Genet* **19**, 148–54.

—— Reinstein, E., Sun, Y., Antalffy, B., Jiang, Y., Ciechanover, A., Orr, H. T., Beaudet, A. L., and Zoghbi, H. Y. (1999). Mutation of the E6-AP ubiquitin ligase reduces nuclear inclusion frequency while accelerating polyglutamine-induced pathology in SCA1 mice. *Neuron* **24**, 879–92.

—— Sun, Y., Opal, P., Antalffy, B., Mestril, R., Orr, H. T., Dillmann, W. H., and Zoghbi, H. Y. (2001). Over-expression of inducible HSP70 chaperone suppresses neuropathology and improves motor function in SCA1 mice. *Hum Mol Genet* **10**, 1511–18.

David, G., Abbas, N., Stevanin, G., Durr, A., Yvert, G., Cancel, G., Weber, C., Imbert, G., Saudou, F., Antoniou, E., Drabkin, H., Gemmill, R., Giunti, P., Benomar, A., Wood, N., Ruberg, M., Agid, Y., Mandel, J. L., and Brice, A. (1997). Cloning of the SCA7 gene reveals a highly unstable CAG repeat expansion. *Nat Genet* **17**, 65–70.

—— Durr, A., Stevanin, G., Cancel, G., Abbas, N., Benomar, A., Belal, S., Lebre, A. S., Abada-Bendib, M., Grid, D., Holmberg, M., Yahyaoui, M., Hentati, F., Chkili, T., Agid, Y., and Brice, A. (1998). Molecular and clinical correlations in autosomal dominant cerebellar ataxia with progressive macular dystrophy (SCA7). *Hum Mol Genet* **7**, 165–70.

Davidson, J. D., Riley, B., Burright, E. N., Duvick, L. A., Zoghbi, H. Y., and Orr, H. T. (2000). Identification and characterization of an ataxin-1-interacting protein: A1Up, a ubiquitin-like nuclear protein. *Hum Mol Genet* **9**, 2305–12.

Davies, S. W., Turmaine, M., Cozens, B. A., DiFiglia, M., Sharp, A. H., Ross, C. A., Scherzinger, E., Wanker, E. E., Mangiarini, L., and Bates, G. P. (1997). Formation of neuronal intranuclear inclusions underlies the neurological dysfunction in mice transgenic for the HD mutation. *Cell* **90**, 537–48.

Dichgans, M., Schols, L., Herzog, J., Stevanin, G., Weirich-Schwaiger, H., Rouleau, G., Burk, K., Klockgether, T., Zuhlke, C., Laccone, F., Riess, O., and Gasser, T. (1999). Spinocerebellar ataxia type 6: evidence for a strong founder effect among German families. *Neurology* **52**, 849–51.

Didierjean, O., Cancel, G., Stevanin, G., Durr, A., Burk, K., Benomar, A., Lezin, A., Belal, S., Abada-Bendid, M., Klockgether, T., and Brice, A. (1999). Linkage disequilibrium at the SCA2 locus. *J Med Genet* **36**, 415–17.

DiFiglia, M., Sapp, E., Chase, K. O., Davies, S. W., Bates, G. P., Vonsattel, J. P., and Aronin, N. (1997). Aggregation of huntingtin in neuronal intranuclear inclusions and dystrophic neurites in brain. *Science* **277**, 1990–3.

Durr, A., Stevanin, G., Cancel, G., Duyckaerts, C., Abbas, N., Didierjean, O., Chneiweiss, H., Benomar, A., Lyon-Caen, O., Julien, J., Serdaru, M., Penet, C., Agid, Y., and Brice, A. (1996). Spinocerebellar ataxia 3 and Machado–Joseph disease: clinical, molecular, and neuropathological features. *Ann Neurol* **39**, 490–9.

Duyao, M., Ambrose, C., Myers, R., Novelletto, A., Persichetti, F., Frontali, M., Folstein, S., Ross, C., Franz, M., Abbott, M., Gray, J., Conneally, P., Young, A., Penney, J., Hollingsworth, Z., Shoulson, I., Lazzarini, A., Falek, A., Koroshetz, W., Sax, D., Bird, E., Vonsattel, J., Bonilla, E., Alvir, J., Bickham Conde, J., Cha, J.-H., Dure, L., Gomez, F., Ramos, M., Sanchez-Ramos, J., Snodgrass, S., de Young, M., Wexler, N., Moscowitz, C., Penchaszadeh, G., MacFarlane, H., Anderson, M., Jenkins, B., Srinifhi, J., Barnes, G., Gusella, J., and MacDonald, M. E. (1993). Trinucleotide repeat length instability and age of onset in Huntington's disease. *Nat Genet* **4**, 387–92.

Duyckaerts, C., Durr, A., Cancel, G., and Brice, A. (1999). Nuclear inclusions in spinocerebellar ataxia type 1. *Acta Neuropathol (Berl)* **97**, 201–7.

Ellerby, L. M., Hackam, A. S., Propp, S. S., Ellerby, H. M., Rabizadeh, S., Cashman, N. R., Trifiro, M. A., Pinsky, L., Wellington, C. L., Salvesen, G. S., Hayden, M. R., and Bredesen, D. E. (1999). Kennedy's disease: caspase cleavage of the androgen receptor is a crucial event in cytotoxicity. *J Neurochem* **72**, 185–95.

Endo, K., Sasaki, H., Wakisaka, A., Tanaka, H., Saito, M., Igarashi, S., Takiyama, Y., Sanpei, K., Iwabuchi, K., Suzuki, Y., Onari, K., Suzuki, T., Weissenbach, J., Weber, J. L., Nomura, Y., Segawa, M., Nishizawa, M., and Tsuji, S. (1996). Strong linkage disequilibrium and haplotype analysis in Japanese pedigrees with Machado–Joseph disease. *Am J Med Genet* **67**, 437–44.

Faber, P. W., Alter, J. R., MacDonald, M. E., and Hart, A. C. (1999). Polyglutamine-mediated dysfunction and apoptotic death of a *Caenorhabditis elegans* sensory neuron. *Proc Natl Acad Sci, USA* **96**, 179–84.

Ferdous, A., Gonzalez, F., Sun, L., Kodadek, T., and Johnston, S. A. (2001). The 19S regulatory particle of the proteasome is required for efficient transcription elongation by RNA polymerase II. *Mol Cell* **7**, 981–91.

Ferlini, A., Patrosso, M. C., Guidetti, D., Merlini, L., Uncini, A., Ragno, M., Plasmati, R., Fini, S., Repetto, M., Vezzoni, P., *et al.* (1995). Androgen receptor gene (CAG)*n* repeat analysis in the differential diagnosis between Kennedy disease and other motoneuron disorders. *Am J Med Genet* **55**, 105–11.

Fernandez-Funez, P., Nino-Rosales, M. L., de Gouyon, B., She, W. C., Luchak, J. M., Martinez, P., Turiegano, E., Benito, J., Capovilla, M., Skinner, P. J., McCall, A., Canal, I., Orr, H. T., Zoghbi, H. Y., and Botas, J. (2000). Identification of genes that modify ataxin-1-induced neurodegeneration. *Nature* **408**, 101–6.

Filla, A., De Michele, G., Santoro, L., Calabrese, O., Castaldo, I., Giuffrida, S., Restivo, D., Serlenga, L., Condorelli, D. F., Bonuccelli, U., Scala, R., Coppola, G., Caruso, G., and Cocozza, S. (1999). Spinocerebellar ataxia type 2 in southern Italy: a clinical and molecular study of 30 families. *J Neurol* **246**, 467–71.

Fujigasaki, H., Martin, J. J., De Deyn, P. P., Camuzat, A., Deffond, D., Stevanin, G., Dermaut, B., Van Broeckhoven, C., Durr, A., and Brice, A. (2001). CAG repeat expansion in the TATA box-binding protein gene causes autosomal dominant cerebellar ataxia. *Brain* **124**, 1939–47.

Gambardella, A., Muglia, M., Labate, A., Magariello, A., Gabriele, A. L., Mazzei, R., Pirritano, D., Conforti, F. L., Patitucci, A., Valentino, P., Zappia, M., and Quattrone, A. (2001). Juvenile Huntington's disease presenting as progressive myoclonic epilepsy. *Neurology* **57**, 708–11.

Gaspar, C., Lopes-Cendes, I., DeStefano, A. L., Maciel, P., Silveira, I., Coutinho, P., MacLeod, P., Sequeiros, J., Farrer, L. A., and Rouleau, G. A. (1996). Linkage disequilibrium analysis in Machado–Joseph disease patients of different ethnic origins. *Hum Genet* **98**, 620–4.

Georgiou, N., Bradshaw, J. L., Chiu, E., Tudor, A., O'Gorman, L., and Phillips, J. G. (1999). Differential clinical and motor control function in a pair of monozygotic twins with Huntington's disease. *Mov Disord* **14**, 320–5.

Geschwind, D. H., Perlman, S., Figueroa, K. P., Karrim, J., Baloh, R. W., and Pulst, S. M. (1997). Spinocerebellar ataxia type 6. Frequency of the mutation and genotype–phenotype correlations. *Neurology* **49**, 1247–51.

Gilman, S., Sima, A. A., Junck, L., Kluin, K. J., Koeppe, R. A., Lohman, M. E., and Little, R. (1996). Spinocerebellar ataxia type 1 with multiple system degeneration and glial cytoplasmic inclusions. *Ann Neurol* **39**, 241–55.

Giunti, P., Stevanin, G., Worth, P. F., David, G., Brice, A., and Wood, N. W. (1999). Molecular and clinical study of 18 families with ADCA type II: evidence for genetic heterogeneity and *de novo* mutation. *Am J Hum Genet* **64**, 1594–603.

Glass, M., Dragunow, M., and Faull, R. L. (2000). The pattern of neurodegeneration in Huntington's disease: a comparative study of cannabinoid, dopamine, adenosine and GABA(A) receptor alterations in the human basal ganglia in Huntington's disease. *Neuroscience* **97**, 505–19.

Goldfarb, L. G., Vasconcelos, O., Platonov, F. A., Lunkes, A., Kipnis, V., Kononova, S., Chabrashvili, T., Vladimirtsev, V. A., Alexeev, V. P., and Gajdusek, D. C. (1996). Unstable triplet repeat and phenotypic variability of spinocerebellar ataxia type 1. *Ann Neurol* **39**, 500–6.

Gomez, C. M. (2001). Polyglutamine aggregates in SCA6 Purkinje cells: a tail of two toxicities. *Neurology* **56**, 1618–19.

Gouw, L. G., Castaneda, M. A., McKenna, C. K., Digre, K. B., Pulst, S. M., Perlman, S., Lee, M. S., Gomez, C., Fischbeck, K., Gagnon, D., Storey, E., Bird, T., Jeri, F. R., and Ptacek, L. J. (1998). Analysis of the dynamic mutation in the SCA7 gene shows marked parental effects on CAG repeat transmission. *Hum Mol Genet* **7**, 525–32.

Gusella, J. F. and MacDonald, M. E. (2000). Molecular genetics: unmasking polyglutamine triggers in neurodegenerative disease. *Nature Rev Neurosci* **1**, 109–15.

Gutekunst, C. A., Li, S. H., Yi, H., Mulroy, J. S., Kuemmerle, S., Jones, R., Rye, D., Ferrante, R. J., Hersch, S. M., and Li, X. J. (1999). Nuclear and neuropil aggregates in Huntington's disease: relationship to neuropathology. *J Neurosci* **19**, 2522–34.

Gwinn-Hardy, K., Singleton, A., O'Suilleabhain, P., Boss, M., Nicholl, D., Adam, A., Hussey, J., Critchley, P., Hardy, J., and Farrer, M. (2001). Spinocerebellar ataxia type 3 phenotypically resembling parkinson disease in a black family. *Arch Neurol* **58**, 296–9.

Harding, A. E. (ed.) (1984) *The hereditary ataxias and related disorders* Churchill Livingston, Edinburgh.

Hashida, H., Goto, J., Kurisaki, H., Mizusawa, H., and Kanazawa, I. (1997). Brain regional differences in the expansion of a CAG repeat in the spinocerebellar ataxias: dentatorubral-pallidoluysian atrophy, Machado–Joseph disease, and spinocerebellar ataxia type 1. *Ann Neurol* **41**, 505–11.

Hayashi, Y., Kakita, A., Yamada, M., Koide, R., Igarashi, S., Takano, H., Ikeuchi, T., Wakabayashi, K., Egawa, S., Tsuji, S., and Takahashi, H. (1998). Hereditary dentatorubral-pallidoluysian atrophy: detection of widespread ubiquitinated neuronal and glial intranuclear inclusions in the brain. *Acta Neuropathol (Berl)* **96**, 547–52.

Hodgson, J. G., Agopyan, N., Gutekunst, C. A., Leavitt, B. R., LePiane, F., Singaraja, R., Smith, D. J., Bissada, N., McCutcheon, K., Nasir, J., Jamot, L., Li, X. J., Stevens, M. E., Rosemond, E., Roder, J. C., Phillips, A. G., Rubin, E. M., Hersch, S. M., and Hayden, M. R. (1999). A YAC mouse model for Huntington's disease with full-length mutant huntingtin, cytoplasmic toxicity, and selective striatal neurodegeneration. *Neuron* **23**, 181–92.

Holbert, S., Denghien, I., Kiechle, T., Rosenblatt, A., Wellington, C., Hayden, M. R., Margolis, R. L., Ross, C. A., Dausset, J., Ferrante, R. J., and Neri, C. (2001). The Gln–Ala repeat transcriptional activator CA150 interacts with huntingtin: neuropathologic and genetic evidence for a role in Huntington's disease pathogenesis. *Proc Natl Acad Sci, USA* **98**, 1811–16.

Holmberg, M., Duyckaerts, C., Durr, A., Cancel, G., Gourfinkel-An, I., Damier, P., Faucheux, B., Trottier, Y., Hirsch, E. C., Agid, Y., and Brice, A. (1998). Spinocerebellar ataxia type 7 (SCA7): a neurodegenerative disorder with neuronal intranuclear inclusions. *Hum Mol Genet* **7**, 913–18.

Holmes, S. E., O'Hearn, E. E., McInnis, M. G., Gorelick-Feldman, D. A., Kleiderlein, J. J., Callahan, C., Kwak, N. G., Ingersoll-Ashworth, R. G., Sherr, M., Sumner, A. J., Sharp, A. H., Ananth, U., Seltzer, W. K., Boss, M. A., Vieria-Saecker, A. M., Epplen, J. T., Riess, O., Ross, C. A., and Margolis, R. L. (1999).

Expansion of a novel CAG trinucleotide repeat in the 5′ region of PPP2R2B is associated with SCA12. *Nat Genet* **23**, 391–2.

Huang, C. C., Faber, P. W., Persichetti, F., Mittal, V., Vonsattel, J. P., MacDonald, M. E., and Gusella, J. F. (1998). Amyloid formation by mutant huntingtin: threshold, progressivity and recruitment of normal polyglutamine proteins. *Somat Cell Mol Genet* **24**, 217–33.

Hughes, R. E., Lo, R. S., Davis, C., Strand, A. D., Neal, C. L., Olson, J. M., and Fields, S. (2001). Altered transcription in yeast expressing expanded polyglutamine. *Proc Natl Acad Sci, USA* **98**, 13201–6.

Huntington's Disease Collaborative Research Group (1993). A novel gene containing a trinucleotide repeat that is expanded and unstable on Huntington's disease chromosomes. The Huntington's Disease Collaborative Research Group [see comments]. *Cell* **72**, 971–83.

Huynh, D. P., Del Bigio, M. R., Ho, D. H., and Pulst, S. M. (1999). Expression of ataxin-2 in brains from normal individuals and patients with Alzheimer's disease and spinocerebellar ataxia 2 [see comments]. *Ann Neurol* **45**, 232–41.

—— Figueroa, K., Hoang, N., and Pulst, S. M. (2000). Nuclear localization or inclusion body formation of ataxin-2 are not necessary for SCA2 pathogenesis in mouse or human. *Nat Genet* **26**, 44–50.

Ichikawa, Y., Goto, J., Hattori, M., Toyoda, A., Ishii, K., Jeong, S. Y., Hashida, H., Masuda, N., Ogata, K., Kasai, F., Hirai, M., Maciel, P., Rouleau, G. A., Sakaki, Y., and Kanazawa, I. (2001). The genomic structure and expression of MJD, the Machado–Joseph disease gene. *J Hum Genet* **46**, 413–22.

Igarashi, S., Tanno, Y., Onodera, O., Yamazaki, M., Sato, S., Ishikawa, A., Miyatani, N., Nagashima, M., Ishikawa, Y., Sahashi, K., *et al.* (1992). Strong correlation between the number of CAG repeats in androgen receptor genes and the clinical onset of features of spinal and bulbar muscular atrophy. *Neurology* **42**, 2300–2.

Ikeda, H., Yamaguchi, M., Sugai, S., Aze, Y., Narumiya, S., and Kakizuka, A. (1996). Expanded polyglutamine in the Machado–Joseph disease protein induces cell death *in vitro* and *in vivo*. *Nat Genet* **13**, 196–202.

Ikeuchi, T., Koide, R., Tanaka, H., Onodera, O., Igarashi, S., Takahashi, H., Kondo, R., Ishikawa, A., Tomoda, A., Miike, T., *et al.* (1995). Dentatorubral-pallidoluysian atrophy: clinical features are closely related to unstable expansions of trinucleotide (CAG) repeat. *Ann Neurol* **37**, 769–75.

—— Takano, H., Koide, R., Horikawa, Y., Honma, Y., Onishi, Y., Igarashi, S., Tanaka, H., Nakao, N., Sahashi, K., Tsukagoshi, H., Inoue, K., Takahashi, H., and Tsuji, S. (1997). Spinocerebellar ataxia type 6: CAG repeat expansion in alpha1A voltage-dependent calcium channel gene and clinical variations in Japanese population. *Ann Neurol* **42**, 879–84.

Imbert, G., Saudou, F., Yvert, G., Devys, D., Trottier, Y., Garnier, J. M., Weber, C., Mandel, J. L., Cancel, G., Abbas, N., Durr, A., Didierjean, O., Stevanin, G., Agid, Y., and Brice, A. (1996). Cloning of the gene for spinocerebellar ataxia 2 reveals a locus with high sensitivity to expanded CAG/glutamine repeats [see comments]. *Nat Genet* **14**, 285–91.

—— Naito, H., Ohama, E., Kawase, Y., Honma, Y., Tokiguchi, S., Hasegawa, S., Tamura, K., Kawai, K., Nagai, H., *et al.* (1990). [A clinical study and neuropathological findings of a familial disease with myoclonus and epilepsy—the nosological place of familial essential myoclonus and epilepsy (FEME)]. *Seishin Shinkeigaku Zasshi* **92**, 1–21.

Inoue, T., Lin, X., Kohlmeier, K. A., Orr, H. T., Zoghbi, H. Y., and Ross, W. N. (2001). Calcium dynamics and electrophysiological properties of cerebellar Purkinje cells in SCA1 transgenic mice. *J Neurophysiol* **85**, 1750–60.

Ishikawa, K., Tanaka, H., Saito, M., Ohkoshi, N., Fujita, T., Yoshizawa, K., Ikeuchi, T., Watanabe, M., Hayashi, A., Takiyama, Y., Nishizawa, M., Nakano, I., Matsubayashi, K., Miwa, M., Shoji, S., Kanazawa, I., Tsuji, S., and Mizusawa, H. (1997). Japanese families with autosomal dominant pure cerebellar ataxia map to chromosome 19p13.1–p13.2 and are strongly associated with mild CAG expansions in the spinocerebellar ataxia type 6 gene in chromosome 19p13.1. *Am J Hum Genet* **61**, 336–46.

Ishikawa, K., Fujigasaki, H., Saegusa, H., Ohwada, K., Fujita, T., Iwamoto, H., Komatsuzaki, Y., Toru, S., Toriyama, H., Watanabe, M., Ohkoshi, N., Shoji, S., Kanazawa, I., Tanabe, T., and Mizusawa, H. (1999). Abundant expression and cytoplasmic aggregations of [alpha]1A voltage-dependent calcium channel protein associated with neurodegeneration in spinocerebellar ataxia type 6. *Hum Mol Genet* **8**, 1185–93.

—— Owada, K., Ishida, K., Fujigasaki, H., Shun Li, M., Tsunemi, T., Ohkoshi, N., Toru, S., Mizutani, T., Hayashi, M., Arai, N., Hasegawa, K., Kawanami, T., Kato, T., Makifuchi, T., Shoji, S., Tanabe, T., and Mizusawa, H. (2001). Cytoplasmic and nuclear polyglutamine aggregates in SCA6 Purkinje cells. *Neurology* **56**, 1753–6.

Jackson, G. R., Salecker, I., Dong, X., Yao, X., Arnheim, N., Faber, P. W., MacDonald, M. E., and Zipursky, S. L. (1998). Polyglutamine-expanded human huntingtin transgenes induce degeneration of *Drosophila* photoreceptor neurons. *Neuron* **21**, 633–42.

Kaemmerer, W. F., Rodrigues, C. M., Steer, C. J., and Low, W. C. (2001). Creatine-supplemented diet extends Purkinje cell survival in spinocerebellar ataxia type 1 transgenic mice but does not prevent the ataxic phenotype. *Neuroscience* **103**, 713–24.

Kao, C. C., Lieberman, P. M., Schmidt, M. C., Zhou, Q., Pei, R., and Berk, A. J. (1990). Cloning of a transcriptionally active human TATA binding factor. *Science* **248**, 1646–50.

Kato, T., Tanaka, F., Yamamoto, M., Yosida, E., Indo, T., Watanabe, H., Yoshiwara, T., Doyu, M., and Sobue, G. (2000). Sisters homozygous for the spinocerebellar ataxia type 6 (SCA6)/CACNA1A gene associated with different clinical phenotypes. *Clin Genet* **58**, 69–73.

Kawaguchi, Y., Okamoto, T., Taniwaki, M., Aizawa, M., Inoue, M., Katayama, S., Kawakami, H., Nakamura, S., Nishimura, M., Akiguchi, I., *et al.* (1994). CAG expansions in a novel gene for Machado–Joseph disease at chromosome 14q32.1 [see comments]. *Nat Genet* **8**, 221–8.

Kawakami, H., Maruyama, H., Nakamura, S., Kawaguchi, Y., Kakizuka, A., Doyu, M., and Sobue, G. (1995). Unique features of the CAG repeats in Machado–Joseph disease [letter; see comments]. *Nat Genet* **9**, 344–5.

Kazantsev, A., Preisinger, E., Dranovsky, A., Goldgaber, D., and Housman, D. (1999). Insoluble detergent-resistant aggregates form between pathological and nonpathological lengths of polyglutamine in mammalian cells. *Proc Natl Acad Sci, USA* **96**, 11404–9.

Kazemi-Esfarjani, P. and Benzer, S. (2000). Genetic suppression of polyglutamine toxicity in *Drosophila*. *Science* **287**, 1837–40.

Kiehl, T. R., Shibata, H., and Pulst, S. M. (2000). The ortholog of human ataxin-2 is essential for early embryonic patterning in *C. elegans*. *J Mol Neurosci* **15**, 231–41.

—— —— Vo, T., Huynh, D. P., and Pulst, S. M. (2001). Identification and expression of a mouse ortholog of A2BP1. *Mamm Genome* **12**, 595–601.

Klement, I. A., Skinner, P. J., Kaytor, M. D., Yi, H., Hersch, S. M., Clark, H. B., Zoghbi, H. Y., and Orr, H. T. (1998). Ataxin-1 nuclear localization and aggregation: role in polyglutamine-induced disease in SCA1 transgenic mice [see comments]. *Cell* **95**, 41–53.

Klockgether, T., Wullner, U., Spauschus, A., and Evert, B. (2000). The molecular biology of the autosomal-dominant cerebellar ataxias. *Mov Disord* **15**, 604–12.

Koide, R., Ikeuchi, T., Onodera, O., Tanaka, H., Igarashi, S., Endo, K., Takahashi, H., Kondo, R., Ishikawa, A., Hayashi, T., *et al.* (1994). Unstable expansion of CAG repeat in hereditary dentatorubral-pallidoluysian atrophy (DRPLA). *Nat Genet* **6**, 9–13.

—— Kobayashi, S., Shimohata, T., Ikeuchi, T., Maruyama, M., Saito, M., Yamada, M., Takahashi, H., and Tsuji, S. (1999). A neurological disease caused by an expanded CAG trinucleotide repeat in the TATA-binding protein gene: a new polyglutamine disease? *Hum Mol Genet* **8**, 2047–53.

Komure, O., Sano, A., Nishino, N., Yamauchi, N., Ueno, S., Kondoh, K., Sano, N., Takahashi, M., Murayama, N., Kondo, I., *et al.* (1995). DNA analysis in hereditary dentatorubral-pallidoluysian atrophy: correlation between CAG repeat length and phenotypic variation and the molecular basis of anticipation. *Neurology* **45**, 143–9.

Koob, M. D., Moseley, M. L., Schut, L. J., Benzow, K. A., Bird, T. D., Day, J. W., and Ranum, L. P. (1999). An untranslated CTG expansion causes a novel form of spinocerebellar ataxia (SCA8). *Nat Genet* **21**, 379–84.

Koyano, S., Uchihara, T., Fujigasaki, H., Nakamura, A., Yagishita, S., and Iwabuchi, K. (1999). Neuronal intranuclear inclusions in spinocerebellar ataxia type 2: triple-labeling immunofluorescent study. *Neurosci Lett* **273**, 117–20.

—— Uchihara, T., Fujigasaki, H., Nakamura, A., Yagishita, S., and Iwabuchi, K. (2000). Neuronal intranuclear inclusions in spinocerebellar ataxia type 2. *Ann Neurol* **47**, 550.

Krobitsch, S. and Lindquist, S. (2000). Aggregation of huntingtin in yeast varies with the length of the polyglutamine expansion and the expression of chaperone proteins. *Proc Natl Acad Sci, USA* **97**, 1589–94.

Kurohara, K., Kuroda, Y., Maruyama, H., Kawakami, H., Yukitake, M., Matsui, M., and Nakamura, S. (1997). Homozygosity for an allele carrying intermediate CAG repeats in the dentatorubral-pallidoluysian atrophy (DRPLA) gene results in spastic paraplegia. *Neurology* **48**, 1087–90.

Lang, A. E., Rogaeva, E. A., Tsuda, T., Hutterer, J., and St George-Hyslop, P. (1994). Homozygous inheritance of the Machado–Joseph disease gene. *Ann Neurol* **36**, 443–7.

La Spada, A. R., Wilson, E. M., Lubahn, D. B., Harding, A. E., and Fischbeck, K. H. (1991). Androgen receptor gene mutations in X-linked spinal and bulbar muscular atrophy. *Nature* **352**, 77–9.

—— Roling D. B., Harding A. E., Warner, C. L., Spiegel, R., Hausmanowa-Petrusewicz, I., Yee, W.-C., and Fischbeck, K. H. (1992). Meiotic stability and genotype-phenotype correlation of the tri-nucleotide repeat in X-linked spinal and bulbar muscular atrophy. *Nat Genet* **2**, 301–4.

—— Fu, Y., Sopher, B. L., Libby, R. T., Wang, X., Li, L. Y., Einum, D. D., Huang, J., Possin, D. E., Smith, A. C., Martinez, R. A., Koszdin, K. L., Treuting, P. M., Ware, C. B., Hurley, J. B., Ptacek, L. J., and Chen, S. (2001). Polyglutamine-expanded ataxin-7 antagonizes crx function and induces cone–rod dystrophy in a mouse model of sca7. *Neuron* **31**, 913–27.

Lebre, A. S., Jamot, L., Takahashi, J., Spassky, N., Leprince, C., Ravise, N., Zander, C., Fujigasaki, H., Kussel-Andermann, P., Duyckaerts, C., Camonis, J. H., and Brice, A. (2001). Ataxin-7 interacts with a Cbl-associated protein that it recruits into neuronal intranuclear inclusions. *Hum Mol Genet* **10**, 1201–13.

Leggo, J., Dalton, A., Morrison, P. J., Dodge, A., Connarty, M., Kotze, M. J., and Rubinsztein, D. C. (1997). Analysis of spinocerebellar ataxia types 1, 2, 3, and 6, dentatorubral-pallidoluysian atrophy, and Friedreich's ataxia genes in spinocerebellar ataxia patients in the UK. *J Med Genet* **34**, 982–5.

Li, H., Li, S. H., Johnston, H., Shelbourne, P. F., and Li, X. J. (2000). Amino-terminal fragments of mutant huntingtin show selective accumulation in striatal neurons and synaptic toxicity. *Nat Genet* **25**, 385–9.

Li, M., Miwa, S., Kobayashi, Y., Merry, D. E., Yamamoto, M., Tanaka, F., Doyu, M., Hashizume, Y., Fischbeck, K. H., and Sobue, G. (1998a). Nuclear inclusions of the androgen receptor protein in spinal and bulbar muscular atrophy. *Ann Neurol* **44**, 249–54.

—— Nakagomi, Y., Kobayashi, Y., Merry, D. E., Tanaka, F., Doyu, M., Mitsuma, T., Hashizume, Y., Fischbeck, K. H., and Sobue, G. (1998b). Nonneural nuclear inclusions of androgen receptor protein in spinal and bulbar muscular atrophy. *Am J Pathol* **153**, 695–701.

Lieberman, A. P. and Fischbeck, K. H. (2000). Triplet repeat expansion in neuromuscular disease. *Muscle Nerve* **23**, 843–50.

Lin, X., Antalffy, B., Kang, D., Orr, H. T., and Zoghbi, H. Y. (2000). Polyglutamine expansion down-regulates specific neuronal genes before pathologic changes in SCA1. *Nat Neurosci* **3**, 157–63.

Lindenberg, K. S., Yvert, G., Muller, K., and Landwehrmeyer, G. B. (2000). Expression analysis of ataxin-7 mRNA and protein in human brain: evidence for a widespread distribution and focal protein accumulation. *Brain Pathol* **10**, 385–94.

Lopes-Cendes, I., Maciel, P., Kish, S., Gaspar, C., Robitaille, Y., Clark, H. B., Koeppen, A. H., Nance, M., Schut, L., Silveira, I., Coutinho, P., Sequeiros, J., and Rouleau, G. A. (1996). Somatic mosaicism in the central nervous system in spinocerebellar ataxia type 1 and Machado–Joseph disease. *Ann Neurol* **40**, 199–206.

Lorenzetti, D., Watase, K., Xu, B., Matzuk, M. M., Orr, H. T., and Zoghbi, H. Y. (2000). Repeat instability and motor incoordination in mice with a targeted expanded CAG repeat in the Sca1 locus. *Hum Mol Genet* **9**, 779–85.

Luthi-Carter, R., Strand, A., Peters, N. L., Solano, S. M., Hollingsworth, Z. R., Menon, A. S., Frey, A. S., Spektor, B. S., Penney, E. B., Schilling, G., Ross, C. A., Borchelt, D. R., Tapscott, S. J., Young, A. B., Cha, J. H., and Olson, J. M. (2000). Decreased expression of striatal signaling genes in a mouse model of Huntington's disease. *Hum Mol Genet* **9**, 1259–71.

Maciel, P., Gaspar, C., DeStefano, A. L., Silveira, I., Coutinho, P., Radvany, J., Dawson, D. M., Sudarsky, L., Guimaraes, J., Loureiro, J. E., *et al.* (1995). Correlation between CAG repeat length and clinical features in Machado–Joseph disease. *Am J Hum Genet* **57**, 54–61.

MacLean, H. E., Choi, W. T., Rekaris, G., Warne, G. L., and Zajac, J. D. (1995). Abnormal androgen receptor binding affinity in subjects with Kennedy's disease (spinal and bulbar muscular atrophy). *J Clin Endocrinol Metab* **80**, 508–16.

Marsh, J. L., Walker, H., Theisen, H., Zhu, Y. Z., Fielder, T., Purcell, J., and Thompson, L. M. (2000). Expanded polyglutamine peptides alone are intrinsically cytotoxic and cause neurodegeneration in *Drosophila*. *Hum Mol Genet* **9**, 13–25.

Martindale, D., Hackam, A., Wieczorek, A., Ellerby, L., Wellington, C., McCutcheon, K., Singaraja, R., Kazemi-Esfarjani, P., Devon, R., Kim, S. U., Bredesen, D. E., Tufaro, F., and Hayden, M. R. (1998). Length of huntingtin and its polyglutamine tract influences localization and frequency of intracellular aggregates. *Nat Genet* **18**, 150–4.

Maruyama, H., Nakamura, S., Matsuyama, Z., Sakai, T., Doyu, M., Sobue, G., Seto, M., Tsujihata, M., Oh-i, T., Nishio, T., *et al.* (1995). Molecular features of the CAG repeats and clinical manifestation of Machado–Joseph disease. *Hum Mol Genet* **4**, 807–12.

Matilla, A., Koshy, B. T., Cummings, C. J., Isobe, T., Orr, H. T., and Zoghbi, H. Y. (1997). The cerebellar leucine-rich acidic nuclear protein interacts with ataxin-1 [published erratum appears in *Nature* 1998; **391** (6669), 818]. *Nature* **389**, 974–8.

—— Roberson, E. D., Banfi, S., Morales, J., Armstrong, D. L., Burright, E. N., Orr, H. T., Sweatt, J. D., Zoghbi, H. Y., and Matzuk, M. M. (1998). Mice lacking ataxin-1 display learning deficits and decreased hippocampal paired-pulse facilitation. *J Neurosci* **18**, 5508–16.

Matsumura, R., Futamura, N., Fujimoto, Y., Yanagimoto, S., Horikawa, H., Suzumura, A., and Takayanagi, T. (1997). Spinocerebellar ataxia type 6. Molecular and clinical features of 35 Japanese patients including one homozygous for the CAG repeat expansion. *Neurology* **49**, 1238–43.

Matsuyama, Z., Kawakami, H., Maruyama, H., Izumi, Y., Komure, O., Udaka, F., Kameyama, M., Nishio, T., Kuroda, Y., Nishimura, M., and Nakamura, S. (1997). Molecular features of the CAG repeats of spinocerebellar ataxia 6 (SCA6). *Hum Mol Genet* **6**, 1283–7.

—— Izumi, Y., Kameyama, M., Kawakami, H., and Nakamura, S. (1999). The effect of CAT trinucleotide interruptions on the age at onset of spinocerebellar ataxia type 1 (SCA1). *J Med Genet* **36**, 546–8.

Mauger, C., Del-Favero, J., Ceuterick, C., Lubke, U., van Broeckhoven, C., and Martin, J. (1999). Identification and localization of ataxin-7 in brain and retina of a patient with cerebellar ataxia type II using anti-peptide antibody. *Brain Res Mol Brain Res* **74**, 35–43.

McCampbell, A., Taylor, J. P., Taye, A. A., Robitschek, J., Li, M., Walcott, J., Merry, D., Chai, Y., Paulson, H., Sobue, G., and Fischbeck, K. H. (2000). CREB-binding protein sequestration by expanded polyglutamine. *Hum Mol Genet* **9**, 2197–202.

Merry, D. E., Kobayashi, Y., Bailey, C. K., Taye, A. A., and Fischbeck, K. H. (1998). Cleavage, aggregation and toxicity of the expanded androgen receptor in spinal and bulbar muscular atrophy. *Hum Mol Genet* **7**, 693–701.

Mhatre, A. N., Trifiro, M. A., Kaufman, M., Kazemi-Esfarjani, P., Figlewicz, D., Rouleau, G., and Pinsky, L. (1993). Reduced transcriptional regulatory competence of the androgen receptor in

X-linked spinal and bulbar muscular atrophy [published erratum appears in *Nat Genet* 1994; **6** (2), 214]. *Nat Genet* **5**, 184–8.

Mizushima, K., Watanabe, M., Abe, K., Aoki, M., Itoyama, Y., Shizuka, M., Okamoto, K., and Shoji, M. (1998). Analysis of spinocerebellar ataxia type 2 in Gunma Prefecture in Japan: CAG trinucleotide expansion and clinical characteristics. *J Neurol Sci* **156**, 180–5.

Monckton, D. G., Cayuela, M. L., Gould, F. K., Brock, G. J., Silva, R., and Ashizawa, T. (1999). Very large (CAG)(n) DNA repeat expansions in the sperm of two spinocerebellar ataxia type 7 males. *Hum Mol Genet* **8**, 2473–8.

Moseley, M. L., Benzow, K. A., Schut, L. J., Bird, T. D., Gomez, C. M., Barkhaus, P. E., Blindauer, K. A., Labuda, M., Pandolfo, M., Koob, M. D., and Ranum, L. P. (1998). Incidence of dominant spinocerebellar and Friedreich triplet repeats among 361 ataxia families. *Neurology* **51**, 1666–71.

Muchowski, P. J., Schaffar, G., Sittler, A., Wanker, E. E., Hayer-Hartl, M. K., and Hartl, F. U. (2000). Hsp70 and hsp40 chaperones can inhibit self-assembly of polyglutamine proteins into amyloid-like fibrils. *Proc Natl Acad Sci, USA* **97**, 7841–6.

Murata, T., Kurokawa, R., Krones, A., Tatsumi, K., Ishii, M., Taki, T., Masuno, M., Ohashi, H., Yanagisawa, M., Rosenfeld, M. G., Glass, C. K., and Hayashi, Y. (2001). Defect of histone acetyl-transferase activity of the nuclear transcriptional coactivator CBP in Rubinstein–Taybi syndrome. *Hum Mol Genet* **10**, 1071–6.

Myers, R. H., MacDonald, M. E., Koroshetz, W. J., Duyao, M. P., Ambrose, C. M., Taylor, S. A., Barnes, G., Srinidhi, J., Lin, C. S., Whaley, W. L., *et al.* (1993). *De novo* expansion of a (CAG)*n* repeat in sporadic Huntington's disease [see comments]. *Nat Genet* **5**, 168–73.

—— Marans, K. S., and MacDonald, M. E. (1998). In *Genetic instabilities and hereditary neurological diseases* (ed. R. D. Wells and S. T. Warren), pp. 301–23. Academic Press, San Diego.

Nagafuchi, S., Yanagisawa, H., Sato, K., Shirayama, T., Ohsaki, E., Bundo, M., Takeda, T., Tadokoro, K., Kondo, I., Murayama, N., *et al.* (1994). Dentatorubral and pallidoluysian atrophy expansion of an unstable CAG trinucleotide on chromosome 12p. *Nat Genet* **6**, 14–18.

Nagai, Y., Azuma, T., Funauchi, M., Fujita, M., Umi, M., Hirano, M., Matsubara, T., and Ueno, S. (1998). Clinical and molecular genetic study in seven Japanese families with spinocerebellar ataxia type 6. *J Neurol Sci* **157**, 52–9.

Nakamura, K., Jeong, S. Y., Uchihara, T., Anno, M., Nagashima, K., Nagashima, T., Ikeda, S., Tsuji, S., and Kanazawa, I. (2001). SCA17, a novel autosomal dominant cerebellar ataxia caused by an expanded polyglutamine in TATA-binding protein. *Hum Mol Genet* **10**, 1441–8.

Norremolle, A., Nielsen, J. E., Sorensen, S. A., and Hasholt, L. (1995). Elongated CAG repeats of the B37 gene in a Danish family with dentato-rubro-pallido-luysian atrophy. *Hum Genet* **95**, 313–18.

Nucifora, F. C. Jr, Sasaki, M., Peters, M. F., Huang, H., Cooper, J. K., Yamada, M., Takahashi, H., Tsuji, S., Troncoso, J., Dawson, V. L., Dawson, T. M., and Ross, C. A. (2001). Interference by huntingtin and atrophin-1 with cbp-mediated transcription leading to cellular toxicity. *Science* **291**, 2423–8.

Okamura-Oho, Y., Miyashita, T., Ohmi, K., and Yamada, M. (1999). Dentatorubral-pallidoluysian atrophy protein interacts through a proline-rich region near polyglutamine with the SH3 domain of an insulin receptor tyrosine kinase substrate. *Hum Mol Genet* **8**, 947–57.

Ophoff, R. A., Terwindt, G. M., Vergouwe, M. N., van Eijk, R., Oefner, P. J., Hoffman, S. M., Lamerdin, J. E., Mohrenweiser, H. W., Bulman, D. E., Ferrari, M., Haan, J., Lindhout, D., van Ommen, G. J., Hofker, M. H., Ferrari, M. D., and Frants, R. R. (1996). Familial hemiplegic migraine and episodic ataxia type-2 are caused by mutations in the Ca^{2+} channel gene CACNL1A4. *Cell* **87**, 543–52.

Ordway, J. M., Tallaksen-Greene, S., Gutekunst, C. A., Bernstein, E. M., Cearley, J. A., Wiener, H. W., Dure, L. S. T., Lindsey, R., Hersch, S. M., Jope, R. S., Albin, R. L., and Detloff, P. J. (1997). Ectopically expressed CAG repeats cause intranuclear inclusions and a progressive late onset neurological phenotype in the mouse. *Cell* **91**, 753–63.

Orr, H. T., Chung, M. Y., Banfi, S., Kwiatkowski, T. J., Jr., Servadio, A., Beaudet, A. L., McCall, A. E., Duvick, L. A., Ranum, L. P., and Zoghbi, H. Y. (1993). Expansion of an unstable trinucleotide CAG repeat in spinocerebellar ataxia type 1. *Nat Genet* **4**, 221–6.

Pareyson, D., Gellera, C., Castellotti, B., Antonelli, A., Riggio, M. C., Mazzucchelli, F., Girotti, F., Pietrini, V., Mariotti, C., and Di Donato, S. (1999). Clinical and molecular studies of 73 Italian families with autosomal dominant cerebellar ataxia type I: SCA1 and SCA2 are the most common genotypes. *J Neurol* **246**, 389–93.

Parker, J. A., Connolly, J. B., Wellington, C., Hayden, M., Dausset, J., and Neri, C. (2001). Expanded polyglutamines in Caenorhabditis elegans cause axonal abnormalities and severe dysfunction of PLM mechanosensory neurons without cell death. *Proc Natl Acad Sci, USA* **98**, 13318–23.

Paulson, H. L., Das, S. S., Crino, P. B., Perez, M. K., Patel, S. C., Gotsdiner, D., Fischbeck, K. H., and Pittman, R. N. (1997a). Machado–Joseph disease gene product is a cytoplasmic protein widely expressed in brain. *Ann Neurol* **41**, 453–62.

——— Perez, M. K., Trottier, Y., Trojanowski, J. Q., Subramony, S. H., Das, S. S., Vig, P., Mandel, J. L., Fischbeck, K. H., and Pittman, R. N. (1997b). Intranuclear inclusions of expanded polyglutamine protein in spinocerebellar ataxia type 3. *Neuron* **19**, 333–44.

Perez, M. K., Paulson, H. L., Pendse, S. J., Saionz, S. J., Bonini, N. M., and Pittman, R. N. (1998). Recruitment and the role of nuclear localization in polyglutamine- mediated aggregation. *J Cell Biol* **143**, 1457–70.

——— —— Pittman, R. N. (1999). Ataxin-3 with an altered conformation that exposes the polyglutamine domain is associated with the nuclear matrix. *Hum Mol Genet* **8**, 2377–85.

Preisinger, E., Jordan, B. M., Kazantsev, A., and Housman, D. (1999). Evidence for a recruitment and sequestration mechanism in Huntington's disease. *Philos Trans R Soc Lond B Biol Sci* **354**, 1029–34.

Pujana, M. A., Corral, J., Gratacos, M., Combarros, O., Berciano, J., Genis, D., Banchs, I., Estivill, X., and Volpini, V. (1999). Spinocerebellar ataxias in Spanish patients: genetic analysis of familial and sporadic cases. The Ataxia Study Group. *Hum Genet* **104**, 516–22.

Pulst, S. M., Nechiporuk, A., Nechiporuk, T., Gispert, S., Chen, X. N., Lopes-Cendes, I., Pearlman, S., Starkman, S., Orozco-Diaz, G., Lunkes, A., DeJong, P., Rouleau, G. A., Auburger, G., Korenberg, J. R., Figueroa, C., and Sahba, S. (1996). Moderate expansion of a normally biallelic trinucleotide repeat in spinocerebellar ataxia type 2 [see comments]. *Nat Genet* **14**, 269–76.

Ranen, N. G., Stine O. C. Abbott, M. H., Sherr M., Codori, A.-M., Franz, M. L., Chao, N. I., Chung, A. S., Pleasant, N., Callahan, C., Kasch, L. M., Ghaffari, M., Chase, G. A., Kazazian, H. H., Brandt, J., Folstein, S. E., and Ross, C. A. (1995). Anticipation and instability of IT-15 (CAG)n repeats in parent–offspring pairs with Huntington's disease. *Am J Hum Genet* **57**, 593–602.

Riess, O., Laccone, F. A., Gispert, S., Schols, L., Zuhlke, C., Vieira-Saecker, A. M., Herlt, S., Wessel, K., Epplen, J. T., Weber, B. H., Kreuz, F., Chahrokh-Zadeh, S., Meindl, A., Lunkes, A., Aguiar, J., Macek, M., Jr., Krebsova, A., Macek, M., Sr., Burk, K., Tinschert, S., Schreyer, I., Pulst, S. M., and Auburger, G. (1997a). SCA2 trinucleotide expansion in German SCA patients. *Neurogenetics* **1**, 59–64.

——— Schols, L., Bottger, H., Nolte, D., Vieira-Saecker, A. M., Schimming, C., Kreuz, F., Macek, M., Jr., Krebsova, A., Macek, M. S., Klockgether, T., Zuhlke, C., and Laccone, F. A. (1997b). SCA6 is caused by moderate CAG expansion in the alpha1A-voltage-dependent calcium channel gene. *Hum Mol Genet* **6**, 1289–93.

Salghetti, S. E., Caudy, A. A., Chenoweth, J. G., and Tansey, W. P. (2001). Regulation of transcriptional activation domain function by ubiquitin. *Science* **293**, 1651–3.

Sanchez, I., Xu, C. J., Juo, P., Kakizaka, A., Blenis, J., and Yuan, J. (1999). Caspase-8 is required for cell death induced by expanded polyglutamine repeats [see comments]. *Neuron* **22**, 623–33.

Sanpei, K., Takano, H., Igarashi, S., Sato, T., Oyake, M., Sasaki, H., Wakisaka, A., Tashiro, K., Ishida, Y., Ikeuchi, T., Koide, R., Saito, M., Sato, A., Tanaka, T., Hanyu, S., Takiyama, Y., Nishizawa, M., Shimizu, N., Nomura, Y., Segawa, M., Iwabuchi, K., Eguchi, I., Tanaka, H., Takahashi, H., and Tsuji, S. (1996). Identification of the spinocerebellar ataxia type 2 gene using a direct identification of repeat expansion and cloning technique, DIRECT [see comments]. *Nat Genet* **14**, 277–84.

Sapp, E., Penney, J., Young, A., Aronin, N., Vonsattel, J. P., and DiFiglia, M. (1999). Axonal transport of N-terminal huntingtin suggests early pathology of corticostriatal projections in Huntington disease. *J Neuropathol Exp Neurol* **58**, 165–73.

Sato, K., Kashihara, K., Okada, S., Ikeuchi, T., Tsuji, S., Shomori, T., Morimoto, K., and Hayabara, T. (1995). Does homozygosity advance the onset of dentatorubral-pallidoluysian atrophy? *Neurology* **45**, 1934–6.

Satyal, S. H., Schmidt, E., Kitagawa, K., Sondheimer, N., Lindquist, S., Kramer, J. M., and Morimoto, R. I. (2000). Polyglutamine aggregates alter protein folding homeostasis in *Caenorhabditis elegans. Proc Natl Acad Sci, USA* **97**, 5750–5.

Saudou, F., Finkbeiner, S., Devys, D., and Greenberg, M. E. (1998). Huntingtin acts in the nucleus to induce apoptosis but death does not correlate with the formation of intranuclear inclusions. *Cell* **95**, 55–66.

Scherzinger, E., Lurz, R., Turmaine, M., Mangiarini, L., Hollenbach, B., Hasenbank, R., Bates, G. P., Davies, S. W., Lehrach, H., and Wanker, E. E. (1997). Huntingtin-encoded polyglutamine expansions form amyloid-like protein aggregates *in vitro* and *in vivo. Cell* **90**, 549–58.

—— Sittler, A., Schweiger, K., Heiser, V., Lurz, R., Hasenbank, R., Bates, G. P., Lehrach, H., and Wanker, E. E. (1999). Self-assembly of polyglutamine-containing huntingtin fragments into amyloid-like fibrils: implications for Huntington's disease pathology. *Proc Natl Acad Sci, USA* **96**, 4604–9.

Schilling, G., Wood, J. D., Duan, K., Slunt, H. H., Gonzales, V., Yamada, M., Cooper, J. K., Margolis, R. L., Jenkins, N. A., Copeland, N. G., Takahashi, H., Tsuji, S., Price, D. L., Borchelt, D. R., and Ross, C. A. (1999). Nuclear accumulation of truncated atrophin-1 fragments in a transgenic mouse model of DRPLA. *Neuron* **24**, 275–86.

—— Jinnah, H. A., Gonzales, V., Coonfield, M. L., Kim, Y., Wood, J. D., Price, D. L., Li, X. J., Jenkins, N., Copeland, N., Moran, T., Ross, C. A., and Borchelt, D. R. (2001). Distinct behavioral and neuropathological abnormalities in transgenic mouse models of HD and DRPLA. *Neurobiol Dis* **8**, 405–18.

Schols, L., Gispert, S., Vorgerd, M., Menezes Vieira-Saecker, A. M., Blanke, P., Auburger, G., Amoiridis, G., Meves, S., Epplen, J. T., Przuntek, H., Pulst, S. M., and Riess, O. (1997). Spinocerebellar ataxia type 2. Genotype and phenotype in German kindreds. *Arch Neurol* **54**, 1073–80.

—— Kruger, R., Amoiridis, G., Przuntek, H., Epplen, J. T., and Riess, O. (1998). Spinocerebellar ataxia type 6: genotype and phenotype in German kindreds. *J Neurol Neurosurg Psychiatry* **64**, 67–73.

Servadio, A., Koshy, B., Armstrong, D., Antalffy, B., Orr, H. T., and Zoghbi, H. Y. (1995). Expression analysis of the ataxin-1 protein in tissues from normal and spinocerebellar ataxia type 1 individuals [see comments]. *Nat Genet* **10**, 94–8.

Shibata, H., Huynh, D. P., and Pulst, S. M. (2000). A novel protein with RNA-binding motifs interacts with ataxin-2. *Hum Mol Genet* **9**, 1303–13.

Shimazaki, H., Takiyama, Y., Sakoe, K., Amaike, M., Nagaki, H., Namekawa, M., Sasaki, H., Nakano, I., and Nishizawa, M. (2001). Meiotic instability of the CAG repeats in the SCA6/CACNA1A gene in two Japanese SCA6 families. *J Neurol Sci* **185**, 101–7.

Shimohata, T., Nakajima, T., Yamada, M., Uchida, C., Onodera, O., Naruse, S., Kimura, T., Koide, R., Nozaki, K., Sano, Y., Ishiguro, H., Sakoe, K., Ooshima, T., Sato, A., Ikeuchi, T., Oyake, M., Sato, T., Aoyagi, Y., Hozumi, I., Nagatsu, T., Takiyama, Y., Nishizawa, M., Goto, J., Kanazawa, I., Davidson, I., Tanese, N., Takahashi, H., and Tsuji, S. (2000). Expanded polyglutamine stretches interact with TAFII130, interfering with CREB-dependent transcription. *Nat Genet* **26**, 29–36.

Shizuka, M., Watanabe, M., Ikeda, Y., Mizushima, K., Okamoto, K., and Shoji, M. (1998). Molecular analysis of a *de novo* mutation for spinocerebellar ataxia type 6 and (CAG)*n* repeat units in normal elder controls. *J Neurol Sci* **161**, 85–7.

Silveira, I., Lopes-Cendes, I., Kish, S., Maciel, P., Gaspar, C., Coutinho, P., Botez, M. I., Teive, H., Arruda, W., Steiner, C. E., Pinto-Junior, W., Maciel, J. A., Jerin, S., Sack, G., Andermann, E., Sudarsky, L., Rosenberg, R., MacLeod, P., Chitayat, D., Babul, R., Sequeiros, J., and Rouleau, G. A. (1996). Frequency of spinocerebellar ataxia type 1, dentatorubropallidoluysian atrophy, and Machado–Joseph disease mutations in a large group of spinocerebellar ataxia patients. *Neurology* **46**, 214–8.

—— Coutinho, P., Maciel, P., Gaspar, C., Hayes, S., Dias, A., Guimaraes, J., Loureiro, L., Sequeiros, J., and Rouleau, G. A. (1998). Analysis of SCA1, DRPLA, MJD, SCA2, and SCA6 CAG repeats in 48 Portuguese ataxia families. *Am J Med Genet* **81**, 134–8.

Sittler, A., Lurz, R., Lueder, G., Priller, J., Hayer-Hartl, M. K., Hartl, F. U., Lehrach, H., and Wanker, E. E. (2001). Geldanamycin activates a heat shock response and inhibits huntingtin aggregation in a cell culture model of Huntington's disease. *Hum Mol Genet* **10**, 1307–15.

Skinner, P. J., Koshy, B. T., Cummings, C. J., Klement, I. A., Helin, K., Servadio, A., Zoghbi, H. Y., and Orr, H. T. (1997). Ataxin-1 with an expanded glutamine tract alters nuclear matrix- associated structures [published erratum appears in *Nature* 1998; **391** (6664), 307]. *Nature* **389**, 971–4.

—— Vierra-Green, C. A., Clark, H. B., Zoghbi, H. Y., and Orr, H. T. (2001). Altered trafficking of membrane proteins in purkinje cells of SCA1 transgenic mice. *Am J Pathol* **159**, 905–13.

Spiegel, R., La Spada, A. R., Kress, W., Fischbeck, K. H., and Schmid, W. (1996). Somatic stability of the expanded CAG trinucleotide repeat in X-linked spinal and bulbar muscular atrophy. *Hum Mutat* **8**, 32–7.

Steffan, J. S., Kazantsev, A., Spasic-Boskovic, O., Greenwald, M., Zhu, Y. Z., Gohler, H., Wanker, E. E., Bates, G. P., Housman, D. E., and Thompson, L. M. (2000). The Huntington's disease protein interacts with p53 and CREB-binding protein and represses transcription. *Proc Natl Acad Sci, USA* **97**, 6763–8.

—— Bodai, L., Pallos, J., Poelman, M., McCampbell, A., Apostol, B. L., Kazantsev, A., Schmidt, E., Zhu, Y. Z., Greenwald, M., Kurokawa, R., Housman, D. E., Jackson, G. R., Marsh, J. L., and Thompson, L. M. (2001). Histone deacetylase inhibitors arrest polyglutamine-dependent neurodegeneration in *Drosophila*. *Nature* **413**, 739–43.

Stenoien, D. L., Cummings, C. J., Adams, H. P., Mancini, M. G., Patel, K., DeMartino, G. N., Marcelli, M., Weigel, N. L., and Mancini, M. A. (1999). Polyglutamine-expanded androgen receptors form aggregates that sequester heat shock proteins, proteasome components and SRC-1, and are suppressed by the HDJ-2 chaperone. *Hum Mol Genet* **8**, 731–41.

Stevanin, G., Cancel, G., Didierjean, O., Durr, A., Abbas, N., Cassa, E., Feingold, J., Agid, Y., and Brice, A. (1995). Linkage disequilibrium at the Machado–Joseph disease/spinal cerebellar ataxia 3 locus: evidence for a common founder effect in French and Portuguese-Brazilian families as well as a second ancestral Portuguese-Azorean mutation. *Am J Hum Genet* **57**, 1247–50.

—— Durr, A., David, G., Didierjean, O., Cancel, G., Rivaud, S., Tourbah, A., Warter, J. M., Agid, Y., and Brice, A. (1997a). Clinical and molecular features of spinocerebellar ataxia type 6. *Neurology* **49**, 1243–6.

—— Lebre, A. S., Mathieux, C., Cancel, G., Abbas, N., Didierjean, O., Durr, A., Trottier, Y., Agid, Y., and Brice, A. (1997b). Linkage disequilibrium between the spinocerebellar ataxia 3/Machado–Joseph disease mutation and two intragenic polymorphisms, one of which, X359Y, affects the stop codon. *Am J Hum Genet* **60**, 1548–52.

—— Giunti, P., Belal, G. D., Durr, A., Ruberg, M., Wood, N., and Brice, A. (1998). *De novo* expansion of intermediate alleles in spinocerebellar ataxia 7. *Hum Mol Genet* **7**, 1809–13.

—— David, G., Durr, A., Giunti, P., Benomar, A., Abada-Bendib, M., Lee, M. S., Agid, Y., and Brice, A. (1999). Multiple origins of the spinocerebellar ataxia 7 (SCA7) mutation revealed by linkage disequilibrium studies with closely flanking markers, including an intragenic polymorphism (G3145TG/A3145TG). *Eur J Hum Genet* **7**, 889–96.

—— Durr, A., and Brice, A. (2000). Clinical and molecular advances in autosomal dominant cerebellar ataxias: from genotype to phenotype and physiopathology. *Eur J Hum Genet* **8**, 4–18.

Suhr, S. T., Senut, M. C., Whitelegge, J. P., Faull, K. F., Cuizon, D. B., and Gage, F. H. (2001). Identities of sequestered proteins in aggregates from cells with induced polyglutamine expression. *J Cell Biol* **153**, 283–94.

Tait, D., Riccio, M., Sittler, A., Scherzinger, E., Santi, S., Ognibene, A., Maraldi, N. M., Lehrach, H., and Wanker, E. E. (1998). Ataxin-3 is transported into the nucleus and associates with the nuclear matrix. *Hum Mol Genet* **7**, 991–7.

Takahashi, H., Egawa, S., Piao, Y. S., Hayashi, S., Yamada, M., Shimohata, T., Oyanagi, K., and Tsuji, S. (2001). Neuronal nuclear alterations in dentatorubral-pallidoluysian atrophy: ultrastructural and morphometric studies of the cerebellar granule cells. *Brain Res* **919**, 12–19.

—— Onodera, O., Takahashi, H., Igarashi, S., Yamada, M., Oyake, M., Ikeuchi, T., Koide, R., Tanaka, H., Iwabuchi, K., and Tsuji, S. (1996). Somatic mosaicism of expanded CAG repeats in brains of patients with dentatorubral-pallidoluysian atrophy: cellular population-dependent dynamics of mitotic instability. *Am J Hum Genet* **58**, 1212–22.

—— Cancel, G., Ikeuchi, T., Lorenzetti, D., Mawad, R., Stevanin, G., Didierjean, O., Durr, A., Oyake, M., Shimohata, T., Sasaki, R., Koide, R., Igarashi, S., Hayashi, S., Takiyama, Y., Nishizawa, M., Tanaka, H., Zoghbi, H., Brice, A., and Tsuji, S. (1998). Close associations between prevalences of dominantly inherited spinocerebellar ataxias with CAG-repeat expansions and frequencies of large normal CAG alleles in Japanese and Caucasian populations. *Am J Hum Genet* **63**, 1060–6.

Takiyama, Y., Igarashi, S., Rogaeva, E. A., Endo, K., Rogaev, E. I., Tanaka, H., Sherrington, R., Sanpei, K., Liang, Y., Saito, M., *et al.* (1995). Evidence for inter-generational instability in the CAG repeat in the MJD1 gene and for conserved haplotypes at flanking markers amongst Japanese and Caucasian subjects with Machado–Joseph disease. *Hum Mol Genet* **4**, 1137–46.

—— Sakoe, K., Namekawa, M., Soutome, M., Esumi, E., Ogawa, T., Ishikawa, K., Mizusawa, H., Nakano, I., and Nishizawa, M. (1998). A Japanese family with spinocerebellar ataxia type 6 which includes three individuals homozygous for an expanded CAG repeat in the SCA6/CACNL1A4 gene. *J Neurol Sci* **158**, 141–7.

Tanaka, F., Doyu, M., Ito, Y., Matsumoto, M., Mitsuma, T., Abe, K., Aoki, M., Itoyama, Y., Fischbeck, K. H., and Sobue, G. (1996a). Founder effect in spinal and bulbar muscular atrophy (SBMA). *Hum Mol Genet* **5**, 1253–7.

—— Sobue, G., Doyu, M., Ito, Y., Yamamoto, M., Shimada, N., Yamamoto, K., Riku, S., Hshizume, Y., and Mitsuma, T. (1996b). Differential pattern in tissue-specific somatic mosaicism of expanded CAG trinucleotide repeats in dentatorubral-pallidoluysian atrophy, Machado–Joseph disease, and X-linked recessive spinal and bulbar muscular atrophy. *J Neurol Sci* **135**, 43–50.

Telenius, H., Kremer, B., Goldberg, Y. P., Theilmann, J., Andrew, S. E., Zeisler, J., Adam, S., Greenberg, C., Ives, E. J., Clarke, L. A., *et al.* (1994). Somatic and gonadal mosaicism of the Huntington disease gene CAG repeat in brain and sperm [published erratum appears in *Nat Genet* 1994; **7** (1), 113]. *Nat Genet* **6**, 409–14.

Trottier, Y., Lutz, Y., Stevanin, G., Imbert, G., Devys, D., Cancel, G., Saudou, F., Weber, C., David, G., Tora, L., *et al.* (1995). Polyglutamine expansion as a pathological epitope in Huntington's disease and four dominant cerebellar ataxias. *Nature* **378**, 403–6.

—— Cancel, G., An-Gourfinkel, I., Lutz, Y., Weber, C., Brice, A., Hirsch, E., and Mandel, J. L. (1998). Heterogeneous intracellular localization and expression of ataxin-3. *Neurobiol Dis* **5**, 335–47.

Tsuji, S. (2000). Dentatorubral-pallidoluysian atrophy (DRPLA). *J Neural Transm Suppl* **58**, 167–80.

Turmaine, M., Raza, A., Mahal, A., Mangiarini, L., Bates, G. P., and Davies, S. W. (2000). Nonapoptotic neurodegeneration in a transgenic mouse model of Huntington's disease. *Proc Natl Acad Sci, USA* **97**, 8093–97.

Ueno, S., Kondoh, K., Kotani, Y., Komure, O., Kuno, S., Kawai, J., Hazama, F., and Sano, A. (1995). Somatic mosaicism of CAG repeat in dentatorubral-pallidoluysian atrophy (DRPLA). *Hum Mol Genet* **4**, 663–6.

Verkerk, A. J. M. H., Pieretti, M., Sutcliffe, J. S., Fu, Y.-H., Kuhl, D. P. A., Pizzuti, A., Reiner, O., Richards, S., Victoria, M. F., Zhang, F., Eussen, B. E., van Ommen, G.-J. B., Blonden, L. A. J., Riggins, G. J., Chastain, J. L., Kunst, C. B., Galjaard, H., Caskey, C. T., Nelson, D. L., Oostra, B. A., and Warren, S. T. (1991). Identification of a gene (FMR-1) containing a CGG repeat coincident with a breakpoint cluster region exhibiting length variation in fragile X syndrome. *Cell* **65**, 905–14.

Vig, P. J., Subramony, S. H., Burright, E. N., Fratkin, J. D., McDaniel, D. O., Desaiah, D., and Qin, Z. (1998). Reduced immunoreactivity to calcium-binding proteins in Purkinje cells precedes onset of ataxia in spinocerebellar ataxia-1 transgenic mice. *Neurology* **50**, 106–13.

—— —— Qin, Z., McDaniel, D. O., and Fratkin, J. D. (2000). Relationship between ataxin-1 nuclear inclusions and Purkinje cell specific proteins in SCA-1 transgenic mice. *J Neurol Sci* **174**, 100–10.

Voges, D., Zwickl, P., and Baumeister, W. (1999). The 26S proteasome: a molecular machine designed for controlled proteolysis. *Annu Rev Biochem* **68**, 1015–68.

Waelter, S., Boeddrich, A., Lurz, R., Scherzinger, E., Lueder, G., Lehrach, H., and Wanker, E. E. (2001). Accumulation of mutant huntingtin fragments in aggresome-like inclusion bodies as a result of insufficient protein degradation. *Mol Biol Cell* **12**, 1393–407.

Wakisaka, A., Sasaki, H., Takada, A., Fukazawa, T., Suzuki, Y., Hamada, T., Iwabuchi, K., Tashiro, K., and Yoshiki, T. (1995). Spinocerebellar ataxia 1 (SCA1) in the Japanese in Hokkaido may derive from a single common ancestry. *J Med Genet* **32**, 590–2.

Wang, G., Ide, K., Nukina, N., Goto, J., Ichikawa, Y., Uchida, K., Sakamoto, T., and Kanazawa, I. (1997). Machado–Joseph disease gene product identified in lymphocytes and brain. *Biochem Biophys Res Commun* **233**, 476–9.

—— Sawai, N., Kotliarova, S., Kanazawa, I., and Nukina, N. (2000). Ataxin-3, the MJD1 gene product, interacts with the two human homologs of yeast DNA repair protein RAD23, HHR23A and HHR23B. *Hum Mol Genet* **9**, 1795–803.

Warner, T. T., Williams, L. D., Walker, R. W., Flinter, F., Robb, S. A., Bundey, S. E., Honavar, M., and Harding, A. E. (1995). A clinical and molecular genetic study of dentatorubropallidoluysian atrophy in four European families. *Ann Neurol* **37**, 452–9.

Warrick, J. M., Paulson, H. L., Gray-Board, G. L., Bui, Q. T., Fischbeck, K. H., Pittman, R. N., and Bonini, N. M. (1998). Expanded polyglutamine protein forms nuclear inclusions and causes neural degeneration in *Drosophila*. *Cell* **93**, 939–49.

—— Chan, H. Y., Gray-Board, G. L., Chai, Y., Paulson, H. L., and Bonini, N. M. (1999). Suppression of polyglutamine-mediated neurodegeneration in *Drosophila* by the molecular chaperone HSP70. *Nat Genet* **23**, 425–8.

Watanabe, H., Tanaka, F., Matsumoto, M., Doyu, M., Ando, T., Mitsuma, T., and Sobue, G. (1998). Frequency analysis of autosomal dominant cerebellar ataxias in Japanese patients and clinical characterization of spinocerebellar ataxia type 6. *Clin Genet* **53**, 13–19.

—— —— Doyu, M., Riku, S., Yoshida, M., Hashizume, Y., and Sobue, G. (2000). Differential somatic CAG repeat instability in variable brain cell lineage in dentatorubral pallidoluysian atrophy (DRPLA): a laser-captured microdissection (LCM)-based analysis. *Hum Genet* **107**, 452–7.

—— —— Abe, K., Aoki, M., Yasuo, K., Itoyama, Y., Shoji, M., Ikeda, Y., Iizuka, T., Ikeda, M., Shizuka, M., Mizushima, K., and Hirai, S. (1996). Mitotic and meiotic stability of the CAG repeat in the X-linked spinal and bulbar muscular atrophy gene. *Clin Genet* **50**, 133–7.

Wexler, N. S., Young, A. B., Tanzi, R. E., Travers, H., Starosta-Rubinstein, S., Penney, J. B., Snodgrass, S. R., Shoulson, I., Gomez, F., Ramos Arroyo, M. A., *et al.* (1987). Homozygotes for Huntington's disease. *Nature* **326**, 194–7.

Wheeler, V. C., White, J. K., Gutekunst, C. A., Vrbanac, V., Weaver, M., Li, X. J., Li, S. H., Yi, H., Vonsattel, J. P., Gusella, J. F., Hersch, S., Auerbach, W., Joyner, A. L., and MacDonald, M. E. (2000). Long glutamine tracts cause nuclear localization of a novel form of huntingtin in medium spiny striatal neurons in HdhQ92 and HdhQ111 knock- in mice. *Hum Mol Genet* **9**, 503–13.

Wood, J. D., Yuan, J., Margolis, R. L., Colomer, V., Duan, K., Kushi, J., Kaminsky, Z., Kleiderlein, J. J., Sharp, A. H., and Ross, C. A. (1998). Atrophin-1, the DRPLA gene product, interacts with two families of WW domain-containing proteins. *Mol Cell Neurosci* **11**, 149–60.

—— Nucifora, F. C., Jr., Duan, K., Zhang, C., Wang, J., Kim, Y., Schilling, G., Sacchi, N., Liu, J. M., and Ross, C. A. (2000). Atrophin-1, the dentato-rubral and pallido-luysian atrophy gene product, interacts with ETO/MTG8 in the nuclear matrix and represses transcription. *J Cell Biol* **150**, 939–48.

Wyttenbach, A., Carmichael, J., Swartz, J., Furlong, R. A., Narain, Y., Rankin, J., and Rubinsztein, D. C. (2000). Effects of heat shock, heat shock protein 40 (HDJ-2), and proteasome inhibition on protein aggregation in cellular models of Huntington's disease. *Proc Natl Acad Sci, USA* **97**, 2898–903.

Wyttenbach, A., Swartz, J., Kita, H., Thykjaer, T., Carmichael, J., Bradley, J., Brown, R., Maxwell, M., Schapira, A., Orntoft, T. F., Kato, K., and Rubinsztein, D. C. (2001). Polyglutamine expansions cause decreased CRE-mediated transcription and early gene expression changes prior to cell death in an inducible cell model of Huntington's disease. *Hum Mol Genet* **10**, 1829–45.

Yabe, I., Sasaki, H., Yamashita, I., Tashiro, K., Takei, A., Suzuki, Y., Kida, H., Takiyama, Y., Nishizawa, M., Hokezu, Y., Nagamatsu, K., Oda, T., Ohnishi, A., Inoue, I., and Hata, A. (2001). Predisposing chromosome for spinocerebellar ataxia type 6 (SCA6) in Japanese. *J Med Genet* **38**, 328–33.

Yamada, M., Tsuji, S., and Takahashi, H. (2000). Pathology of CAG repeat diseases. *Neuropathology* **20**, 319–25.

—— Sato, T., Shimohata, T., Hayashi, S., Igarashi, S., Tsuji, S., and Takahashi, H. (2001). Interaction between neuronal intranuclear inclusions and promyelocytic leukemia protein nuclear and coiled bodies in CAG repeat diseases. *Am J Pathol* **159**, 1785–95.

Yamamoto, A., Lucas, J. J., and Hen, R. (2000). Reversal of neuropathology and motor dysfunction in a conditional model of Huntington's disease [see comments]. *Cell* **101**, 57–66.

Yanagisawa, H., Bundo, M., Miyashita, T., Okamura-Oho, Y., Tadokoro, K., Tokunaga, K., and Yamada, M. (2000). Protein binding of a DRPLA family through arginine–glutamic acid dipeptide repeats is enhanced by extended polyglutamine. *Hum Mol Genet* **9**, 1433–42.

Yasuda, S., Inoue, K., Hirabayashi, M., Higashiyama, H., Yamamoto, Y., Fuyuhiro, H., Komure, O., Tanaka, F., Sobue, G., Tsuchiya, K., Hamada, K., Sasaki, H., Takeda, K., Ichijo, H., and Kakizuka, A. (1999). Triggering of neuronal cell death by accumulation of activated SEK1 on nuclear polyglutamine aggregations in PML bodies. *Genes Cells* **4**, 743–56.

Yazawa, I., Nukina, N., Hashida, H., Goto, J., Yamada, M., and Kanazawa, I. (1995). Abnormal gene product identified in hereditary dentatorubral-pallidoluysian atrophy (DRPLA) brain [see comments]. *Nat Genet* **10**, 99–103.

Young, A. B. (1998). In *Molecular neurology* (ed. J. B. Martin), pp. 35–54. Scientific American Inc, New York.

Yue, S., Serra, H. G., Zoghbi, H. Y., and Orr, H. T. (2001). The spinocerebellar ataxia type 1 protein, ataxin-1, has RNA-binding activity that is inversely affected by the length of its polyglutamine tract. *Hum Mol Genet* **10**, 25–30.

Yvert, G., Lindenberg, K. S., Picaud, S., Landwehrmeyer, G. B., Sahel, J. A., and Mandel, J. L. (2000). Expanded polyglutamines induce neurodegeneration and trans-neuronal alterations in cerebellum and retina of SCA7 transgenic mice. *Hum Mol Genet* **9**, 2491–506.

—— Lindenberg, K. S., Devys, D., Helmlinger, D., Landwehrmeyer, G. B., and Mandel, J. L. (2001). SCA7 mouse models show selective stabilization of mutant ataxin-7 and similar cellular responses in different neuronal cell types. *Hum Mol Genet* **10**, 1679–92.

Zhang, L., Fischbeck, K. H., and Arnheim, N. (1995). CAG repeat length variation in sperm from a patient with Kennedy's disease. *Hum Mol Genet* **4**, 303–5.

Zhou, Y. X., Wang, G. X., Tang, B. S., Li, W. D., Wang, D. A., Lee, H. S., Sambuughin, N., Zhou, L. S., Tsuji, S., Yang, B. X., and Goldfarb, L. G. (1998). Spinocerebellar ataxia type 2 in China: molecular analysis and genotype–phenotype correlation in nine families. *Neurology* **51**, 595–8.

Zhuchenko, O., Bailey, J., Bonnen, P., Ashizawa, T., Stockton, D. W., Amos, C., Dobyns, W. B., Subramony, S. H., Zoghbi, H. Y., and Lee, C. C. (1997). Autosomal dominant cerebellar ataxia (SCA6) associated with small polyglutamine expansions in the alpha 1A-voltage-dependent calcium channel. *Nat Genet* **15**, 62–9.

Zuhlke, C., Hellenbroich, Y., Dalski, A., Kononowa, N., Hagenah, J., Vieregge, P., Riess, O., Klein, C., and Schwinger, E. (2001). Different types of repeat expansion in the TATA-binding protein gene are associated with a new form of inherited ataxia. *Eur J Hum Genet* **9**, 160–4.

Section 6   Therapeutic interventions

15 Comprehensive care in Huntington's disease

Martha A. Nance and Beryl Westphal

Introduction

Huntington's disease (HD) is at once a genetic disease and a neurodegenerative disorder, affecting individuals ranging in age from young children to elderly adults over a course of many years. The issues that confront HD families span the expertise of many medical professionals, and are best met by a coordinated team of professionals. We describe below a set of algorithms for the comprehensive management of HD, emphasizing an integrated approach to care that focuses on the impact that HD has on the daily lives of affected individuals and their care-givers. Until there is a preventive or curative treatment for HD, the goals of management must be to reduce symptoms, decrease disability, and improve quality of life. While pharmacological therapies for neurological and psychiatric symptoms provide the cornerstones of medical management, the contributions of the nurse, social worker, dietitian, genetic counsellor, therapists, and other health professionals to an improved quality of life for HD families should not be underestimated. The approaches and principles described below have evolved over two decades of experience in the Hennepin County Medical Center HD Clinic, and should be taken as a framework, rather than as a rigid protocol. Few pharmacological or non-pharmacological treatments have proven efficacy in HD, leaving room for creative problem-solving in the management of today's patients, and for development and rigorous study of improved treatments for the patients of tomorrow.

Multidisciplinary care teams

Because of the long duration of the disease and its wide range of clinical and psychosocial effects, HD families benefit from a multidisciplinary team of care-providers (Kallail *et al.* 1989; Klimek *et al.* 1997; Haskins and Harrison 2000). The specialties represented in the HD Clinic at Hennepin County Medical Center, and their roles, are shown in Table 15.1. HD specialty clinics in other locations might benefit from the involvement of specialists in dentistry, internal medicine, psychiatry, physical therapy, obstetrics and gynaecology, hospice care, and other therapists (art, music, recreation). Families benefit particularly from longitudinal case management, which can be provided by a nurse (Shakespeare and Anderson 1993; Van der Weyden 1994).

Principles of care

In order to improve function, reduce disability, and improve quality of life, the health care team must first characterize the individual medical, neurological, psychiatric, and functionally disabling aspects of the patient's disease, and then fit these pieces into the overall context of

Table 15.1 Team management of HD at Hennepin County Medical Center

Specialty	Role
Neurology	Diagnosis, counselling, symptom management, make appropriate referrals, coordinate and supervise team
Nursing	Case management: answer questions, triage problems, follow-up on care plan; education of patient, family, and outside facilities, programmes, and care-givers
Research Nursing	Coordinate clinical research activities
Neuropsychology	Cognitive assessment, counselling about compensatory strategies, recommendations regarding vocational, legal, competency issues
Psychology	Supportive counselling; family and relationship counselling; behavioural modification strategies; counselling of predictive testing applicants
Genetic counselling	Take family history; counsel patient and family about genetic risks; counsel at-risk and affected individuals about reproductive options; coordinate predictive testing programme
Social services	Assist with financial, vocational, housing, legal problems; assist with disability, guardianship, other proxy procedures; identify resources for in-home, respite, day, or long-term care
Physical therapy	Exercise programme; gait training and safety; train with assistive devices; strategies for wheelchair, seating, and bed positioning and safety
Occupational therapy	Safety evaluation and counselling; assistive devices
Speech therapy	Baseline and follow-up assessment of dysphagia; counselling about swallowing techniques, feeding strategies, food textures, gastrostomy tube placement; assessment of communication, compensatory strategies, assistive communication devices
Dietary	Baseline and follow-up assessment of nutritional status and counselling about weight maintenance or weight-gain strategies; identification of behavioural or psychosocial problems influencing nutrition; recommendations following dysphagia assessment, coordinated with speech pathologist
Chaplaincy	Support patient and family, identify spiritual resources, grief counselling, assist with Advance Care Directives
Volunteers from lay organization	Provide educational and support materials, engage patient and family in lay organization activities
HD long-term care unit leadership	Facilitate care for institutionalized patients; in-service education for other skilled nursing facilities

the patient's disease stage, life history, and social situation, to create a coherent treatment plan. The multitude of medical, social, and psychological issues commonly addressed over the course of the disease are grouped into categories in Table 15.2. We first discuss the management of individual problems within a category, and then present algorithms depicting how these individual problems typically fit together in the early, middle, and late stages of HD. HD care is discussed in more detail in a clinical manual, *The physician's guide to Huntington's disease* (Rosenblatt *et al.* 1999).

Categories of symptom management in HD

Movement disorder

A wide range of arrhythmic involuntary movements can be seen in HD, ranging from high-amplitude ballistic movements to writhing, dystonic postures, to brief, almost tic-like

Table 15.2 Management issues in HD

Management issues	Management issues
Movement disorder	**Mania**
Chorea	Explosive and impulsive behaviour
Impaired volitional movements	Resistive behaviour
Gait disorder	Substance abuse
Dystonia and rigidity	Sexual disorders
Positioning in bed and chair	**Support for the care-giver**
Oral motor disorder	Adjustment to the diagnosis
Speech and communication problems	Relationship changes
Dysphagia	Coping with disease progression
Cognitive disorder	Family disagreements
Vocational impairment and disability	Preparing for death
Home safety	**Social issues**
Ability to perform self-care	Work and disability
Miscellaneous medical issues	Driving
Weight loss/malnutrition	Financial and insurance concerns
Sleep disturbance	Accessing community services
General medical and dental care	Placement outside the home
Complications of late-stage HD	**Educational issues**
Regurgitation	Diagnosis and the diagnostic process
Screaming	Facts about disease course and treatment
Delirium	Genetic counselling
Fever	Accessing educational resources and materials
Cachexia	Educating the extended family
Infections	Educating health care professionals
Terminal care	Educating other professionals
Behavioural and psychiatric disorder	Research opportunities
Depression and suicidality	**Special issues**
Anxiety	Juvenile-onset HD
Obsessions and compulsions	Managing at-risk individuals
Delusions and hallucinations	Predictive and prenatal genetic testing

movements. The nature of the involuntary movements does not have any proven therapeutic relevance. Early in the disease, chorea is often of more cosmetic than functional significance. Chorea that is severe, embarrassing, or functionally limiting can be treated with dopamine-blocking or -depleting drugs, such as haloperidol, tetrabenazine, or one of the atypical antipsychotics such as risperidone or olanzapine (Shoulson 1981; Girotti *et al.* 1984; Parsa *et al.* 1997; Jankovic and Beach 1997; Van Vugt *et al.* 1997; Dallocchio *et al.* 1999; Dipple 1999; Grove *et al.* 2000). The benefits of drug therapy are usually modest, although an occasional patient will have dramatic benefits. Neuroleptics must be used with the understanding that they may worsen or hasten the development of hypokinesia, which develops anyway as the disease progresses, and which is more highly correlated to gait disturbance and functional disability than chorea (Koller and Trimble 1985; van Vugt *et al.* 1996). Benzodiazepines such as clonazepam may calm chorea by reducing anxiety, or may have direct motor effects (Peiris *et al.* 1976). Other drugs with reported beneficial effects on chorea in clinical trials include tiapride and apomorphine (Dose and Lange 2000; Albanese *et al.* 1995). A trend toward improvement in chorea was seen in recent studies of lamotrigine and riluzole, in which the main aim was to evaluate the effects of the medication on disease progression (Kremer *et al.* 1999; Rosas *et al.* 1999).

Medications do not improve upon the disturbance of voluntary motor function, which is typically characterized by difficulty initiating, sequencing, and persisting with motor actions or tasks. An exercise programme may help the patient to maintain strength, flexibility, and stamina, while counselling the patient, family, and employers to adjust home and job duties appropriately can reduce anxiety and stress. Intensive gait training may improve some aspects of gait disturbance (Thaut *et al.* 1999). The use of warm pool therapy has been reported (Sheaff 1990).

The emergence of truncal rigidity in the middle stages of the disease increases the risk of falls, which can lead to lacerations, traumatic bursitis, limb fractures, or subdural haematomas. Severe chorea can also result in falls or repeated trauma to joints or limbs that are not padded adequately. Whereas canes or wheeled walkers may benefit patients who have rigidity alone, the simultaneous presence of chorea and rigidity reduces their utility in most HD patients. An occasional patient benefits from a merrywalker (essentially a wheeled ring, in the centre of which the patient stands), but these devices are somewhat unwieldy. Padding the body parts that tend to be injured during falls (typically the elbows, knees, or head) and attending to safety measures in the home (installing grab bars and railings, reducing the number of trips up and down stairs) may postpone the need for a wheelchair. Adapted wheelchairs and reclining chairs that can withstand choreiform movements without restricting the patient dangerously may be necessary, and periodic adjustment or additional adaptations are often required as the patient loses postural control or has changes in chorea or rigidity. Manufacturers of specialty equipment for patients with chorea are listed in publications of the Huntington Disease Society of America (www.hdsa.org) and through several Internet resources (see Table 15.3).

In the later stages, chorea often gives way to severe rigidity and dystonia, and then to a state characterized by what we call 'postural and limb dyscontrol', in which voluntary movements are few and ballistic, and the ability to maintain an erect head and trunk posture is lost. Patients with postural and limb dyscontrol are at high risk for restraint-related injury or death, as ballistic movements propel them under the headboard of a bed or through a siderail, or scissor them over a lap or chest restraint (Miles and Irvine 1992; Nance and Sanders 1996). Safety can be improved by means of creative sleeping arrangements, such as large swaddling

Table 15.3 Internet resources

Address	Comments
www.huntington-assoc.com	International Huntington Association; has links to other national HD organizations
www.hdsa.org	Huntington's Disease Society of America
www.hsc-ca.org	Huntington Society of Canada
www.had.org.uk	Huntington's Association of the United Kingdom
www.hdfoundation.org	Hereditary Disease Foundation; funds HD research
www.huntington-study-group.org	Huntington Study Group, an international, multicentre clinical trials group
www.wemove.org	Worldwide Education and Awareness for Movement Disorders; directed primarily towards professionals
www.kumc.edu/hospital/huntingtons	University of Kansas HD Clinic website; has information and links
www.hdac.org	HD Advocacy Center; many useful links for patients and families

hammocks, queen-sized floor mattresses with padded bumpers, or a low open bed with an adjacent padded floor. We have not generally found medications to be beneficial in reducing stiffness in late HD, but antispasticity or anti-parkinsonian drugs may have modest benefits in some patients. Although its use has not been reported, it is possible that injection of botulinum toxin might benefit a patient with particularly disabling dystonia of a small muscle amenable to injection (for example, jaw dystonia).

Oral motor disturbance

Communication becomes increasingly difficult as HD progresses, and in the late stages patients are mute. Early introduction of assistive communication devices, at a time when patients have the cognitive ability to learn how to use them, can be helpful. Simple devices, such as word boards, may be more useful than technologically sophisticated but physically small electronic devices, which are difficult for individuals with chorea to use. A speech therapist can instruct care-givers in strategies for assisting the impaired speaker, including cueing, spelling words, providing word choices, and allowing enough time for the speaker to complete a thought (Seidman-Carlson and Wells 1998). Behavioural problems often increase as speech becomes incomprehensible, seemingly as an attempt by the patient to vent frustration and to control the environment around him.

Dysphagia is a major contributor to the disability and morbidity of late-stage HD. Mealtimes can be frightening to patient and care-givers as the risk of choking increases. Inability to eat safely or independently contributes to low self-esteem and depression, increases the level of care needed, and ultimately leads to weight loss and the risk of aspiration pneumonia. A team approach to dysphagia is beneficial, including baseline assessment of swallow function and counselling by the speech pathologist in tandem with specific dietary goals and recommendations by the dietitian. Poor dentition, unusual food-related behaviours (such as obsessive intake of certain foods or drinks, food refusals, binging, or purging), mood disturbance, and medications can all influence nutritional status and should be identified and treated. Patients may need financial or personal assistance in order to get access to and prepare nutritionally adequate foods. The physician, nurse, and counsellor should encourage the patient and family to discuss their attitudes toward gastrostomy tube feedings at an early stage of the disease, when the patient is able to articulate his desires clearly. The diagnosis and management of dysphagia in HD has been discussed (Lavers 1982; Folstein *et al.* 1983; Leopold and Kagel 1985; Hunt and Walker 1989; Kagel and Leopold 1992.

Cognitive disturbance

The neuropsychological aspects of the dementia in HD are discussed in Chapter 3. From a functional perspective, cognitive changes are reflected first in impairments in vocational and domestic function (which in turn lead to changes in relationships with spouse and family, and impaired self-esteem) and later in concerns about safety in the home and ability to perform self-cares such as bathing, toileting, grooming, dressing, and feeding.

Formal assessment of cognitive function helps the physician or neuropsychologist to give specific recommendations regarding employment and disability, legal and financial competence, and other social issues. Repeated assessments at intervals allow the health care team to appreciate the trajectory of a particular patient's disease, and therefore to provide appropriate prognostic information and recommendations. No medications are known to reduce or slow the dementia of HD.

In the middle stages of HD, home safety often becomes a major concern for families, as the affected person becomes less attentive to himself and his environment. An in-home assessment of safety and provision of assistive devices to help with eating, dressing, bathing, and walking, can make care easier and safer. Creating simple means for the patient to access emergency services, such as a speed-dial option on the telephone, an emergency whistle, or other signalling device, can relieve concerns when the care-giver is away or unavailable. Identification bracelets or wallet cards indicating the patient's diagnosis can be helpful. Some communities have a 'Meals on Wheels' service which provides lunches to homebound individuals who cannot prepare their own meals.

In the late stages, HD-affected individuals are prone to having episodes of delirium related to concomitant illness, medications, or undefined causes. Reduction of scheduled central nervous system (CNS)-active medications is desirable at this time and may be possible, as patients may be less able to generate the aggressive or disruptive behaviours that required their use months or years earlier. Evaluation for intercurrent injury, illness, or infection is important in any patient who has an abrupt change in cognitive or functional status.

Behavioural/psychiatric disturbance

A wide variety of psychological and psychiatric problems can be seen in individuals with HD, as was more fully discussed in Chapter 3. While some patients in supportive environments have almost no behavioural problems, the other extreme seems to be more common, including severe degrees of depression, anxiety, obsessiveness, and explosive, resistive, and impulsive behaviour. We have seen substance abuse, sexual disorders, and eating disorders, which may wax and wane as part of a more general tendency toward obsessive or impulsive behaviours. Mania, paranoid or delusional behaviour, and hallucinations are somewhat less common but can be severe.

The management of behavioural and psychiatric disturbances includes medications, counselling (for patients in earlier stages, and care-givers at any time), and modification of the environment. The role of the nurse in identifying and managing psychiatric symptoms has been discussed (Hofmann 1999). Published studies on the pharmacological management of psychiatric symptoms in HD have been reviewed recently (Leroi and Michalon 1998). A wide variety of medications have been used, most with little more than anecdotal evidence of efficacy in this population. In our own clinical practice, we have largely replaced the older antipsychotics with the newer atypical antipsychotics such as risperidone, olanzapine, and quetiapine, and the tricyclic antidepressants with serotonin re-uptake inhibitors. In both cases the newer drugs have an improved side-effect profile as well as seemingly better efficacy in controlling explosive or impulsive behaviours (Ranen *et al.* 1996). Clozapine has been studied, with mixed results (Bonuccelli *et al.* 1994; Colosimo *et al.* 1995). Severe anxiety may require large doses of anti-anxiety agents and, in our experience, may still be inadequately controlled. Propranolol, valproate, carbamazepine, or benzodiazepines can help to decrease impulsive, aggressive, or explosive behaviour (Findling 1993; Stewart 1993; Bhandary and Masand 1997; Grove *et al.* 2000). In the late stages we often use benzodiazepines or opiates to calm agitated patients with screaming or severe ballistic movements. A few reports have documented benefits from hypnosis (Witz and Kahn 1991) and from electroconvulsive therapy (ECT) (Ranen *et al.* 1994; Lewis *et al.* 1996; Beale *et al.* 1997) in treatment-resistant HD patients. The successful use of leuprolide acetate to treat exhibitionism has been reported (Rich and Ovsiew 1994).

Other neurological and medical issues

Weight loss

Weight loss in HD is multifactorial, relating partly to increased resting energy expenditure, but also to dysphagia, unusual behaviours or obsessions related to food, and psychosocial factors limiting access to high-quality foods (Sanberg *et al.* 1981; Nance and Sanders 1996; Pratley *et al.* 2000). Slower progression of HD has been associated with higher premorbid body mass index (Myers *et al.* 1991). Early and continued attention to dysphagia and nutrition, including the use of high-calorie supplements, treatment of food obsessions and caffeine, alcohol, or cigarette addictions, and engagement of the patient and family in identifying and utilizing food preferences, can help patients to maintain weight, to appear healthier, and perhaps to improve function. Caloric needs for HD-affected individuals are commonly given at 4000–5000 calories per day, although there is little scientific evidence for this specific calorie range. Nutritional recommendations must be combined with an assessment of dysphagia and appropriate changes in food texture and eating style. When, despite attempts to improve oral caloric intake, a patient continues to lose weight, a discussion about gastrostomy tube feedings is appropriate. If the patient has previously written Advance Care Directives, the family's decisions about this and other late- or terminal-stage care issues are much easier.

Sleep

Few studies have discussed sleep disturbances in HD, although in our experience they are common. Reported problems include reduced sleep efficiency, frequent nocturnal awakenings, decreased slow-wave sleep, and increased sleep spindling (Hansotia *et al.* 1985; Emser *et al.* 1988; Wiegand *et al.* 1991; Taylor and Bramble 1997). We would add to this list sleep phase disturbances, severe anxiety related to insomnia, and sleep state misperception. Involuntary movements may occur during sleep arousals, and complaints of excessive sleep-related movements, although uncommon, can occur. We have not seen clinically significant rapid-eye-movement (REM) sleep behaviour disorder or restless legs syndrome. Management of sleep disorders includes counselling of patient and family about sleep hygiene, treatment of any ongoing mood disturbance or anxiety, and the judicious use of a hypnotic agent.

Dental and general medical care

We emphasize the importance of aggressive dental care and age-appropriate general medical care in patients with HD. Neglect of oral hygiene and medication-induced xerostomia can lead to dental decay, which in turn worsens dysphagia and dysarthria, and can lead to food refusal and emergence of food-related behaviours. Involuntary movements make dental work difficult, and poor oral motor control impairs patients' ability to control dental plates and dentures (Feeney 1985; Kieser *et al.* 1999).

   Although chronic medical co-morbidity is relatively mild (in comparison to neurodegenerative disorders affecting an older population, such as Alzheimer's disease and parkinsonism), 20–40 percent of patients eventually die of causes unrelated to HD (Sorenson and Fenger 1992; Nance and Sanders 1996). Because of the typical onset age and long duration of HD, it is important not to neglect general age-appropriate health care.

Medical complications of late-stage HD

Problem-focused medical care is necessary in the late stages, when medical complications supervene. Postprandial regurgitation often emerges as a problem shortly after patients have become unable to feed themselves. Other causes of regurgitation must be ruled out before assuming that this is due to HD, and care-givers should be counselled to give smaller meals and to feed the patient more slowly. Later in the disease, severe dysphagia leads to aspiration pneumonias and cachexia, while the bedridden state predisposes to infections, decubitus ulcers, and delayed healing of injuries. Delirium and episodes of fever, often without obvious inciting cause, can occur. Neuroleptic malignant syndrome and catatonia have been reported, presumably in response to medications or changes in medications (Mateo *et al.* 1992). In the last weeks of life, some patients have a noticeable increase in agitation, frequently accompanied by unprovoked screaming. Utilization of Advance Care Directives, empiric use of sedatives, pain relievers, antidepressants, or narcotics, and involvement of hospice nursing care ease the suffering of the patient, family, care-givers, and health care team in these last weeks.

Support for the care-giver: education

The health of the patient with HD depends heavily on the medical and psychological health and stamina of the care-givers. Thus, care of the patient must take into account the effects of HD on relationships within the family, as well as the ability of the care-giver and family to cope with the progression of the disease. While the physician often has his or her hands full managing the medical aspects of the patient's disease, the nurse, social worker, psychologist, or spiritual counsellor or adviser can help to address the problems of the care-givers, including financial and employment issues, disagreements among family members, and varying styles and degrees of adaptation to the diagnosis, progression, and ultimately fatal nature of the disease (Kessler and Bloch 1989; Jolley 1990). In many areas, support groups are available and, where they are not, the Internet can provide access to others with similar concerns. Useful Internet resources for patients and health professionals are shown in Table 15.3.

Opportunities for education about HD abound. Because the disorder is uncommon and complex, the symptoms, course, and management may be unfamiliar even to health professionals, let alone employers, insurers, law enforcement officials, and others in the community. Misunderstandings about the genetic aspects of HD are still common, and families remain unsure how to access accurate information about the course of the disease, its treatment, and research opportunities. A genetic counsellor can explain genetic aspects of the disorder and coordinate any requests for predictive or prenatal testing. Involvement of lay organizations or nursing staff to assist with education can remove some of the educational burden from the physician. The lay HD organizations provide an important resource of accurate and timely web-accessible information about the disease. The Huntington Disease Society of America has established a network of regional HD 'Centers of Excellence' in the USA, at which comprehensive care and education are available. The organization, WE MOVE (Worldwide Education and Awareness for Movement Disorders; www.wemove.org) provides information and educational materials, primarily directed towards health professionals, about HD and other movement disorders.

Social issues

From the very beginning of the illness, when effects on work and interpersonal relationships are just beginning, to the later stages, when the family considers care alternatives for a person who can no longer walk, talk, feed, dress, or bathe him- or herself, the financial, emotional, and logistical impact of HD on the immediate and extended family is enormous. This complex aspect of HD responds best to longitudinal case management by a knowledgeable nurse or social worker. Early in the disease, inability to maintain gainful employment causes financial stresses as well as stresses on family relationships. For patients in the USA, driving often becomes a contentious issue, and approaches to the assessment of driving capacity have been published (Rubin 1994; Rebok *et al.* 1995). Securing disability benefits and finding appropriate noncompetitive work or voluntary activities can decrease irritable or aggressive behaviour in the early- to mid-stage patient who is unable to maintain competitive work. Insurability is a major concern for at-risk individuals and, in the USA, lack of medical insurance may limit access to services or treatments for some affected individuals. The role of social services and support systems in helping the affected individual, spouse, and family address various aspects of the disease has been discussed (Sands 1984; Kessler and Bloch 1989; Kessler 1993; Jarka *et al.* 1996).

In the middle stages of the disease, when patients begin to require assistance with activities of daily living, community programmes that provide meals, domestic or personal care services, day care programmes, and respite care might be appropriate. As personal care needs increase in the later stages, placement in a skilled nursing facility is often necessary. Characteristics of individuals in long-term care have been reviewed (Nance and Sanders 1996). In a few locations, specialized long term care 'HD units' exist but, in most communities, the family and health care team will have to work together with the staff of the local or regional nursing facility to ensure that the special needs of the HD-affected individual are met.

Team management of HD

Recognizing the stage of the disease

After a patient's individual problems are identified and before a care plan is devised, it is useful to determine the stage of the disease. Although several different functional scales have been developed (Bylsma *et al.* 1993; Myers *et al.* 1988), we find the Total Functional Capacity Scale (TFC; Shoulson and Fahn 1979; Shoulson 1981) to be the most useful in clinical practice. Points are assigned in the TFC according to an individual's ability to work, to manage money, to perform household chores, to perform activities of daily living, and to live at home or in supervised care. Possible scores range from 0 to 13 points, and five disease stages are assigned on the basis of the point total, with stages 1 (11–13 points) and 2 (7–10 points) representing the early stages and stages 4 (1–2 points) and 5 (0 points) representing the late stages of the disease. This scale provides a view not only of the progression of the disease itself, but also of its psychosocial and functional effects on the patient and his family. Patients progress gradually down the TFC, losing approximately 0.6–0.7 points per year in the early years (Feigin *et al.* 1995; Marder *et al.* 2000). In stages 1 and 2, patients are often still able to work or drive, or at least to travel and enjoy volunteer and leisure activities. By stages 4 and 5, 24-hour supervision and significant assistance with personal cares and daily life activities are necessary. Stage 3 is a time of transition, as the patient moves from independent living to an increasing need for assistance and supervision.

Three practical limitations to the TFC should be mentioned. Although it is a marker of disease progression that is not generally subject to significant daily or weekly fluctuation, an occasional patient with psychiatric symptoms out of proportion to motor or cognitive symptoms may score poorly on the TFC because potentially reversible depression, obsessions, delusions, or anxiety are interfering with the ability to work or care for oneself.

The TFC is difficult to apply to children or young adults with HD, who may never have had the ability to work, manage money, or perform household chores in the first place. Although we have suggested an adaptation of the TFC for use in children (Nance 2001), the adapted scale has not been validated and must be used with caution.

Finally, because the TFC was designed as a tool to be used in therapeutic trials, it is more sensitive to changes in early HD, and less sensitive to the changes that occur in the late stages. It is not helpful, for instance, in assessing the level of care needs for patients in long-term care. The Physical Disability and Independence Scale (Myers *et al.* 1988) is not subject to the floor effects of the TFC and may be more useful in evaluating late-stage patients, but this scale also lacks detail about specific areas of functioning that might be helpful to care-providers.

HD care algorithms

The diagnosis of HD

Although the development of a simple and accurate genetic test has greatly simplified the diagnosis of HD, a gene test is not a replacement for clinical evaluation of the patient. The appropriate management of the patient depends on the current symptoms, functional restrictions, and psychosocial complications, which only become apparent as the clinician interacts with the patient and his care-givers. The differential diagnosis of HD is discussed in Chapter 2. An algorithm for the diagnostic evaluation of a patient suspected to have HD is shown in Fig. 15.1.

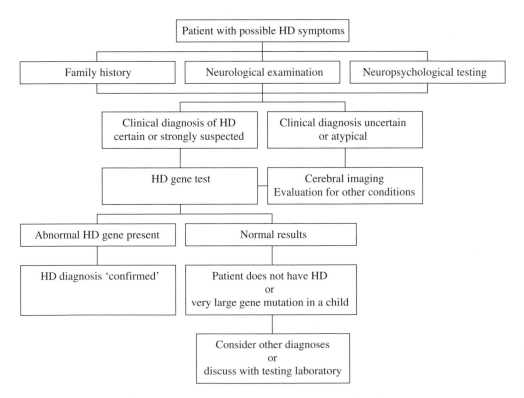

Fig. 15.1 Evaluation of a patient suspected to have HD.

Formal neuropsychological assessment may not always be necessary prior to diagnostic gene testing but, if the clinical diagnosis is uncertain or if cognitive complaints are prominent, a cognitive battery can be helpful for diagnosis and also for management purposes, to assist with counselling about work, driving, or financial or legal competency.

The HD gene test must be used carefully, as the presence of the gene does not necessarily mean that a patient's symptoms are due to HD. However, in the proper clinical context, a positive gene test permits the physician to make the diagnosis of HD with confidence and to move on to treatment and management issues.

When the clinical presentation is atypical or the family history absent, a more extensive diagnostic evaluation or cerebral imaging might be indicated to rule out other genetic or acquired disorders, but eventually a gene test is required for confirmation of the diagnosis of HD. On the other hand, when the family is well known to the examiner and the clinical diagnosis is obvious, genetic testing may be superfluous. At this time, neither the size nor the parental origin of the gene mutation is known to have any therapeutic significance.

The gene test has close to 100 per cent accuracy in an affected individual, as it is a specific assay for the only gene mutation known to cause HD. A few unusual cases have been reported in which polymorphisms elsewhere in the patient's HD gene, or limitations of routinely used laboratory techniques, led to a false-negative result (Gellera *et al.* 1996; Nance *et al.* 1999; L.C. Williams *et al.* 2000). This concern is particularly relevant to the testing of children, as gene mutations of the very large size that may be associated with very early onset of HD symptoms may not be detectable using standard clinical laboratory assays. A normal gene test result in a patient with a clinical diagnosis of HD should prompt a discussion between the clinician and the testing laboratory, or a reassessment of the clinical diagnosis.

The diagnosis of HD should be accompanied by counselling about the disease and its expected course, genetic aspects, and general and patient-specific therapeutic and management strategies. When the family and the patient differ widely in their perception of the disease symptoms or acceptance of the diagnosis, separate counselling sessions may be appropriate.

Management of early HD

Algorithms for the medical and psychosocial care of early HD are presented in Figs 15.2 and 15.3. Medical management typically includes baseline assessment of cognitive function, nutritional state, and dysphagia, with appropriate counselling. Age-appropriate medical and dental care and an exercise programme should be established. Attention should be given to psychosocial issues, such as vocational and financial concerns, adjustment to diagnosis, and the concerns and questions of the care-givers and family.

Patients who are aware of a family history of HD often do not seek medical attention until a social crisis forces them to. Thus, the first task for the health care team after diagnosis may be crisis intervention with housing authorities, child or adult protection workers, the legal or judicial system, or an employer. Psychological or psychiatric disturbance may be prominent at initial presentation. Stabilization of mood, irritable or explosive behaviour, anxiety, or paranoid or delusional thoughts may lead to marked improvement in a patient's ability to function at work or home. Involuntary movements usually do not require pharmacological treatment at this stage, but changes in voluntary motor control may already cause functional impairment. Patients whose occupations require physically or cognitively demanding or time-constrained activities may no longer be able to continue in their jobs and should be helped to seek disability benefits.

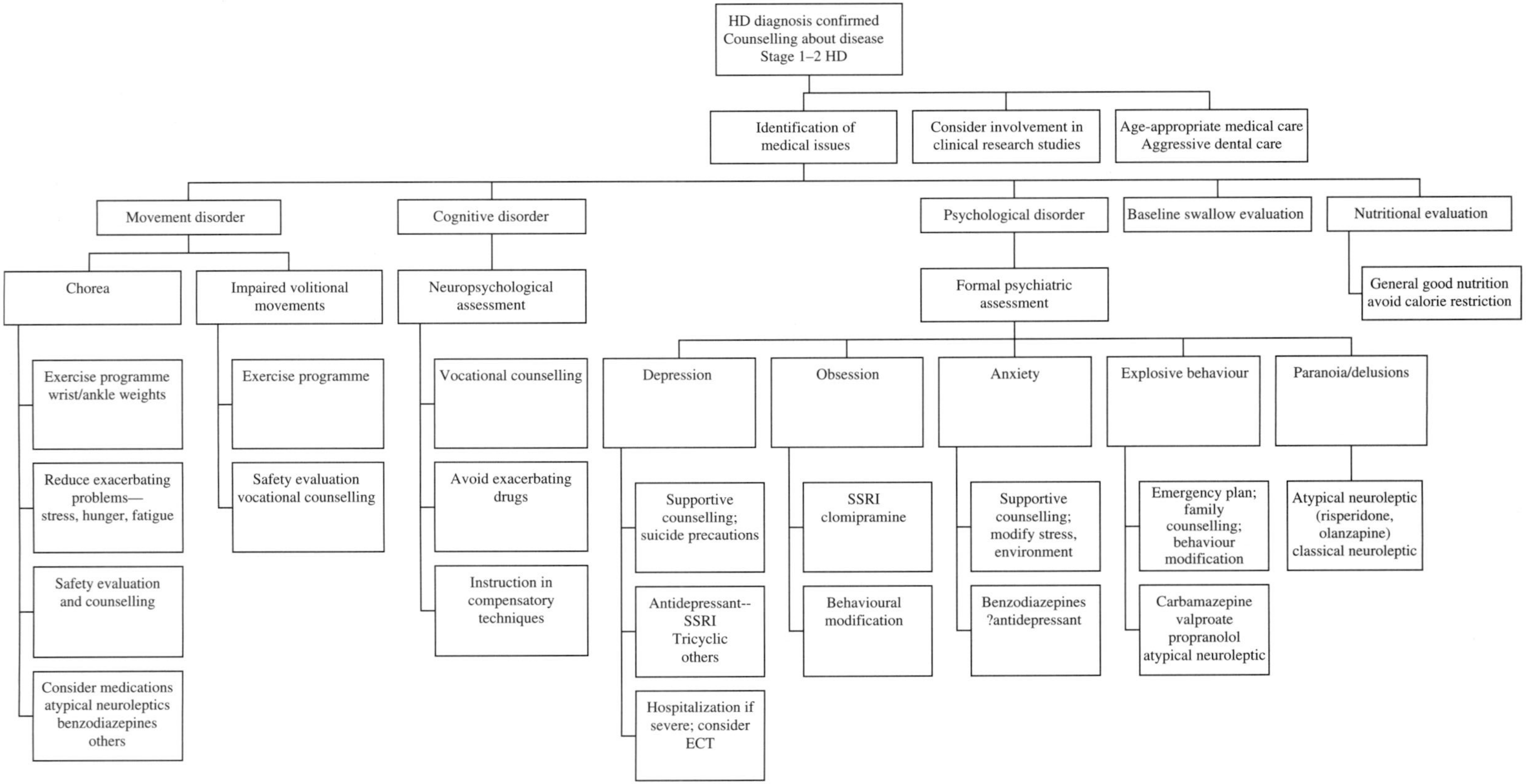

Fig. 15.2 Medical management of early (stage 1–2) HD.

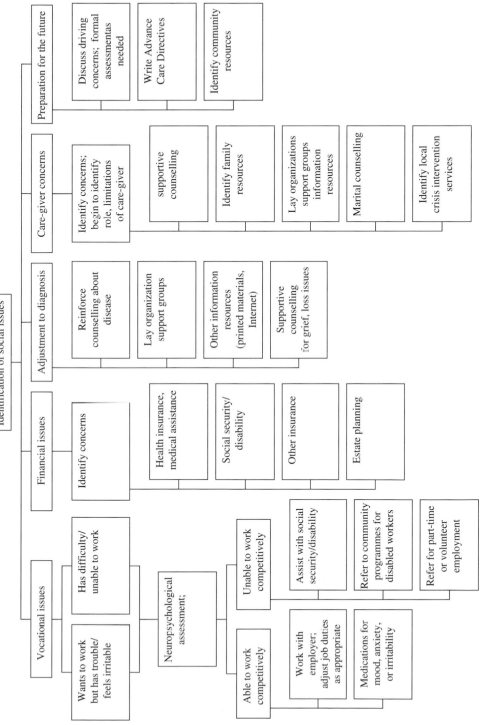

Fig. 15.3 Social management of early (stage 1–2) HD.

Patients who live alone or who lack family support should be identified even at this early time as being vulnerable, and should be followed closely by the team or care coordinator.

The era of experimental therapeutic research in HD has arrived. Research into new treatments typically focuses on patients in the early stages of HD, and involvement in research can infuse a struggling patient or family with enthusiasm and hope. Affected individuals should be encouraged to participate in appropriate research trials.

Management of the middle stages

Stage 3 on the TFC corresponds to the middle stage of HD, a time of major transition for affected individuals. Entering stage 3, individuals are ambulatory, able to communicate and care for themselves, and able to enjoy leisure or volunteer activities. Leaving stage 3, they need substantial assistance with personal care, 24-hour supervision, and often have difficulty ambulating or communicating.

Figures 15.4 and 15.5 show algorithms for the medical and psychosocial management of mid-stage HD. By this time, the movement disorder has progressed so that walking, swallowing, and speech are significantly impaired and benefit from a team evaluation. Rigidity/dystonia may emerge, chorea may become severe, or both. Weight loss is usually apparent, but even at this stage can respond to aggressive management with high-calorie foods, nutritional supplements, or changes in the texture of food, style of eating (for example, finger foods or having a care-giver feed the patient), and reduction of related obsessions or habits such as smoking, substance abuse, or caffeine abuse.

The cognitive disorder has certainly led to retirement from gainful employment and probably from volunteer work by the time the patient enters stage 3. If driving privileges have not already been suspended, they must be at this point. Increasing levels of supervision are necessary, as patients become increasingly limited in their ability to feed, dress, and clean themselves, and to respond appropriately to novel situations or emergencies. Care-givers require help, either from other family members, or from community-based care programmes, to manage care needs. Respite care can help restore a physically or emotionally fatigued care-giver, and support groups may help them to gain support and useful suggestions from other care-givers. Patients who do not have a family care-giver often fail in independent living at this time, although they probably do not have care needs that qualify them for admission to a skilled nursing care facility. In some communities, assisted living residences or group homes are available, but this can be a difficult time, particularly for patients who are suspicious or who do not accept medical or social interventions easily.

Some individuals with HD are prone to episodes of aggressive or explosive behaviour. We often design with the care-giver and the patient an emergency behaviour plan, so that both parties agree in advance what steps are to be taken in these situations. Although spouses have often adjusted to the altered relationship that comes with HD by the time the affected person enters the middle stages, more complex family conflicts sometimes emerge as the children become adolescents or young adults. At-risk children vary widely in their desire to involve themselves with their affected parent or even to learn about HD, and young adult children may develop strong opinions about the parent's care that differ from the spouse's views or plans. The situation becomes even more complex if one or more of the children develop symptoms of HD, or if some undergo predictive genetic testing and others do not. Education, counselling, and support for all parties are needed, although often impossible to achieve.

It is important to discuss late-stage care issues when the affected person is in the early to middle stages of the disease and is still able to communicate his wishes. It has become popular

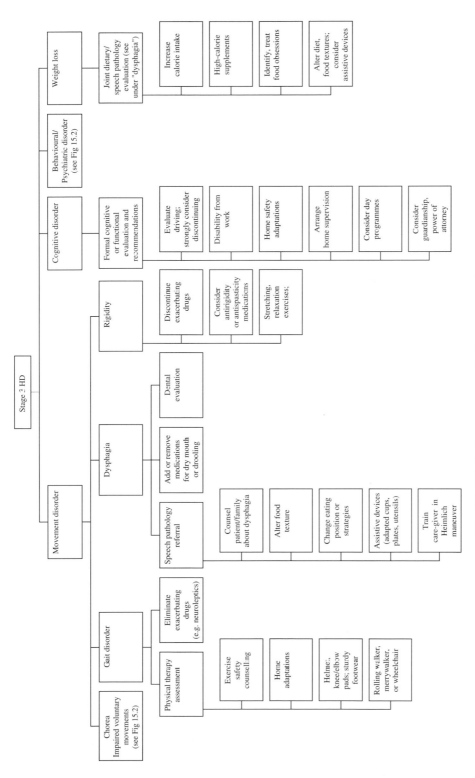

Fig. 15.4 Medical management of mid-stage (stage 3) HD.

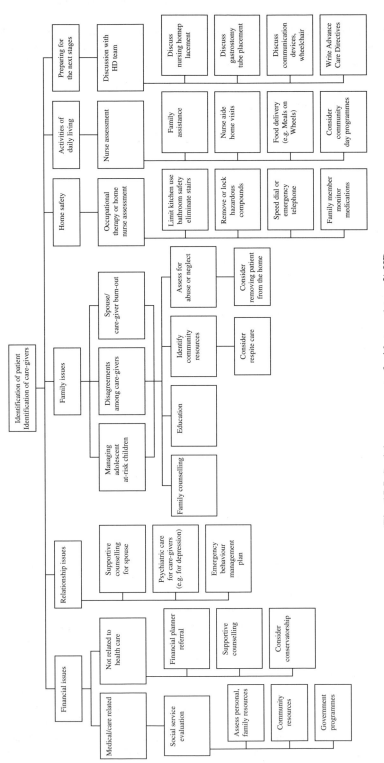

Fig. 15.5 Social management of mid-stage (stage 3) HD.

in the USA for patients to write Advance Care Directives, which detail how they wish to be cared for under specified circumstances, in the event that they are not then able to communicate their desires. Families must also be counselled about the anticipated complications and time course of functional decline, so that they can prepare financially and emotionally for the late stages.

Management of the late stages
In the late stages of HD, affected persons have marked restrictions in all aspects of daily life. The main goals of management at this time are to reduce pain and suffering, and to provide compassionate nursing care to reduce medical complications and maintain as much dignity as possible. Figures 15.6 and 15.7 present algorithms for care in the late stages of HD. The family often becomes less involved when the affected person enters a long-term care facility; it may be very difficult emotionally for an at-risk person to visit an affected parent in this stage. The new care-givers must acknowledge this difficulty without prejudice, and support the family while caring for the affected individual.

Dementia is probably severe by this stage, but becomes difficult to assess because communication has become difficult or impossible. Troublesome aggressive behaviour may diminish as the patient loses the ability to act on impulses or frustrations; however, resistive behaviours emerge as patients struggle to maintain some control over their environment. In our experience, conflicts over meals, bathing, and cigarettes are common in the nursing home, and are best managed by a high degree of patience among care-providers, and by negotiation and environmental and behavioural modification strategies, rather than by medications. We have recently seen a marked reduction in smoking-related behaviour problems in the nursing home, as well as improved safety and nursing staff satisfaction, since the introduction of smokeless nicotine inhalers.

Dysphagia and consequent choking, weight loss, or recurrent pneumonias must eventually be addressed in all patients. Advance directives from the patient regarding the implementation of gastrostomy tube feedings, hospitalization for acute infections, and emergency resuscitation measures relieve the family of the burden of making decisions on behalf of the patient. Trained hospice nursing staff can help ease the terminal days for both patient and family. The cause of death in HD-affected individuals is usually HD or a recognizable terminal infection.

Special situations

Juvenile HD
Juvenile-onset HD accounts for about 10 per cent of HD-affected individuals (Hayden and Beighton 1977; Siesling *et al.* 1997). Both the clinical symptoms and the family issues can differ significantly from those typically seen in adult-onset patients (Siesling *et al.* 1997; Nance 1997, 2001). Chorea is less common the younger the patient is at symptom onset, while rigidity and dystonia are more common and severe earlier in the disease. Epileptic seizures, which may present a significant management problem, are seen in up to 25 per cent of patients. Behavioural problems can be very severe, particularly in adolescents.

Families that include a person with juvenile HD are often headed by single, divorced, widowed, or married but overburdened women, as it is usually the male parent who has HD, and at a relatively young age. The psychosocial issues include management at the same time of two generations of affected people, maintaining normalcy for the rest of the family, school-related concerns, financial planning, care-giver burn-out, and, later on, out-of-home placement of a child or young adult. In some ways, the psychosocial needs of the juvenile HD family are

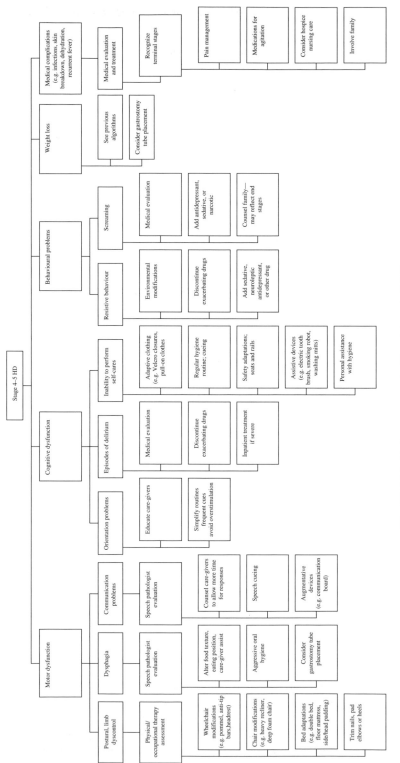

Fig. 15.6 Medical management of late (stage 4–5) HD.

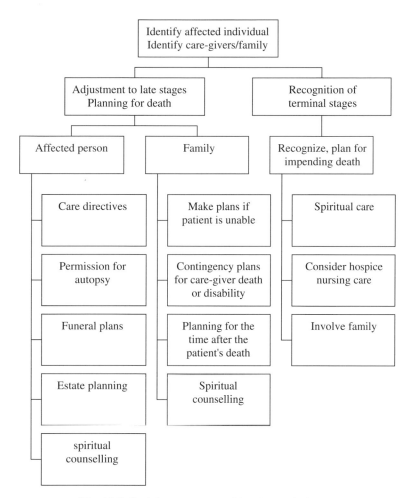

Fig. 15.7 Social management of late (stage 4–5) HD.

closer to those of families with children with other neurodegenerative diseases than to those of adult HD families. Thus, if HD-specific resources are unavailable in a particular community, drawing on experiences or resources utilized by children with other chronic mental, behavioural, or neurological disorders can be helpful.

At-risk individuals
Individuals at-risk for HD range in age from 0 to 90 years, and have a wide-range of experience with HD, knowledge about the disease, life experiences, and interest in speaking with medical professionals about their at-risk status. The existence of a gene test allows the possibility of presymptomatic, or predictive, testing. Studies have suggested that a minority of at-risk individuals—4 to 24 per cent—choose to have a predictive gene test (Taylor 1994; Laccone *et al.* 1999; Maat-Kievit *et al.* 2000; Harper *et al.* 2000). Many issues confront the at-risk individual in addition to the question of whether or not to have a predictive test. The management of an at-risk individual is driven by the medical, psychological, or social issues

that the particular individual presents with. Some common concerns of at-risk individuals and approaches to their management are shown in Table 15.4.

Predictive and prenatal testing
The discovery of the HD gene allowed at-risk individuals the opportunity to determine, long in advance of any symptoms, whether they carry the gene that will one day cause HD. This ability to perform 'predictive' or 'presymptomatic' genetic testing has raised numerous ethical, legal, and social concerns, which have been the subject of numerous scientific and lay publications over the years prior to and since the discovery of the gene. Presymptomatic testing in HD is discussed in detail in Chapter 7. We will restrict ourselves to a brief discussion of issues directly related to clinical care of HD patients and families.

The predictive gene test for HD currently has no therapeutic implications (that is, there is no drug that a person should take based solely on the knowledge of being a gene carrier), so that the only potential benefits are psychosocial. The International Huntington Association, World Federation of Neurology, and Huntington's Disease Society of America have all established guidelines for predictive testing in an effort to ensure that those who are considering undergoing a predictive test are counselled appropriately about the possible risks and benefits of the test, and to minimize the occurrence of adverse psychological or social outcomes of the test process or its results (Anonymous 1994; Huntington's Disease Society of America 1994). In fact, the risk of severe psychological morbidity or mortality from predictive testing appears to be less than 1 per cent (Almqvist *et al.* 1999). However, changes in self-perception, relationships with family and friends, and moderate changes in mood are common (Quaid and Wesson 1995; Broadstock *et al.* 2000; Meiser and Dunn 2000), as are effects on other family members (Sobel and Cowan 2000, J.K. Williams *et al.* 2000). Social complications such as loss of insurance or loss of employment or promotion appear to be uncommon so far, but represent an ongoing long-term risk. It is unknown whether patients who undergo predictive testing without the counselling and support outlined in the guidelines mentioned above have a higher risk of psychological or social distress than those who undergo testing at a centre with expertise in

Table 15.4 Management of individuals at-risk for HD

Issue	Management
Concern about symptoms clearly unrelated to HD	Reassurance; referral for medical evaluation
Concern about possible HD symptoms	Neurological or neuropsychologic evaluation
Coping with parent's illness	Supportive counselling; spiritual support and counselling
Psychological concerns (relationships, recovery from abuse, substance abuse, etc.)	Psychological evaluation and treatment
Psychiatric disturbance (e.g. depression, anxiety)	Psychiatric evaluation, medication
Financial planning/insurance concerns	Discussion with social worker or financial planner
Poor understanding of /misunderstandings about disease	Educational counselling; referral to lay group literature or meetings
Questions about risk to self or children; reproductive options	Genetic counselling
Desire for predictive or prenatal testing	Referral to genetic counsellor or centre specializing in HD predictive and prenatal testing
Involvement in research	Referral to HD clinical research centre

genetic and psychological counselling of individuals at-risk for HD. In the USA, centres with expertise in this area are listed on the website of the Huntington Disease Society of America; in other countries, access to predictive and prenatal testing for HD is often restricted to genetics centres. Predictive testing of minors has been discouraged in the past (Bloch and Hayden 1990; Clarke 1994), but may be considered on a case-by case basis in the case of adolescents (Binedell *et al.* 1996).

Health professionals who intend to perform gene tests for HD must be prepared for situations that test their own moral boundaries or present ethical conflicts. Does the desire of one twin to be tested outweigh the right of the other twin not to be tested? What about the individual who wants testing whose at-risk parent does not (Maat-Kievit *et al.* 1999b; Benjamin and Lashwood 2000)? Should the symptomatic patient who unexpectedly has two abnormally expanded genes be told the whole result or just the part that relates to his or her own disease status? On what ethical basis does one refuse to test a minor whose parent requests a test, or a minor who wants a test with or without parental agreement? When a woman wants a prenatal test that her at-risk husband does not want, whose interests take priority? How should the health professional manage a patient who remains 'anonymous' (Burgess *et al.* 1997), or who refuses to participate in certain routine parts of the pre-test assessment, such as providing a family history, or undergoing genetic or psychological counselling?

The uptake of prenatal testing for HD is low throughout the world (Mandich *et al.* 1998; Maat-Kievit *et al.* 1999a; Kromberg *et al.* 1999). Complications of prenatal testing, other than those related to the procedure itself, relate primarily to the unusual circumstances that sometimes surround the request, such as a pregnant at-risk minor, prenatal testing against the wishes of an at-risk father, or testing of a twin pregnancy. Preimplantation testing for HD has been discussed and performed (Evers-Kiebooms *et al.* 1996; Schulman *et al.* 1996; Braude *et al.* 1998; Stern *et al.* 2000).

Conclusions

The keys to successful management of an HD family are a sensitive and patient ear, a multi-faceted approach, and creativity. By working together with the patient and family to identify and address problems, the health care team can improve the quality of life for those facing this difficult disease.

Acknowledgements

Wayne Brass, Jeff Boyd, Carol Ludowese, Carole Roth, Mary Morgan, Susan Braun-Johnson, Naomi Lundeen, David Tupper, Brian McNeill, and Scott Bundlie all contributed to this chapter.

References

Albanese A., Cassetta E., Carretta D., Bentivoglio A.R., and Tonali P. (1995). Acute challenge with apomorphine in Huntington's disease: a double-blind study. *Clin. Neuropharmacol.* **18**, 427–434.

Almqvist E.W., Bloch M., Brinkman R., Craufurd D., and Hayden M.R. (1999). A worldwide assessment of the frequency of suicide, suicide attempts, or psychiatric hospitalization after predictive testing for Huntington disease. *Am. J. Hum. Genet.* **64**, 1293–1304.

Anonymous (1994). Guidelines for the molecular genetics predictive test in Huntington's disease. *Neurology* **44**, 1533–1536.

Beale M.D., Kellner C.H., Gurecki P., and Pritchett J.T. (1997). ECT for the treatment of Huntington's disease: a case study. *Convulsive Ther.* **13**, 108–112.

Benjamin C.M. and Lashwood A. (2000). United Kingdom experience with presymptomatic testing of individuals at 25 per cent risk for Huntington's disease. *Clin. Genet.* **58**, 41–49.

Bhandary A.N. and Masand P.S. (1997). Buspirone in the management of disruptive behaviours due to Huntington's disease and other neurological disorders. *Psychosomatics* **38**, 389–391.

Binedell J., Soldan J.R., Scourfield J., and Harper P.S. (1996). Huntington's disease predictive testing: the case for an assessment approach to requests from adolescents. *J. Med. Genet.* **33**, 912–918.

Bloch M. and Hayden M.R. (1990). Opinion: predictive testing for Huntington disease in childhood: challenges and implications. *Am. J. Hum. Genet.* **46**, 1–4.

Bonuccelli U., Ceravolo R., Maremmani C., Nuti A., Rossi G., and Muratorio A. (1994). Clozapine in Huntington's chorea. *Neurology* **44**, 821–823.

Braude P.R., DeWert G.M., Evers-Kiebooms G., Pettigrew R.A., and Geraedts J.P. (1998). Non-disclosure preimplantation genetic diagnosis for Huntington's disease: practical and ethical dilemmas. *Prenatal Diagnos.* **18**, 1422–1426.

Broadstock M., Michie S., and Marteau T. (2000). Psychological consequences of predictive genetic testing: a systematic review. *Eur. J. Hum. Genet.* **8**, 731–738.

Burgess M.M., Adam S., Bloch M., and Hayden M.R. (1997). Dilemmas of anonymous predictive testing for Huntington disease: privacy vs. optimal care. *Am. J. Med. Genet.* **71**, 197–201.

Bylsma F.W., Rothlind J., Hall M.R., Folstein S.E., and Brandt J. (1993). Assessment of adaptive functioning in Huntington's disease. *Movement Dis.* **8**, 183–190.

Clarke A. The genetic testing of children. Working Party of the Clinical Genetics Society (UK) (1994). *J. Med. Genet.* **31**, 785–797.

Colosimo C., Cassetta E., Bentivoglio A.R., and Albanese A. (1995). Clozapine in Huntington's disease. *Neurology* **45**, 1023–1024.

Dallocchio C., Buffa C., Tinelli C., and Mazzarello P. (1999). Effectiveness of risperidone in Huntington chorea patients. *J. Clin. Psychopharmacol.* **19**, 101–103.

Dipple H.C. (1999). The use of olanzapine for movement disorder in Huntington's disease: a first case report. *J. Neurol. Neurosurg. Psychiatry* **67**, 123–124.

Dose M. and Lange H.W. (2000). The benzamide tiapride: treatment of extrapyramidal and other clinical syndromes. *Pharmacopsychiatry* **33**, 19–27.

Emser W., Brenner M., Stober T., and Schimrigk K. (1988). Changes in nocturnal sleep in Huntington's and Parkinson's disease. *J. Neurol.* **235**, 177–179.

Evers-Kiebooms G., Fryns J.P., Demyttenaere K., Decruyenaere M., Boogaerts A., Cloostermans T., Cassiman J.J., Dom R., and Van den Berghe H. (1996). Predictive and preimplantation genetic testing for Huntington's disease and other late onset dominant disorders: not in conflict but complementary. *Clin. Genet.* **50**, 275–276.

Feeney A.W. (1985). Dental treatment considerations for patients with Huntington's disease. *J. Conn. State Dent. Assoc.* **59**, 118–123.

Feigin A., Keiburtz K., Bordwell K., Como P., Steinberg K., Sotack J., Zimmerman C., Hickey C., Orme C., and Shoulson I. (1995). Functional decline in Huntington's disease. *Movement Dis.* **10**, 211–214.

Findling R.L. (1993). Treatment of aggression in juvenile-onset Huntington's disease with buspirone. *Psychosomatics* **34**, 460–461.

Folstein S.E., Chandler E., and Ravich W. (1983). Mealtime manual for Huntington disease patients. *Huntington Rev. Inherited Neuropsychiatr. Dis.* **2**, 1–11.

Gellera C., Meoni C., Castellotti B., Zappacosta B., Girotti F., Taroni F., and DiDonato S. (1996). Errors in Huntington's disease diagnostic test caused by trinucleotide deletion in the IT15 gene. *Am. J. Hum. Genet.* **59**, 475–477.

Girotti F., Carella F., Scigliano G., Grassi M.P., Soliveri P., Giovannini P., Parati E., and Caraceni T. (1984). Effect of neuroleptic treatment on involuntary movements and motor performances in Huntington's disease. *J. Neurol., Neurosurg., Psychiatry* **47**, 848–852.

Grove V.E. Jr., Quintanilla J., and DeVaney G.T. (2000). Improvement of Huntington's disease with olanzapine and valproate. *New Engl. J. Med.* **343**, 973–974.

Hansotia P., Wall R., and Berendes J. (1985). Sleep disturbances and severity of Huntington's disease. *Neurology* **35**, 1672–1674.

Harper P.S., Lim C., and Craufurd D. (2000). Ten years of presymptomatic testing for Huntington's disease: the experience of the UK Huntington's Disease Prediction Consortium. *J. Med. Genet.* **37**, 567–571.

Haskins B.A. and Harrison M.B. (2000). Huntington's disease. *Curr. Treatment Opt. Neurol.* **2**, 243–262.

Hayden M.R. and Beighton P. (1977). Huntington's chorea in the Cape coloured community of South Africa. *S. Afr. Med. J.* **52**, 886–888.

Hofmann N. (1999). Understanding the neuropsychiatric symptoms of Huntington's disease. *J. Neurosci. Nursing* **31**, 309–313.

Hunt V.P. and Walker F.O. (1989). Dysphagia in Huntington's disease. *J. Neurosci. Nursing* **21**, 92–95.

Huntington's Disease Society of America (1994). *Guidelines for predictive testing*. New York: Huntington's Disease Society of America.

Jankovic J. and Beach J. (1997). Long-term effects of tetrabenazine in hyperkinetic movement disorders. *Neurology* **48**, 358–362.

Jarka M., Brosig B., and Richter H.E. (1996). Psychosocial problems in Huntington chorea: 1: overview, project description, social, and illness-related data. *Psychiatria Praxis* **23**, 117–120.

Jolley A. (1990). Easing the inevitable. *Nursing Times* **22**, 36–38.

Kagel M.C. and Leopold N.A. (1992). Dysphagia in Huntington's disease: a 16 year retrospective. *Dysphagia* **7**, 106–114.

Kallail K.J., Godfrey N.E., Suter G., and Anthimides L. (1989). A multidisciplinary approach to the management of Huntington's disease. *Kansas Med.* **90**, 309–311.

Kessler S. (1993). Forgotten person in the Huntington disease family. *Am. J. Med. Genet.* **15**, 145–150.

—— and Bloch M. (1989). Social system responses to Huntington disease. *Fam. Processes* **28**, 59–68.

Kieser J., Jones G., Borlase G., and MacFadyen E. (1999). Dental treatment of patients with neurodegenerative disease. *NZ Dent. J.* **95**, 130–134.

Klimek M.L., Rohs G., Young L., Suchowersky O., and Trew M. (1997). Multidisciplinary approach to management of a hereditary neurodegenerative disorder: Huntington disease. *Axone* **19**, 34–38.

Koller W.C. and Trimble J. (1985). The gait disorder of Huntington's disease. *Neurology* **35**, 1450–1454.

Kremer B., Clark C.M., Almqvist E.W., Raymoond L.A., Graf P., Jacova C., Mezei M., Hardy M.A., Snow B., Martin W., and Hayden M.R. (1999). Influence of lamotrigine on progression of early Huntington disease: a randomized clinical trial. *Neurology* **53**, 1000–1001.

Kromberg J.G., Krause A., Spurdle A.B., Temlett J.A., Lucas M., Rodseth D., Stevens G., and Jenkins T. (1999). Utilisation of predictive, prenatal and diagnostic testing for Huntington's disease in Johannesburg. *S. Afr. Med. J.* **89**, 774–778.

Laccone F., Engel U., Holinski-Feder E., Weigell-Weber M., Marczinek K., Nolte D., Morris-Rosendahl D.J., Zuhlke C., Fuchs K., Weirich-Schwaiger H., Schluter G., von Beust G., Vicira-Sacckcr A.M., Weber B.H., and Riess O. (1999). DNA analysis of Huntington's disease: five years of experience in Germany, Austria, and Switzerland. *Clin. Genet.* **53**, 801–806.

Lavers A. (1982). Feeding difficulties in patients with Huntington's chorea. *Nursing Times* **78**, 920–921.

Leopold N.A. and Kagel M.C. (1985). Dysphagia in Huntington's disease. *Arch. Neurol.* **42**, 57–60.

Leroi I. and Michalon M. (1998). Treatment of the psychiatric manifestations of Huntington's disease: a review of the literature. *Can. J. Psychiatry* **43**, 933–940.

Lewis C.F., DeQuardo J.R., and Tandon R. (1996). ECT in genetically confirmed Huntington's disease. *Neuropsychiatry Clin. Neurosci.* **8**, 209–210.

Maat-Kievit A., Vegter-van der Vlis M., Zoeteweij M., Losekoot M., van Haeringen A., Kanhai H., and Roos R. (1999a). Experience in prenatal testing for Huntington's disease in The Netherlands: procedures, results and guidelines (1987–1997). *Prenatal Diagnos.* **19**, 450–457.

Maat-Kievit A., Vegter-van der Vlis M., Zoeteweij M., Losekoot M., van Haeringen A., and Roos R.A. (1999b). Predictive testing of 25 percent at-risk individuals for Huntington disease (1987–1997). *Am. J. Med. Genet.* **88**, 662–668.

—— —— —— —— —— —— (2000). Paradox of a better test for Huntington's disease. *J. Neurol., Neurosurg. Psychiatry* **69**, 579–583.

Mandich P., Jacopini G., Di Maria E., Sabbadini G., Chimirri F., Bellone E., Novelletto A., Ajmar F., and Frontali M. (1998). Predictive testing for Huntington's disease: ten years' experience in two Italian centres. *Ital. J. Neurol. Sci.* **19**, 68–74.

Marder K., Zhao H., Myers R.H., Cudkowicz C., Kayson E., Kieburtz K., Orme C., Paulsen J., Penney J.B., Siemers E., Shoulson I., and the Huntington Study Group. (2000). Rate of functional decline in Huntington's disease. *Neurology* **54**, 452–458.

Mateo D., Munoz-Blanco J.L., and Giminez-Roldan S. (1992). Neuroleptic malignant syndrome related to tetrabenazine introduction and haloperidol discontinuation in Huntington's disease. *Clin. Neuropharmacol.* **15**, 63–68.

Meiser B. and Dunn S.(2000). Psychological impact of genetic testing for Huntington's disease: an update of the literature. *J. Neurol., Neurosurg. Psychiatry* **69**, 574–578.

Miles S.H. and Irvine P. (1992). Deaths caused by physical restraints. *Gerontologist* **32**, 762–766.

Myers R.H., Vonsattel J.P., Stevens T.J., Cupples L.A., Richardson E.P., Martin J.B., and Bird E.D. (1988). Clinical and neuropathological assessment of severity in Huntington's disease. *Neurology* **38**, 341–347.

—— Sax D.S., Koroshetz W.F., Mastromauro C., Cupples L.A., Kiely D.K., Pettingill F.K., and Bird E.D. (1991). Factors associated with slow progression in Huntington's disease. *Arch. Neurol.* **48**, 800–804.

Nance MA, for the Huntington disease Genetic Testing Group. (1997). Genetic testing of children at-risk for Huntington disease. *Neurology* **49**, 1048–1053.

—— (2001). *Juvenile Huntington's disease—a handbook*. New York: Huntington's Disease Society of America.

—— Sanders G. (1996). Characteristics of Huntington disease-affected individuals in the nursing home. *Movement Dis.* **11**, 542–548.

—— Mathias-Hagen V., Breningstall G., Wick M.J., and McGlennan R.C. (1999). Molecular diagnostic analysis of a very large trinucelotide repeat in a patient with juvenile Huntington disease. *Neurology* **52**, 392–394.

Parsa M.A., Szigethy E., Voci J.M., and Meltzer H.Y. (1997). Risperidone in treatment of choreoathetosis of Huntington's disease. *J. Clin. Psychopharmacol.* **17**, 134–135.

Peiris J.B., Boralessa H., and Lionel N.D. (1976). Clonazepam in the treatment of choreiform activity. *Med. J. Australia* **1**, 225–227.

Pratley R.E., Salbe A.D., Ravussin E., and Caviness J.N. (2000). Higher sedentary energy expenditure in patients with Huntington's disease. *Ann. Neurol.* **47**, 64–70.

Quaid K.A. and Wesson M.K. (1995). Exploration of the effects of predictive testing for Huntington on intimate relationships. *Am. J. Med. Genet.* **57**, 46–51.

—— Peyser C.E., and Folstein S.E. (1994). ECT as a treatment for depression in Huntington's disease. *J. Neuropsychiatry Clin. Neurosci.* **6**, 154–159.

Ranen N.G., Lipsey J.R., Treisman G., and Ross C.A. (1996). Sertraline in the treatment of severe aggressiveness in Huntington's disease. *J. Neuropsychiatry Clin. Neurosci.* **8**, 338–340.

Rebok G.W., Bylsma F.W., Keyl P.M., Brandt J., and Folstein S.E. (1995). Automobile driving in Huntington's disease. *Movement Dis.* **10**, 778–787.

Rich S.S. and Ovsiew F. (1994). Leuprolide acetate for exhibitionism in Huntington's disease. *Movement Dis.* **9**, 353–357.

Rosas H.D., Koroshetz W.J., Jenkins B.G., Chen Y.I., Hayden D.L., Beal M.F., and Cudkowicz M.E. (1999). Riluzole therapy in Huntington's disease. *Movement Dis.* **14**, 326–330.

Rosenblatt A., Ranen N.G., Nance M.A., and Paulsen J.S. (1999). *A physician's guide to the management of Huntington's disease*, 2nd edn. New York: Huntington's Disease Society of America.

Rubin A.J. (1994). *Evaluating driving capacity in HD*. New York: Huntington Disease Society of America.

Sanberg P.R., Fibiger H.C., and Mark R.F. (1981). Body weight and dietary factors in Huntington's disease patients compared with matched controls. *Med. J. Australia* **1**, 407–409.

Sands R.G. (1984). Social work with victims of Huntington's disease. *Soc. Work Hlth Care* **9**, 63–71.

Schulman J.D., Black S.H., Handyside A., and Nance W.E. (1996). Preimplantation testing for Huntington's disease and certain other dominantly inherited disorders. *Clin. Genet.* **49**, 57–58.

Seidman-Carlson R. and Wells D.L. (1998). The ability to comprehend affective communication in individuals with Huntington's disease. *J. Gerontol. Nursing* **24**,16–23.

Shakespeare J. and Anderson J. (1993). Huntington's disease—falling through the net. *Hlth Trends* **25**, 19–23.

Sheaff F. (1990). Hydrotherapy in Huntington's disease. *Nursing Times* **86**, 46–49.

Shoulson I. (1981). Huntington disease: functional capacities in patients treated with neuroleptic and antidepressant drugs. *Neurology* **31**, 1333–1335.

—— Fahn S. (1979). Huntington's disease: clinical care and evaluation. *Neurology* 29: 1–3.

Siesling S., Vegter-van der Vlis M., and Roos R.A. (1997). Juvenile Huntington disease in the Netherlands. *Ped. Neurol.* **17**, 37–43.

Sobel S.K. and Cowan D.B. (2000). Impact of genetic testing for Huntington disease on the family system. *Am. J. Med. Genet.* **90**, 49–59.

Sorenson S.A. and Fenger K. (1992). Causes of death in patients with Huntington's disease and in unaffected first degree relatives. *J. Med. Genet.* **29**, 911–914.

Stern H.J., Harton G.L., Sisson M.E., Jones S.L., Fallon L.A., Thorsell L.P., Getlinger M.E., Black S.H., and Schulman J.D. (2000). Non-disclosing preimplantation genetic diagnosis for Huntington disease *Am. J. Hum. Genet.* **67** (suppl.), A 42.

Stewart J.T. (1993). Huntington's disease and propranolol. *Am. J. Psychiatry* **150**, 166–167.

Taylor N. and Bramble D. (1997). Sleep disturbance and Huntington's disease. *Br. J. Psychiatry* **171**, 393.

Taylor S.D. (1994). Demand for predictive genetic testing for Huntington's disease in Australia, 1987 to 1993. *Med. J. Australia* **161**, 254–255.

Thaut M.H., Miltner R., Lange H.W., and Hoemberg V. (1999). Velocity modulation and rhythmic synchronization of gait in Huntington's disease. *Movement Dis.* **14**, 808–819.

Van der Weyden R. (1994). Caring for a patient with Huntington's disease. *Nursing Times* **90**, 33–35.

Van Vugt J.P., van Hilten B.J., and Roos R.A. (1996). Hypokinesia in Huntington's disease. *Movement Dis.* **11**, 384–388.

—— Siesling S., Vergeer M., van der Velde E.A., and Roos R.A. (1997). Clozapine versus placebo in Huntington's disease: a double blind randomised comparative study. *J. Neurol., Neurosurg. Psychiatry* **63**, 35–39.

Wiegand M., Moller A.A., Lauer C.J., Stolz S., Schreiber W., Dose M, and Krieg J.C. (1991). Nocturnal sleep in Huntington's disease. *J. Neurol.* **238**, 203–208.

Williams J.K., Schutte D.L., Holkup P.A., Evers C., and Muilenburg A. (2000). Psychosocial impact of predictive testing for Huntington disease support persons. *Am. J. Med. Genet.* **96**, 353–359.

Williams L.C., Hegde M.R., Nagappan R., Faull R.L., Giles J., Winship I., Snow K., and Love D.R. (2000). Null alleles at the HD locus: implications for diagnostics and CAG repeat instability. *Genet. Testing* **4**, 55–60.

Witz M. and Kahn S. (1991). Hypnosis and the treatment of Huntington's disease. *Am. J. Clin. Hypnosis* **34**, 79–90.

16 Therapeutic trials in Huntington's disease

Karl Kieburtz and Ira Shoulson

Introduction

Huntington's disease (HD) is an autosomal dominant, adult-onset, neurodegenerative disorder that results from the unstable expansion of the trinucleotide CAG repeat within the coding region of the mutant gene on chromosome 4. The cardinal clinical features of HD include a movement disorder characterized initially by chorea and later by dystonia and parkinsonism, progressive cognitive decline, and disordered behaviour, particularly depression and agitation. These signs and symptoms typically emerge in adulthood and progress relentlessly, leading to increasing functional disability and eventual death over a period of approximately 15–20 years. More details of the clinical aspects of the disease are given in Chapter 2.

HD is an illness with characteristic clinical features, high diagnostic precision, and profound and progressive functional disability. Identification of the mutant gene and its CAG expansion has enabled testing of individuals at risk for HD in order to determine their gene carrier status. Much has been learned of the pathogenetic basis of the neuronal degeneration and gliosis underlying this degenerative disorder (see Chapters 11–13), making HD ripe for experimental therapeutics. Clinical trials provide the best evidence with respect to therapeutic effects. Uncontrolled, or open-label, treatment reports are considered relatively poor evidence. Controlled trials, where the intervention studied is compared to an active or inactive (placebo) comparator, provide better evidence. These trials can be parallel group design (one group receives one intervention, the other group receives the comparator) or cross-over design (each participant receives both interventions). The best evidence of therapeutic effects is derived from randomized (assignment to intervention is by random chance), controlled, double-blind (neither the subject nor investigator know the actual intervention assignment) clinical trials. Herein, we review the evidence from clinical trials about treatment of the clinical features of HD (symptomatic therapy), the progression of illness (neuroprotective therapy), and the early strategies to postpone the onset of illness (preventive therapy).

In the context of HD, *symptomatic therapy* refers to interventions that ameliorate the clinical features of illness, but where the benefits are only temporary in the setting of progressive neurodegeneration. In contrast, *neuroprotective therapy* represents an enduring treatment that favourably influences the genetic aetiology or neuropathogenesis of HD and slows functional decline in patients with manifest illness. *Preventive therapy* represents an intervention that forestalls the clinical onset of illness in presymptomatic gene carriers. *Restorative therapies* are treatments that rejuvenate or replace failing neuronal populations and thereby restore function. Restorative therapies are considered in the next chapter on cell transplants. All types of therapy may be associated with short-term symptomatic improvement or worsening in clinical signs or symptoms.

Symptomatic therapy

Movement disorders

Chorea is considered one of the cardinal signs of HD and because of its conspicuous nature is often the target of therapeutic intervention. As HD progresses, other movement disorders, particularly dystonia and parkinsonism, develop and may be a greater part of the cause of functional disability than chorea. Clinicians have used dopamine receptor antagonists, such as haloperidol, to control chorea. The anti-choreic effect of haloperidol is widely accepted to be swift and profound. However, the complications of aggravated parkinsonism, impaired balance, difficulties with swallowing, apathy, and dysphoria, limit the utility of this palliative approach in most patients with HD. However, dopamine receptor antagonists are one of the most commonly prescribed medications for individuals with HD. Fahn (1973) conducted one of the few placebo-controlled studies of the dopamine antagonist perphenazine, involving a cross-over design in eight patients with HD, and found this neuroleptic to exert significant anti-choreic effects over a 4-week period of observation. However, the long-term benefits of this approach have never been assessed systematically. There is no evidence that the common use of neuroleptic treatment has any beneficial effect on the course of HD (Shoulson and Kieburtz 1997).

There is also a reported experience with tetrabenazine, a synthetic benzoquinolizine, that both depletes presynaptic storage of monoamines and blocks postsynaptic dopamine receptors (Jankovic and Beach 1997). A potential advantage of tetrabenazine over dopamine receptor antagonists is that tetrabenazine is not known to cause tardive dyskinesias. Jankovic and Beach (1997) reported that approximately 80 per cent of HD patients experienced an initial anti-choreic response on tetrabenazine at an average dosage of 150–200 mg per day. The initial benefit seems to be sustained in most patients. Common adverse effects of tetrabenazine include drowsiness, parkinsonism, and depression. There have been no placebo-controlled investigations of tetrabenazine.

Van Vugt and colleagues (1997) conducted a placebo-controlled trial of clozapine, a non-neuroleptic dopamine receptor antagonist, and found it to have modest anti-choreic effects. An open-label study of clozapine, at dosages ranging from 25 to 150 mg per day, reported a moderate to marked reduction in choreic movements in five patients, with somnolence the only reported adverse effect (Bonuccelli *et al.* 1994). Although tetrabenazine and clozapine may be effective in the short term in reducing chorea in patients who are particularly troubled or limited by these movements, the functional benefits, potential risks, and long-term adverse events are unknown. Most authorities advise against routine use of anti-choreic agents unless the choreic movements are sufficiently severe and disabling, and the long-term effects can be supervised and assessed. Since chorea tends to diminish over time in the setting of progressive neuronal degeneration, it is sensible to re-evaluate the effectiveness of anti-choreic therapy in the context of the known risks of such interventions.

On the basis of preclinical studies suggesting relative functional deficits of acetylcholine and gamma aminobutyric acid (GABA) in the HD post-mortem brain, cholinergic and GABAergic pharmacological strategies have been explored. Cholinergic interventions have included the administration of choline (Growden *et al.* 1977) and deanol, which is converted peripherally to choline (Tarsy and Bralower 1977). Open-label administration of choline to ten patients with HD resulted in no sustained impact on motor features (Growden *et al.* 1977). Deanol acetomidobenzoate was administered to three HD patients in a placebo-controlled, cross-over design without impact on chorea (Tarsy and Bralower 1977). GABAergic strategies have included muscimol, a potent GABA-mimetic agonist (Shoulson *et al.* 1978), and L-acetyl-carnitine, which increases central levels of GABA (Goetz *et al.* 1990). Muscimol was given in a placebo-controlled, double-blind cross-over design to 10 HD patients and found to reduce chorea in the most severely affected patients but also to heighten dystonia, particularly in the early-onset patients who had predominant parkinsonian and dystonic features (Shoulson *et al.* 1978). No impact on motor function was observed in a 1-week, double-blind, placebo-controlled cross-over study of L-acetyl-carnitine in ten HD patients. The effects of ketamine, an *N*-methyl-D-aspartate (NMDA)-type glutamate receptor antagonist, was assessed in a double-blind, cross-over design in 10 HD patients, but no improvement in chorea and some worsening of other motor features were found (Murman *et al.* 1997). Dextromethorphan, a weak NMDA-type glutamate receptor agonist, was examined in an open-label study in 10 HD patients without beneficial impact on chorea or motor function (Walker and Hunt 1989).

Cognitive impairment

There are no interventions that ameliorate the cognitive impairment of HD. A small open-label study of donepezil, a piperidine-based reversible acetylcholinesterase inhibitor used in Alzheimer's disease, found no evidence of cognitive improvement in 8 HD patients and a 50 per cent withdrawal rate largely due to intolerance (Fernandez *et al.* 2000). Cognitive features were also assessed in four of the aforementioned trials examining anti-choreic effects. Both muscimol and ketamine exerted mild adverse effects on cognition and function (Shoulson *et al.* 1978; Murman *et al.* 1997) while L-acetyl-carnitine and dextromethorphan showed no effect on cognition or behaviour (Goetz *et al.* 1990; Walker and Hunt 1989).

Behavioural manifestations

Depression, apathy, and irritability are the most common behavioural manifestations of HD (see Chapter 3). Standard antidepressant medications, including tricyclics and selective seratonin re-uptake inhibitors (SSRIs), have been used in HD. Few controlled studies have been performed to confirm their effectiveness. Fluoxetine, an SSRI that is widely held to exert antidepressant effects in depressed HD patients, did not improve functional capacity in a placebo-controlled trial of 30 nondepressed HD patients over an average 48 days of observation (Como *et al.* 1997).

In a report of six HD patients with pharmacotherapy-refractory depression, electroconvulsive therapy was found to be effective, especially in the two patients who had prominent delusions (Ranen *et al.* 1994). With advancing HD, irritability, aggressiveness, and impulsiveness may become troublesome. Case reports suggest that sertraline and the combination of valproate and olanzapine may be helpful for agitation and aggressiveness (Ranen *et al.* 1996a; Grove *et al.* 2000). However, there is a major unmet need and lack of well-controlled, prospective studies examining agents that might ameliorate depression, anxiety, and aggressiveness in HD.

Neuroprotective therapy

Neuroprotective treatment strategies have been based on evolving theories of the neuropathogenesis of HD, including the roles of excitatory neurotransmission and abnormal bioenergetic function in the process of neuronal degeneration. These two mechanisms may be interdependent such that cells with bioenergetic defects may be more prone to excitatory-related neurotoxic injury. Both mechanisms may also lead to increased oxidative stress and free radical production (Chapters 8, 10, and 12). Most neuroprotective studies to date have employed interventions that attenuate or modulate glutamatergic neurotransmission, enhance bioenergic mechanisms, or exert anti-oxidative properties.

Studies of feasibility and tolerability

Because HD is a slowly progressive neurodegenerative disorder, neuroprotective interventions may need to be administered for several years to detect the desired slowing of disease. Such interventions should have a satisfactory tolerability profile, particularly if their use is also anticipated for preventive effects in healthy individuals at risk for HD. Short-term tolerability trials are essential in establishing the necessary confidence limits for safety and tolerability and doses. This initial clinical experience, especially if carried out in a placebo-controlled design, also allows an assessment of the short-term symptomatic benefits of the intervention on the clinical features of HD.

Anti-glutamatergic drugs have been assessed in short-term trials. In a 4-week study of the glutamate receptor ion channel blocker, remacemide hydrochloride (200 and 600 mg per day), good safety and tolerability were found in association with modest anti-choreic effects (Kieburtz et al. 1996). In an open-label 6-week trial of riluzole (Rosas et al. 1999), 50 mg twice daily of this glutamate release inhibitor was well tolerated and was associated with a reduction in chorea. A recently completed 8-week, placebo-controlled trial by the Huntington Study Group (2001), involving 63 HD patients, found riluzole at a dosage of 200 mg/day to be generally well tolerated and to have lessened the severity of chorea without improving function capacity (Huntington Study Group 2001a). A longer-term trial of riluzole in HD is underway in Europe.

Coenzyme Q_{10} is a cofactor of complex I in the mitochondrial electron chain cascade and also exerts antioxidant properties. At dosages ranging from 600 to 1200 mg per day, coenzyme Q10 was well tolerated, but there was no apparent impact on motor or cognitive features of the illness (Feigin et al. 1996). The potent free-radical scavenger, OPC-14,117, was evaluated in a 12-week, placebo-controlled study using a range of dosages involving 64 HD patients. A modest reduction in plasma and cerebrospinal fluid (CSF) indices of oxidative stress was observed but without benefits on motor or cognitive function (The Huntington Study Group 1998). Elevations of hepatic transaminase in several subjects treated with OPC-14,117 emphasized the need for adequate safety and tolerability studies before embarking on long-term neuroprotective trials.

A pilot placebo-controlled trial of creatine was undertaken by the Huntington Study Group based on the evidence that creatine, like coenzyme Q10, enhanced mitochondrial oxidative functions defective in HD. Dosages of up to 5 g daily for 2 months were well tolerated, and had no short-term impact on the clinical features of HD (The Huntington Study Group 2001b).

Neuroprotection trials

There have been four relatively large, long-term trials of putative neuroprotective interventions in HD. Two clinical trials of free-radical scavengers have been carried out. A placebo-controlled trial of alpha-tocopherol (3000 IU per day) for 1 year in 73 HD patients did not show clear-cut benefits, but possible slowing of progression in the early stages of HD was suggested by a *post hoc* analysis (Peyser *et al.* 1995). A placebo-controlled trial of the antioxidant idebenone, 180 mg/day, 90 mg twice a day, in 91 HD patients for 1 year failed to show any beneficial impact on the progression of HD (Ranen *et al.* 1996b).

Two studies have pursued anti-glutamatergic strategies. Baclofen and lamotrigine are thought to diminish glutamate neurotransmission by inhibiting corticostriatal glutamate release. A placebo-controlled trial of baclofen (60 mg per day) in 60 patients for up to 42 months failed to show any benefit to the progression of functional decline in HD (Shoulson *et al.* 1989). A placebo-controlled trial of lamotrigine (400 mg per day) in 64 patients followed for 30 months showed no clear evidence of slowing of the progression of functional decline in HD, although there was a trend towards decreased chorea in the treated group (Kremer *et al.* 1999).

Despite the disappointing results of these studies, they yielded valuable information, indicating that functional measurements, such as the Total Functional Capacity (TFC) scale (Shoulson and Fahn 1979), are sensitive to clinical decline in early HD patients. These studies also indicated that larger studies of a total sample size of 300–400 subjects would be necessary to detect benefits that would be of great clinical relevance, such as a slowing of functional decline (Shoulson *et al.* 1989).

The CARE HD trial and future directions

Participants in the Huntington Study Group have carried out a multicentre controlled trial to examine the effects of the glutamate antagonist, remacemide, and the enhancer of mitochondrial bioenergetics, coenzyme Q_{10} (CoQ), in patients with HD. This study evaluated 347 ambulatory patients with HD who were enrolled at 23 investigative sites in the USA and Canada. Research participants in the early stages of HD were randomized to one of four treatment arms using a factorial design (placebo, CoQ alone, remacemide alone, and the combination of CoQ and remacemide). The 2×2 factorial design provided for the assessment of the independent and combined efficacy of remacemide, 600 mg/day, and CoQ, also 600 mg/day, in slowing the functional decline of HD. After randomization, subjects were followed prospectively for 30 months, assessed by the Unified Huntington Disease Rating Scale (UHDRS; Matthews *et al.* 1998) using the TFC scale as the primary outcome measure. Secondary measures included several clinical efficacy measures derived from the UHDRS and a supplemental neuropsychological test battery (Kieburtz 1999; Huntington Study Group 2001).

A report of the CARE-HD study has recently been published (Huntington Study Group 2001). Although the 13 per cent slowing of total functional capacity over 30 months in the Co Q-treated subjects was not statistically significant ($p=0.15$), other functional measures were internally consistent and showed a similar magnitude of slowing of decline. Remacemide exerted anti-choreic effects without benefit to functional capacity or cognitive performance. Both CoQ and remacemide were well tolerated over the 30 month period of observation. These data suggest that CoQ may have modest neuroprotective benefits in slowing the decline of HD, but they need further confirmation in randomized studies.

Possible new interventions

With the development of transgenic mouse and fly models of HD, new possibilities for therapeutic interventions have emerged. Both creatine and minocycline, an inhibitor of caspase and neuronal apoptosis, have been demonstrated to decrease mortality and slow motor decline in transgenic mouse models of HD (Matthews *et al.* 1998; Chen *et al.* 2000). The same models also suggest that remacemide and coenzyme Q_{10} may be protective (R. Ferrante, M. F. Beal, personal communication). Histone deacetylase (HDAC) inhibitors have been shown to exert both neuroprotective and restorative effects in a *Drosophila* transgenic model of HD and some of these compounds are already being used in clinical trials for cancers (Steffan *et al.* 2001). The Huntington Study Group is commencing pilot tolerability trials of these interventions in preparation for larger-scale neuroprotective studies.

Preventive therapeutic trials

Discovery of the fundamental genetic defect underlying HD has greatly enriched our knowledge of the molecular genetics and pathogenesis of this neurodegenerative disease. In turn, this knowledge has improved prospects for developing rational therapies aimed at preventing or delaying the clinical onset of HD. While the CAG repeat length is a relatively precise measure, determination of the clinical onset of HD is a relatively imprecise measure (Huntington Study Group 1996), which has not been examined prospectively, especially with an eye towards therapeutic trials.

HD gene expression and subtle neuropathological changes may begin as early as during development (Gomez-Tortosa *et al.* 2001). The clinical abnormalities seem to evolve and emerge gradually over many years of a poorly understood prodromal phase, culminating in what is considered manifest illness or the 'onset of HD'. The diagnosis of manifest HD rests largely on clinical assessment, often confirmed in hindsight months or years after the first signs have appeared and functional capacity has become impaired (Greenamyre and Shoulson 1994). The issues surrounding the definition of age of onset are discussed in Chapters 2, 3, and 7. Small-cohort studies and retrospective clinical experience suggest that either motor, cognitive, or behavioural abnormalities may be the earliest signs of HD (Harper 1996; Hayden 1981; Folstein 1989). Some early clinical features, particularly in the behavioural sphere, may represent nonspecific manifestations of 'being at risk for HD' rather than a consequence of mutant gene expression (Folstein *et al.* 1983). Prior to the initiation of any clinical trial with an agent intended to delay the onset of HD in a clinically unaffected population, it is essential to establish well-defined criteria for the clinical onset of HD.

Although there have been many reports examining the early clinical characteristics of HD in at-risk individuals and in asymptomatic gene carriers (listed in Table 16.1), these studies have been relatively small, employing retrospective or cross-sectional analyses of selected motor, cognitive, and psychiatric measures and largely involving adults at risk for HD who are undergoing predictive gene testing. Although subtle motor and cognitive abnormalities have been suggested as being the earliest markers of HD, the accuracy of these findings has not been confirmed, and false-positive rates (abnormalities in individuals who do not carry the HD gene) have been reported to be as high as 8 per cent (Siemers *et al.* 1996; McCusker *et al.* 2000).

In 1999, the Huntington Study Group began a major collaborative project to characterize and measure the clinical onset of HD in a diverse cohort of individuals who were at immediate risk for having inherited the HD gene. The Prospective Huntington At Risk Observational Study (PHAROS) cohort will eventually include 1000 healthy adults, aged 30–55 years, who have not undergone testing for the HD gene and wish to remain unaware of their HD gene

Table 16.1 Some studies of the early clinical characteristics of HD

Beenen *et al.* 1986
Young *et al.* 1987
Collewijn *et al.* 1988
Jason *et al.* 1988
Coleman *et al.* 1990
Penney *et al.* 1990
Strauss and Brandt 1990
Baxter *et al.* 1992
Bradshaw *et al.* 1992
Bylsma *et al.* 1992
Diamond *et al.* 1992
Rothlind *et al.* 1993
Shiwach and Norbury 1994
Blackmore *et al.* 1995
Foroud *et al.* 1995
Giordani *et al.* 1995
Rosenberg *et al.* 1995
ampodonico *et al.* 1996
Siemers *et al.* 1996
Jason *et al.* 1997
de Boo *et al.* 1997a,b, 1999
Hahn-Barma *et al.* 1998
Kirkwood *et al.* 1999, 2000a,b
McCusker *et al.* 2000

status, yet desire to contribute to knowledge about HD by participating in research. To date, 600 eligible research participants have been enrolled in PHAROS, which involves a stringent arrangement that conceals genetic (DNA) information and protects confidentiality. A blood sample is obtained from consenting research participants to measure the CAG repeat length of the HD gene, an individual finding that will never be disclosed to the research participant nor to any other party.

In PHAROS, standardized clinical assessments are carried out at about 9-month intervals for up to 7 years of prospective observation by investigators, who are also kept unaware of HD gene status, in order to define the early, HD-gene-specific signs predictive of manifest disease. PHAROS is intended to provide objective knowledge about the positive predictive value and reliability of early clinical signs of HD and their relationship to CAG repeat length and other genetic and environmental modifiers.

Although only 3 per cent of the adults in the USA who are at immediate risk of developing HD have chosen to undergo presymptomatic predictive testing for the HD gene, relatively little is known about the 97 per cent who have not. PHAROS will also lead to an understanding of the feasibility, psychosocial, ethical, confidentiality, and legal issues relevant to this under-studied majority of at-risk individuals who have chosen not to learn of their HD fate.

The Huntington Study Group has also planned and designed the PREDICT-HD (Neurobiological Predictors of HD) study to identify radiographic biomarkers and subtle cognitive changes possibly antedating the clinical onset of HD, over a 3–5 year period of observation, in a cohort of individuals who have undergone presymptomatic predictive testing and are aware of their HD gene status. Supported by a grant from the US National Institutes of Health,

PREDICT-HD seeks to enroll 500 unaffected adults who have undergone presymptomatic DNA testing and have thereby been informed that they carry the HD gene. Like PHAROS, PREDICT-HD will follow research participants prospectively to assess the early clinical changes paralleling the onset of HD. PREDICT-HD will also involve sophisticated and standardized measures of cognitive performance and volumetric assessment of serial brain magnetic resonance images.

Conclusions

The experimental therapeutics of HD has a long way to go in developing effective symptomatic, neuroprotective, and preventive treatments. These therapeutics will only be capable of assessment in the light of detailed longitudinal clinical studies of the type described above, giving a clear picture of the onset and progression of HD. The quantum advances in understanding the aetiology and pathogenesis of HD and the steady, incremental gains being achieved in clinical trials hold promise for addressing the manifold unmet needs of HD patients and their families.

References

Baxter LRJ, Mazziotta JC, Pahl JJ, Grafton ST, St. George-Hyslop P, Haines JL, *et al.* (1992). Psychiatric, genetic, and positron emmission tomographic evaluation of persons at risk for Huntington's disease. *Archives of General Psychiatry* **49** (2), 148–154.

Beenen N, Buttner U, and Lange HW (1986). The diagnostic value of eye movement recordings in patients with Huntington's disease and their offspring. *Electroencephalography and Clinical Neurophysiology* **63** (2), 119–127.

Blackmore L, Simpson SA, and Crawford JR (1995). Cognitive performance in UK sample of presymptomatic people carrying the gene for Huntington's disease. *Journal of Medical Genetics* **32** (5), 358–362.

Bonuccelli U, Ceravolo R, Maremmani C, Nuti A, Rossi G, and Muratorio A (1994). Clozapine in Huntington's chorea. *Neurology* **44**, 821–823.

Bradshaw JL, Phillips JG, Dennis C, Mattingley JB, Andrewes D, Chiu E, *et al.* (1992). Initiation and execution of movement sequences in those suffering from and at-risk of developing Huntington's disease. *Journal of Clinical and Experimental Neuropsychology* **14** (2), 179–192.

Bylsma FW, Brandt J, and Strauss ME (1992). Personal and extrapersonal orientation in Huntington's disease patients and those at risk. *Cortex* **28** (1), 113–122.

Campodonico JR, Codori AM, and Brandt J (1996). Neuropsychological stability over two years in asymptomatic carriers of the Huntington's disease mutation. *Journal of Neurology, Neurosurgery and Psychiatry* **61** (6), 621–624.

Chen M, Ona VO, Li M, Ferrante RJ, Fink KB, Zhu S, Bian J, Guo L, Farrell LA, Hersch SM, Hobbs W, Vonsattel JP, Cha JHJ, and Friedlander RM (2000). Minocycline inhibits caspase-1 and caspase-3 expression and delays mortality in a transgenic mouse model of Huntington's disease. *Nature Medicine* **6**, 797–801.

Coleman R, Anderson D, and Lovrien E (1990). Oral motor dysfunction in individuals at risk of Huntington disease. *American Journal of Medical Genetics* **37** (1), 36–39.

Collewijn H, Went LN, Tamminga EP, and Vegter-Van der Vlis M (1988). Oculomotor deficits in patients with Huntington's disease and their offspring. *Journal of Neuroscience* **86** (2–3), 307–320.

Como PG, Rubin AJ, O'Brien CF, Lawler K, Hickey C, Rubin AE, Henderson R, McDermott MP, McDermott M, Steinberg K, and Shoulson I (1997). A controlled trial of fluoxetine in non-depressed patients with Huntington's disease. *Movement Disorders* **12**, 397–401.

de Boo GM, Tibben A, Lanser JB, Jennekens-Schinkel A, Hermans J, Maat-Kievit A, *et al.* (1997a). Early cognitive and motor symptoms in identified carriers of the gene for Huntington disease. *Archives of Neurology* **54** (11), 1353–1357.

de Boo G, Tibben A, Lanser JB, Jennekens-Schinkel A, Hermans J, Vegter-Van der Vlis M, *et al.* (1997b). Intelligence indices in people with a high/low risk for developing Huntington's disease. *Journal of Medical Genetics* **54**, 564–568a.

de Boo GM, Tibben A, Hermans JA, Jennekens-Schinkel A, Maat-Kievit A, and Roos RA (1999). Memory and learning are not impaired in presymptomatic individuals with an increased risk of Huntington's disease. *Journal of Clinical and Experimental Neuropsychology* **21** (6), 831–836.

Diamond R, White RF, Myers RH, Mastromauro C, Koroshetz WJ, Butters N, *et al.* (1992). Evidence of presymptomatic cognitive decline in Huntington's disease. *Journal of Clinical and Experimental Neuropsychology* **14** (6), 961–975.

Fahn S (1973). Treatment of choreic movements with perphenazine. In *Advances in neurology*, Vol. 1 (eds, A Barbeau, T Chase, GW Paulson), pp. 755–764. Raven Press, New York.

Feigin A, Kieburtz K, Como P, Hickey C, Claude K, Abwender D, Zimmerman C, Steinberg K, and Shoulson I (1996). Assessment of coenzyme Q10 tolerability in Huntington's disease. *Movement Disorders* **11**, 321–323.

Fernandez HH, Friedman JH, Grace J, and Beason-Hazen S. (2000). Donepezil for Huntington's disease. *Movement Disorders* **15**, 173–176.

Folstein SE (1989). *Huntington's disease: a disorder of families*. Johns Hopkins University Press, Baltimore.

Folstein SE, Franz ML, Jensen BA, Chase GA, and Folstein MF (1983). Conduct disorder and affective disorder among the offspring of patients with Huntington's disease. *Psychological Medicine* **13** (1), 45–52.

Foroud T, Siemers E, Kleindorfer D, Bill DJ, Hodes ME, Norton JA, *et al.* (1995). Cognitive scores in carriers of Huntington's disease gene compared to non-carriers. *Annals of Neurology* **37** (5), 657–664.

Giordani B, Berent S, Boivin MJ, Penney JB, Lehtinen S, Markel D, *et al.* (1995). Longitudinal neuropsychological and genetic linkage analysis of persons at risk for Huntington's disease. *Archives of Neurology* **52** (1), 59–64.

Goetz CG, Tanner CM, Cohen JA, Thelen JA, Carroll VS, Klawans HL, and Fariello RG (1990). L-acetyl-carnitine in Huntington's disease: Double-blind placebo controlled crossover study of drug effects on movement disorder and dementia. *Movement Disorders* **5**, 263–264.

Gomez-Tortosa E, MacDonald ME, Friend JC, Taylor SAM, Weiler LJ, Cupples LA, *et al.* (2001). Quantitative neuropathological changes in presymptomatic Huntington's disease. *Annals of Neurology* **49**, 29–34.

Greenamyre JT and Shoulson I (1994). Huntington's disease. In *Neurodegenerative diseases* (ed. D. Calne), pp. 685–704. W.B. Saunders, Philadelphia.

Grove VE, Quintanilla J, and DeVaney GT (2000). Improvement of Huntington's disease with olanzapine and valproate. *New England Journal of Medicine* **343**, 973–974.

Growdon JH, Cohen EL, and Wurtman RJ (1977). Huntington's disease: clinical and chemical effects of choline administration. *Annals of Neurology* **1**, 418–422.

Hahn-Barma V, Deweer B, Durr A, Dode C, Feingold J, Pillon B, *et al.* (1998). Are cognitive changes the first symptoms of Huntington's disease? A study of gene carriers. *Journal of Neurology, Neurosurgery and Psychiatry* **62** (2), 172–177.

Harper PS (ed.) (1996). *Huntington's disease*, 2nd edn. W.B. Saunders, London.

Hayden MR (1981). *Huntington's chorea*. Springer-Verlag, Berlin.

Huntington Study Group (FJ Marshal, primary author) (1996). Inter-laboratory variability of (CAG)n determinations in Huntington's disease (HD). *Neurology* **46**, A258.

—— (Marshall F, primary author) (1998). Safety and tolerability of the free-radical scavenger OPC-14117 in Huntington's disease. *Neurology* **50**, 1366–1373.

Huntington Study Group (Marshall F, primary author) (2001a). Riluzole dosing in Huntington's disease (RID-HD). Abstract of a paper presented at the 19th International Meeting of the World Federation of Neurology Research Group on Huntington's Disease, August 25–28, 2001, Copenhagen, Denmark.

—— (K Kieburtz, primary author) (2001b). Placebo-controlled trial of creatine in Huntington's disease. *Neurology* **56**, A386.

—— (K Kieburtz, primary author (2001). A randomized, placebo-controlled trial of co enzyme Q10 and remacemide in Huntington's disease (CARE-HD). *Neurology* **57**, 376–397.

Jankovic J and Beach J (1997). Long-term effects of tetrabenazine in hyperkinetic movement disorders. *Neurology* **48**, 358–362.

Jason GW, Pajurkova EM, Suchowersky O, Hewitt J, Hilbert C, and Hayden MR (1988). Presymptomatic neuropsychological impairment in Huntington's disease. *Archives of Neurology* **45** (7), 769–773.

Jason GW, Suchowersky O, Pajurkova EM, Graham L, Klimek ML, Garber AT, *et al.* (1997). Cognitive manifestations of Huntington disease in relation to genetic structure and clinical onset. *Archives of Neurology* **54** (9), 1081–1088.

Kieburtz K (1999). Antiglutamate therapies in Huntington's disease. *Journal of Neural Transmission* **55**, 97–102.

Kieburtz K, Feigin A, McDermott M, Como P, Abwender D, Zimmerman C, Hickey C, Orme C, Claude K, Sotack J, Greenamyre JT, Dunn C, and Shoulson I (1996). A controlled trial of remacemide hydrochloride in Huntington's disease. *Movement Disorders* **11**, 273–277.

Kirkwood SC, Siemers E, Stout JC, Hodes ME, Conneally PM, Christian JC, *et al.* (1999). Longitudinal cognitive and motor changes among presymptomatic Huntington disease gene carriers. *Archives of Neurology* **56** (5), 563–568.

Kirkwood SC, Siemers E, Bond C, Conneally PM, Christian JC, and Foroud T (2000a). Confirmation of subtle motor changes among presymptomatic carriers of the Huntington disease gene. *Archives of Neurology* **57** (7), 1040–1044.

Kirkwood SC, Siemers E, Hodes ME, Conneally PM, Christian JC, and Foroud T (2000b). Subtle changes among presymptomatic carriers of the Huntington's disease gene. *Journal of Neurology, Neurosurgery and Psychiatry* **69**, 773–779.

Kremer B, Clark CM, Almqvist EW, Raymond LA, Graf P, Jacova C, Mezei M, Hardy MA, Snow B, Martin W, and Hayden MR (1999). Influence of lamotrigine on progression of early Huntington disease. A randomized clinical trial. *Neurology* **53**, 1000–1011.

Matthews RT, Yang L, Jenkins BG, Ferrante RJ, Rosen BR, Kaddurah-Daouk R, and Beal MF (1998). Neuroprotective effects of creatine and cyclocreatine in animal models of Huntington's disease. *Journal of Neuroscience* **18**, 156–163.

McCusker E, Richards F, Sillence D, Wilson M, and Trent RJ (2000). Huntington's disease: neurological assessment of potential gene carriers presenting for predictive DNA testing. *Journal of Clinical Neuroscience* **7** (1), 38–41.

Murman DL, Giordani B, Mellow AM, Johanns JR, Little RJA, Hariharan M, and Foster NL (1997). Cognitive, behavioral, and motor effects of the NMDA antagonist ketamine in Huntington's disease. *Neurology* **49**, 153–161.

Penney JB, Young BM, Shoulson I, Starosta-Rubinstein S, Snodgrass SR, Sanchez-Ramos J, *et al.* (1990). Huntingon's disease in Venezuela: 7 years of follow-up on symptomatic and asymptomatic individuals. *Movement Disorders* **5** (2), 93–99.

Peyser CE, Folstein M, Chase GA, Starkstein S, Brandt J, Cockrell JR, Bylsma F, Coyle JT, McHugh PR, and Folstein SE (1995). Trial of d-α-tocopherol in Huntington's disease. *American Journal of Psychiatry* **152**, 1771–1775.

Ranen NG, Peyser CE, and Folstein SE (1994). ECT as a treatment for depression in Huntington's disease. *Journal of Neuropsychiatry and Clinical Neurosciences* **6**, 154–159.

—— Lipsey JR, Treisman G, and Ross CA (1996a). Sertraline in the treatment of severe aggressiveness in Huntington's disease. *Journal of Neuropsychiatry and Clinical Neurosciences* **8**, 338–340.

—— Peyser CE, Coyle JT, Bylsma FW, Sherr M, Day L, Folstein MF, Brandt J, Ross CA, and Folstein SE (1996b). A controlled trial of idebenone in Huntington's disease. *Movement Disorders* **11**, 549–554.

Rosas HD, Koroshetz WJ, Jenkins BG, Chen YI, Hayden DL, Beal MF, and Cudkowicz ME (1999). Riluzole therapy in Huntington's disease (HD). *Movement Disorders* **14**, 326–330.

Rosenberg NK, Sorenson SA, and Christensen AL (1995). Neuropsychological characteristics of Huntington's disease carriers: a double blind study. *Journal of Medical Genetics* **32** (8), 600–604.

Rothlind JC, Brandt J, Zee D, Codori AM, and Folstein S (1993). Unimpaired verbal memory and oculomotor control in asymptomatic adults with the genetic marker for Huntington's disease. *Archives of Neurology* **50** (8), 799–802.

Shiwach RS and Norbury CG (1994). A controlled psychiatric study of individuals at risk for Huntington's disease. *British Journal of Psychiatry* **165** (4), 500–505.

Shoulson I and Fahn S (1979). Huntington's disease: clinical care and evaluation. *Neurology* **29**, 1–3.

—— Kieburtz K (1997). Neuroprotective therapy for Huntington's disease. In *Neuroprotection: fundamental and clinical aspects* (ed. PR Bär and MF Beal), pp 457–464. Marcel Dekker, Inc., New York.

—— Goldblatt D, Charlton M, and Joynt RJ (1978). Huntington' disease: treatment with muscimol, a GABA-mimetic drug. *Annals of Neurology* **4**, 279–284.

—— Odoroff C, Oakes D, Behr J, Goldblatt D, Caine E, Kennedy J, Miller C, Bamford K, Rubin A, Plumb S, and Kurlan R (1989). A controlled clinical trial of baclofen in early Huntington's disease. *Annals of Neurology* **25**, 252–259.

Siemers E, Foroud T, Bill DJ, Sorbel J, Norton JA, Jr., Hodes ME, *et al.* (1996). Motor changes in presymptomatic Huntington disease gene carriers. *Archives of Neurology* **53** (6), 487–492.

Steffan JS, Bodai L, Pallos J, Poelman M, McCampbell A, Apostol BL, Kazantsev A, Schmidt E, Zhu YZ, Greenwald M, Kurokawa R, Housman DE, Jackson GR, Marsh JL, and Thompson LM (2001). Histone deacetylase inhibitors arrest polyglutamine-dependent neurodegeneration in *Drosophila. Nature* **413**, 739–743.

Strauss ME and Brandt J (1990). Are there neuropsychologic manifestations of the gene for Huntington's disease in asymptomatic, at-risk individuals? *Archives of Neurology* **47** (8), 905–908.

Tarsy D and Bralower M (1977). Deanol acetamidobenzoate treatment in choreiform movement disorders. *Archives of Neurology* **343**, 756–758.

Van Vugt JP, Siesling S, Vergeer M, van der Velde EA, and Roos RA (1997). Clozapine versus placebo in Huntington's disease: a double blind randomized comparative study. *Journal of Neurology, Neurosurgery and Psychiatry* **63**, 35–39.

Walker FO and Hunt VP (1989). An open label trial of dextromethorphan in Huntington's disease. *Clinical Neuropharmacology* **12**, 322–330.

Young AB, Penney JB, Starosta-Rubenstein S, Markel D, Berent S, Rothley J, *et al.* (1987). Normal caudate glucose metabolism in persons at risk for Huntington's disease. *Archives of Neurology* **44** (3), 254–257.

17 Cell and tissue transplantation

Stephen B. Dunnett and Anne E. Rosser

Introduction

While medical strategies are available to alleviate some symptoms of Huntington's disease (HD), such as the use of neuroleptics or antidepressants for particular psychiatric/behavioural deficits or special diets for the weight loss, it remains the case that the fundamental progressive neurodegenerative process is essentially untreatable medically. It is in this context that new therapies for cellular repair are now under active exploration at the research level. These novel strategies essentially fall into two distinct classes: (1) neuroprotection to slow or halt the progression of the neurodegenerative disease process and (2) cell transplantation to surgically replace essential striatal circuit neurones once lost. These two techniques are not themselves mutually exclusive, since the problems of delivering trophic factors into the central nervous system (CNS) can be facilitated using implants of engineered cells as vectors for their delivery to precisely targeted sites, and grafted cells themselves require appropriate trophic support in order to survive and function appropriately (Dunnett and Mayer 1992). In this chapter we will provide an overview of cell-based repair strategies for HD, which have progressed in recent years from promising animal models to the first clinical trials in patients.

Principles of cell transplantation in the CNS

Although there have been sporadic attempts at transplantation of neuronal cells into the adult mammalian CNS since the beginning of the twentieth century, with variable success, the basic conditions for reliable neural transplantation were finally established in the 1970s and the techniques have been subsequently refined over the last two decades (for a historical account, see Björklund and Stenevi (1985)). Essentially, the fundamental requirements for successful engraftment are to identify a suitable source of donor cells, to employ a transplantation technique that does not excessively traumatize these cells, and to select a target site in the host brain that can nourish and support them.

Sources of donor cells

The most widely studied and successful cells for transplantation are primary embryonic neurones, that is, neurones taken directly from the developing brain and transplanted without any period of further division in culture. The phenotypic fate of such developing neurones is determined at the time of uterine implantation so that they express by default the particular phenotypes of experimental or therapeutic interest. However, primary neurones only survive well following transplantation if they are taken during the restricted time window in development when the cells are first born. At this time their fate is determined, and they are actively expressing their ontogenetic programmes for axonal growth and appropriate target connection. For most populations of neuronal cells, the critical time window is restricted to a few days in the second half of embryonic development (in mouse or rat), although it can extend into the first week of postnatal life for late differentiating cell populations, such as are found in the neocortex, cerebellum, and dentate gyrus (Dunnett and Björklund 1992; Olson *et al.* 1983). Having identified the critical developmental age for a particular donor cell population, the relevant tissues need to be identified and accurately dissected (Brundin and Strecker 1991; Dunnett and Björklund 1992). In humans, the equivalent stages of development are typically of 2–3 weeks duration and reached at 6–12 weeks of gestation, depending on the particular cell population under consideration (Butler and Juurlink 1987).

As long as clinical transplantation remains dependent on primary human embryonic cells, applications will always be restricted due to the limited availability of donor tissue, the practical difficulties in standardization of techniques, and the ethical issues that surround any use of human foetal tissues. Consequently, there has been a vigorous search over the last decade for alternatives that are more readily available and less ethically controversial. Such alternatives include xenotransplantation from non-human species, and laboratory-maintained and expanded cells such as can be derived from stem cells. These alternatives will be considered in more detail after reviewing what can be achieved with primary embryonic neurones, which provide the 'gold standard' for cell-based repair strategies in a variety of neurodegenerative diseases.

Host sites

Isolated cells and tissues require suitable support and nourishment, especially during the first few days after transplantation. 'Solid' grafts of small pieces of embryonic tissue, in particular, need to be implanted into a richly vascularized site where they can rapidly become incorporated into the host vascular circulation. A few natural sites are available that accommodate this need, such as the epithelial surfaces of the lateral and third ventricles or the choroidal fissure above the thalamus (Stenevi *et al.* 1976). Alternatively, a suitable artificial site can be created, for example, by the delayed cavitation method, in which an aspirative cavity is made in the cortex followed by an interval of several weeks (during which a new highly vascularized pial lining forms over the floor and walls of the cavity) before implantation of the grafted tissue (Stenevi *et al.* 1985). More recently, the development of cell suspension methods, whereby cells for transplantation are prepared as dissociated suspensions and then injected stereotaxically into deep brain sites, have circumvented the need for generation of transplantation cavities (Fig. 17.1; Schmidt *et al.* 1981). Unlike solid grafts, dissociated cells can integrate directly into the host parenchyma (Björklund *et al.* 1983; Schmidt *et al.* 1981). Moreover, the cell suspension method allows single or multiple deposits to be placed throughout the neuraxis (Björklund and Dunnett 1992). Implants made into adults by-and-large survive equivalently from youth through to old age (Gage *et al.* 1983; Lund *et al.* 1987), although there is evidence that implants into the developing brain can migrate further and exhibit greater plasticity than when transplanted into adult hosts (Lund and Yee 1992; Olsson *et al.* 1997).

Immunological factors

Experience with organ transplantation might suggest that immunological factors would provide a critical barrier for transplantation in the brain as they do elsewhere in the body. In fact,

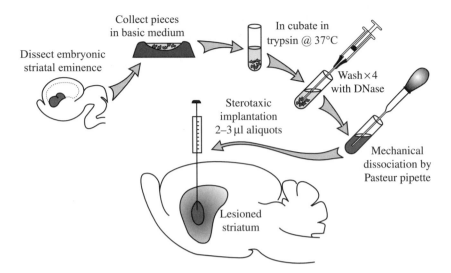

Fig. 17.1 Schematic illustration of techniques for cell suspension grafting in the rodent CNS.

the brain has long been known to be an 'immunologically privileged' site, in the sense that allografts of skin or other tissues (and, in particular, nerve cells) into the brain do not suffer the same process of rejection that would take place if the same tissue were implanted into most other sites in the body (Lund and Bannerjee 1992). The reason for this privilege is still only partially understood, although factors known to be of importance include the following.

- The blood–brain barrier protects the brain from circulating cells and molecules of the immune system, making the efferent arm of the immune response weak.
- Major and minor histocompatability molecules are expressed at only low levels on the cell surface of neurones, although glia (and in particular activated glia) do exhibit higher levels of expression.
- Lymphatic drainage from the brain is limited so that the afferent arm of the immune response is weak.
- Cell suspensions have no donor-derived microvasculature and exhibit no hyperacute rejection response.

As a consequence, neuronal allografts (that is, where donor and host are of the same species) exhibit long-term survival and no overt signs of rejection, without any special treatment. Nevertheless, the immunological privilege of the brain is partial and is exaggerated once we cross species barriers, so that xenografts are typically rejected, although even xenografts may be protected to an extent using a variety of immunosuppression strategies (Lund and Bannerjee 1992; Watts and Dunnett 2000).

Striatal grafts in experimental rats

The basis for recent clinical trials of cell transplantation in HD derives first and foremost from the demonstration that striatal tissues survive transplantation and function so as to alleviate both motor and cognitive deficits in experimental models of the disease in rats. A variety of different experimental model systems have been used.

- Excitotoxic lesions made by stereotaxic injection of excitatory amino acids (kainic acid, ibotenic acid, or quinolinic acid) directly into the striatum (Dunnett *et al.* 2000; Sanberg and Coyle 1984). This has been the most commonly used model for studies of grafting in rodents.
- Striatal ischaemia made by occlusion of the middle cerebral artery (Nishino *et al.* 1992; Zhou *et al.* 1991).
- Metabolic lesions of the striatum using the mitochondrial toxins malonate and 3-nitropropionic acid (Borlongan *et al.* 1995).
- R6/2 transgenic mice that overexpress exon 1 of the HD gene with a greatly expanded CAG repeat length (Mangiarini *et al.* 1996; Dunnett *et al.* 1998).

Graft survival and internal organization

In virtually all studies, the striatal grafts are made by dissection of the ganglionic eminence from developing embryos of 13–17 days of embryonic age (E13–E17), pooling of the tissue pieces from multiple donors, enzymatic digestion and dissociation of the cells, and stereotaxic injection of the dissociated suspensions directly into the striatal parenchyma (Fig. 17.1). When the host animals are killed several weeks or months later and processed for routine histological visualization (Fig. 17.2), the grafts typically show good survival, having grown several-fold in volume over that initially injected.

An immediately distinctive feature of striatal grafts, when visualized using a variety of staining methods characteristic of striatal tissues, is their patchy internal organization. This is illustrated in Fig. 17.2 for acetylcholinesterase (AChE), a strong marker of striatal neuropil

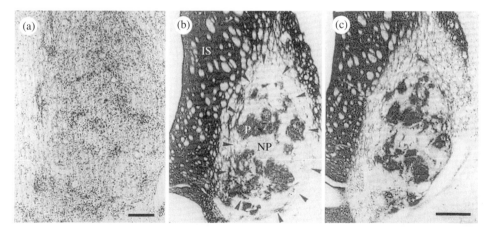

Fig 17.2 Photomicrographs of survival and internal organization of striatal grafts in the adult rat striatum. (a) Cresyl violet stain for Nissl substance to visualize cell bodies. Note healthy grafts comprising predominantly neurones and the relative absence of glial or inflammatory reactions at the graft–host borders. (b) Acetylcholinesterase histochemistry, shows patchy organizations of striatal-like neuropil IS, intact striatum. (c) DARPP-32 immunohistochemistry stains striatal medium spiny projection neurones. P, Patch; NP, non-patch compartments of striatal grafts. Scale bars: (a) 50 μm; (b),(c) 200 μm.

(Graybiel *et al.* 1989; Isacson *et al.* 1987b), but is equally apparent when using other striatal specific markers such as the dopamine and adenylate cyclase receptor related phosphoprotein DARPP-32 (Doucet *et al.* 1989; Fricker *et al.* 1997a; Labandeira-Garcia *et al.* 1991), striatal enriched phosphoprotein STEP (Fricker *et al.* 1994, 1997a), or the dopamine D1 and D2 receptors (Deckel *et al.* 1988; Isacson *et al.* 1987a; Liu *et al.* 1990). These patches do not correspond to the patch versus matrix organization of the neostriatum. Rather, the patches represent zones of strong staining with a variety of markers of striatal neurones, neuropil, or receptors (the so-called 'P zones'; Graybiel *et al.* 1989), interspersed with areas that exhibit features characteristic of nonstriatal neurones (the so-called 'NP zones'), including distinctive cellular morphology of cortical pyramidal cells by Golgi staining (Clarke *et al.* 1994), of pallidal cells by enkephalin and calbindin immunohistochemistry (Graybiel *et al.* 1989, 1990) and by expression of cholecystokinin mRNA characteristic of the neocortex (Sirinathsinghji *et al.* 1993). This combination of phenotypes is due to the fact that striatal neurones differentiate alongside many other cell types in the germinal cell layer of the ventricular zone of the ganglionic eminence, from where the cells migrate through the subventricular zone to deep and remote sites (Fig. 17.3). The neurones destined to form the developing striatum stop in the area underlying the subventricular zone, whereas other cells continue to migrate through this area to form and populate other telencephalic sites such as the lateral cortex, globus pallidus, and amygdala (De Carlos *et al.* 1996; Smart and Sturrock 1979). It is, therefore, not

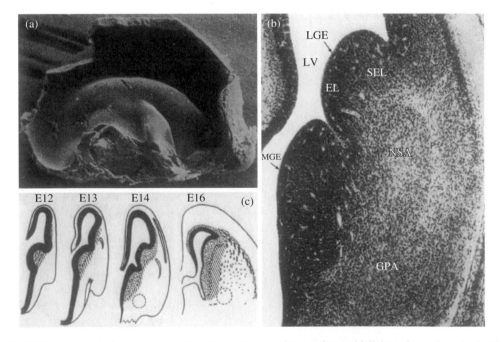

Fig. 17.3 Embryonic development of the rat ganglionic eminence, from which the striatum is derived. (a) Scanning electron micrograph. (b) Nissl-stained frozen sections. (c) Schematic illustration of the development over E12–E16 days of gestation. lGE, Lateral ganglionic eminence; MGE, medial ganglionic eminence; EL, ependymal layer; GPA, globus pallidus anlage; LV, lateral ventricle; NSA, neostriatal anlage; SEL, subependymal layer. (Collated from Smart and Sturrock (1979) with permission.)

possible to undertake a selective dissection that harvests only striatal precursors or newly differentiated striatal neurones, and the grafts inevitably comprise both striatal and nonstriatal populations.

Since the grafts are prepared as a dissociated cell suspension, one surprising feature is that they do develop into such well-demarcated P and NP zones. It is not just the cell types that become separated; the afferent and efferent connections that subsequently develop with the host brain also respect the same boundaries within the grafts (see below). This could come about by several different processes (Barker and Dunnett 1999).

- Striatal and nonstriatal cells migrate and self-aggregate into clusters of cells of similar type based on competition between attractive and repulsive cell surface markers.

- Selective cell death of neurones whose neighbours are of a dissimilar type, resulting in selective survival of similar cells.

- The phenotype of each cell is itself determined by its neighbours, resulting in plasticity of each cell to match that which predominates in its surroundings.

At present we have no data to distinguish these alternative hypotheses, but their resolution would open new ways to control the differentiation and plasticity of striatal neurones both for, and within, transplants. In the meantime, the composition of the grafts is largely determined by two factors: the age of the donor and the precise dissection of the donor tissue.

Striatal neurones differentiate predominantly at days E12–E15, and tissue dissected from the whole ganglionic eminence harvested at this age gives rise to grafts comprising 30–50 per cent of striatal-like P zones. By contrast, tissue harvested from later embryos gives rise to grafts that are not only smaller and show less cellular expansion, but in which the proportion of P zones is also substantially reduced (Fricker *et al.* 1997a; Watts *et al.* 2000b). This is not surprising in light of the fact that cortical components of the ganglionic eminence differentiate during this later period.

Second, there has been a considerable debate about whether improved grafts—based on the criterion of the proportion of the graft that comprises striatal-like P-zone tissues—can be derived from a selective dissection of the ganglionic eminence. Isacson and colleagues have argued that, since DARPP-32 striatal projection neurones derive primarily from the lateral ridge of the ganglionic eminence (LGE), more selective grafts could be achieved by taking a dissection restricted to the LGE. They have described grafts based on this restricted dissection in which the P zones (by AChE and DARPP-32 staining) comprise 70–90 per cent of total graft volume tissues (Deacon *et al.* 1994). Based on similar reasoning, Freeman has gone one step further and argued for a far-lateral dissection (Freeman *et al.* 1995). However, although the LGE is indeed the primary source of striatal projection neurones and grafts restricted to the medial ridge of the ganglionic eminence (MGE) exhibit a minimal P-zone compartment, nevertheless, the MGE does give rise to other populations of striatal interneurones that may be critical for proper striatal development (Olsson *et al.* 1998). Thus, although the proportion of P zone derived from an LGE dissection is higher, both the overall survival as well as the total volume of the P-zone compartment is significantly greater when tissue from the whole ganglionic eminence (WGE) is included in the grafts (Watts *et al.* 2000b). Ultimately, however, the choice of dissection for clinical trials in patients will depend on which works best in a variety of functional tests, and functional efficacy has so far only been well studied and demonstrated for the whole dissection method.

Graft–host connections

When implanted into the denervated striatum at the appropriate developmental age, striatal grafts give rise to extensive tissue connections with the host brain. This has been most extensively studied by Wictorin and colleagues using a variety of antergorade and retrograde tracing techniques, as illustrated in Fig. 17.4 (Wictorin 1992). To summarize a large series of studies, striatal grafts routinely establish projections to the globus pallidus, the proximal target of normal striatal neurones in the intact brain, and many grafts send longer-distance projections to remote targets, in particular, the substantia nigra pars reticulata (Pritzel *et al.* 1986; Wictorin *et al.* 1989b, 1991). Retrograde tracing reveals that these efferent projections derive from medium-sized neurones in the striatal-like P-zone compartments of the grafts (Wictorin *et al.* 1989a). Reciprocally, the grafts receive afferent connections from all major populations of neurones of the host brain that would normally project into the intact striatum, including the neocortex, thalamus, substantia nigra pars compacta, and raphe nucleus (Wictorin *et al.* 1988; Wictorin and Björklund 1989). The substantia nigra is particularly straightforward to visualize using sensitive tyrosine hydroxylase immunohistochemistry, which again confirms that the afferent fibres penetrate throughout the grafts but only undergo extensive terminal ramification in the P zones, in which appropriate target neurones are located (Wictorin *et al.* 1989a).

The selectivity of connections has been confirmed at the ultrastructural level (Clarke and Dunnett 1993). In this study, we identified afferent cortical inputs by first making cortical lesions and then looking for degenerating terminals. Dopaminergic terminals were visualized by gold labelling of a tyrosine hydroxylase antibody binding. Cortical and dopaminergic inputs made symmetric and asymmetric synaptic contacts, respectively, on to the heads and the necks of the dendritic spines of γ-aminobutyric acid (GABA)ergic, medium spiny, projection

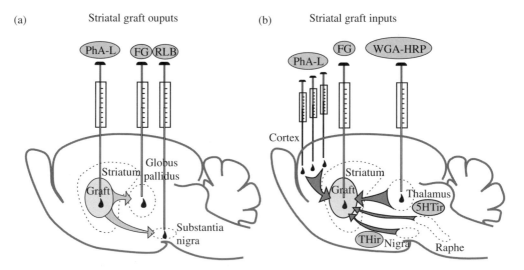

Fig. 17.4 Afferent and efferent connections of striatal grafts. Schematic illustration of the connections of striatal grafts, indicating the major projections and the tracing methods used for their visualization. (Redrawn from Wictorin (1992) with permission). FG, fluorogold; PhA-L, Phaseolus leucoagglutinin; RLB, rhodamine labelled beads; ir, immunoreactivity; WGA-HRP, wheat germ agglutinin-horse radish peroxidase.

neurones (identified by immunohistochemistry for the synthetic enzyme, glutamic acid decar-boxylase (GAD), Golgi staining, and retrograde transport of the retrograde tracer wheat germ agglutinin–horseradish peroxidase from the globus pallidus, respectively). This study demon-strated that neurones in striatal grafts re-establish both inputs and outputs necessary to become properly integrated into the host basal ganglia circuitry, although, of course, electron microscopy provides little quantitative information and the density of appropriate connections almost certainly does not return to normal.

Thus, although the graft comprises a mixed population of both striatal-like and non-striatal-like neurones, afferent and efferent connections appear to be selectively and specifically established with the P-zone compartment. This selective reorganization and reconstruction of an appropriate striatal circuitry by the grafts in the host brain may explain how we see functionally beneficial effects of the grafts on a range of behavioural assessments (see below).

Neurochemical indices of function

Early studies of striatal lesions monitored the decline of GAD and choline acetyltransferase (ChAT) activities as key indicators of loss of the GABAergic medium spiny projection neurones and the giant cholinergic interneurones of the striatum, respectively (Coyle and Schwarcz 1976). Activity of both enzymes is restored in the grafted striatum when assayed biochemically at post-mortem (Isacson *et al.* 1985; Schmidt *et al.* 1981), in accord with the histochemical evidence of survival of the associated populations of neurones within the grafts.

A comparable situation has been determined in the living brain using implanted microdial-ysis and push–pull perfusion probes for recording GABA turnover *in vivo*. The excitotoxic lesions reduce GABA overflow by 60–80 per cent in the striatum and by approximately 90–95 per cent in the target areas of the globus pallidus and substantia nigra. GABAergic turnover returns to the normal range in the grafted striatum, as recorded by microdialysis (Campbell *et al.* 1993), and turnover returns to 34 and 60 per cent of normal levels in the nigra and pallidum, respectively, as recorded by push–pull perfusion (Sirinathsinghji *et al.* 1988).

These *in vivo* monitoring methods can provide additional information on functional activity of the grafts. Thus, the study by Campbell *et al.* (1993) indicated that graft-derived GABA turnover was derived from normal vesicular release since potassium-induced surge in release was calcium-dependent. Moreover, the turnover from pallidal axon terminals shows the same magnitude of response to amphetamine in grafted and normal animals, suggesting that affer-ent dopaminergic stimulation can be transduced by grafted medium spiny neurones that carry the dopamine receptors and that these neurones respond with appropriate change in inhibitory GABA release in their projection targets in the host pallidum (Sirinathsinghji *et al.* 1988).

Electrophysiological indices of function

Electrophysiological studies indicate that neurones of the grafted striatum are spontaneously active, respond to a range of host-derived inputs, and influence their host targets in a similar way to normal striatal neurones, but differ in a variety of details. Thus, in *in vitro* slices, all grafted neurones exhibited a slowly inactivating potassium current resembling the delayed rectifier characteristic of mature striatal neurones, suggesting that they express the normal complement of depolarization-activated potassium channel proteins (Surmeier *et al.* 1992). However, they also expressed a number of abnormal features, including higher input resist-ances, longer time constants, and increased sensitivity to direct application of glutamate or *N*-methyl-D-aspartate (NMDA) (Siviy *et al.* 1993; Walsh *et al.* 1988).

Grafted striatal neurones exhibit monosynaptic responses to stimulation of inputs, either in adjacent areas of the host striatum or in the cortex and thalamus, both *in vitro* (Rutherford *et al.* 1987) and *in vivo* (Xu *et al.* 1991), and the activation of grafted neurones following cortical stimulation has been confirmed anatomically by visualization of the induction of the immediate early gene c-*fos* (Labandeira-Garcia and Guerra 1994). However, again, membrane conductances, input resistances, and time constants differed from those seen in the normal striatum, suggesting a sparseness of synaptic connections and changes in lateral inhibition between graft neurones (Rutherford *et al.* 1987; Xu *et al.* 1991).

Grafted neurones project to the host globus pallidus, and this is found to reverse the lesion-induced increase in spontaneous firing of pallidal neurones, suggesting the restitution of inhibitory influences associated with GABA release in the reformed pathway (Nakao *et al.* 1999). Moreover, systemic administration of apomorphine induces an increase in spontaneous activity in the globus pallidus, which is mediated via the striatopallidal projection since the response is blocked by quinolinic acid striatal lesions. The physiological response of pallidal neurones is restored after implantation of striatal grafts (Nakao *et al.* 2000), providing physiological evidence of transduction of dopaminergic signals in striatal neurones in grafts to the host pallidal targets, in direct parallel with the *in vivo* neurochemical studies (Sirinathsinghji *et al.* 1988) described in the previous section. What remains to be established, and for which there is at present no data, is whether changes in cortical activity can also be transduced by the graft and can restore a functional corticostriatopallidal circuit relayed through the graft (Dunnett *et al.* 2000).

Behavioural indices of function

HD in man produces a complex array of motor, cognitive, and psychiatric symptoms. Both motor and cognitive features of the disease can be well represented in animal models involving striatal lesions (Sanberg and Coyle 1984). By contrast, evaluation of psychiatric symptoms in experimental animals, in particular rodents, is necessarily problematic, although there has been some recent progress in tackling this issue through evaluation of motivational deficits in animals' sensitivity to changes in reward (Eagle *et al.* 1999a,b), and in the expression of disgust reactions to aversive tastes (Eagle *et al.* unpublished observations). Striatal grafts have been seen to alleviate both motor and cognitive deficits in experimental rats and primates, whereas the motivational aspects have not yet been directly evaluated. We will only summarize these studies here (see Table 17.1), since a more comprehensive recent review is available elsewhere (Dunnett *et al.* 2000).

Bilateral striatal lesions induce marked hyperactivity in rats which is reversed by striatal grafts. The deficits, and the corresponding graft-derived effects, are greater if the tests are conducted during the active night period, when the animals are food-deprived, or when the lesions target more ventral areas of the striatum (Deckel *et al.* 1983; Isacson *et al.* 1984, 1986; Reading and Dunnett 1995). Unilateral striatal lesions induce whole-body motor asymmetries and other turning biases (in particular when the animals are activated by dopaminergic drugs), which may also be alleviated by striatal grafts (Borlongan *et al.* 1998; Dunnett *et al.* 1988). The grafts are also competent to alleviate more complex motor behaviours. For example, rats have good manual dexterity for picking up and manipulating food, and unilateral striatal lesions produce an inability to use the contralateral paw, that is, the paw on the opposite side of the body (since descending motor pathways cross the midline at the level of the hindbrain,

Table 17.1 Behavioural studies of striatal transplants

Function	Test	First reports of recovery with striatal grafts
Locomotor activity	Digiscan activity monitor	Deckel *et al.* 1983
	Photocell open field	Isacson *et al.* 1984
	Photocell cages	Isacson *et al.* 1986
Coordination and balance	Omnitech rotarod	Giordano *et al.* 1990
	Paw reaching tray test	Dunnett *et al.* 1988
	Paw reaching staircase test	Montoya *et al.* 1990
Rotation and turning	Rotometer bowls	Dunnett *et al.* 1988
	Elevated body swing test	Borlongan *et al.* 1995
Memory	Step through passive avoidance	Piña *et al.* 1994a
	Step down passive avoidance	Koide *et al.* 1993
	Radial maze	Koide *et al.* 1993
Cognition	T maze delayed alternation	Isacson *et al.* 1986
	Morris water maze	Aihara *et al.* 1994
	Operant DRL schedule*	Reading and Dunnett 1995
Motor habit learning	9-hole box operant tasks	Mayer *et al.* 1992
	Skinner box operant task	Döbrössy and Dunnett 1998

the contralateral paw is under the control of the ipsilateral hemisphere, that is, the side damaged by the lesion, and thus is the side on which motor deficits are manifest), to reach grasp and retrieve pieces of food from tubes, trays, or wells (Montoya *et al.* 1990; Whishaw *et al.* 1986). Such deficits in skilled reaching are alleviated by striatal grafts (Dunnett *et al.* 1988; Montoya *et al.* 1990). Interestingly, this is one class of striatal behaviours that is also disrupted by dopamine-denervating nigrostriatal lesions, but which is not alleviated by dopamine-rich nigral grafts (Dunnett *et al.* 1987; Montoya *et al.* 1990). To explain this difference we have hypothesized that, whereas both types of graft replace lost neurones, nigral grafts need to be placed ectopically in order to reinnervate the striatum whereas striatal grafts can connect appropriately when placed homotopically. Thus, functional recovery is seen only in the condition in which the neuronal circuitry, on which the behaviour is dependent, is reconstructed (that is, with striatal grafts).

There has been less extensive analysis of the effects of striatal grafts on cognitive functions, but here also the results are clear-cut (Table 17.1). Striatal grafts have been seen to alleviate deficits in rats with bilateral striatal lesions on a variety of cognitive tasks, including delayed spatial alternation in T mazes (Deckel *et al.* 1986; Isacson *et al.* 1986), spatial learning in Morris water maze (Aihara *et al.* 1994), step-through and step-down passive avoidance (Giordano *et al.* 1998; Piña *et al.* 1994b), and operant differential reinforcement of low rates of responding in an operant chamber (Reading and Dunnett 1995). A feature of these various tests is that they are all also sensitive to cortical lesions, and recovery suggests reconstruction of cortical basal-ganglia loops responsible for the control of complex behaviours, in particular of the frontal type (Dunnett *et al.* 2000).

Mechanisms of functional recovery

The motor and cognitive aspects of striatal function converge in the analysis of habit learning, and studies designed to look at rats' abilities to acquire and relearn specific lateralized stimulus–response ('S–R') associations have been particularly informative in revealing important aspects of graft function.

In the 1980s, Trevor Robbins, Mirjiana Carli, and colleagues introduced a novel operant apparatus, one wall of which contains a horizontal array of nine holes (see Fig. 17.5). Behind each hole is both a light that can be illuminated and a photocell beam that detects whether the animal pokes its nose into that hole. This is then used to test whether rats can detect and respond rapidly to brief lights flashed in one or other of the holes in the array. In the standard 'Carli' task, only three holes are used. Rats are trained to poke and hold their nose in the

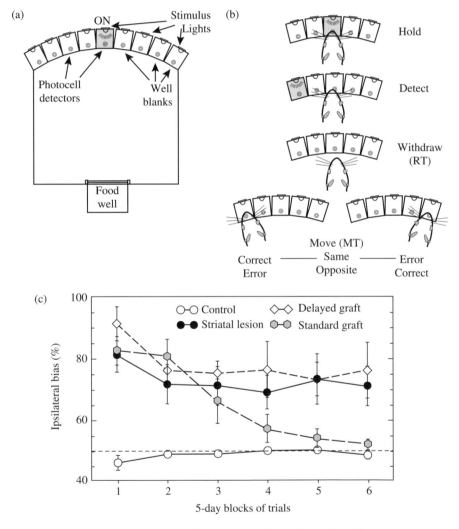

Fig. 17.5 Learning to use to transplant. (a) Schematic illustration of the '9-hole box' operant test apparatus. (b) Sequence of events comprising a discrete trial in the 'Carli' task. (c) RT, reaction time Performance of control, striatal lesioned, and striatal grafted rats in the task. (See text for details; data from Brasted *et al.* (2000) with permission.)

central hole until a light flashes briefly in one of the side holes. Some animals are trained to respond in the illuminated hole ('same' group) whereas others are trained to respond in the symmetrical hole on the other side ('opposite' group). Unilateral lesions of the dopamine input to the striatum on one side impaired animals' responding in the hole on the contralateral side (Carli *et al*. 1985). Since this response was to be made to contralateral stimuli in the 'same' group and ipsilateral stimuli in the 'opposite' group, the lesion is not causing a sensory deficit or neglect of contralateral stimuli, but rather the deficit is in response space. Moreover, the lesioned rats had a selective impairment in their latencies to withdraw the nose from the central hole (initiation or reaction time) with no change in the time taken to make the lateralized movement (response or execution time), indicating that the impairment involved a selective deficit in initiating the lateralized response, not in executing the movement itself (Carli *et al*. 1985). A similar deficit has since been reported in rats with striatal lesions (Mittleman *et al*. 1988).

Mayer *et al*. (1992) first sought to evaluate whether striatal grafts could alleviate deficits in the operant version of the Carli lateralized discrimination and reaction time task. Separate groups were pre-trained to criterion before receiving striatal lesions, lesions plus additional striatal grafts, or sham surgery, and then a 4-month interval was allowed for the grafts to grow and become re-established in the host brain before retesting. When they were finally returned to the test, control animals remembered well and could immediately continue performing on both sides to a high level of accuracy, whereas both the lesion and the graft groups showed profound impairment on the contralateral side. However, whereas the lesion animals remained permanently impaired, with repeated testing the grafted animals relearned the task over 3 weeks. This profile of effects has now been replicated several times (see Fig. 17.5; Brasted *et al*. 1999a,b, 2000). It is not sufficient for a graft to be present and connected with the host brain (which would have been fully established by the time testing recommenced). Rather, the animals must 'learn to use the grafts'. This implies that the grafts are not just providing a motor gate or switch that allows functional capacities mediated elsewhere to be revealed in performance. Rather, it has been proposed that the striatum is the substrate for mediating S–R habit formation, and the present results suggest that the neurones and connections of the graft actually contribute to the neural circuitry that underlies the learning and performance of those motor habits. When intrinsic striatal neurones are lost and replaced in the grafts, the neuronal pathways and synaptic circuits representing those motor associations need to be re-established through experience, which is represented at the functional level by relearning of the lost motor skills (Brasted *et al*. 1999a).

Notwithstanding the mechanism, the 'learning to use the transplant' phenomenon identified in these experiments suggests that a planned programme of rehabilitation will be an important component in maximizing the functional efficacy of grafts in developing a clinically effective therapy for HD patients.

Preclinical studies in animals

We can conclude from the above studies that striatal grafts have the capacity to provide functional repair of striatal damage, at least as caused by excitotoxic lesions of the striatum in experimental animals. We may therefore ask what additional information would be necessary or desirable to have prior to commencing clinical trials to test whether a similar surgical strategy might be of benefit in patients with striatal degeneration, in particular in HD (Peschanski *et al.* 1995, 1996; Shannon and Kordower 1996). A range of issues needs to be addressed, relating to the ethics and safety of human foetal donor tissues, the optimal age and preparation of human striatal tissue grafts, scaling up to the primate brain, determining efficacy in potentially more valid transgenic models of human disease, and validating key aspects of *in vivo* assessment by positron emission tomography (PET) scanning.

Transgenic mice hosts

Grafts may survive and function in the striatum of rats with excitotoxic, metabolic, or ischaemic lesions, but these are acute challenges and differ both in genetic causation and rate of progress from the human disease. There exist a number of transgenic, knock-in, and inducible models of the human gene defect, involving insertion of the full length or fragments of the huntingtin gene carrying CAG repeats expanded into the disease range, and some lines of these mice exhibit profound neurodegenerative and neurological deficits that are similar in several important respects to those seen in the human disease (see Chapter 13). Only one study has so far investigated implantation of striatal grafts into R6/2 transgenic mice, and reported good survival of the grafts comparable to that seen in normal mice (Dunnett *et al.* 1998). Only limited behavioural effects were seen, and then only early in the expression of disease phenotype. The grafts did not alleviate the precipitous loss of body weight from 12 weeks of age in these mice that leads to their death by approximately 15 weeks. However, this may not be surprising since the inclusion pathology in the mice is far more widespread than is seen in the human disease, affecting hypothalamus, hippocampus, and cortex among other areas, which would not be affected by selective striatal transplantation. What the results do indicate is that the grafted tissues are not subject to the same disease process leading to inclusion formation and subsequent progressive brain atrophy that is seen in the brains of host mice carrying the mutant transgene (Dunnett *et al.* 1998), giving optimism that striatal grafts may survive similarly well in patients.

Primate hosts

If we are to transplant striatal tissues in humans, we need confidence that the procedures that work in rats can be scaled up to the primate basal ganglia, which differs not only in the scale over which growth and integration will be required but also in anatomical differentiation into discrete caudate nucleus and putamen. The first studies of striatal grafts in primates were conducted by xenotransplantation of embryonic rat ganglionic eminence into the baboon striatum. The grafts were seen to survive and promote modest recovery on the animals' dyskinetic responses to low-dose apomorphine (Hantraye *et al.* 1992; Isacson *et al.* 1989). This was closely followed by detailed characterization of survival, and morphological differentiation, of striatal neurones in allografts in the rhesus striatum (Helm *et al.* 1992). However, the grafts did not survive well long-term in this model (Helm *et al.* 1993), most probably because the cells were prepared as a cell suspension by mechanical dissociation without enzymatic digestion, a protocol that is profoundly detrimental to cell survival in rats (Watts *et al.* 2000a). More recently, better long-term survival has been achieved with enzymatically dissociated cell suspensions of striatal allografts (Kendall *et al.* 1998; Palfi *et al.* 1998) and these two studies also demonstrated for the first time functional recovery in striatally grafted monkeys, in skilled reaching and barrier detour tasks, respectively. Critically, the grafts were seen to develop an appropriate internal morphological organization and both afferent and efferent connections with the host brain, similar to that which has been well established in the rat, giving credence to plans for scaling up to humans.

Human-to-rat xenografts

Studies of primate allografts employed donor tissues from embryos at stages of morphological development (equivalent to Carnegie stages 19–23; Butler and Juurlink 1987) similar to those that had been established empirically as optimal in rodents. A similar principle would provide an initial provisional estimate of 7–9 weeks of gestation for dissection of striatal tissues from human donors. This estimate has been validated by xenotransplantation of human striatal grafts into immunosuppressed rat hosts (Grasbon-Frodl *et al*. 1996; Pundt *et al*. 1994). Although the grafts survive well, differentiate to exhibit a variety of striatal transmitter phenotypes (Pundt *et al*. 1996b, 1997), and are able to alleviate some behavioural deficits in the host rats (Pundt *et al*. 1996a), there have been concerns about whether human and rodent tissues are comparable for two reasons. First, the human xenografts typically exhibit a rather low proportion of AChE- and DARPP-32-rich P zones (Brundin *et al*. 1996; Grasbon-Frodl *et al*. 1996). Second, there are occasional cases in which the grafts grow very large (Grasbon-Frodl *et al*. 1996), raising fears of potential for uncontrolled overgrowth. Such concerns have waned with the recent reports of appropriate morphological development and functional recovery in primate allografts. Human tissue takes much longer than rat or subhuman primate to develop, which suggests that the limited differentiation is due to the short survival of the human tissue in the rat. Moreover, 'overgrowth' may simply be due to the small size of the rat brain compared to that of the human from which the grafted tissue was derived. Finally, many of the signals necessary to regulate both growth and differentiation may be species-specific and not well regulated in the xenograft situation, although the molecular identities of those signalling mechanisms are still poorly defined.

Imaging

It will not be possible in clinical trials to collect the detailed morphological data relating to the survival, growth, and connections of the grafts that can be collected from systematic post-mortem analyses in experimental animals. Consequently, the development of sensitive and selective scanning protocols to assess graft survival and integration *in vivo* is likely to be important for interpretation of clinical outcomes. Although the gross atrophy of the striatum in HD can be well monitored by magnetic resonance imaging (MRI), it was not known whether this would be sensitive enough to detect and resolve graft tissues, or to determine whether the grafts comprised healthy or dying, striatal or nonstriatal neurones. Consequently, several labs have sought to validate alternative methods for functional imaging of striatal grafts *in vivo*. The two basic strategies are structural and functional MRI and PET using a variety of metabolic and receptor-specific ligands. These need to be considered in turn.

Early attempts to visualize striatal lesions and grafts in rat brain turned up difficulties in resolving striatal grafted tissue from the background with either T1- or T2-weighting or gadolinium enhancement, although the enlarged ventricles induced by the lesions and the growth of glioma cell grafts could be clearly detected (Norman *et al*. 1989a,b). A recent study has been a little more successful, in particular with T1-weighting (Guzman *et al*. 1999), suggesting that the survival and development of the grafts could at least be detected, even if not studied in detail. By contrast, the enlarged scale provided by MRI of primate brain has yielded more clear-cut resolution of striatal grafts in T1-weighted MRI (Denys *et al.* 1992; Kendall *et al.* 2000).

Although it has lower spatial and temporal resolution than MRI, greater definition of striatal grafts has been achieved using PET (Fig. 17.6). Using a small animal scanner for rats, Torres

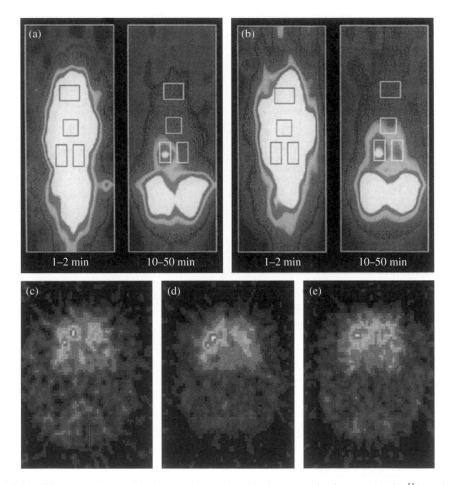

Fig. 17.6 PET scans of striatal lesions and striatal grafts in rats and primates. (a),(b) ^{11}C-raclopride imaging of the rat brain. The short latency (1–2min) scan indicates nonspecific binding throughout the brain (horizontal section: anterior down, posterior up), on to which is placed a mask for unbiased location of the striatum bilaterally, thalamus, and cerebellum. The later (10–30min) scan indicates specific binding retained in the intact striatum, (a) lost in the lesioned striatum (a), and (b) partially restored in the grafted striatum (b). (c)–(e) ^{11}C-raclopride imaging of the marmoset brain. (c) The caudate and putamen are seen in resolvable signals in the left hemisphere, but binding is markedly reduced in the lesioned right hemisphere (c). (d) No restitution of signal in the grafted right striatum in a lesioned monkey that did not recover in a skilled reaching task. (e) Significant restitution of the raclopride binding signal in the grafted right striatum in a lesioned monkey that showed good recovery in the behavioural task. (Data from Torres *et al.* (1995) and Besret *et al.* (2000) with permission.)

et al. (1995) have shown that striatal grafts could be clearly demarcated using the D2 receptor ligand raclopride, which provides greater discrimination of the grafts from background than either the D1 ligand SCH-23390 or the metabolic marker 2-fluorodeoxyglucose. Moreover, the technique clearly distinguished striatal graft tissues from control grafts of cortical tissue, and the raclopride signal correlated highly with post-mortem measurement of P-zone volume in the grafts (Torres *et al.* 1995). In a subsequent study, comparing different ages of donor tissue, there was again a close relationship between the degree of restoration of the PET raclopride binding constant in the grafted striatum and recovery of skilled paw reaching (Fricker *et al.* 1997b). Preliminary data have recently been accumulated to replicate this method in primates (Besret *et al.* 2000; Kendall *et al.* 2000). As a consequence of the animal studies, the use of longitudinal PET scans with raclopride is now recommended as a core component of the CAPIT (core assessment protocol for transplantation) longitudinal assessment protocol for clinical trials in HD.

Clinical transplantation trials

Implantation of foetal tissues in Parkinson's disease (PD) can yield significant clinical benefit in a substantial proportion of patients, provided the surgical methods are based on a sound biological foundation (Lindvall and Hagell 2000). Studies in experimental animals indicate that a similar strategy may be effective in HD, and the preclinical studies reviewed in the previous section have resolved a series of issues that were of potential concern prior to their experimental investigation. On this basis a number of centres have taken the decision to commence clinical trials of foetal striatal tissue transplantation in HD patients (Table 17.2).

Ethical issues

For trials of human neural transplantation the ethical debate focuses on two areas: the collection and use of human foetal tissues for research and clinical use, and the issues associated with experimental surgery in HD patients.

Table 17.2 Clinical trials of cell transplantation in HD

	n	First operation	First full publication
Cuba & Czechoslovakia.	2	1989	Sramka *et al.* 1992
Mexico City, Mexico	2	1990	Madrazo *et al.* 1993
Los Angeles, USA	≥14	1995	Philpott *et al.* 1997
Boston, USA*	12	1997	Fink *et al.* 2000
University of Southern Florida, Tampa, USA	6	1998	Freeman *et al.* 2000
Créteil, France	5	1997	Bachoud-Levy, 2000a,b
King's College London, UK	2	1999	—
NEST-UK	4	2000	NEST-UK collaborative group 2002

*Porcine cells.

The ethics of human foetal tissue collection

The legality of performing elective surgical termination of pregnancy varies worldwide. However, it is legal in most parts of the Western world and then the debate focuses on the collection and use of the foetal tissues. The main thrust of recent debate has centred on the possibility that the wish of researchers and clinicians to use foetal tissues could influence the decision to proceed with an abortion and the methods by which this may take place (Boer 1994, 1999; Burd *et al.* 1998; de la Cuetara-Bernal 1998; Turner and Kearney 1993). In most European countries, the grounds for approving each individual case of induced abortion involve a process of balancing the interests and well-being of the women against those of the foetus. Needless to say, views differ as to how this balance should be weighted. Concerns have centred around the possibilities, first, that a woman's choice on whether to seek or proceed with a termination might be influenced by the perception that it could aid others, and, second, that the medical decisions on the treatment of the woman and whether, when, and how to undertake the termination might be influenced by the potential subsequent use of the tissue. To address these concerns, a consortium of NECTAR (the Network of European CNS Transplantation and Restoration) generated a detailed set of guidelines for ethical tissue collection (Boer 1994) that were adopted for self-regulation by all participating European neural transplantation centres. Subsequent discussions at national and international levels have led to most countries now formally adopting similar regulations or guidelines. For example, in the UK, guidelines were proposed in a Royal Commission chaired by the Reverend Polkinghorne (Polkinghorne *et al.* 1989) and subsequently clarified by guidance notes from the UK Department of Health (1995). In essence these guidelines set out to ensure separation of the medical process of elective termination of pregnancy from the process of collecting and using the foetal tissues, with the aim that neither a woman's decision nor the medical practice to terminate a pregnancy should in any way be influenced by the decision to donate the tissue for purposes of research or treatment.

The ethics of experimental surgery

The ethics of experimental surgery are concerned with a number of issues directed at protection and management of the patients in experimental trials of neural transplantation in HD. Two concerns have dominated this discussion: the nature of informed consent and the use of sham surgery as a control procedure.

As with any experimental procedure, it is essential that the patients are fully informed and that they are able to consider and understand properly all the issues surrounding the operation before giving consent. In the case of a highly experimental intervention, such as neural transplantation, at this stage of its development, most authorities would agree that full informed consent must be given by the patient at the time of surgery, and that consent in advance of the procedure, or consent by proxy is not sufficient. The consenting procedure requires special attention in conditions such as HD in which cognitive decline is part of the disease. Thus, it is important that the patient's cognitive and psychiatric status are carefully assessed and that the physician in charge is fully convinced that the patient is capable of making an informed decision. For this reason the European groups contributing to the multicentre development of a core assessment protocol for transplantation in Huntington's disease (CAPIT-HD) elected to restrict experimental trials of neural transplantation in HD to early to moderate stages of the disease (Quinn *et al.* 1996).

A second group of ethical issues relates to study design. How can we produce meaningful results with the minimum number of volunteers whilst avoiding the bias of placebo effects?

These design issues require application of meticulous and adequate data collection, and the selection of sensitive and valid end points. An issue peculiar to surgical interventions is whether or not to include sham surgery, that is, a double-blind placebo group in which surgery is performed but the potentially modifying intervention is not delivered. The proponents of sham surgery argue that meaningful results cannot be obtained without proper blinding of both the patient and the researcher so that surgical studies conform to the principles that govern the execution of large drug trials (Freeman *et al.* 1997). In the one PD study so far conducted using sham surgery (Freed *et al.* 2000), control patients were administered a general anaesthetic and a burr hole was performed, but the dura was not penetrated and the cells were not delivered. One could argue, therefore, that this did not constitute a proper sham operation and that the patients themselves could infer whether they had received a graft from the duration of the operation, although in practice this does not appear to have happened. However, others have argued that sham surgery, even with general anaesthetic alone, involves significant risk and that the first ethical imperative is to do no harm, at the level of the individual patient as well as the group (Boer 1999). Although placebo trials may be appropriate in the future once the techniques are finally established, they are not so at present while neural transplantation techniques are still in evolution (Dunnett *et al.* 2001; Widner *et al.* 1994).

Safety issues

Neural transplantation of human foetal tissue involves harvesting of the tissue, cell preparation, and stereotaxic placement of the tissue into the appropriate striatal target(s). The risks are difficult to quantify *a priori*, and most centres have embarked on small safety studies prior to starting larger efficacy studies (Bachoud-Lévy *et al.* 2000a; Kopyov *et al.* 1998b). We will consider safety issues pertaining first to the collection of human foetal tissues and second to the neurosurgical procedures.

Human foetal CNS tissue must be collected and processed under sterile conditions. Details of collection will vary from place to place and the collection procedures described here are largely with reference to our own experience (Rosser and Dunnett 2001). In our hands, and those of a number of other centres, collection has most successfully been achieved under ultrasound guidance during routine elective termination of pregnancy (Nauert and Freeman 1994). It is an ethical imperative that the surgical process of uterine evacuation should not be modified from normal routine procedures. The collection of suitable tissue for transplantation is therefore a matter of careful tissue handling and experience on the part of the surgeon. Tissue is collected under sterile conditions on ice and dissected in a tissue culture hood using a dissecting microscope. Foetal tissue is always to some extent fragmented at collection, but provided this is not extreme striatal tissue can be identified in approximately 30–40 per cent of cases. The correct anatomical identification of striatal tissue is critical both for reasons of safety and for the transplant to be effective. The inclusion of nonstriatal tissue could potentially lead to abnormalities of tissue growth, as has already been reported for inappropriate dissection of the mesencephalon for transplants in PD (Folkerth and Durso 1996; Mamelak *et al.* 1998). To date, there have been no reports of tissue overgrowth following implantation of human foetal tissue into patients with HD, although the number of transplants done for HD worldwide is still relatively small and more are needed before we can be confident that this will not be a problem.

The second potential risk is the transfer of donor infections, although this risk is smaller for neural transplantation than in whole-organ transplants from cadavers because the foetus is protected by the placental barrier. In our own study, foetal tissue assessment is undertaken primarily by screening maternal blood a week prior to tissue collection. Screening can only be performed, of course, for a defined list of pathogens for which effective tests are available and is not undertaken for other pathogens for which this does not apply, for example, prion diseases. In addition, for some tests there is a small risk that the patient has become infected too recently to have yet mounted a detectable antibody response. So, although the risk of passing on an infection through foetal tissue implantation is believed to be low, it does exist and must be explained as part of the consenting procedure to potential tissue recipients.

Following dissection, the tissue is prepared for implantation either as a suspension or as minced tissue pieces. Sterility of the technique and purity of the reagents used to digest the tissue (in the case of a suspension) must be considered for tissue safety. Once implanted, the cells must survive, grow, and make connections. Cell death or rejection of the graft tissue does not appear to cause any adverse effects as the debris appears to be rapidly and efficiently cleared without signs of accompanying inflammation or significant scarring.

Stereotaxic implantation of the injection needle itself carries a defined but small neurosurgical risk of haemorrhage, which is generally assessed, from extensive experience with similar methods in biopsy surgery, as less than 1 per cent per needle pass.

It is clear that, of the several hundred patients worldwide who have received transplants for PD, serious perioperative complications are rare. Indeed, for the vast majority of patients who have received intrastriatal human foetal tissue there have been few reports of any adverse effects. However, the consequences of an adverse surgical outcome may be devastating and the potential risks include intracranial haemorrhage and stroke, although these should be small risks in centres in which there is established expertise in stereotaxic surgery.

The need for immunosuppression has not been proven, although most centres have decided to give immunosuppression for a period of months to cover the likely period in which the blood–brain barrier will be open, during which the graft is theoretically most vulnerable to immune attack (Widner 1998). The most common approach is to treat with the 'triple' therapy of cyclosporin, azathioprine, and prednisolone, at relatively low levels in comparison to those received by whole-organ transplant patients. The effects of immunosuppression are now well known and, if serious side-effects occur, the immunosuppression can be discontinued in the knowledge that this does not necessarily condemn the graft to rejection.

Clinical assessment of the effects of transplantation

It is essential that effective methods are available to assess the progress of a disease so that the effects of an intervention can be measured and, the greater the potential risk of the intervention, the more important it becomes to have an accurate read-out of benefit in order to make an accurate risk–benefit assessment. Neural transplantation imposes additional constraints on clinical data collection, because the limitations of tissue collection dictate that only small numbers of patients can be transplanted in any one centre at any one time. Thus, in order to acquire large enough numbers for meaningful analysis, multicentre trials are required. Assessment protocols must be standardized so that comparisons can be made across time and between examiners. Such an approach has an inherent problem in that there is variability between different examiners, and in order to minimize such variability a number of standardized protocols have now been developed and validated. The elements that make up a research protocol must be relatively easy to apply and quantify, and sensitive to the core pathogenic events as well as the therapeutic intervention.

The Huntington's Study Group (HSG) in the USA has developed and validated one of the major assessment tools for HD, the UHDRS (Unified Huntington'Disease Rating Scale; Kieburtz *et al.* 1996). It has been used for assessment in reported studies of drug intervention in HD (Shoulson *et al.* 1998; Van Vugt *et al.* 1997) as well as the natural history of the condition (Siesling *et al.* 1998). The UHDRS comprises four domains of clinical performance in HD: motor function; functional capacity; cognitive functions; and psychiatric abnormalities. The way in which answers are recorded (yes/no or a number on a scale) makes transfer of information to a computerized database straightforward.

The major European NECTAR centres have cooperated to develop and validate protocols designed for the assessment of intracerebral transplantation and other related neurosurgical interventions in PD (Langston *et al.* 1992) and more recently for HD, that is the 'Core assessment protocol for intracerebral transplantation in Huntington's disease' (CAPIT-HD; Quinn *et al.* 1996). The CAPIT-HD battery consists of the UHDRS, which, as described above, is largely concerned with motor and functional assessment, an extensive battery of neuropsychological tests, comprehensive neuropsychiatric tests, and imaging; each to be undertaken at defined intervals (Fig. 17.7). In particular, the imaging component comprises mandatory PET and MRI undertaken immediately preoperatively and at 2 years, and ideally also 12 months preoperatively. This imaging is to study the anatomical integrity of the graft (MRI) as well as functional measures such as the extent of dopamine receptor binding (for example, raclopride binding on PET scanning). The latter measure is especially helpful as it gives an *in situ* measure of the functional capacity of the graft to restore and repair neuropharmacological systems, which in the case of PD has been shown to correlate well with functional recovery as assessed clinically.

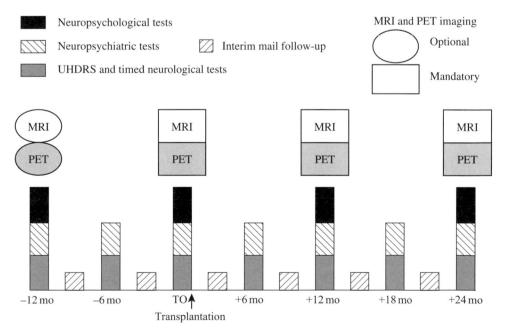

Fig. 17.7 The Core Assessment Protocol for Intracerebral Transplantation in HD (CAPIT-HD). Schematic illustration of the timing of the individual tests in each functional domain.

The tests that form the core assessment programme need to be applied longitudinally in patients whilst minimizing any practice effect. The initial assessment requires a relatively long run-in period in order that a stable baseline can be obtained, given that most patients with neurological disorders show day-to-day variability. Furthermore, the tests should ideally be given under similar conditions. Thus the complete assessment protocol involves a series of different approaches including historical information, clinical examination with neuropsychological and neuropsychiatric assessments where appropriate, along with imaging and neurophysiological measures.

Clinical trials in progress

A small number of centres world-wide have embarked on clinical studies of neural transplantation in HD (Table 17.2). The first report was of four patients with 'severe HD' transplanted bilaterally into the caudate with human foetal mesencephalic tissue, the reasons for using mesencephalic tissue remaining unexplained in the paper (Sramka *et al.* 1992). There are essentially no data relating to patient outcome other than a brief statement to the effect that the patients showed some improvement in terms of the hyperkinesia. Madrazo and colleagues (1995) reported two patients, one with severe and one with mild HD, who received unilateral implants of human foetal striatal tissue pieces into a surgically created cavity in the ventricular wall of the caudate nucleus. Patient assessment was more detailed, although still rather limited, using one scale for abnormal movements and three scales for disability. The assessment period was for 10 months preoperatively and 16 and 33 months postoperatively. With the variable nature of the data, it is unfortunately not possible to draw any firm conclusions from this study other than the absence of serious adverse effects.

An initial safety evaluation was published on the first three patients from the Los Angeles team (Kopyov *et al.* 1998b). Each patient received bilateral grafts from multiple foetal donors in a single-stage operation. The grafts survived in all patients, as assessed by MRI, and grew within the implanted striatum without causing any displacement of surrounding tissue over a 1-year follow-up period. No patients demonstrated any adverse effects of the surgery or the associated cyclosporine immunosuppression, nor did any patient exhibit deterioration following the procedure. The authors concluded that 'the limited experience provided by these three patients indicates that foetal tissue transplantation can be performed in HD patients without unexpected complications'. The authors present data showing that UHDRS overall motor and behavioural scores were improved at 6 and 12 months compared to preoperatively. However, the variable nature of the disease requires that longer assessments be performed in order to confirm such reports. Functional scores did not show consistent changes. The same authors have also demonstrated magnetic resonance spectroscopy (MRS) evidence of graft survival (Ross *et al.* 1999) and have published efficacy data in chapter form (Kopyov *et al.* 1998a), but not as peer-reviewed full-length papers. A group of transplanted HD patients in Tampa, Florida, included one patient who died 18 months after transplantation (from cardiovascular disease) and postmortem histology demonstrated surviving transplanted cells with typical morphology of the developing striatum (Fig 17.9), and no evidence of immune rejection.

At the time of writing, other centres involved in neural transplantation trials include a multicentre European consortium in which the two most active groups are one in Créteil, France, who have performed transplants (see below), and a multicentre UK group (NEST-UK) who have recently completed the first phase of a safety trial; and a further UK group at Kings College, London, who have launched an independent programme.

The Créteil group have published both safety and efficacy reports on their first five patients and are about to launch a large-scale multicentre transplantation programme. The safety report was based on at least 2 years of preoperative assessment and 1 year of postoperative follow-up following unilateral foetal tissue implants into the caudate and putamen (Bachoud-Lévy *et al*. 2000a). Assessments were performed using the CAPIT-HD battery plus a number of additional tests. They reported no major adverse effects, although they did note some minor psychological problems in both patients and carer, and some compliance difficulties with the immunosuppression. The efficacy report was of the same five patients following transplantation into the contralateral striatum and was based on the same period of preoperative assessment and 1 year of postoperative assessment following the second transplant (Bachoud-Lévy *et al*. 2000b). Three of the five patients showed evidence of improved function, and corresponding increased striatal metabolic activity on ^{18}F-fluorodeoxyglucose PET scans (Fig. 17.8). In particular, these same three patients either maintained or improved scores on a number of cognitive tests, in contrast to the two patients with no increased PET signal and a group of 22 non-transplanted HD patients at a similar stage of the disease who continued to decline. The three positive patients also all improved on functional assessments of daily living and on a subset of electrophysiological tests, in particular the bilateral N20 wave of the somatosensory-evoked potential. This latter result is particularly dramatic because it has never previously been reported to recover once lost in HD. The psychiatric scores for the improved patients have apparently remained stable. One of the patients who failed to show long-term improvement was particularly instructive; he showed clinical and electrophysiological improvement until 5 months after the second implant after which time his performance

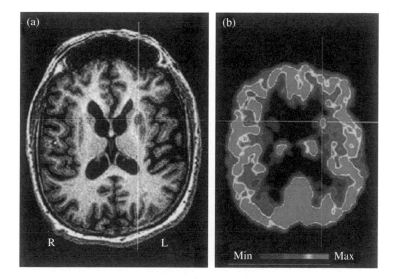

Fig. 17.8   MRI and PET imaging of cell transplantation in HD. (a) MRI from a patient in the Créteil series indicating surviving graft tissue in the caudate putamen on the left caudate putamen. (b) Restitution of cellular metabolism in graft in the same patient, visualized by fluorodeoxyglucose PET scan. The location of the graft in the PET scan can be determined by co-registration with the MRI (cross-hairs in each panel). (From Bachoud-Levi *et al*. (2000b) with permission.)

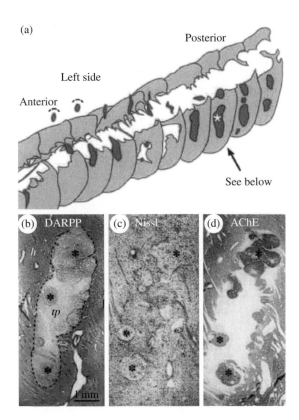

Fig. 17.9 Post-mortem histology of striatal transplant in HD. (a) Camera lucida tracings of the location of the transplanted tissues (red) in the left caudate and putamen. (From Freeman et al. (2000) with permission.) (b)–(d) Photomicrographs of the graft (marked with asterisk in (a) stained with (b) DARPP-32 to visualize striatal projection neurones (b), (c) with cresyl violet to visualize all cells (c), and (d) with AChE to visualize striatal-like neuropil. tp, transplant; h, host.

declined, and this corresponded with the appearance of a left putamen cyst on MRI and loss of the grafts. The authors therefore suggested that this patient's transplants were originally responsible for the clinical improvement but recovery was lost following graft destruction (most likely due to an infection and immunological reaction), further supporting the notion that there is a direct relationship between graft survival and improved function.

Long-term prospects

Although primary foetal ganglionic eminence tissues allografted to the isotopic sites in the brain (with attention to the various methodological requirements described above) provide the gold standard for demonstrating the benefit of striatal transplants, the ethical and practical difficulties of collecting foetal tissue and coordinating these collections with neurosurgery are significant and, indeed, seriously limit the widespread application of this technology. It is crucial, therefore, to seek to identify suitable alternative cell sources for transplantation. Moreover, if it were possible to maintain, store, and expand cells for transplantation in the laboratory, donor cells could then be made available as and when required by the neurosurgical schedule rather than *vice versa*. The donor materials would be available for systematic selection, characterization, manipulation, and screening, markedly enhancing the standardization and safety of the preparation protocols. However, there is the requirement that any alternative cell source should be at least equal to primary tissue in terms both of safety and efficacy.

A number of theoretical alternatives have been identified. Here we will briefly consider stem cell technologies and xenografts, as these appear to us to be the most likely sources to have the potential for translation to clinical trials in the foreseeable future.

Stem cells

The term 'stem cell' is often used indiscriminately to describe any of a wide variety of cells with proliferative potential. Definitions vary but, in general, a neural stem cell can be considered to be one that has self-renewing capacity, but is also able to differentiate into alternative lineage-restricted precursors that can eventually produce fully differentiated cell types (Fig. 17.10). The particular interest in stem cells as a source of cells for neural transplantation derives from the notion that they can be stimulated to divide exponentially in the laboratory to produce large numbers of progeny. A variety of potential sources of stem cell can be considered, but with the proviso that it must be possible to achieve differentiation of the progeny along the particular neuronal pathways into the mature CNS cell types required for transplantation.

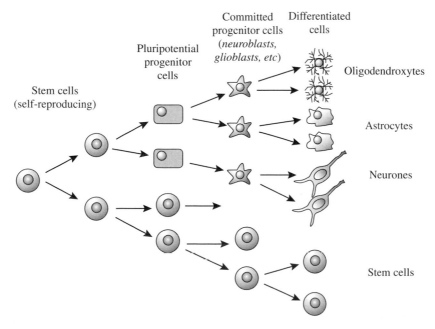

Fig. 17.10 Schematic lineages of stem, progenitor, committed precursor, and differentiated cell types comprising the CNS.

Neural stem cells are most easily isolated from the developing brain and expanded *in vitro* in response to mitogens, such as epidermal growth factor (EGF) and fibroblast growth factor-2 (FGF-2). Once the mitogens have been withdrawn, the neural stem cells' default pathway for differentiation is into neural cells. Although our understanding of neural stem cells is rapidly evolving (Alvarez-Buylla *et al.* 2001; Morshead and Van der Kooy 2001), there is some evidence of greater plasticity than previously thought (Bjornson *et al.* 1999). The capacity of human neural stem cells to differentiate into different neuronal cell types has been noted following their transplantation into the developing brain (Brustle *et al.* 1998; Flax *et al.* 1998; Rosser *et al.* 2000). However, the situation is less clear following transplantation into the adult brain where cell survival and neuronal differentiation appear to be poor. Thus, the major challenge for the application of this technology is how best to control the differentiation of the specific neuronal phenotypes required in the adult brain environment.

A second source is embryonic stem (ES) cells, which are isolated at the blastula stage and grown in the laboratory using a feeder cell layer. The proliferative potential of these cells appears to be enormous, and the cells are truly totipotent in that they can, in principle, produce all cell types in the human body. They need to be considered seriously as a potential cell source for transplantation (Svendsen and Smith 1999), although it has been difficult until recently to isolate and grow these cells from human blastulas (Thomson *et al.* 1998). It is likely that the main challenge facing human neural stem cells, that of controlling neuronal differentiation, will apply equally to ES cells, although there is one recent report of ES cells being induced to form dopamine neurones (Kawasaki *et al.* 2000).

With the possibility that many cells, and in particular many varieties of stem cells, have a greater plasticity in terms of their final differentiated phenotype than was originally suspected, comes the possibility that neural cells could be developed from many other tissue types. For example, the possibility has been mooted that bone marrow stem cells could be persuaded down a neuronal lineage (Brazelton *et al.* 2000; Mezey *et al.* 2000; Woodbury *et al.* 2000). However, these studies so far have been proof of principle only and it is likely that these sources, whilst circumventing the problems of immune rejection, will still be subject to the problem of controlling their differentiation potential.

Xenografts

The problem of tissue availability may also eventually be circumvented by transplanting primary embryonic tissue from another species—the most likely choice being the pig. The reasons for using porcine tissue are that the pig brain is of a comparable size and has a similar rate of development to that of the human, pigs have large litters and can be bred in pathogen-free conditions, and transgenic technology is available for pig so that the future potential for genetic manipulation of the tissue is already in place. The two main issues to be resolved prior to clinical use of such tissue are the identification of effective immunotherapy strategies for overcoming the immune rejection, which remains problematic with xenografts, and the safety concerns about transfer of pig endogenous retroviruses (PERVs) to the human population (Barker 2000; Larsson and Widner 2000; Widner 1998).

Clinical trials using porcine donor tissue transplants have commenced in Boston, USA, in both HD and PD patients. There is a report of survival of at least a limited number of xenografted cells in a post-mortem study involving one of the patients in the PD series (Deacon *et al.* 1997), whereas a preliminary report of porcine tissue transplantation in the HD patient series has shown no evidence of clinical recovery (Fink *et al.* 2000). However, the survival of tissue in these studies was poor, and in our judgement improved strategies for immunosuppression are required before further trials should be conducted.

Conclusion

Studies in experimental animals have demonstrated the viability of transplanting foetal neural tissues into the adult brain to repair the damage and alleviate motor and cognitive symptoms associated with focal striatal lesions. These have provided the basis for initial clinical trials in patients. Although the outcomes appear promising, the dependence of present protocols on foetal donor tissues will always restrict widespread availability of transplantation therapies. Consequently, there is active investigation of alternative sources of cells for transplantation, of which the two most promising at present appear to be to use expanded neural stem cells or xenografts of foetal striatal tissues. However, significant problems with each remain to be solved, and clinical trials with these alternative sources are not yet warranted.

References

Aihara, N., Mizukawa, K., Koide, K., Mabe, H., and Nishino, H. (1994). Striatal grafts in infarct stri-atopallidum increase GABA release, reorganize GABA$_A$ receptor and improve water-maze learning in the rat. *Brain Research Bulletin* **33**, 483–488.

Alvarez-Buylla, A., Garcia-Verdugo, J. M., and Tramontin, A. D. (2001). A unified hypothesis on the lineage of neural stem cells. *Nature Reviews, Neuroscience* **2**, 287–293.

Bachoud-Lévy, A. C., Bourdet, C., Brugières, P., Nguyen, J. P., Grandmougin, T., Haddad, B., Jény, R., Bartolomeo, P., Boissé, M. F., Dalla Barba, G., Degos, J. D., Ergis, A. M., Lefaucheur, J. P., Lisovoski, F., Pailhous, E., Rémy, P., Palfi, S., Defer, G. L., Césaro, P., Hantraye, P., and Peschanski, M. (2000a). Safety and tolerability assessment of intrastriatal neural allografts in Huntington's disease patients. *Experimental Neurology* **161**, 194–202.

—— Rémy, P., Nguyen, J. P., Brugières, P., Lefaucheur, J. P., Bourdet, C., Baudic, S., Gaura, V., Maison, P., Haddad, B., Boissé, M. F., Grandmougin, T., Jény, R., Bartolomeo, P., Dalla Barba, G., Degos, J. D., Lisovski, F., Ergis, A. M., Pailhous, E., Césaro, P., Hantraye, P., and Peschanski, M. (2000b). Motor and cognitive improvements in patients with Huntington's disease after neural transplantation. *Lancet* **356**, 1975–1979.

Barker, R. A. (2000). Porcine neural xenografts: what are the issues? *Ciba Foundation Symposia* **231**, 184–196.

—— and Dunnett, S. B. (1999). *Neural repair transplantation and rehabilitation*. The Psychology Press, Hove, UK.

Besret, L., Kendall, A. L., and Dunnett, S. B. (2000). Aspects of PET imaging relevant to the assessment of striatal transplantation in Huntington's disease. *Journal of Anatomy* **196**, 597–607.

Björklund, A. and Dunnett, S. B. (1992). Neural transplantation in adult rats. In *Neural transplantation: a practical approach* (ed. S. B. Dunnett and A. Björklund), pp. 57–78. IRL Press, Oxford.

—— Stenevi, U. (1985). Intracerebral neural grafting: a historical perspective. In *Neural grafting in the mammalian CNS* (ed. A. Björklund and U. Stenevi), pp. 3–14. Elsevier, Amsterdam.

—— —— Schmidt, R. H., Dunnett, S. B., and Gage, F. H. (1983). Intracerebral grafting of neuronal cell suspensions. II. Survival and growth of nigral cell suspensions implanted in different brain sites. *Acta Physiologica Scandinavica* **522** (suppl.), 9–18.

Bjornson, C. R. R., Rietze, R. L., Reynolds, B. A., Magli, M. C., and Vescovi, A. L. (1999). Turning brain into blood: a hematopoietic fate adopted by adult neural stem cells *in vivo*. *Science* **283**, 534–537.

Boer, G. J. (1994). Ethical guidelines for the use of human embryonic or foetal tissue for experimental and clinical neurotransplantation and research. *Journal of Neurology* **242**, 1–13.

—— (1999). Theoretical issues in neurografting of human embryonic cells. *Theor. Med. Bioeth.* **20**, 461–475.

Borlongan, C. V., Cahill, D. W., and Sanberg, P. R. (1995). Asymmetrical behavior in rats following striatal lesions and foetal transplants: the elevated body swing test. *Restorative Neurology and Neuroscience* **9**, 15–19.

—— Poulos, S. G., Cahill, D. W., and Sanberg, P. R. (1998). Effects of foetal striatal transplants on motor asymmetry in ibotenic acid model of Huntington's disease. *Psychobiology* **26**, 49–52.

Brasted, P. J., Watts, C., Robbins, T. W., and Dunnett, S. B. (1999a). Associative plasticity in striatal transplants. *Proceedings of the National Academy of Sciences of the United States of America* **96**, 10524–10529.

—— Watts, C., Torres, E. M., Robbins, T. W., and Dunnett, S. B. (1999b). Behavioural recovery following striatal transplantation: effects of postoperative training and P zone volume. *Experimental Brain Research* **128**, 535–538.

—— Robbins, T. W., and Dunnett, S. B. (2000). Behavioral recovery after transplantation into a rat model of Huntington's disease requires both anatomical connectivity and extensive postoperative training. *Behavioral Neuroscience* **111**, 139–151.

Brazelton, T. R., Rossi, F. M. V., Keshet, G. I., and Blau, H. M. (2000). From marrow to brain: expression of neuronal phenotypes in adult mice. *Science* **290**, 1775–1779.

Brundin, P. and Strecker, R. E. (1991). Preparation and intracerebral grafting of dissociated foetal brain tissue in rats. In *Methods in neuroscience. Vol. 7. Lesions and transplantation*, (ed. P. M. Conn), pp. 305–326. Academic Press, New York.

—— Fricker, R. A., and Nakao, N. (1996). Paucity of P-zones in striatal grafts prohibit commencement of clinical trials in Huntington's disease. *Neuroscience* **71**, 895–897.

Brustle, O., Choudhary, K., Karram, K., Huttner, A., Murray, K., Dubois-Dalcq, M., and McKay, R. D. G. (1998). Chimeric brains generated by intraventricular transplantation of foetal human brain cells into embryonic rats. *Nature Biotechnology* **16**, 1040–1044.

Burd, L., Gregory, J. M., and Kerbeshian, J. (1998). The brain–mind quiddity: ethical issues in the use of human brain tissue for therapeutic and scientific purposes. *Journal of Medical Ethics* **24**, 118–122.

Butler, H. and Juurlink, B. H. J. (1987). *An atlas for staging mammalian and chick embryos.* CRC Press, Boca Raton.

Campbell, K., Kalén, P., Wictorin, K., Lundberg, C., Mandel, R. J., and Björklund, A. (1993). Characterization of GABA release from intrastriatal striatal transplants: dependence on host-derived afferents. *Neuroscience* **53**, 403–415.

Carli, M., Evenden, J. L., and Robbins, T. W. (1985). Depletion of unilateral striatal dopamine impairs initiation of contralateral actions and not sensory attention. *Nature* **313**, 679–682.

Clarke, D. J. and Dunnett, S. B. (1993). Synaptic relationships between cortical and dopaminergic inputs and intrinsic GABAergic systems within intrastriatal striatal grafts. *Journal of Chemical Neuroanatomy* **6**, 147–158.

Clarke, D. J., Wictorin, K., Dunnett, S. B., and Bolam, J. P. (1994). Internal composition of striatal grafts: light and electron microscopy. In *The basal ganglia* IV. *New ideas on structure and function* (ed. G. Percheron, J. S. McKenzie, and J. Féger), pp. 189–196. Plenum Press, New York.

Coyle, J. T. and Schwarcz, R. (1976). Lesions of striatal neurones with kainic acid provides a model for Huntington's chorea. *Nature* **263**, 244–246.

Deacon, T., Schumacher, J., Dinsmore, J., Thomas, C., Palmer, P., Kott, S., Edge, A., Penney, D., Kassissieh, S., Dempsey, P., and Isacson, O. (1997). Histological evidence of foetal pig neural cell survival after transplantation into a patient with Parkinson's disease. *Nature Medicine* **3**, 350–353.

Deacon, T. W., Pakzaban, P., and Isacson, O. (1994). The lateral ganglionic eminence is the origin of cells committed to striatal phenotypes: neural transplantation and developmental evidence. *Brain Research* **668**, 211–219.

De Carlos, J. A., Lopez-Mascaraque, L., and Valverde, F. (1996). Dynamics of cell migration from the lateral ganglionic eminence in the rat. *Journal of Neuroscience* **16**, 6146–6156.

Deckel, A. W., Robinson, R. G., Coyle, J. T., and Sanberg, P. R. (1983). Reversal of long-term locomotor abnormalities in the kainic acid model of Huntington's disease by day 18 foetal striatal implants. *European Journal of Pharmacology* **92**, 287–288.

—— Moran, T. H., Coyle, J. T., Sanberg, P. R., and Robinson, R. G. (1986). Anatomical predictors of behavioral recovery following foetal striatal transplants. *Brain Research* **365**, 249–258.

—— Moran, T. H., and Robinson, R. G. (1988). Receptor characteristics and recovery of function following kainic acid lesions and foetal transplants of the striatum. 2. Dopaminergic systems. *Brain Research* **474**, 39–47.

de la Cuetara-Bernal, K. (1998). Foetal nerve tissue, ethics and transplants. *Revue Neurologique* **27**, 1043–1049.

Denys, A., Leroy-Willig, A., Riche, D., and Hantraye, P. (1992). MR appearance of neural grafts in a primate model of Huntington disease. *American Journal of Roentgenology* **158**, 215–216.

Department of Health (UK) (1995). Guidance on the supply of foetal tissue for research, diagnosis and therapy. *Guidance Notes* 1–3.

Döbrössy, M. D., and Dunnett, S. B. (1998). Striatal grafts alleviate deficits in response execution in a lateralised reaction time task. *Brain Research Bulletin* **47**, 585–593.

Doucet, G., Murata, Y., Brundin, P., Bosler, O., Mons, N., Geffard, M., Ouimet, C. C., and Björklund, A. (1989). Host afferents into intrastriatal transplants of foetal ventral mesencephalon. *Experimental Neurology* **106**, 1–9.

Dunnett, S. B. and Björklund, A. (1992). Staging and dissection of rat embryos. In *Neural transplantation: a practical approach* (ed. S. B. Dunnett and A. Björklund), pp. 1–19. IRL Press, Oxford.

—— Mayer, E. (1992). Neural grafts, growth factors and trophic mechanisms of recovery. In *Neurodegeneration* (ed. A. J. Hunter and M. Clarke), pp. 183–217. Academic Press, New York.

Dunnett, S. B., Whishaw, I. Q., Rogers, D. C., and Jones, G. H. (1987). Dopamine-rich grafts ameliorate whole body motor asymmetry and sensory neglect but not independent limb use in rats with 6-hydroxydopamine lesions. *Brain Research* **415**, 63–78.

—— Isacson, O., Sirinathsinghji, D. J. S., Clarke, D. J., and Björklund, A. (1988). Striatal grafts in rats with unilateral neostriatal lesions. III. Recovery from dopamine-dependent motor asymmetry and deficits in skilled paw reaching. *Neuroscience* **24**, 813–820.

—— Carter, R. J., Watts, C., Torres, E. M., Mahal, A., Mangiarini, L., Bates, G., and Morton, A. J. (1998). Striatal transplantation in a transgenic mouse model of Huntington's disease. *Experimental Neurology* **154**, 31–40.

Dunnett, S. B., Nathwani, F., and Björklund, A. (2000). The integration and function of striatal grafts. *Progress in Brain Research* **127**, 345–380.

—— Björklund, A., and Lindvall, O. (2001). Cell therapy in Parkinson's disease—stop or go? *Nature, Reviews Neuroscience* **2**, 365–369.

Eagle, D. M., Humby, T., Dunnett, S. B., and Robbins, T. W. (1999a). Effects of regional striatal lesions on motor, motivational and executive aspects of progressive ratio performance in rats. *Behavioral Neuroscience* **113**, 716–731.

—— Humby, T., Howman, M., Reid-Henry, A., Dunnett, S. B., and Robbins, T. W. (1999b). Differential effects of ventral and regional dorsal striatal lesions on sucrose drinking and affective contrast in rats. *Psychobiology* **27**, 267–276.

Fink, J. S., Schumacher, J. M., Ellias, S. A., Palmer, E. P., Saint-Hilaire, M., Shannon, K., Penn, R., Starr, P., Van Horne, C., Kott, H. S., Dempsey, P. K., Fischman, A. J., Raineri, R., Manhart, C., Dinsmore, J., and Isacson, O. (2000). Porcine xenografts in Parkinson's disease and Huntington's disease patients: preliminary results. *Cell Transplantation* **9**, 273–278.

Flax, J. D., Aurora, S., Yang, C. H., Simonin, C., Wills, A. M., Billinghurst, L. L., Jendoubi, M., Sidman, R. L., Wolfe, J. H., Kim, S. U., and Snyder, E. Y. (1998). Engraftable human neural stem cells respond to developmental cues, replace neurons, and express foreign genes. *Nature Biotechnology* **16**, 1033–1039.

Folkerth, R. D. and Durso, R. (1996). Survival and proliferation of non-neural tissues, with obstruction of cerebral ventricles, in a parkinsonian patient treated with foetal allografts. *Neurology* **46**, 1219–1225.

Freed, C. R., Breeze, R. E., and Fahn, S. (2000). Placebo surgery in trials of therapy for Parkinson's disease. *New England Journal of Medicine* **342**, 353–354.

Freeman, T. B., Sanberg, P. R., and Isacson, O. (1995). Development of the human striatum: implications for foetal striatal transplantation in the treatment of Huntington's disease. *Cell Transplantation* **4**, 539–545.

—— Vawter, D., Goetz, C. G., Leaverton, P. E., Hauser, R. A., Sanberg, P. R., Godbold, J. H., and Olanow, C. W. (1997). Toward the use of surgical placebo-controlled trials. *Transplantation Proceedings* **29**, 1925.

—— Cicchetti, F., Hauser, R. A., Deacon, T. W., Li, X. J., Hersch, S. M., Nauert, G. M., Sanberg, P. R., Kordower, J. H., Saporta, S., and Isacson, O. (2000). Transplanted foetal striatum in Huntington's disease: phenotypic development and lack of pathology. *Proceedings of the National Academy of Sciences of the United States of America* **97**, 13877–13882.

Fricker, R. A., Torres, E. M., Lombroso, P. J., and Dunnett, S. B. (1994). STEP, a novel striatal marker to distinguish patch/non-patch organisation of embryonic striatal transplants in the ibotenic acid lesioned neostriatum of the rat. *NeuroReport* **5**, 2638–2640.

—— Sirinathsinghji, D. J. S., Torres, E. M., Hume, S., and Dunnett, S. B. (1997a). The effects of donor stage on the survival and function of embryonic striatal grafts. I. Anatomy and development of the grafts. *Neuroscience* **79**, 695–710.

—— Torres, E. M., Hume, S. P., Myers, R., Opacka-Juffry, J., Ashworth, S., and Dunnett, S. B. (1997b). The effects of donor stage on the survival and function of embryonic striatal grafts. II. Correlation between positron emission tomography and reaching behaviour. *Neuroscience* **79**, 711–722.

Gage, F. H., Björklund, A., Stenevi, U., and Dunnett, S. B. (1983). Intracerebral grafting of neuronal cell suspensions. VIII. Survival and growth of implants of nigral and septal cell suspensions in intact brains of aged rats. *Acta Physiologica Scandinavica* **522** (suppl.), 67–75.

Giordano, M., Ford, L. M., Shipley, M. T., and Sanberg, P. R. (1990). Neural grafts and pharmacological intervention in a model of Huntington's disease. *Brain Research Bulletin* **25**, 453–465.

—— Salado-Castillo, R., Sánchez-Alavez, M., and Prado-Alcalá, R. A. (1998). Striatal transplants prevent AF64A-induced retention deficits. *Life Sciences* **63**, 1953–1961.

Grasbon-Frodl, E. M., Nakao, N., Lindvall, O., and Brundin, P. (1996). Phenotypic development of the human embryonic striatal primordium: a study of cultured and grafted neurons from the lateral and medial ganglionic eminence. *Neuroscience* **73**, 171–183.

Graybiel, A. M., Liu, F. C., and Dunnett, S. B. (1989). Intrastriatal grafts derived from foetal striatal primordia. 1. Phenotypy and modular organization. *Journal of Neuroscience* **9**, 3250–3271.

—— —— —— (1990). Cellular reaggregation *in vivo*: modular patterns in intrastriatal grafts derived from foetal striatal primordia. *Progress in Brain Research* **82**, 401–405.

Guzman, R., Meyer, M., Lövblad, K. O., Ozdoba, C., Schroth, G., Seiler, R. W., and Widmer, H. R. (1999). Striatal grafts in a rat model of Huntington's disease: time course comparison of MRI and histology. *Experimental Neurology* **156**, 180–190.

Hantraye, P., Riche, D., Mazière, M., and Isacson, O. (1992). Intrastriatal transplantation of cross-species foetal striatal cells reduces abnormal movements in a primate model of Huntington disease. *Proceedings of the National Academy of Sciences of the United States of America* **89**, 4187–4191.

Helm, G. A., Palmer, P. E., Simmons, N. E., DiPierro, C., and Bennett, J. P. (1992). Descriptive morphology of developing foetal neostriatal allografts in the rhesus monkey: a correlated light and electron microscopic Golgi study. *Neuroscience* **50**, 163–179.

—————— (1993). Degeneration of long-term foetal neostriatal allografts in the rhesus monkey: an electron microscopic study. *Experimental Neurology* **123**, 174–180.

Isacson, O., Brundin, P., Kelly, P. A. T., Gage, F. H., and Björklund, A. (1984). Functional neuronal replacement by grafted striatal neurons in the ibotenic acid lesioned rat striatum. *Nature* **311**, 458–460.

—— —— Gage, F. H., and Björklund, A. (1985). Neural grafting in a rat model of Huntington disease: progressive neurochemical changes after neostriatal ibotenate lesions and striatal tissue grafting. *Neuroscience* **16**, 799–817.

Isacson, O., Dunnett, S. B., and Björklund, A. (1986). Graft-induced behavioral recovery in an animal model of Huntington disease. *Proceedings of the National Academy of Sciences of the United States of America* **83**, 2728–2732.

—— Dawbarn, D., Brundin, P., Gage, F. H., Emson, P. C., and Björklund, A. (1987a). Neural grafting in a rat model of Huntington's disease: striosomal-like organization of striatal grafts as revealed by acetylcholinesterase histochemistry, immunocytochemistry and receptor autoradiography. *Neuroscience* **22**, 481–497.

—— Pritzel, M., Dawbarn, D., Brundin, P., Kelly, P. A. T., Wiklund, L., Emson, P. C., Gage, F. H., Dunnett, S. B., and Björklund, Λ. (1987b). Striatal neural transplants in the ibotenic acid-lesioned rat neostriatum—cellular and functional aspects. *Annals of the New York Academy of Sciences* **495**, 537–555.

—— Riche, D., Hantraye, P., Sofroniew, M. V., and Mazière, M. (1989). A primate model of Huntington's disease: cross-species implantation of striatal precursor cells to the excitotoxically lesioned baboon caudate–putamen. *Experimental Brain Research* **75**, 213–220.

Kawasaki, H., Mizuseki, K., Nishikawa, S., Kaneko, S., Kuwana, Y., Nakanishi, S., Nishikawa, S. I., and Sasai, Y. (2000). Induction of midbrain dopaminergic neurons from ES cells by stromal cell-derived inducing activity. *Neuron* **28**, 31–40.

Kendall, A. L., Hantraye, P., and Palfi, S. (2000). Striatal tissue transplantation in non-human primates. *Progress in Brain Research* **127**, 381–401.

—— Rayment, F. D., Torres, E. M., Baker, H. F., Ridley, R. M., and Dunnett, S. B. (1998). Functional integration of striatal allografts in a primate model of Huntington's disease. *Nature Medicine* **4**, 727–729.

Kieburtz, K., Penney, J. B., Como, P., Ranen, N., Shoulson, I., Feigin, A., Abwender, D., Greenamyre, J. T., Higgins, D., Marshall, F. J., Goldstein, J., Steinberg, K., Shih, C., Richard, I., Hickey, C., Zimmerman, C., Orme, C., Claude, K., Oakes, D., Sax, D. S., Kim, A., Hersch, S., Jones, R., Auchus, A., Olsen, D., Bissey-Black, C., Rubin, A., Schwartz, R., Dubinsky, R., Mallonee, W., Gray, C., Godfrey, N., Suter, G., Shannon, K. M., Stebbins, G. T., Jaglin, J. A., Marder, K., Taylor, S., Louis, E., Moskowitz, C., Thorne, D., Zubin, N., Wexler, N., Swenson, M. R., Paulsen, J., Swerdlow, N. R., Albin, R., Wernette, C., Walker, F., Hunt, V., Roos, R., Young, AB., Koroshetz, W., Bird, E., Myers, C., Cudkowicz, M., Guttman, M., StCyr, J., Burkholder, J., Lundin, A., Ashizawa, T., Jankovic, J., Siemers, E., Quaid, K., Martin, W., Sanchez-Ramos, J., Facca, A., Rey, G., Suchowersky, O., Rohs, G., Klinek, M. L., Ross, C., Bylsma, F. W., Sherr, M., Hayden, M. R., Raymond, L., Clark, C., and Kremer, B. (1996). Unified Huntington's disease rating scale: reliability and consistency. *Movement Disorders* **11**, 136–142.

Koide, K., Hashitani, T., Aihara, N., Mabe, H., and Nishino, H. (1993). Improvement of passive avoidance task after grafting of foetal striatal cell suspensions in ischemic striatum in the rat. *Restorative Neurology and Neuroscience* **5**, 205–214.

Kopyov, O. V., Jacques, S., Kurth, M., Philpott, L. M., Lee, A., Patterson, M., Duma, C., Lieberman, A., and Eagle, K. S. (1998a). Foetal transplantation for Huntington's disease: clinical studies. In *Cell transplantation for neurological disorders* (ed. T. B. Freeman and J. H. Kordower), pp. 95–134. Humana Press, Totowa, New Jersey.

—— —— Lieberman, A., Duma, C. M., and Eagle, K. S. (1998b). Safety of intrastriatal neurotransplantation for Huntington's disease patients. *Experimental Neurology* **119**, 97–108.

Labandeira-Garcia, J. L. and Guerra, M. J. (1994). Cortical stimulation induces fos expression in intrastriatal striatal grafts. *Brain Research* **652**, 87–97.

—— Wictorin, K., Cunningham, E. T., and Björklund, A. (1991). Development of intrastriatal striatal grafts and their afferent innervation from the host. *Neuroscience* **42**, 407–426.

Langston, J. W., Widner, H., and Goetz, C. G. (1992). Core assessment program for intracerebral transplantation (CAPIT). *Movement Disorders* **7**, 2–13.

Larsson, L. C. and Widner, H. (2000). Neural tissue xenografting. *Scandinavian Journal of Immunology* **52**, 249–256.

Lindvall, O. and Hagell, P. (2000). Clinical observations after neural transplantation in Parkinson's disease. *Progress in Brain Research* **127**, 299–320.

Liu, F. C., Graybiel, A. M., Dunnett, S. B., and Baughman, R. W. (1990). Intrastriatal grafts derived from foetal striatal primordia. 2. Reconstitution of cholinergic and dopaminergic systems. *Journal of Comparative Neurology* **295**, 1–14.

Lund, R. D. and Bannerjee, R. (1992). Immunological considerations in neural transplantation. In *Neural transplantation: a practical approach* (ed. S. B. Dunnett and A. Björklund), pp. 161–176. IRL Press, Oxford.

—— Yee, K. T. (1992). Intracerebral transplantation to immature hosts. In *Neural transplantation: a practical approach* (ed. S. B. Dunnett and A. Björklund), pp. 79–91. IRL Press, Oxford.

—— Rao, K., Hankin, M. H., Kunz, H. W., and Gill, T. J. (1987). Transplantation of retina and visual-cortex to rat brains of different ages—maturation, connection patterns, and immunological consequences. *Annals of the New York Academy of Sciences* **495**, 227–241.

Madrazo, I., Cuevas, C., Castrejon, H., Guizar-Sahagun, G., Franco-Bourland, R., Ostrosky-Solis, F., Aguilera, M., and Magallon, E. (1993). The first homotopic foetal homograft of the striatum in the treatment of Huntington's disease [in Spanish]. *Gac. Med. Mex.* **129**, 109–117.

—— Franco-Bourland, R. E., Castrejon, H., Cuevas, C., and Ostrosky-Solis, F. (1995). Foetal striatal homotransplantation for Huntington's disease: First two case reports. *Neurological Research* **17**, 312–315.

Mamelak, A. N., Eggerding, F. A., Oh, D. S., Wilson, E., Davis, R. L., Spitzer, R., Hay, J. A., and Caton, W. L. III (1998). Fatal cyst formation after foetal mesencephalic allograft transplant for Parkinson's disease. *Journal of Neurosurgery* **89**, 592–598.

Mangiarini, L., Sathasivam, K., Seller, M., Cozens, B., Harper, A., Hetherington, C., Lawton, M., Trottier, Y., Lehrach, H., Davies, S. W., and Bates, G. P. (1996). Exon 1 of the HD gene with an expanded CAG repeat is sufficient to cause a progressive neurological phenotype in transgenic mice. *Cell* **87**, 493–506.

Mayer, E., Brown, V. J., Dunnett, S. B., and Robbins, T. W. (1992). Striatal graft-associated recovery of a lesion-induced performance deficit in the rat requires learning to use the transplant. *European Journal of Neuroscience* **4**, 119–126.

Mezey, E., Chandross, K. J., Harta, G., Maki, R. A., and McKercher, S. R. (2000). Turning blood into brain: cells bearing neuronal antigens generated *in vivo* from bone marrow. *Science* **290**, 1779–1782.

Mittleman, G., Brown, V. J., and Robbins, T. W. (1988). Intentional neglect following unilateral ibotenic acid lesions of the striatum. *Neuroscience Research Communications* **2**, 1–8.

Montoya, C. P., Astell, S., and Dunnett, S. B. (1990). Effects of nigral and striatal grafts on skilled forelimb use in the rat. *Progress in Brain Research* **82**, 459–466.

Morshead, C. M. and Van der Kooy, D. (2001). A new 'spin' on neural stem cells? *Current Opinion in Neurobiology* **11**, 59–65.

Nakao, N., Ogura, M., Nakai, K., and Itakura, T. (1999). Embryonic striatal grafts restore neuronal activity of the globus pallidus in a rodent model of Huntington's disease. *Neuroscience* **88**, 469–477.

—— Nakai, K., and Itakura, T. (2000). Foetal striatal transplants reinstate the electrophysiological response of pallidal neurons to systemic apomorphine challenge in rats with excitotoxic striatal lesions. *European Journal of Neuroscience* **12**, 3426–3432.

Nauert, G. M. and Freeman, T. B. (1994). Low-pressure aspiration abortion for obtaining embryonic and early gestational foetal tissue for research purposes. *Cell Transplantation* **3**, 147–151.

NEST-UK collaborative group (2002). Unilateral transplantation of human primary foetal tissue in four patients with Huntington's disease: NEST-UK safety report. *Journal of Neurology Neurosurgery and Psychiatry*, (in press).

Nishino, H., Koide, K., Aihara, N., Mitzukawa, K., and Nagai, H. (1992). Striatal grafts in infarct striatum after occlusion of the middle cerebral artery improve passive avoidance/water maze learning, GABA release and GABAa receptor deficits in the rat. *Restorative Neurology and Neuroscience* **4**, 178.

Norman, A. B., Thomas, S. R., Pratt, R. G., Samaratunga, R. C., and Sanberg, P. R. (1989a). A magnetic resonance imaging contrast agent differentiates between the vascular properties of foetal striatal tissue transplants and gliomas in rat brain *in vivo*. *Brain Research* **503**, 156–159.

—— —— —— —— —— (1989b). Magnetic resonance imaging of rat brain following kainic acid-induced lesions and foetal striatal tissue transplants. *Brain Research* **483**, 188–191.

Olson, L., Seiger, Å., and Strömberg, I. (1983). Intraocular transplantation in rodents: a detailed account of the procedure and examples of its use in neurobiology with special reference to brain tissue grafting. *Advances in Cellular Neurobiology* **4**, 407–442.

Olsson, M., Bentlage, C., Wictorin, K., Campbell, K., and Björklund, A. (1997). Extensive migration and target innervation by striatal precursors after grafting into the neonatal striatum. *Neuroscience* **79**, 57–78.

—— Björklund, A., and Campbell, K. (1998). Early specification of striatal projection neurons and interneuronal subtypes in the lateral and medial ganglionic eminence. *Neuroscience* **84**, 867–876.

Palfi, S., Condé, F., Riche, D., Brouillet, E., Dautry, C., Mittoux, V., Hantraye, P., and Peschanski, M. (1998). Foetal striatal allografts reverse cognitive deficits in a primate model of Huntington's disease. *Nature Medicine* **4**, 963–966.

—— Césaro, P., and Hantraye, P. (1995). Rationale for intrastriatal grafting of striatal neuroblasts in patients with Huntington's disease. *Neuroscience* **68**, 273–285.

—— Césaro, P., and Hantraye, P. (1996). What is needed versus what would be interesting to know before undertaking neural transplantation in patients with Huntington's disease. *Neuroscience* **71**, 899–900.

Philpott, L. M., Kopyov, O. V., Lee, A. J., Jacques, S., Duma, C. M., Caine, S., Yang, M., and Eagle, K. S. (1997). Neuropsychological functioning following foetal striatal transplantation in Huntington's chorea: three case presentations. *Cell Transplantation* **6**, 203–212.

Piña, A. L., Ormsby, C. E., and Bermúdez-Rattoni, F. (1994a). Differential recovery of inhibitory avoidance learning by striatal, cortical, and mesencephalic foetal grafts. *Behavioral and Neural Biology* **61**, 196–201.

—— —— Miranda, M. I., Jiménez, N., Tapia, R., and Bermúdez-Rattoni, F. (1994b). Graft-induced recovery of inhibitory avoidance conditioning in striatal lesioned rats is related to choline acetyltransferase activity. *Journal of Neural Transplantation and Plasticity* **5**, 11–16.

Polkinghorne, J., Hoffenberg, R., Kennedy, I., and Macintyre, S. (1989). *Review of the guidance on the research use of foetuses and foetal material*. HMSO, London.

Pritzel, M., Isacson, O., Brundin, P., Wiklund, L., and Björklund, A. (1986). Afferent and efferent connections of striatal grafts implanted into the ibotenic acid lesioned neostriatum in adult rats. *Experimental Brain Research* **65**, 112–126.

Pundt, L. L., Kondoh, T., and Low, W. C. (1994). Transplantation of human foetal striatal brain tissue from spontaneous abortuses into a rodent model of Huntington's disease. *Cell Transplantation* **3**, 212.

Pundt, L. L., Kondoh, T., Conrad, J. A., and Low, W. C. (1996a). Transplantation of human foetal striatum into a rodent model of Huntington's disease ameliorates locomotor deficits. *Neuroscience Research* **24**, 415–420.

—— —— —— —— (1996b). Transplantation of human striatal tissue into a rodent model of Huntington's disease: phenotypic expression of transplanted neurons and host-to-graft innervation. *Brain Research Bulletin* **39**, 23–32.

—— Narang, N., Kondoh, T., and Low, W. C. (1997). Localization of dopamine receptors and associated mRNA in transplants of human foetal striatal tissue in rodents with experimental Huntington's disease. *Neuroscience Research* **27**, 305–315.

Quinn, N. P., Brown, R., Craufurd, D., Goldman, S., Hodges, J. R., Kieburtz, K., Lindvall, O., MacMillan, J. C., and Roos, R. A. C. (1996). Core assessment programme for intracerebral transplantation in Huntington's disease (CAPIT-HD). *Movement Disorders* **11**, 143–150.

Reading, P. J. and Dunnett, S. B. (1995). Embryonic striatal grafts ameliorate the disinhibitory effects of ventral striatal lesions. *Experimental Brain Research* **105**, 76–86.

Ross, B. D., Hoang, T. Q., Bluml, S., Dubowitz, D. J., Kopyov, O. V., Jacques, D. B., Lin, A., Seymour, K., and Tan, J. (1999). *In vivo* magnetic resonance spectroscopy of human foetal neural transplants. *Nuclear Magnetic Resonance in Biomedicine* **12**, 221–236.

Rosser, A. E. and Dunnett, S. B. (2001). Neural transplantation for the treatment of Huntington's disease. In *Movement disorders surgery* (ed. J. K. Krauss, J. Jankovic, and R. G. Grossman), pp. 353–373. Lippincott, Williams, and Wilkins, Philadelphia.

—— Tyers, P., and Dunnett, S. B. (2000). The morphological development of neurons derived from EGF- and FGF-2-driven human CNS precursors depends on their site of integration in the neonatal rat brain. *European Journal of Neuroscience* **12**, 2405–2413.

Rutherford, A., Garcia-Muñoz, M., Dunnett, S. B., and Arbuthnott, G. W. (1987). Electrophysiological demonstration of host cortical inputs to striatal grafts. *Neuroscience Letters* **83**, 275–281.

Sanberg, P. R. and Coyle, J. T. (1984). Scientific approaches to Huntington's disease. *CRC Critical Reviews in Clinical Neurobiology* **1**, 1–44.

Schmidt, R. H., Björklund, A., and Stenevi, U. (1981). Intracerebral grafting of dissociated CNS tissue suspensions: a new approach for neuronal transplantation to deep brain sites. *Brain Research* **218**, 347–356.

Shannon, K. M. and Kordower, J. H. (1996). Neural transplantation for Huntington's disease: Experimental rationale and recommendations for clinical trials. *Cell Transplantation* **5**, 339–352.

Shoulson, I., Penney, J. B., Kieburtz, K., Oakes, D., Chase, T., Choi, D., Marder, K., Moskowitz, C., Zubin, N., Ventura, P., Feigin, A., Hickey, C., Como, P., Richard, I. H., Goldstein, J., Hersch, S., Bissey-Black, C., Jones, R., Swenson, M. R., Bell, J., Paulsen, J. S., Swenson, A., Tawfik-Reedy, Z., and Orme, C. (1998). Safety and tolerability of the free-radical scavenger OPC-14117 in Huntington's disease. *Neurology* **50**, 1366–1373.

Siesling, S., Van Vugt, J. P. P., Zwinderman, K. A. H., Kieburtz, K., and Roos, R. A. C. (1998). Unified Huntington's disease rating scale: a follow up. *Movement Disorders* **13**, 915–919.

Sirinathsinghji, D. J. S., Dunnett, S. B., Isacson, O., Clarke, D. J., Kendrick, K., and Björklund, A. (1988). Striatal grafts in rats with unilateral neostriatal lesions. II. *In vivo* monitoring of GABA release in globus pallidus and substantia nigra. *Neuroscience* **24**, 803–811.

—— Mayer, E., Fernandez, J. M., and Dunnett, S. B. (1993). The localisation of CCK mRNA in embryonic striatal tissue grafts: further evidence for the presence of non-striatal cells. *NeuroReport* **4**, 659–662.

Siviy, S. M., Walsh, J. P., Radisavljevic, Z., Cohen, R. W., Buchwald, N. A., and Levine, M. S. (1993). Evidence for enhanced synaptic excitation in transplanted neostriatal neurons. *Experimental Neurology* **123**, 222–234.

Smart, I. H. M. and Sturrock, R. R. (1979). Ontogeny of the neostriatum. In *The neostriatum* (ed. I. Divac and R. G. E. Öberg), pp. 127–146. Pergamon Press, New York.

Sramka, M., Rattaj, M., Molina, H., Vojtassak, J., Belan, V., and Ruzicky, E. (1992). Stereotactic technique and pathophysiological mechanisms of neurotransplantation in Huntington's chorea. *Stereotactic and Functional Neurosurgery* **58**, 79–83.

Stenevi, U., Björklund, A., and Svendgaard, N.-A. (1976). Transplantation of central and peripheral monoamine neurons to the adult rat brain: techniques and conditions for survival. *Brain Research* **114**, 1–20.

—— Kromer, L. F., Gage, F. H., and Björklund, A. (1985). Solid neural grafts in intracerebral transplantation cavities. In *Neural grafting in the mammalian CNS* (ed. A. Björklund and U. Stenevi), pp. 41–49. Elsevier, Amsterdam.

Surmeier, D. J., Xu, Z. C., Wilson, C. J., Stefani, A., and Kitai, S. T. (1992). Grafted neostriatal neurons express a late-developing transient potassium current. *Neuroscience* **48**, 849–856.

Svendsen, C. N. and Smith, A. G. (1999). New prospects for human stem-cell therapy in the nervous system. *Trends in Neurosciences* **22**, 357–364.

Thomson, J. A., Itskovitz-Eldor, J., Shapiro, S. S., Waknitz, M. A., Swiergiel, J. J., Marshall, V. S., and Jones, J. M. (1998). Embryonic stem cell lines derived from human blastocysts. *Science* **282**, 1145–1147.

Torres, E. M., Fricker, R. A., Hume, S., Myers, R., Opacka-Juffry, J., Ashworth, S., Brooks, D. J., and Dunnett, S. B. (1995). Assessment of striatal graft viability in the rat *in vivo* using a small diameter PET scanner. *NeuroReport* **6**, 2017–2021.

Turner, D. A. and Kearney, W. (1993). Scientific and ethical concerns in neural foetal tissue transplantation. *Neurosurgery* **33**, 1031–1037.

Van Vugt, J. P., Siesling, S., Vergeer, M., Van der Velde, E. A., and Roos, R. A. (1997). Clozapine versus placebo in Huntington's disease: A double blind randomised comparative study. *Journal of Neurology, Neurosurgery and Psychiatry* **63**, 35–39.

Walsh, J. P., Zhou, F. C., Hull, C. D., Fisher, R. S., Levine, M. S., and Buchwald, N. A. (1988). Physiological and morphological characterization of striatal neurons transplanted into the striatum of adult rats. *Synapse* **2**, 37–44.

Watts, C. and Dunnett, S. B. (2000). Immunoprotection of cell and tissue implants in the central nervous system. In *Neuromethods 36: neural transplantation methods* (ed. S. B. Dunnett, A. A. Boulton, and G. B. Baker), pp. 477–501. Humana Press, Totowa, New Jersey.

—— Brasted, P. J., and Dunnett, S. B. (2000a). The morphology, integration and functional efficacy of striatal grafts differs between cell suspensions and tissue pieces. *Cell Transplantation* **9**, 395–407.

—— —— Eagle, D. M., and Dunnett, S. B. (2000b). Embryonic donor age and dissection influence striatal graft development and functional integration in a rodent model of Huntington's disease. *Experimental Neurology* **163**, 85–97.

Whishaw, I. Q., O'Connor, W. T., and Dunnett, S. B. (1986). The contributions of motor cortex, nigrostriatal dopamine and caudate–putamen to skilled forelimb use in the rat. *Brain* **109**, 805–843.

Wictorin, K. (1992). Anatomy and connectivity of intrastriatal striatal transplants. *Progress in Neurobiology* **38**, 611–639.

Wictorin, K. and Björklund, A. (1989). Connectivity of striatal grafts implanted into the ibotenic acid-lesioned striatum. 2. Cortical afferents. *Neuroscience* **30**, 297–311.

—— Isacson, O., Fischer, W., Nothias, F., Peschanski, M., and Björklund, A. (1988). Connectivity of striatal grafts implanted into the ibotenic acid-lesioned striatum. 1. Subcortical afferents. *Neuroscience* **27**, 547–562.

—— Ouimet, C. C., and Björklund, A. (1989a). Intrinsic organization and connectivity of intrastriatal striatal transplants in rats as revealed by DARPP-32 immunohistochemistry: specificity of connections with the lesioned host brain. *European Journal of Neuroscience* **1**, 690–701.

—— Simerly, R. B., Isacson, O., Swanson, L. W., and Björklund, A. (1989b). Connectivity of striatal grafts implanted into the ibotenic acid-lesioned striatum. 3. Efferent projecting graft neurons and their relation to host afferents within the grafts. *Neuroscience* **30**, 313–330.

Wictorin, K., Lagenaur, C. F., Lund, R. D., and Björklund, A. (1991). Efferent projections to the host brain from intrastriatal striatal mouse-to-rat grafts: time course and tissue-type specificity as revealed by a mouse specific neuronal marker. *European Journal of Neuroscience* **3**, 86–101.

Widner, H. (1998). Immunological issues in rodent and primate transplants. In *Cell transplantation for neurological disorders* (ed. T. B. Freeman and H. Widner), pp. 171–187. Humana Press, Totowa, New Jersey.

—— Albanese, A., Aebischer, P., Annett, L. E., Björklund, A., Boer, G. J., Brundin, P., Césaro, P., Dunnett, S. B., Hantraye, P., Lindvall, O., López-Lozano, J. J., Oertel, W. H., Olson, L., Peschanski, M., Quinn, N. P., Sawle, G. V., Staal, M. J., Steinbusch, H. W. M., Wolters, E. C., and Zimmer, J. (1994). NIH neural transplantation funding [letter]. *Science* **263**, 737.

Woodbury, D., Schwarz, E. J., Prockop, D. J., and Black, I. B. (2000). Adult rat and human bone marrow stromal cells differentiate into neurons. *Journal of Neuroscience Research* **61**, 364–370.

Xu, Z. C., Wilson, C. J., and Emson, P. C. (1991). Synaptic potentials evoked in spiny neurons in rat neostriatal grafts by cortical and thalamic stimulation. *Journal of Neurophysiology* **65**, 477–493.

Zhou, F. C., Pu, C. F., and Finger, S. (1991). Nimodipine-enhanced survival of suboptimal neural grafts. *Restorative Neurology and Neuroscience* **3**, 211–215.

Index